COMPREHENSIVE MEDICAL ASSISTING EXAM REVIEW

THIRD EDITION

COMPREHENSIVE MEDICAL ASSISTING EXAM REVIEW

THIRD EDITION

PREPARATION FOR THE CMA, RMA, AND CMAS EXAMS

J.P. CODY, MPH, MBA, CMA (AAMA)
INSTRUCTOR AND PRACTICUM COORDINATOR
MEDICAL OFFICE ADMINISTRATION
WILLIAM RAINEY HARPER COLLEGE
PALATINE, ILLINOIS

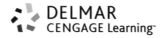

DELMAR
CENGAGE Learning™

Australia • Brazil • Japan • Korea • Mexico • Singapore • Spain • United Kingdom • United States

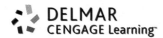

DELMAR
CENGAGE Learning

Comprehensive Medical Assisting Exam Review: Preparation for the CMA, RMA, and CMAS Exams, Third Edition
J.P. Cody

Vice President, Career and Professional Editorial: Dave Garza

Director of Learning Solutions: Matthew Kane

Senior Acquisitions Editor: Rhonda Dearborn

Managing Editor: Marah Bellegarde

Senior Product Manager: Sarah Prime

Editorial Assistant: Chiara Astriab

Vice President, Career and Professional Marketing: Jennifer Baker

Marketing Director: Wendy Mapstone

Senior Marketing Manager: Nancy Bradshaw

Marketing Coordinator: Erica Ropitzky

Production Director: Carolyn Miller

Senior Content Project Manager: Ken McGrath

Senior Art Director: Jack Pendleton

Technology Project Manager: Erin Zeggert

Library of Congress Control Number: 2009944000

ISBN-13: 978-1-4354-9914-0
ISBN-10: 1-4354-9914-X

Delmar
5 Maxwell Drive
Clifton Park, NY 12065-2919
USA

Cengage Learning is a leading provider of customized learning solutions with office locations around the globe, including Singapore, the United Kingdom, Australia, Mexico, Brazil, and Japan. Locate your local office at: **international.cengage.com/region**

Cengage Learning products are represented in Canada by Nelson Education, Ltd.

To learn more about Delmar, visit **www.cengage.com/delmar**
Purchase any of our products at your local college store or at our preferred online store **www.CengageBrain.com**

Notice to the Reader
Publisher does not warrant or guarantee any of the products described herein or perform any independent analysis in connection with any of the product information contained herein. Publisher does not assume, and expressly disclaims, any obligation to obtain and include information other than that provided to it by the manufacturer. The reader is expressly warned to consider and adopt all safety precautions that might be indicated by the activities described herein and to avoid all potential hazards. By following the instructions contained herein, the reader willingly assumes all risks in connection with such instructions. The publisher makes no representations or warranties of any kind, including but not limited to, the warranties of fitness for particular purpose or merchantability, nor are any such representations implied with respect to the material set forth herein, and the publisher takes no responsibility with respect to such material. The publisher shall not be liable for any special, consequential, or exemplary damages resulting, in whole or part, from the readers' use of, or reliance upon, this material.

Printed in the United States of America
3 4 5 6 7 12 11

Table of Contents

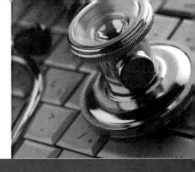

SECTION III: GENERAL MEDICAL KNOWLEDGE

SECTION IV: ADMINISTRATIVE KNOWLEDGE

SECTION V: CLINICAL KNOWLEDGE

SECTION VI: PRACTICE EXAMS

Dedicated to

My students
who have helped me learn
the art of teaching.

J.P. Cody

Preface

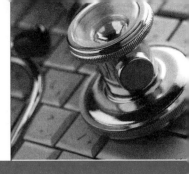

This book is written to achieve three main purposes:

1. To assist students to study and learn the myriad concepts found in an accredited program.
2. To help prepare students for the type of tests they are likely to encounter in their training.
3. To serve as a valuable guide in preparing for the CMA, RMA, and CMAS exams.

Consistent with these purposes, the text will describe these three certification exams, discuss various study and test-taking strategies for the course content candidates are likely to encounter in general, and the certification exams in particular, as well as cover material typically included in an accredited program. The text provides practice tests to assess knowledge weaknesses and monitor improvements, as well as provide guidelines on how to score the practice exams to approximate an actual exam score.

OUTSTANDING FEATURES

The features that distinguish this review book from others in the market include the following:

Single, Comprehensive Study Source. As a study tool, *Comprehensive Medical Assisting Exam Review* is designed to serve as a single, comprehensive source of study material. In fact, it is the most comprehensive book on the market, thus ensuring you do not miss any important test information. Rather than studying multiple texts to ensure a comprehensive review, candidates can effectively rely on this one text to meet their review needs. Material from a wide variety of sources has been brought together so that students do not have to read over a large stack of reference books, thus saving time and effort learning and memorizing the many concepts required to prepare for, and pass, the certification exam.

Study Outline Format. From many sources, exam content has been compiled, organized, condensed, and streamlined in an outline format, thus eliminating the bulk of nonessential information typically included in course textbooks. This facilitates the learning, retention, and recall of the many facts and concepts included in the certification exam.

Diagnostic Practice Tests. Unlike any other review book on the market, *Comprehensive Medical Assisting*

Exam Review contains pre-tests and posttests that are designed to identify subject matter weaknesses, to focus student review, and to monitor learning progress. An Exam Practice CD is also included in the back of this book for computer-generated and scored practice tests.

Exam Scoring. *Comprehensive Medical Assisting Exam Review* is the only book on the market that provides a scoring approximation to determine whether you are likely to pass or fail the actual certification exam. With other review books, the best you can determine is whether your score improves. Unfortunately, an improved score may still be a failing score. Without this feedback, you are unable to gauge the real effectiveness of your study efforts.

Course and Text Supplement. Students can use this book to assist them in learning course material as a supplement to course lectures and readings. Given that certification often is a prerequisite to employment, passing the certification exam the first time may serve to avoid delays in employment. Using the text early in the curriculum increases the likelihood of passing the certification exam on the first attempt.

Primary Course Text. *Comprehensive Medical Assisting Exam Review* is an ideal text for use in certification review seminars or courses.

Outcome Evaluation. The practice exams allow educators to assess student preparedness for certification as well as program effectiveness associated with learning outcomes.

Curriculum Reference. Educators can use the text as a reference for designing or improving program curricula, lecture material, or evaluation instruments consistent with programmatic accreditation criteria and certification exam content.

NEW TO THE THIRD EDITION

Although its purpose has not changed since first published, myriad developments have occurred requiring a number of changes and updates. This third edition reflects these changes as summarized below:

- Chapters 1 and 3 describe the new CMA exam format and testing protocol as well as updates to the RMA exam content distribution.

- Chapters 6 through 9 have undergone a major reorganization. Chapter 6 content is devoted to human development and Chapter 7 focuses on professionalism and the patient-provider relationship including new content on workplace etiquette and seeking employment. Chapter 8 addresses the legal aspects of health care; while Chapter 9, the ethical aspects.
- Chapters 10 through 15 have also been reorganized. Chapter 10 includes new content on writing mechanics and informational brochures. Chapter 13 includes both medical coding and insurance claims processing that was formerly in separate chapters. Chapter 14 now focuses on facilities management issues with new content in office design, office safety, and accessibility. Chapter 15 includes new content on opening a medical practice.
- Chapters 16 through 21 have been significantly reorganized, as well. Chapter 16 now includes material that was formerly distributed among three chapters with new content on pulmonary function tests. Chapter 18 has been updated to include the 50 most common drugs and a section on intravenous therapy. Chapter 19 has been significantly revised to reflect the most recent changes in CPR and first aid protocol. Chapter 20 includes the laboratory science material that was formerly distributed among four chapters.
- Finally, the pre- and post practice exams have been updated to reflect the new organization of the text, as well as the changes in the exam protocols.

SUPPLEMENTS

Exam Practice CD. Found in the back of this book, the Exam Practice CD contains over 1,600 questions to practice for your certification exam. The Exam Practice CD allows you to practice single topics or take full tests that simulate the exam experience. Brief rationales for the correct answer are included for each question. Exam Practice CD content prepared by Lynn G. Slack, BS, CMA (AAMA).

Web Tutor Advantage Course Cartridge. The Web Tutor Advantage course cartridge has been developed to supplement the textbook and enhance the learning experience. It provides rich communication tools for instructors and students, including a course calendar, chat, e-mail, threaded discussions, web links and a white board. Web Tutor content prepared by Tricia Berry, MATL, OTR/L.

Each chapter includes:
- Electronic book chapters for self-paced online study or review
- Animations and video clips to illustrate difficult or visual topics
- Chapter quizzes with certification-style questions to reinforce learning, provide important practice for the exams, and clarify why answers are—or aren't—correct

- Flash cards of important terminology covering the material
- Links to certification organization web sites

Medical Assisting Exam Review On The Go. Download quizzes to practice "on the go" for your certification exam using your cell phone or other mobile device. Quizzes are organized by major exam topic—General, Administrative, and Clinical. Quiz content prepared by Tricia Berry, MATL, OTR/L.

Download Medical Assisting Exam Review On The Go from your cell phone at:
http://www.m.healthcare.delmar.cengage.com.

1. Open your web browser on your cell phone.
2. Navigate to the URL input field (this is different on all cell phones).
3. Using your keypad, type in the URL listed above.
4. The mobile game page will prompt you to accept to download the game.
5. Click "OK" to download.
6. You will find the game in your "downloads" or "games" area on your cell phone (this is different on all cell phones).

Service & Software Requirements:
- Medical Assisting Exam Review On The Go works on the following mobile services: AT&T (most phones, except the Apple iPhone), Verizon Wireless (with JAVA installed), Sprint & T-Mobile.
- The cell phone must be web-enabled to access the Internet.
- The cell phone must have JAVA installed; must allow 3rd party JAVA applications to be installed; must be compatible with JAVA applications.

For more information on how to use the mobile media, go to www.podcasts.cengage.com/healthcare. IMPORTANT NOTE: The use of Medical Assisting Exam Review On The Go is free of charge. However, you may incur a fee from your mobile phone provider for the data that is used to download the game. Please contact your provider for your specific service options. Delmar is not responsible for any charges associated with this download.

ACKNOWLEDGMENTS

Successfully preparing a book revision, as with many things in life, requires a team effort. As such, the following persons deserve my thanks and appreciation:

Dianna J. Cody
President
Cardinal Carriers Logistics
West Union, Illinois

Janet Thomas, BS, RHIT, CCS
Associate Professor
Health Information Management
Vincennes University
Vincennes, Indiana

The following reviewers also deserve my appreciation. Without them, truth, accuracy, and relevance would have been compromised:

Reviewers
Tricia Berry, MATL, OTR/L
Assistant Dean of Clinical Placement
School of Health Sciences
Kaplan University
Davenport, IA

Cheryl Bordwine, BS, HCA, NCICS
College of the Mainland
La Marque, Texas

Dahn Brown
Ridley-Lowell Business and Technical Institute
Binghamton, NY

Betsy Cavanaugh, BSN, CMA (AAMA)
Hesser College
Keene, NH

Cherika DeJesus, AAS, CMA (AAMA)
Medical Assistant Chair Minnesota School of Business
Maple Grove, MN

Teresa England Lewis
North Montco Technical Career Center
Lansdale, PA

Rhonda Epps, CMA (AAMA), RT, AS
Director of Healthcare Education National College
Knoxville, TN

Suzanne Fisher, RN
San Joaquin Valley College
Rancho Cordova, CA

Kathryn A. Kalanick, CMA (AAMA), NCPT
Educational Pathways
Nephi, UT

Lisa S. Nagle, CMA (AAMA)
Medical Assisting Program Director
Augusta Technical College
Augusta, GA

Lynn G. Slack, BS, CMA (AAMA)
Medical Programs Director
Kaplan Career Institute
Pittsburgh, PA

Marilyn Turner, RN, CMA (AAMA)
Medical Assisting Program Director Ogeechee Technical College
Statesboro, GA

Lori Warren, RN, CPC, CCP, CLNC
Medical Assisting Program Director
Spencerian College
Louisville, KY

ABOUT THE AUTHOR

John P. Cody, MPH, MBA, CMA (AAMA), has acquired nearly 30 years of health care and adult education experience. His health care experience began while serving as a general duty Hospital Corpsman in the U.S. Navy. During his military service, he completed training and gained experience as an emergency medical technician, medical laboratory technician, clinical and laboratory supervisor, and administrative supervisor. Shortly before being honorably discharged from the Navy, John completed his B.S. degree in Health Care Management from Southern Illinois University. Being a strong advocate of higher education, John subsequently completed a master's degree in public health administration, as well as one in business management from the University of Minnesota. Concomitantly, John has served as a professor of health sciences, program director, and academic administrator in business and allied health education. John lives with his family in East, Central Illinois.

INTRODUCTION

The third edition of *Medical Assisting Exam Review* reflects the continuing evolution of medical assisting practice. As it was true in the introductory remarks of earlier editions, medical assistant certification continues to be an important milestone in one's professional development as an allied health professional. And equally as true, certification is being required by greater numbers of organizations that employ them. Given the new developments in health services delivery and the requisite skills and knowledge required to effectively deliver these services as an allied health practitioner, my convictions as an allied health educator and the intent of the book have not changed. The many changes and updates in the third edition reflect this. As before, to all of you who have chosen to embark upon the path of professional certification, I wish you fair winds and following seas.

J. P. Cody

HOW TO USE THE EXAM PRACTICE CD

The Exam Preparation Program provides you with hundreds of multiple choice questions similar to the ones you will find on the CMA, RMA and CMAS exams. The Exam Practice CD is organized into two parts: a Study Mode and a Practice Test Mode.

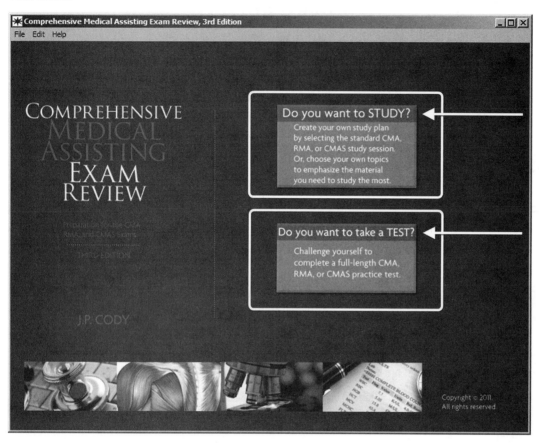

In Study Mode, you can pick the specific topics you need to emphasize and select how many questions you want to attempt.

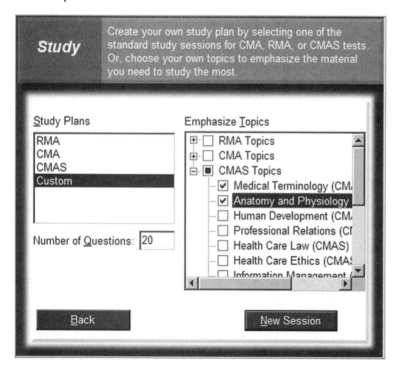

During the study session, you get immediate feedback about your answer choice.

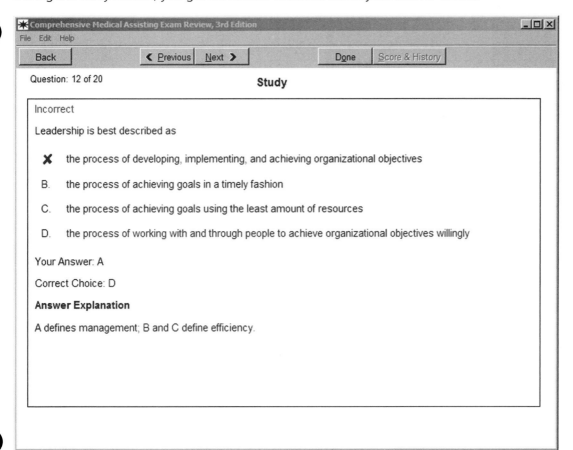

When your study session is complete, you will get an extensive assessment of your results including the questions you answered correctly, incorrectly, or left blank as well as your performance organized by topics covered.

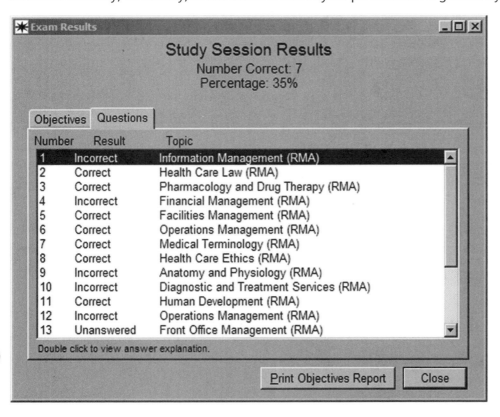

In Practice Test Mode, you will take simulated full-length exams for CMA, RMA, and CMAS. Once you have answered all the questions, you will get a detailed, printable report of your results.

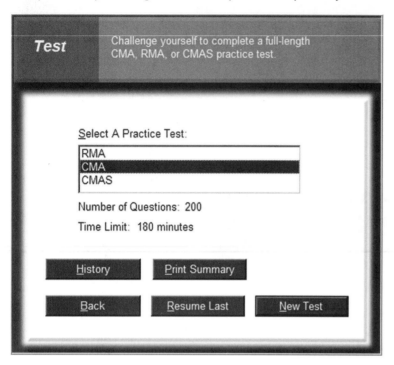

SECTION I

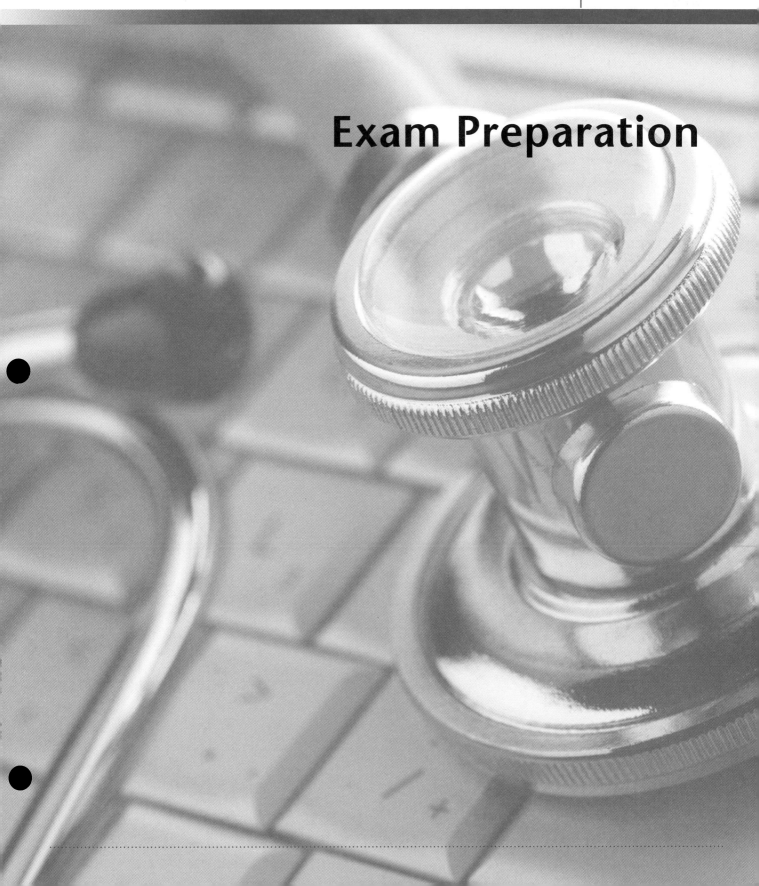

Exam Preparation

CHAPTER 1

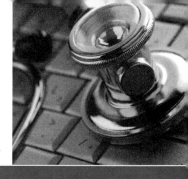

The Examinations

INTRODUCTION

The purpose of this manual is to assist you, the student, in preparing for exams you are likely to encounter in your training, as well as the medical assistant certification (CMA [AAMA]), registration (RMA [AMT]), or medical administrative specialist (CMAS [AMT]) exam. The manual is arranged according to the content of these exams and is divided into five sections. Section I comprises this and two other chapters, and provides general information about studying, test-taking, and the organization and format of the certification exams. This chapter describes the prescribed exams, the question types, and how to score the practice tests according to their respective scoring criteria. Chapters 2 and 3 discuss basic study and test-taking strategies to familiarize you with the mechanics of the testing process and to help overcome test anxiety. At the end of Section I, an abbreviated comprehensive pre-test for each of the three exams addressed in this book; the CMA (AAMA), RMA (AMT), and CMAS (AMT) certification exams, is provided to assess your medical assistant knowledge base. Its purpose is to identify any knowledge weaknesses you may have and to direct you to the appropriate chapters for further study. Sections II, III, and IV outline the subject areas arranged in chapters of the general, administrative, and clinical exam components, respectively. Section V consists of a full comprehensive post-test for each of the three exams. These practice tests are designed to further assess test performance, identify knowledge weakness, and provide guidance on continued study.

To study while you are taking classes, it is recommended that you do the following:

1. Read Chapters 1 through 3.
2. Review the appropriate chapters or sections of chapters corresponding to the required texts being studied or the classes or topics within the classes you are taking.
3. As you prepare for in-class medical assistant tests, review Chapters 2 and 3; employ any or all of the study or test-taking suggestions that will be of use.
4. Use the outlines in the chapters you are studying as a tool to prepare for the test. Augment the outlines

with other information emphasized by the instructor or texts being used.

To prepare for a certification exam, it is recommended that you follow a process of organized study as follows:

1. If you have used this text during the course of your medical assistant training, most or all of the chapters will be familiar to you.
2. Read Chapters 1 through 3.
3. Take the pre-test at the end of Section I, keeping within the prescribed time limit. Score the test and calculate the score described later in this chapter.
4. Depending on which component has the lowest score—general, administrative, or clinical—turn to the appropriate section of the manual and study the outline using the appropriate suggestions discussed in Chapter 2.
5. Attend to the weaker of the remaining two sections as described above.
6. Eventually, you may wish to browse through all the chapters in each section, studying specific areas in detail as warranted.
7. Take the appropriate test found in Section V or on the CD provided in the back of the book. In any event, it is suggested that you take at least a post-test before writing the actual certification exam.

CMA (AAMA) EXAM DESCRIPTION

The CMA (AAMA) certification examination is a computer based test that is arranged by appointment at sites throughout the country, and can be taken by individuals who meet the training and experience requirements for medical assistant certification as determined by the American Association of Medical Assistants (AAMA).

The CMA (AAMA) exam is a 200-question, multiple-choice test, covering three broad areas: general medical knowledge, administrative knowledge, and clinical knowledge. Of the 200 questions, 180 questions will be scored and count toward the final score. The other 20 questions will be tested for use in future exams and will not count toward the final score. These 20 test questions will be randomly distributed throughout the exam and will be indistinguishable from those that will be scored. The subject material includes the following:

CMA (AAMA) Exam Content Outline
I. General (Transdisciplinary) 33.3% (60 questions)
Chapters 4–9

II. Administrative 33.3% (60 questions)
Chapters 10–15

III. Clinical 33.3% (60 questions)
Chapters 16–21

The complete CMA (AAMA) Exam Outline is available to view at the AAMA web site, www.aama-ntl.org.

RMA (AMT) AND CMAS (AMT) EXAM DESCRIPTIONS

The RMA (AMT) and CMAS (AMT) exams can be taken by individuals who meet the training and experience requirements of the American Medical Technologists (AMT). The RMA (AMT) exam is available in computerized or pencil and paper formats. The computerized exam is offered by appointment Monday through Saturday at various testing sites throughout the United States. Pencil and paper exams, however, are generally offered by sponsoring schools and are scheduled when a sufficient number of applicants have made application. Both exams consist of 200 to 210 multiple-choice questions covering the content as outlined below.

RMA (AMT) Exam Content Outline
I. General Medical Assisting Knowledge 41% (82 questions)
A. Anatomy and Physiology (Ch. 5)

B. Medical Terminology (Ch. 4)

C. Medical Law (Ch. 8)

D. Medical Ethics (Ch. 9)

E. Human Relations (Ch. 7)

F. Patient Education (Ch. 7)

II. Administrative Medical Assisting 24% (48 questions)
A. Insurance (Ch. 13)

B. Finance and Bookkeeping (Ch. 12)

C. Medical Receptionist/Secretarial/Clerical (Ch. 10–11, 14–15)

III. Clinical Medical Assisting 35.0% (70 questions)
A. Asepsis (Ch. 16)

B. Sterilization (Chs. 16 and 17)

C. Instruments (Ch. 16–17)

D. Vital Signs and Mensurations (Ch. 16)

E. Physical Examinations (Ch. 16)

F. Clinical Pharmacology (Ch. 18)

G. Minor Surgery (Ch. 17)

H. Therapeutic Modalities (Ch. 16)

I. Laboratory Procedures (Ch. 20)

J. Electrocardiography (Ch. 16)

K. First Aid and Emergency Response (Ch. 19)

Courtesy of the American Medical Technologists

CMAS (AMT) Exam Content Outline
I. Medical Assisting Foundation 13% (26 questions)
A. Medical Terminology (Ch. 4)

B. Basic Anatomy and Physiology (Ch. 5)

C. Legal and Ethical Considerations (Chs. 8 and 9)

D. Professionalism (Ch. 7)

II. Basic Clinical Medical Office Assisting 8% (16 questions)
A. Basic Health History Interview (Ch. 16)

B. Basic Charting (Ch. 16)

C. Vital Signs and Measurements (Ch. 16)

D. Asepsis in the Medical Office (Ch. 16)

E. Examination Preparation (Ch. 16)

F. Medical Office Emergencies (Ch. 19)

G. Pharmacology (Ch. 18)

III. Medical Office Clerical Assisting 10% (20 questions)
A. Appointment Management and Scheduling (Ch. 11)

B. Reception (Ch. 11)

C. Communication (Ch. 7)

D. Patient Information and Community Resources (Chs. 10 and 15)

IV. Medical Records Management 14% (28 questions)

A. Systems (Ch. 10)

B. Procedures (Ch. 10)

C. Confidentiality (Chs. 8 and 10)

V. Health Care Insurance Processing, Coding, and Billing 17% (34 questions)

A. Insurance Processing (Ch. 13)

B. Coding (Ch. 13)

C. Insurance Billing Finances (Chs. 12 and 13)

VI. Medical Office Financial Management 17% (34 questions)

A. Fundamental Financial Management (Ch. 12)

B. Patient Accounts (Ch. 12)

C. Banking (Ch. 12)

D. Payroll (Ch. 12)

VII. Medical Office Information Processing 7% (14 questions)

A. Fundamentals of Computing (Ch. 10)

B. Medical Office Computer Applications (Ch. 10)

VIII. Medical Office Management 14% (28 questions)

A. Office Communications (Ch. 10)

B. Business Organizational Management (Ch. 15)

C. Human Resources (Ch. 15)

D. Safety (Ch. 14)

E. Supplies and Equipment (Ch. 14)

F. Physical Office Plant (Ch. 14)

G. Risk Management and Quality Assurance (Ch. 15)

Courtesy of the American Association of Medical Technologists

EXAM QUESTION FORMAT

All three certification exams consist of A-type multiple-choice questions. The following describes the significant features of the A-type multiple-choice question.

Components of a Multiple-Choice Question

A multiple-choice question is commonly called an item; it has two parts: a stem and a list of response options. The stem is that part of an item that poses a question, problem, or incomplete statement. The stem can have either positive or negative polarity. A stem that is positively polarized arranges the question in the context of what is true; for example, "Which of the following procedures requires informed consent?" A stem that is negatively polarized arranges the question in the context of what is false; for example, "All of the following procedures require informed consent except:". Likewise, the stem can be either a complete sentence or an incomplete sentence. Complete stems are statements or questions that contain a complete thought and can be answered before reviewing the response options. A response option is paired with the stem that either answers the question or is strongly associated with it. Incomplete stems present a portion of a statement or incomplete thought that must be paired with a response option to complete a sentence or thought.

The response options represent the possible answers to an item posed by the stem. There must be at least three options to be considered in a multiple-choice question; however, most items contain four or five options. Options are usually identified by a letter (lowercase or uppercase) or a number. One of the options represents the best response, whereas the others, called distracters, represent less desirable responses and are considered incorrect. Options can be presented in four grammatical arrangements: a sentence, a completion of a stem, an incomplete sentence, or a single word.

Positive Polarity. This is the most common multiple-choice question arrangement. It consists of a stem and five lettered options for the CMA (AAMA) exam (one best answer and four distracters), and four lettered options for the RMA (AMT) and CMAS (AMT) exams (one best answer and three distracters). The candidate is required to select the one best answer. For example:

Which of the following is a function of the skeletal system?

a. absorption of nutrients

b. homeostasis

c. sensation

d. framework for support

e. elimination of waste

Negative Polarity. A format commonly found in each exam presents a stem that generally calls for what is false. Stems having negative polarity generally include the term "**EXCEPT**" capitalized and bold-faced. The question, therefore, calls for the exception. For example:

Each of the following is a function of the skeletal system ***EXCEPT***

    a. framework for support
    b. blood cell production
    c. protection of internal organs
    d. sensation
    e. site of attachment of muscles

In both examples, D is the correct response, whereas A, B, C, and E are distracters.

SCORING THE EXAM

The following sections discuss how to score the practice exams found in this book to approximate the score one might receive on an actual certification exam. The formulae given represent rough approximations determined through statistical analysis of past student test performance. One's true test performance represents a range of scores. For example, a CMA (AAMA) score of 500 means that one's score is likely to be somewhere between 475 and 525. An RMA (AMT) or CMAS (AMT) score of 82 means that one's score is likely to be between 77 and 87.

The CMA (AAMA) Exam

The CMA (AAMA) examination consists of 60 scored and a few unscored questions in each of three content sections (general, administrative, and clinical) for a total of 200 questions. The CMA candidate is allowed 160 minutes (2 hours, 40 minutes) to complete the exam. The exam is scheduled in two 80 minute segments with an optional 20 minute break in between. There are no penalties for guessing because the exam is scored according to the number of correct responses out of the total number of questions possible. Each question is assigned equal weight regardless of the section in which it is found. The candidate must achieve a minimum score to receive certification.

The CMA (AAMA) exam results provided to the candidate will indicate the candidate's score, the minimum passing score, and certification status (pass or fail). The pass/fail determination is based on a standardized score. Accordingly, the raw score (the number of correct responses) is rescaled; that is, mathematically converted to a standard score. In this case, the mean number of questions answered correctly by past candidates was set to 500. This standardization allows future exam scores to be directly comparable to past scores. The pass/fail decision is based on a single score according to the candidate's performance on the entire examination. The minimum passing standard score is 445. To be awarded certification, the candidate must achieve a minimum standard score of 445.

As a means of assisting CMA (AAMA) candidates in preparing for this important examination, the following information is provided to permit candidates to convert their raw scores to standard scores. Candidates can then compare their standard score to the minimum passing score of 445 to learn whether they passed or failed. Knowing what constitutes a passing and failing score is an essential measure to assess a candidate's overall performance, as well as provide valuable feedback for continued improvement. The following formula, therefore, can be used to convert a raw test score, expressed as a percent of the questions answered correctly, to a standard score to approximate the score one would likely receive on the actual CMA (AAMA) examination.

CMA (AAMA) EXAM SCORING FORMULA

■ **(Raw Score $\times$ 10) $-$ 200**

Example 1: Raw score = 72% (130 correct out of a possible 180 questions)

$$(72 \times 10) - 200$$

Step 1:	72×10	= 720
Step 2:	$720 - 200$	= 520

The standard score is 520, which is passing ($520 > 445$).

Example 2: Raw score = 46% (41 correct out of a possible 90 questions)

$$(46 \times 10) - 200$$

Step 1:	46×10	= 460
Step 2:	$460 - 200$	= 260

The standard score is 260, which is failing ($260 < 445$).

When preparing for the CMA (AAMA) exam, use the above formula throughout this manual to convert raw scores of practice tests to standard scores. If a score exceeds 800, consider the score to be 800; likewise, if a score is below 200, consider it to be 200.

The RMA (AMT) and CMAS (AMT) Exams

The RMA (AMT) and CMAS (AMT) exams each consist of 200 to 210 questions according to the topical areas presented earlier. Unlike the CMA (AAMA) exam, each question is weighted according to difficulty and is not computed on a curve, but is converted to a scaled score. The minimum passing scaled score is 70. The score of 70 does not represent the number or percentage of questions answered correctly.

As a means of determining whether a practice-test score represents a passing score or not, the following formula can be used to convert a raw test score, expressed as a percent of the questions answered correctly, to a scaled score to approximate the total score one might receive on the actual exam.

RMA (AMT) AND CMAS (AMT) EXAM SCORING FORMULA

■ **(Raw Score × 0.6) + 40**

<u>Example 1:</u> Raw score = 72% (144 correct out of a possible 200 questions)

$$(72 \times 0.6) + 40$$

| Step 1: | 72×0.6 | = 43.2 |
| Step 2: | $43.2 + 40$ | = 83.2 |

The scaled score is 83, which is passing (83 > 70).

<u>Example 2:</u> Raw score = 46% (23 correct out of a possible 50 questions)

$$(46 \times 0.6) + 40$$

| Step 1: | 46×0.6 | = 27.6 |
| Step 2: | $27.6 + 40$ | = 67.6 |

The scaled score is 67.6, which is failing (67.6 < 70).

When preparing for the RMA (AMT) or CMAS (AMT) exams, use the above formula throughout this manual to convert raw scores of practice tests to scaled scores. If a score exceeds 100, consider the score to be 100.

The next two chapters discuss useful techniques in studying medical assistant course information and the specific information included in the various examinations. These chapters also include useful test-taking tips to successfully pass medical course quizzes and tests, as well as these certification exams.

CERTIFICATION EXAM APPLICATIONS

Information and applications for the certification exams discussed in this book can be acquired from the following organizations:

CMA (AAMA) Exam
AAMA Certification
7999 Eagle Way
Chicago, Illinois 60678-1079
800-228-2262
http://www.aama-ntl.org

RMA (AMT) and CMAS (AMT) Exams
American Medical Technologists
10700 W. Higgins Road, Suite 150
Rosemont, Illinois 60018
847-823-5169
http://www.amt1.com

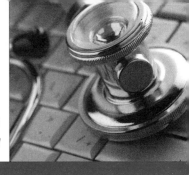

CHAPTER 2

Study Techniques

STUDY METHODS

Successfully preparing and passing a written test, whether it is a test given in a medical assisting course or a certification examination, requires the ability to learn and recall information. Therefore, the intent of this chapter is to provide some guidance for developing test preparation and study skills.

Note-Taking

Note-taking is an important component of effective learning. It is the means by which one records and organizes information for later review and study. Although taking notes is typically performed during a lecture to capture the information provided by an instructor or speaker, note-taking techniques can similarly be used while studying written material as a means of recording and organizing its important concepts. The development of note-taking skills, therefore, will serve you well in your education and certification test preparation. Regardless of the method used, the critical aspect of effective note-taking is keeping the information organized so that subordinate points are placed in close proximity to the concepts they support or illuminate so that these relationships are visibly apparent. The major portions of this text, for example, are organized in an outline format to do just that. This organized way to record or present information clarifies the interrelationships within the information as a whole, as well as the detail necessary to sustain these relationships. This permits the student or examinee to not only learn the details of a given subject, but to understand how these details are related to one another to create a unified subject. The three most common methods of taking notes include the outline format, mind-mapping format, and Cornell format. These methods are discussed in the following sections.

Outline format (see Figure 2-1). This format, preferred by the author and extensively used throughout this text, organizes information using headings, subheadings, and subordinate points. A systematic labeling system using Roman numerals (I, II, III. . .), Arabic numerals (1, 2, 3. . .), and lowercase and uppercase letters keeps the headings and subordinate information organized so that

---

I. **Nervous System**
  A. Function
  B. Organization
    1. Central Nervous System
    2. Peripheral Nervous System
      a. Afferent (Sensory) Nervous System
      b. Efferent (Motor) Nervous System
        (1) Somatic Nervous System
        (2) Autonomic Nervous System
          (a) Sympathetic Nervous System
          (b) Parasympathetic Nervous System
            i) Promotes digestion and elimination funcions.
            ii) Restores normal resting function after episodes of stress.
II. **Sensory System**
  A. Function
  B. Organization

Figure 2-1

Outline format. Delmar/Cengage Learning.

---

the important note-taking features described above are maintained.

Mind-mapping (see Figure 2-2). A more creative variation of the outline format, mind-mapping is often preferred by students who think and process information outside the linear constraints of strict outlining. The note-taker typically begins by recording the main topic or idea at the center of the page. From the central main idea, the student records the subordinate or supporting information as an extension or branch of the main idea. Information subordinate to these branchings is recorded as further extensions much like the limbs and branches of a tree. Like outlining, mind-mapping organizes information so that the details of a subject clearly demonstrate its unifying features.

Cornell format (see Figure 2-3). This note-taking method is used by drawing a vertical line from the top to the bot-

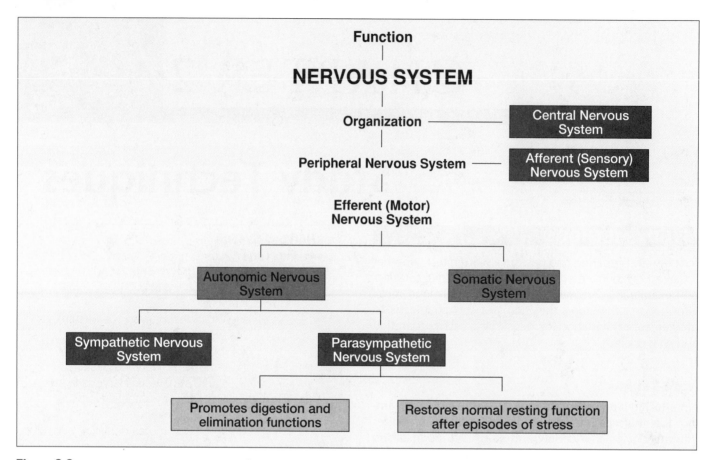

Figure 2-2

Mind-mapping format. Delmar/Cengage Learning.

tom of the note-page approximately two inches from the left edge. Written notes are recorded to the right of the line, perhaps using either the outline or mind-mapping format, or any format the student chooses. The space to the left of the vertical line is used to record any information the student chooses to enhance organization, topic integration, and the like. This may include highlighting key terms or main ideas, as well as references to written sources such as texts and periodicals. Additionally, this space may be used to record other information while the student studies the notes, such as questions, examples, supporting concepts, information from other sources that clarify the notes, etc.

Effective note-taking, especially the methods discussed above, forces students to organize the information as it is heard or read. This permits greater concentration on the subject matter and enhances the cognitive processes vital to comprehension and memory. The following points discuss additional guidelines to consider when taking notes.

- Record your name, the date, and the page number on each page of your notes.
- Attempt to prepare your notes in your own words rather than in the speaker's or author's.
- Record only the information that makes the concepts understandable, not everything you hear or read.
- Ask the lecturer to clarify anything said or written on the board that you do not understand.

- Instead of recording all information shown on overheads and slides, request copies, or offer to make copies for your notes if appropriate.
- Avoid using a recording device unless it clearly improves your note-taking or learning. It is a courtesy to speakers to seek permission to record their lectures.
- Record your notes clearly enough the first time to avoid recopying them later. Your time is better spent studying your notes rather than rewriting them.
- Avoid using the notes of others. It is useful, however, to compare your notes with those of others to identify any important concepts that you may have missed or misinterpreted.
- Use shorthand techniques, standardized or ones of your own design, for frequently occurring words such as *the, and, by, with, of,* etc. The use of medical shorthand, abbreviations, and acronyms can be valuable in quickly and accurately recording information.
- Concepts repeated or written on the board are usually important and should be included in your notes.
- Participate by asking questions and contributing ideas, especially if they clarify your notes.

See p. 22 of text	**NERVOUS SYSTEM**
	Function:
	Organization:
Brain/spinal cord	Central Nervous System
	Peripheral Nervous System
Sends sensory	Afferent (Sensory) Nervous System
information to brain.	
Sends signals to	Efferent (Motor) Nervous System
organs and body	Somatic Nervous System
Confusing (?)	Autonomic Nervous System
	Sympathetic Nervous System
	Parasympathetic Nervous System:
Clarify	Promotes digestion and elimination funcions.
	Restores normal resting function after episodes of stress.
	SENSORY SYSTEM
Read next week	
	Function:
	Organization:

Figure 2-3

Cornell format. Delmar/Cengage Learning.

- If a lecturer has a tendency to skip around, leave plenty of space in your notes for additions.
- If important information is repeated that has been recorded earlier, use connecting arrows instead of recording the information again.
- Use pencil or erasable ink when recording notes so that errors can be easily and neatly corrected.
- Record references to authors, texts, and other sources in the margins of your notes.

Time Management

Lack of time is the most common excuse for poor test performance. More often than not, it is not a lack of time but a lack of time management. Just getting started and beginning the study process tends to be more difficult than studying itself; however, delaying your study activities will only interfere with your ability to effectively prepare for an exam. This is especially crucial with regard to certification exams because they may be infrequently administered. The following are some basic tips for organizing your study time:

- Study difficult or boring subjects first. Students generally find the administrative component the least interesting, and anatomy and physiology the most difficult; perhaps these are good places to start.
- Avoid cramming by spacing out your study time. Attempt to devote a specific time each day or week for study.

- Study during the time of day when you function best. Some are naturally morning people, others are night people; keep this in mind when scheduling your study time.
- Study material organized on three–by–five–inch index cards (or a cassette recorder) during waiting periods. When you are waiting for the bus or in line at the theater, keep material on hand to study while you wait.
- Negotiate an agreement with significant others concerning your study time.
- Do not permit others to interfere with your study time: learn to say "NO."
- Attempt to accomplish one more thing in the time allotted.
- In the event of time constraints, perfection cannot be a high priority.

Developing Discipline

Effective study requires discipline. One method you can exercise to develop greater discipline is described as follows:

Study as long as you are interested, but no longer. Once you have become uninterested or bored, make the commitment to stop; however, read one more page or solve one more problem; then stop, even if your interest is renewed. During the next study session, take the same approach, but this time complete two study units before stopping. In the following study session, complete three study units before quitting, and so on. Using this technique helps you to develop greater discipline in the effective use of study time.

An additional method is the common "To Do" list. In planning your test preparation activities and study time, itemize all of the things you need to do to prepare for the exam. Organize this list by prioritizing each activity into one of three categories: A, B, and C. The A category represents tasks that are the most important and must be completed first. Category B items have intermediate importance and will ultimately fall into the A category as A tasks are completed. Category C items have the least importance and are routinely completed as time permits. As a rule of thumb, you should spend 80% of your time attending to the top 20% of your objectives; that is, category A items. Likewise, you should spend the other 20% of your time on the remaining 80% of your objectives; that is, category B and C items.

SQ3R Method

SQ3R is a five-step guide to assist in the study of any subject. SQ3R is shorthand for SQRRR—an acronym that means Survey, Question, Read, Recite, and Review. This method is useful because it organizes the study process into manageable steps to facilitate learning. The following is a brief description of each step:

Survey. To survey the material you are studying, scan the table of contents, paragraph headings, illustrations, examples, summaries, and sample questions to get a sense of the basic content of the material and its organization.

Question. Based on the content just surveyed, formulate in your mind questions that might be answered within the material. Or, read any review or discussion questions at the end of each chapter as a stimulus for pinpointing important concepts and information in the chapter. Write down the questions on paper or in the margins of the text, referring to them as needed.

Read. Read the material and focus your energies on understanding the subject matter while attempting to answer the questions created in the previous step.

Recite. Attempt to recite aloud the material you recall from the reading. Review the questions posed earlier to stimulate recall.

Review. Review the material to identify information gaps and to clarify poorly understood concepts. Repeat the process until you are satisfied with your performance.

This can be an especially effective technique because it allows for the creation of associations and relationships within the material as a means of improving understanding and recall. The chapters of this manual are organized in a manner suitable to the SQ3R methodology.

Study Groups

Studying in groups can enhance the learning process by making the study process more enjoyable and more energetic. By studying in a group arrangement, students are permitted to exchange ideas and impressions, thereby confirming or questioning each other's understanding. Group study requires more participative activity and is much less passive than independent study. It is recommended, however, that you limit your study group to three to five members; larger groups often lead to excessive socializing. Group study requires greater logistical commitment than does studying alone, so it is important that group members agree to, and adhere to, the study group's objectives. The following are some suggestions concerning study groups:

1. Formulate and agree on the study group's purpose and ultimate objective. The group must agree on what it wishes to accomplish. In studying for a course test or certification exam, the group's ultimate objective would naturally be to pass the test. Whatever the case, members may have different goals. One member may wish to concentrate on a single portion of the exam, whereas others may wish to concentrate on other areas. To be effective, however, the group must agree on the goals it wishes to pursue and attempt to align each member's agenda to the group's overall study plan. If there is wide disparity, perhaps it is best to form smaller study groups or seek other group members with parallel needs.

2. Schedule the study sessions and establish an agenda for each. Agree on meeting times and places as well as a tentative agenda for each meeting. It is important to maintain a certain level of flexibility because subsequent meeting agendas may be affected by what occurred in the preceding study session; adjust the schedule accordingly to meet each member's needs while focusing on the study group's goals.

3. Test each other through questions. Questioning is an effective way of assessing what you know and remember. There are a variety of ways of approaching this step; one way would be to ask selected members specific questions soliciting the assistance of others as needed. Another technique would be to ask open-ended questions of the group in general to stimulate discussion and to explore new ways of looking at different concepts.

4. Practice teaching each other. One of the most effective ways to learn something is to have to teach it. Within a group, each member has a favorite topic or commands a certain level of expertise in a particular subject area. By taking advantage of this, members can choose an area and give a lecture or some form of presentation to help other members organize or learn that subject. Another approach is to have members who are weak in a given subject give a presentation on that subject. Discussing techniques each uses to help remember certain facts or concepts is valuable as well.

5. Conduct open-ended discussions. It may be very useful, as well as helpful to clarify one's own understanding, to discuss and debate selected issues, especially if these issues are controversial. Legal and ethical issues are particularly suitable to this forum.

6. Rely on each other for support. If you have a particular skill that others lack, such as dosage calculations, attempt to make yourself available to tutor one of your group members. Help each other out; not only in study but in other areas as well, such as day care and transportation.

Cramming

Cramming, although pedagogically unsound, is sometimes necessary. When confronted with the need to cram, students are often tempted to learn everything lightly; however, this approach allows for marginal recall. First, it is better to focus on your weakest areas. Taking the practice tests will permit you to identify your weakest subject areas. It is recommended that you spend 25% of your time learning the material and the remaining 75% drilling yourself on that material. Second, use outlines, flash cards, or a cassette recorder as resources for your study drills. Reading material repeatedly is an inefficient means of studying; instead, recite the material aloud to imprint the information in your memory. Last, avoid studying the day before the exam to allow your batteries to recharge. Relax and avoid any pretest anxiety.

Memory Techniques

A considerable number of questions on medical assistant tests and on certification exams are knowledge-based questions requiring the recall of facts and information. The vast majority of your study time, therefore, will probably be devoted to memorizing facts, terminology, principles, concepts, and theories. There are a number of devices that have been developed to assist you in memorizing and recalling information. Some of these devices are described below.

Repetition. Memorization is imprinting information in the brain through repetitive processes for later recall. The more senses employed in this process, the more effective the recall. Repetition techniques reinforce learning, retention, and recall; however, this form of learning is rote in nature, having little impact on comprehension. Selected repetition techniques are described as follows:

- Index cards are an excellent tool for memorizing information through repetition. They can be used to learn terminology, steps in a procedure, or any information of a factual nature.
- Digital recorders are effective tools as well. Suppose, for example, you want to remember the five basic functions of the skeletal system as outlined in the anatomy and physiology chapter:

Anatomy and Physiology

A. Skeletal system functions
  1. Framework for support
  2. Protection of internal organs
  3. Blood cell production
  4. Attachment for muscles
  5. Calcium and phosphorous storage and release

You might record the following statement: "The five functions of the skeletal system are . . ." Now pause long enough to list them in your mind. Then record the functions by stating them out loud. Continue doing this with the outlines as appropriate. Play back the recording, attempting to recite the answers before they are given. Continue this process as needed to memorize the material.

Pegword System. The pegword system was introduced in England by John Sanbrook in 1879. It is a powerful method of memorizing items on a list. The author has found it particularly useful in memorizing the instruments arranged in various surgical packs. The items on a list are associated with a series of numbered objects shown below:

One: Bun
Two: Shoe
Three: Tree
Four: Door
Five: Hive
Six: Sticks
Seven: Heaven
Eight: Gate
Nine: Wine
Ten: Hen

For example, suppose you want to remember the following list:

1. car
2. knife
3. stethoscope
4. apple
5. girl
6. window
7. box
8. book
9. pencil
10. shirt

Now read back over the list and attempt to memorize them for a moment. Next, without peeking, attempt to write down as many items as you can remember. Most people rarely recall all of them. Now visualize the matchup of the items in the list with the numbered objects shown above as follows:

One: A *car* sitting in a *bun*.
Two: A *knife* sticking out of a *shoe*.
Three: A *stethoscope* hanging from a *tree*.
Four: An *apple* wedged in a *door*.
Five: A *girl* holding a *beehive*.
Six: A *window* surrounded by *sticks*.
Seven: A *box* floating in *heaven*.

Eight: A *book* balanced on a *gate.*
Nine: A *pencil* floating in *wine.*
Ten: A *shirt* worn by a *hen.*

Visualize these paired images for a moment, attempting to memorize them. Now, without peeking, write down, in order, the items from the list. If done properly, you should have been able to remember all of them. Not only can you list the items in order with this technique, but you can identify, out of order, each item by number. The key is to create a mental image of the items to be remembered. Because this technique allows you to organize the information in your memory, research has demonstrated an increase in recall ability by a factor of two to four. The nice thing about this method is that the imagery need not make any sense; according to experts, the more absurd the association, the stronger the recall.

Rhyming. Rhyming, an ancient technique, can be a useful device to improve memory. Examples include eight times eight fell on the floor, picked it up with sixty-four ($8 \times 8 = 64$); in fourteen hundred ninety-two, Columbus sailed the ocean blue; thirty days hath September, April, June, and November, all the rest are thirty-one, but for February the excepted one. A clever variation to this technique can be used to prevent confusing carpals (handbones) with tarsals (footbones): Hands steer a car(pals), feet step on tar(sals).

Alpha Prompts. Associating information with letters of the alphabet can be helpful. Reciting the names of the fifty states, for example, is easier when listed alphabetically. The ABCs of basic life support is a common example: A-airway, B-breathing, and C-circulation. The classic signs for diabetes mellitus are the three Ps: polyuria, polydipsia, and polyphagia.

Acrostics. Acrostics are devices such as acronyms and related arrangements that aid information recall. An acronym is a mnemonic device that uses the first letter of a series of words. Examples include: ROY G. BIV to remember the colors of the visible light spectrum—Red, Orange, Yellow, Green, Blue, Indigo, and Violet; HOMES to remember the names of the Great Lakes—Huron, Ontario, Michigan, Erie, and Superior. Another acrostic arrangement uses the first letter of the words in a phrase or saying to provide a memory cue. Examples include: *Kings Play Cards On Fairly Good Satin* to remember the taxonomic organization of organisms—Kingdom, Phylum, Class, Order, Family, Genus, and Species; *All Dieters Eat Kilocalories* to remember the fat-soluble vitamins A, D, E, and K.

Comprehension, Application, and Analysis

Methods of exercising and testing the comprehension, application, and analysis of information are best conducted during group study sessions described earlier. The majority of techniques discussed thus far apply to knowledge questions: those that require recall of facts and information. Comprehension questions, on the other hand, not only require information recall, but require understanding of the information as well as its significance. Comprehension is demonstrated when one can summarize, paraphrase, interpret, or translate the information, as well as determine the implications, consequences, or effects of the information. A technique useful in developing comprehension that is appropriate to group study is to examine how and why an issue or concept of discussion is important or relevant. For example, when learning that trauma can lead to shock, it is important to know why this occurs. When injury occurs, the autonomic nervous system responds by constricting blood vessels, creating inadequate peripheral blood flow and causing insufficient return of blood to the heart for subsequent transport of oxygen to body cells and tissues. Application questions not only require remembering and comprehending information, but also require the ability to take the underlying theories or principles supporting the information and apply them to other situations or scenarios. Application questions force the student to use the information, not just remember and understand it. A useful exercise is to attempt to associate new information to what is already known. For example, when reviewing the principles of surgical asepsis, attempt to recall the last time you performed such a procedure and relate the principles and theories that support your actions step by step. Another useful exercise employs identifying principles or theories common to more than one situation. For example, the principle of capillary action is common to many medical procedures and interventions.

Analysis questions require the ability to recall, understand, and apply information as well as the ability to dissect and evaluate its arrangement, structure, and organization. Analysis allows you to differentiate among the various theoretical and principal components of a concept to identify any underlying interrelationships and significance. For example, when studying disease processes, it is learned that there are myriad causes for hepatitis. Analytical skills can be exercised by attempting to identify the various reasons hepatitis occurs, given different clinical pictures.

SUMMARY

To perform well on a course exam or a certification exam requires greater than minimal commitment to organized study. Your task, therefore, is to develop a study plan that identifies the subject areas to be studied, as well as the time commitment needed for each. Once you have organized your study plan and a timetable, you must then exercise discipline and adhere to the plan. There are no clear shortcuts, so make the commitment to study for the exam no matter how difficult, and follow the advice of Winston Churchill: "Never! Never! Never! Never give up!"

CHAPTER 3

Test-Taking Techniques

By themselves, test-taking techniques are poor substitutes for lack of knowledge; however, medical assistant programs that require a wide variety of coursework, as well as broad-based tests like most certification exams make it difficult to know all of the material well. Employing a test-taking principle here and a technique there improves the probability of increasing one's test score, especially for those who are predisposed to test anxiety. Test-taking is a skill distinct from recalling, understanding, applying, and analyzing information; therefore, learning how to take a test is an integral component of the test-taking challenge. Whether you are preparing for a certification exam or a test in a medical assistant course, the following are some suggestions and advice on successfully taking tests.

Tips on Multiple-Choice Questions

As discussed in Chapter 1, the exams consist of multiple-choice questions. These questions consist of a stem and four or five lettered response options; that is, three or four distracters and "one best answer." Consider the following suggestions when answering this question type:

- Read the question carefully before jumping to the response options.
- Identify whether the question is asking for the true response (positive polarity) or the false response (exception—negative polarity).
- Do not read into the question information that is not provided. Likewise, do not dismiss information that is provided.
- Attempt to answer the question in your mind before reviewing the options.
- If the answer you have determined is not among the response options, choose the best available option or attempt to identify the correct option by eliminating the distracters.
- Always stick with your initial response unless you have made an obvious error and you are certain of the correct response.
- If the options cover a wide range of quantities and you do not know the correct option, choose one in the middle of the range.

- After eliminating as many distracters as you can, and the remaining options are similar except for a word or two, choose the one that has the greatest complexity or wordiness.
- In sentence completion questions, eliminate the grammatically incorrect options (unusual for certification exams).
- Do not choose an option that is partially true or partially false.
- Heed terms that are underlined, *italicized,* CAPITALIZED, or in **bold type.**
- Options associated with patient-relation questions that imply all is well, deny patient feelings, change the subject raised by patients, encourage cheerfulness, or renounce professional responsibility usually represent distracters; avoid choosing them.
- If a question totally confounds you, mark it with a "?" and skip it. If time permits return to the question and do the following:
  - Choose one of two options that are similar, except for a word or two.
  - Choose one of two options that sound or look similar.
  - If two quantities are approximately equal, choose one.
  - Choose the option that appears to have the greatest detail, complexity, or wordiness.
  - Two or more options that are plausible where no one is clearly better than the others are usually distracters; eliminate them.
  - Choose the option that uses the same terms or language found in the stem.
  - If two options are opposites, choose one.
  - Choose one of the central options avoiding the first or last option.
- If none of the above suggestions help you narrow down the possibilities, answer all the questions marked "?" with the same letter. This will increase the statistical chances of choosing the correct response option.
- If very little time remains, quickly mark the unanswered questions with the same letter as described above.

True-False Questions

Although simple true-false questions will not be found in any of the certification exams, they may be used in a medical assistant course. Simply stated, a true-false question is usually a statement regarding a concept, fact, or state of affairs; the student is to determine whether the statement, as it is written, is either true or false. If a test consists of a variety of question types to include true-false questions, and depending on the complexity of the test and time allotted to complete it, it is advisable to answer true-false questions quickly because they generally are awarded the least number of points; this should make intuitive sense because guessing will provide a 50% probability of being right. If, on the other hand, a test is composed of entirely true-false questions, answer each one carefully. There are two other points to bear in mind: (1) if any part of a true-false statement is false, the whole statement must be considered false, and (2) absolute qualifiers such as always; never, all, and none generally make the statement false.

True-false substitution questions are an interesting variation of the simple true-false type that may be used as a testing instrument in a medical assisting course. A statement is made with one or more words underlined. If the statement is true, the student simply marks it true; however, if the statement is false, the student must substitute the underlined word(s) with a word or phrase that will make the statement true. This question type is more difficult and offers a smaller probability of guessing correctly than does the simple true-false question:

_____ The neuron is the functional physiologic unit of the kidney.

This statement as it is presented is false, the neuron is not the functional unit of the kidney; it is a nerve cell. If the underlined word were replaced with the word *nephron* in the space provided, the statement would then be true.

Fill-in-the-Blank and Essay Questions

Fill-in-the-blank items are equally common question types in medical assisting courses. This question type consists of a sentence containing a blank space for insertion of a word or phrase to correctly complete the sentence. Preparing for fill-in-the-blank questions often demands over-learning because of the specificity required in answering such a question correctly.

Essay questions are considered among most students to be the most difficult testing format. Fortunately, this format is not found on any of the certification exams; however, essay questions are common in medical assisting courses. Unlike a multiple-choice question in which the question and answer are clearly stated, and the student merely recognizes and selects the correct option, essay questions require the student to verbalize an answer without reference to any source other than one's own memory and comprehension. Students clearly realize that studying for an essay test is a whole different matter when compared to a multiple-choice test. As an evaluation instrument, essay questions are designed to test the student's knowledge, comprehension, application, and analysis of the subject matter as described in Chapter 2. Often, essay questions also allow the instructor to evaluate a student's writing or communication skills. According to education psychologists, having knowledge and understanding of a subject is a skill distinct from the ability to explain this knowledge and understanding. This is often frustrating to students who, having the proper knowledge of a concept, experience great difficulty in explaining the concept to another. This text was designed not only for the purpose of helping candidates prepare for certification exams, but to be used as a study aid to help students prepare for medical assistant course exams as well. The following advice, therefore, is provided to assist students in answering essay-type questions:

- Become familiar with the meaning of key words commonly found in essay questions (see Figure 3-1).
- Mentally, or on your paper, prepare a mind-map or brief outline to organize your thoughts. Writing your outline on paper may earn some points even if you do not have time to prepare a formal answer.
- Leave plenty of space between the points and sub-points of your outline for later inclusions.
- Think about the question further while you refer to your outline; include additional points that come to mind in the spaces left in your outline.
- Once you are satisfied with the organization of your thoughts on paper, prepare the written response to the question while referring to the outline to keep your writing organized.
- Write neatly and legibly.
- Avoid writing any introductory information, and get directly to the point. Although this is an essay question, it is not an essay. Avoid filler sentences that add useless information to your answer.
- Time permitting, review your writing for errors and clarity.

Attitude

Test scores are not a measure of self-worth; however, we often associate our sense of worthiness with our performance on an exam. Thoughts such as "If I don't pass this test, I'm a failure" are mental traps not rooted in truth. Failing a test is failing a test, nothing more. It is in no way descriptive of your value as a person or as a health-care professional. Believing that test performance is a reflection of your virtue places unreasonable pressure on your performance. Not passing the certification test only means that your certification status has been delayed. Maintaining a positive attitude is therefore important. If you have studied hard, reaffirm this mentally and believe that you will do well. If, on the other hand, you did not study as hard as you should have or wanted to, accept

- Analyze — Identify the parts of a concept, explaining each along with their interrelationship.
- Compare — Explain the similarities among two or more things. Contrasting may be implied.
- Contrast/Distinguish — Explain the differences among two or more things. Comparisons may be implied.
- Criticize/Evaluate — Formulate an evaluation or judgment regarding the merits of the issue in question.
- Define — Provide a meaning for a term or concept. Do not rely on examples only.
- Describe — Identify the characteristics, traits, or qualities, or formulate a mental picture of the issue in question.
- Discuss — To examine or explain the importance or relevance of the issue in question.
- Enumerate — List the issues in question.
- Illustrate — Provide examples of the issue in question.
- Interpret — Provide an explanation of an issue's meaning according to one's or another's understanding,
- Outline — List the important features, concepts, or parts of the issue in question.
- Prove — Provide valid reasons and evidence to support the issue in question.
- State — Directly identify the issue in question.
- Summarize — Provide a brief account or explanation of the important points of the issue in question.
- Trace — Identify the sequence, progress, or order of the issue in question.

Figure 3-1

Essay questions key words. Delmar/Cengage Learning.

that as beyond your control for now and attend to the task of doing the best you can. If things do not go well this time, you know what needs to be done in preparation for the next exam. Talk to yourself in positive terms. Avoid rationalizing past or future test performance by placing the blame on secondary variables. Thoughts such as, "I didn't have enough time," or "I should have . . .," only compound the stress of test-taking. Take control by affirming your value, self-worth, and dedication to meeting the test challenge head on. Repeat to yourself "I can and I will pass this exam."

Exagiophobia

Exagiophobia (Cody, 1991) is a term the author coined to describe the abnormal fear of tests; it is derived from the Greek *exagion* meaning a weighing, as in a test or trial, and the Greek *phobos* meaning fear. Exagiophobia, or test anxiety, is a common occurrence and sometimes can be manifested in phobic proportions. Fear creates unwanted tension and unclear thinking and ultimately prevents success on exams by predisposing your mind to failure. Desensitizing yourself to the fear response can be an effective means of overcoming and controlling your fear of the test situation. A common method psychologists use to help clients overcome anxieties and phobias is through phobic desensitization. The patient is taught to relax while gradually re-entering the phobic situation. This is done first through imagination and later in reality, all the while keeping the anxiety and fear response to a minimum. This method is effective when relaxation

becomes associated with the anxiety or fear response. To attempt phobic desensitization, practice the following steps:

Develop and practice a method of relaxation. Any method that works for you will do fine; for example,

1. get comfortable and loosen any tight clothing
2. contract your toe muscles and count to 10
3. relax your toes and enjoy the release of tension
4. do the same with your feet muscles and continue on up your body to the facial muscles
5. close your eyes taking a deep breath for as long as it takes to naturally count to 5
6. hold your breath for approximately 5 more seconds
7. exhale slowly to a count of 5.

Practice a desensitization routine. Once you have developed a relaxation technique that works for you, practice desensitizing yourself to the fear response. You can do this by imagining a testing situation as vividly as you can. If you become anxious or uneasy, clear your mind and proceed through the relaxation process. Once relaxed, attempt to visualize a testing situation for 30 seconds without any feelings of anxiety. Again, if you become uncomfortable, exercise the relaxation technique you have chosen. Periodically continue this exercise until you can imagine a testing situation for 3 minutes or longer without any feelings of uneasiness. Once this is accomplished, take the practice test at the end of this book or on the CD using your relaxation technique as warranted.

Remember, the CMA (AAMA) exam is a 160 minute, 200-item test, while the RMA (AMT) and CMAS (AMT) exams are 3-hour, 200- to 210-item tests. It has been the author's experience that the vast majority of examinees spend no more than 85% of the available time to complete either exam, so take your time and use whatever methods seem appropriate to gain control of the test situation. A few minutes periodically devoted to phobic desensitization will probably not cause you to go over time.

Beginning Your Medical Assistant Education

As you embark on your training as a medical assistant, it is recommended that you refer to this review guide as you study and prepare for medical assistant course exams and ultimately a certification exam. As you read your course texts and classroom notes, refer to the appropriate chapters in this text to help you understand and highlight important concepts and principles. Information in this guide that clarifies your reading or notes should be recorded in the margins or spaces of your text or in your notes to promote comprehension and recall abilities. If this guide was not available early in your training, but near the end, review your class notes and corresponding chapters in this guide as described above. This may include your course texts as well. Therefore, be willing to do what is necessary, according to your own preferences and idiosyncrasies, to nurture comprehension and recall abilities.

Months Before the Certification Exam

The earlier you start preparing for the exam the better. It is recommended that you begin your preparatory activities no later than 4 months before the exam date. This allows approximately 4 to 5 months to prepare. Spend the first 2 months studying the material you are weakest in (general, administrative, or clinical), devote half of the remaining time to the next weakest area, and the latter half of the remaining time briefly going over your strongest area. Be sure to exercise test-taking techniques by completing some practice tests. Attempt to plan and adhere to a study schedule identifying microgoals along the way. Weeks one and two, for example, may have as a goal the memorization of all word parts found in Chapter 4 that are not readily recognizable to you. You might prepare for this activity by constructing flash cards to help memorize these word parts.

Weeks Before the Certification Exam

If you are unfamiliar with the location of the test site take the time to travel to the test site so that you do not get lost or delayed on exam day. It is recommended that you arrive 30 minutes before the scheduled test time. Candidates are generally not allowed to sit for the exam if they arrive more than 15 to 30 minutes after the scheduled test time. If you are late but admissible, you will not be permitted to make up any lost time.

The Day Before the Exam

The day before the exam, follow your normal routine. Take time to assemble the materials you will need for the exam by placing them in a readily accessible location. You will need your scheduling permit or authorization to test document, two forms of identification—one with a picture and signature, two or more No. 2 pencils (for RMA/CMAS paper exams), erasers, and perhaps a small pencil sharpener in the event one is not available at the test facility (calculators are prohibited). Avoid any study activity and attempt to get a good night's rest. Set your alarm to allow you to get to the test facility at least 30 minutes before the exam.

Exam Day

What to expect. Arrive at least 30 minutes before the exam time. You will register with the test site administrator by presenting the appropriate authorization document and proper identification. Depending on the testing service, you may sign in and have a digital photograph taken. You will then secure any personal belongings in an assigned locker. You may also be given an access code to begin the computer-based test. The test may begin with an optional tutorial before the test is administered. For the CMA exam the first 100 questions will be given for 80 minutes, after which time you may elect to take up to a 20-minute break. The second set of 100 questions will then be given over 80 minutes as well. Upon completing the exam, you may be given an unofficial pass/fail result. You will then check out with the test site administrator.

Manage the test. Once you begin the test, progress from the simple to the complex; turn to the section that you feel most confident about. Employ any of the test-taking techniques mentioned previously, as needed. Answer the easy questions first, skipping over the more difficult ones until later. Move on to the section with the next level of difficulty, and leave the most difficult section for last. There should be enough time to go over the entire exam to answer the questions you skipped over. For paper exams, once all items have been answered, go over the answer sheet to ensure that all the circles are filled in properly and extraneous marks erased.

SUMMARY

Test-taking skills are an important component of the examination challenge. By becoming familiar with the test format and various discriminatory techniques, you can avoid unnecessary distractions and neutralize any potentially negative effects the test arrangement may have on your score. As you prepare for and take practice tests, attempt to use whatever techniques seem appropriate. The reasons for taking practice tests are threefold: Developing familiarity with the exam format, exercising test-taking techniques, and identifying knowledge weaknesses. It is up to you, so take control and succeed. Good luck to you, CMA/RMA/CMAS-to-be!

SECTION II

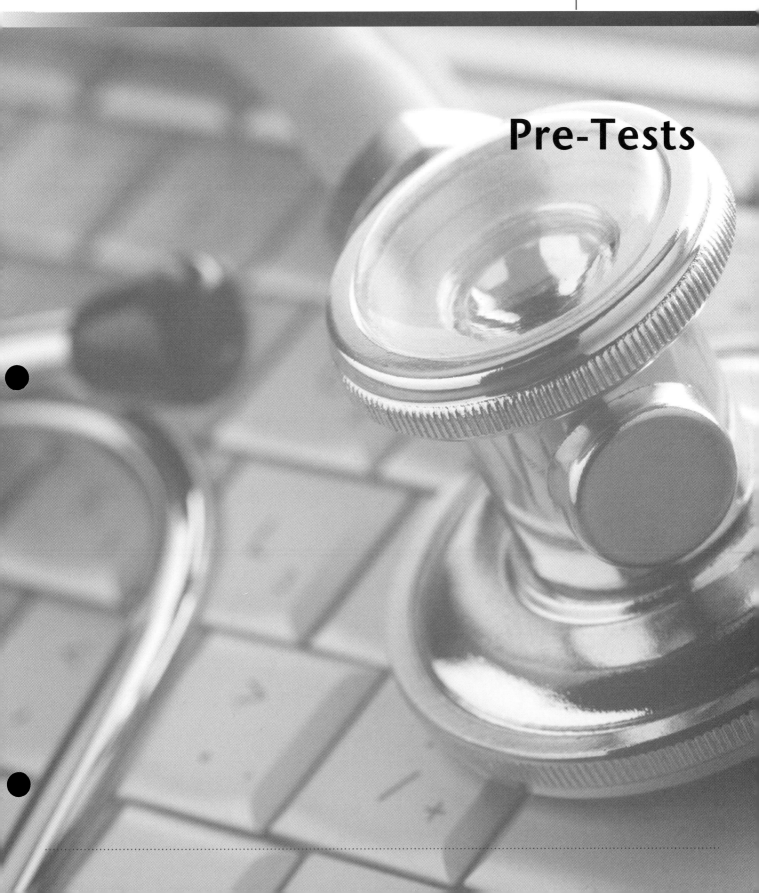

Pre-Tests

CMA SIMULATION TEST

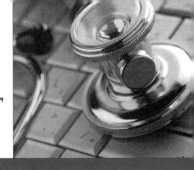

Pre-Test

90-question, 80 minute, timed diagnostic exam

PART 1: GENERAL

DIRECTIONS

Each of the questions or incomplete statements below is followed by five suggested answers or completions. Select the *one* answer or completion that is *best* in each case and fill in the circle containing the corresponding letter on the answer sheet. Perforated answer sheets are located at the back of the book.

1. The suffix -osis means
   a. blood condition
   b. destruction
   c. condition of
   d. drooping
   e. inflammation

2. Blood returning from the body to the heart enters the
   a. left atrium
   b. right atrium
   c. left ventricle
   d. right ventricle
   e. aorta

3. Represents physical changes with accompanying increase in size.
   a. Growth
   b. Development
   c. Personality
   d. Id
   e. Ego

4. The communication process includes all of the following elements **EXCEPT**
   a. source
   b. message
   c. channel
   d. receiver
   e. jargon

5. "Let the master answer" describes the legal doctrine
   a. res ipsa loquitur
   b. respondeat superior
   c. informed consent
   d. res judicata
   e. non suis juris

6. Confidentiality is ethically supported by the concept of
   a. beneficence
   b. nonmalfeasance
   c. fidelity
   d. all of the above
   e. none of the above

7. Which of the following combining forms means "eyelid"?
   a. cost/o
   b. or/o
   c. ocul/o
   d. blephar/o
   e. nas/o

8. The twelfth cranial nerve is the
   a. acoustic
   b. trigeminal
   c. olfactory
   d. hypoglossal
   e. facial

9. A behavioral aspect that is characterized by an increase in the complexity of function and skill.
   a. Growth
   b. Development
   c. Personality
   d. Id
   e. Ego

10. In Abraham Maslow's Hierarchy of Needs, the need to be respected describes the
    a. physiological need
    b. safety need
    c. social need
    d. self-esteem need
    e. self-actualization need

11. A consent form is not required if the patient is
    a. a minor
    b. elderly
    c. incompetent
    d. unconscious and critically injured
    e. an attorney

12. A standard or principle that guides our behavior regarding what is right and what is wrong is a(n)
    a. norm
    b. moral
    c. morale
    d. ethic
    e. virtue

13. The most common connecting vowel found in combining forms is
    a. a
    b. e
    c. i
    d. o
    e. u

14. The structure that prevents material from entering the windpipe is the
    a. trachea
    b. epiglottis
    c. bronchus
    d. alveolus
    e. pharynx

15. Proximodistal growth and development progresses from:
    a. head to toe.
    b. the center outward.
    c. the front to the rear.
    d. the left to the right.
    e. earlier to later.

16. Exhibiting immature behavior as a result of stress or anxiety describes
    a. regression
    b. denial
    c. sublimation
    d. repression
    e. none of the above

17. If a patient refuses consent to treatment, the medical assistant should
    a. coerce the patient into consenting
    b. explain to the patient that refusing consent will result in termination of care
    c. delay treatment and consult the health care provider
    d. force treatment on the patient for his or her own good
    e. dismiss the patient and schedule another appointment

18. Telling the truth best defines
    a. beneficence
    b. nonmalfeasance
    c. justice
    d. veracity
    e. fidelity

19. The term tachycardia is synonymous with
    a. fast heart rate
    b. slow heart rate
    c. normal heart rate
    d. irregular heart rate
    e. sluggish heart rate

20. The wristbones are collectively known as
    a. metatarsals
    b. tarsals
    c. metacarpals
    d. carpals
    e. digitals

21. According to Sigmund Freud, which of the following is **NOT** a personality level?
    a. Id
    b. Ego
    c. Superego
    d. Libido
    e. None of the above

22. An unconscious defense mechanism characterized by behavior that is the opposite of one's true feelings describes
    a. introjection
    b. dissociation
    c. rationalization
    d. projection
    e. reaction formation (compensation)

23. Failing to act when one has the duty to act describes the tort
    a. nonfeasance
    b. misfeasance
    c. malfeasance
    d. negligence
    e. malpractice

24. Positive character traits are
    a. duties
    b. virtues
    c. justice
    d. ethics
    e. rights

25. Balanitis refers to which body system?
    a. nervous system
    b. reproductive system
    c. digestive system
    d. circulatory system
    e. respiratory system

26. The tube extending from the kidney to the bladder is the
    a. ureter
    b. urethra
    c. epididymis
    d. seminal vesicle
    e. vas deferens

27. Erik Erikson is credited with formulating which of the following theories?
    a. Psychosexual development
    b. Cognitive development
    c. Psychosocial development
    d. Moral development
    e. Spiritual development

28. Elisabeth Kübler-Ross is credited with establishing the
    a. elements of the communication process
    b. steps in dealing with the emotionally distressed patient
    c. five stages of dying
    d. philosophical principles of nursing practice and patient care
    e. development of the unconscious defense mechanisms

29. Defamation of character employing the written word describes
    a. invasion of privacy
    b. libel
    c. slander
    d. embezzlement
    e. fraud

30. Disclosing unpleasant information to a patient is best supported by the ethical concept of
    a. veracity
    b. right
    c. nonmalfeasance
    d. justice
    e. duty

PART 2: ADMINISTRATIVE

DIRECTIONS

Each of the questions or incomplete statements below is followed by five suggested answers or completions. Select the *one* answer or completion that is *best* in each case, and fill in the circle containing the corresponding letter on the answer sheet.

1. When using a typewriter to complete selected forms, pica pitch consists of what number of characters per inch?
    a. 8
    b. 9
    c. 10
    d. 11
    e. 12

2. Scheduling the number of patients who can be seen in 1 hour based on the average appointment time describes the
    a. time specified system
    b. wave system
    c. modified wave system
    d. double-booking system
    e. clustering (grouping) system

3. The bank is also known as the
    a. drawee
    b. drawer
    c. payee
    d. payor
    e. endorser

4. Which of the following would require an ICD-9 (or 10) CM code?
    a. hysterosalpingo-oophorectomy
    b. cystopexy
    c. cleidorrhaphy
    d. glossitis
    e. tracheostomy

5. A purchase agreement provision that covers the cost of repair resulting from faulty design or manufacturing is the
    a. service agreement
    b. garnishee
    c. guarantee
    d. warranty
    e. quarantine

6. The meeting chairperson is responsible for which of the following?
   a. developing the meeting agenda
   b. determining who should be present
   c. informing the members of the meeting logistics
   d. deciding on the meeting time, place, and duration
   e. all of the above

7. The number of lines separating the inside address and the salutation is
   a. 2
   b. 3
   c. 4
   d. 15
   e. none of the above

8. All of the following should be considered when scheduling appointments **EXCEPT**
   a. patient need
   b. provider preference
   c. available facilities
   d. scheduling system
   e. day of the week

9. The bank statement shows a balance of $4,050.00. Outstanding deposits total $1,025.00 and outstanding checks total $700.00. The checkbook balance should be
   a. $2,325.00
   b. $3,725.00
   c. $4,050.00
   d. $4,375.00
   e. $5,775.00

10. All of the following would require a CPT code **EXCEPT**
    a. myringotomy
    b. atherosclerosis
    c. herniorrhaphy
    d. appendectomy
    e. rhinoplasty

11. A gratuitous payment for professional services for which custom or propriety forbids a price to be set is a(n)
    a. professional fee
    b. honorarium
    c. gratuity
    d. tip
    e. bribe

12. Protocol regarding who reports to whom within an organization's hierarchy is the
    a. chain of custody
    b. organizational chart
    c. chain of authority
    d. article of incorporation
    e. chain of infection

13. The tab key allows one to
    a. set the margins
    b. move the cursor a predetermined number of spaces to the right
    c. center the cursor
    d. return the cursor to the left margin
    e. count the number of spaces across a page

14. Scheduling patients with similar diagnoses, treatments, or needs within a specified time frame describes
    a. double-booking
    b. grouping (clustering)
    c. time specified
    d. time management
    e. wave

15. Categorizing accounts according to the number of days the account is pastdue describes
    a. aging accounts receivable
    b. accounts receivable categorization
    c. accounts receivable turnover
    d. accounts receivable analysis
    e. none of the above

16. A health care entitlement program for the indigent that is funded by both state and federal revenues but is administered by the state is
    a. Medicare
    b. Medicaid
    c. Blue Cross
    d. Blue Shield
    e. Tricare

17. The amount of supplies used as a buffer while awaiting receipt of additional supplies is called
    a. safety stock
    b. stock-out
    c. replenishment
    d. inventory
    e. back-order

18. When hiring a new employee, the medical assistant should consider all of the following **EXCEPT**
    a. demeanor
    b. appearance
    c. credentials
    d. experience
    e. marital status

19. Open punctuation refers to
    a. placing a comma after the complimentary close
    b. placing a semicolon after the complimentary close
    c. placing a colon after the salutation
    d. placing a semicolon after the salutation
    e. placing no punctuation after the salutation

20. To mitigate potential legal difficulties, appointments should be recorded in
    a. indelible ink
    b. erasable ink
    c. pencil
    d. any of the above
    e. none of the above

21. A medical assistant who is compensated every other Friday is being paid
    a. semimonthly
    b. biweekly
    c. bimonthly
    d. semiweekly
    e. semiannually

22. An amount that is paid on an insurance contract before the payment of benefits is
    a. deductible
    b. coinsurance
    c. assignment
    d. exclusion
    e. prepaid fee

23. According to the Americans with Disabilities Act (ADA), outpatient facilities should provide how many accessible parking spaces?
    a. One for every 25 or fewer spaces
    b. Two for every 26 to 50 spaces
    c. 10% of available spaces
    d. 20% of available spaces
    e. None of the above

24. In preparing for air travel, luggage should be checked-in at least _____ hour(s) before scheduled takeoff.
    a. 0.5
    b. 1.0
    c. 1.5
    d. 2.0
    e. 2.5

25. What number of lines of text represent 1 inch?
    a. 5
    b. 6
    c. 7
    d. 8
    e. 9

26. When it is 2:00 p.m. in Minnesota, it is _____ in Georgia.
    a. 12:00 p.m.
    b. 1:00 p.m.
    c. 2:00 p.m.
    d. 3:00 p.m.
    e. 4:00 p.m.

27. A property or right owned by a business defines
    a. capital
    b. liability
    c. asset
    d. revenue
    e. expense

28. A prepaid health plan that emphasizes health prevention and promotion is a(n)
    a. HMO
    b. PPO
    c. IPA
    d. IVP
    e. PID

29. Assuming a clinic has five entrances, how many must be accessible according to federal law?
    a. One
    b. Two
    c. Three
    d. Four
    e. Five

30. A job description usually includes all of the following **EXCEPT**
    a. job title
    b. to whom the position reports
    c. job duties
    d. payroll guidelines
    e. who reports to the position

PART 3: CLINICAL

DIRECTIONS

Each of the questions or incomplete statements below is followed by five suggested answers or completions. Select the *one* answer or completion that is *best* in each case and fill in the circle containing the corresponding letter on the answer sheet.

1. The acronym PERRLA is typically recorded in what part of the Review of Systems?
    a. head and neck
    b. cardiovascular
    c. respiratory
    d. urinary
    e. gastrointestinal

2. Instruments designed to grasp objects are
    a. scissors
    b. forceps
    c. scopes
    d. probes
    e. sounds

3. Tylenol is an example of a(n)
   a. generic name
   b. chemical name
   c. synthetic name
   d. trade name
   e. anticoagulant

4. During two-rescuer CPR, the compression to ventilation ratio for children is
   a. 15:1
   b. 15:2
   c. 30:1
   d. 30:2
   e. 30:18

5. Which of the following is a cardiac enzyme?
   a. glucose
   b. coagulase
   c. lipase
   d. amylase
   e. CPK

6. A nutrient that yields 4 kilocalories per gram is
   a. carbohydrates
   b. fats
   c. vitamin A
   d. sodium
   e. iron

7. The position of choice for orthopnea is
   a. lithotomy
   b. dorsal recumbent
   c. Fowler's
   d. prone
   e. supine

8. Which of the following is a physical disinfection agent?
   a. boiling water
   b. alcohol
   c. Betadine
   d. iodine
   e. bleach

9. A subcutaneous injection typically employs a
   a. 1.5-inch needle
   b. ¾-inch needle
   c. ⅝-inch needle
   d. ¼-inch needle
   e. none of the above

10. In adult CPR, the depth of chest compressions is
    a. 0.5 to 1.0 inches
    b. 1.0 to 1.5 inches
    c. 1.5 to 2.0 inches
    d. 2.0 to 2.5 inches
    e. 2.5 to 3.0 inches

11. The presence of hemoglobin in the urine is most likely indicative of
    a. UTI
    b. glomerulonephritis
    c. hydronephrosis
    d. urinary hemorrhage
    e. pyelonephritis

12. Proteins consist of the following **EXCEPT**
    a. carbon
    b. potassium
    c. hydrogen
    d. oxygen
    e. nitrogen

13. The three-point gait describes the use of which device?
    a. walker
    b. wheelchair
    c. crutches
    d. cane
    e. braces

14. The medical assistant's responsibilities in surgical care and treatment include
    a. preparing the room
    b. preparing the patient
    c. assisting the health care provider
    d. reinforcing postsurgical instructions
    e. all of the above

15. The provider orders 600 mg Augmentin. Augmentin, 200 mg per 0.5 mL, is available. The medical assistant should administer
    a. 0.5 mL
    b. 0.75 mL
    c. 1 mL
    d. 1.5 mL
    e. 2 mL

16. When encountering an unconscious person, the medical assistant should *first*
    a. assess the victim's responsiveness
    b. call for help
    c. administer artificial respirations
    d. splint any broken bones
    e. control any bleeding

17. Normally, the hematocrit is approximately
    a. one-third the hemoglobin
    b. two-thirds the hemoglobin
    c. twice the hemoglobin
    d. three times the hemoglobin
    e. four times the hemoglobin

18. All of the following are minerals **EXCEPT**
    a. sodium
    b. hydrogen
    c. copper
    d. iron
    e. calcium

19. The "S" of SOAP notes represents
    a. data acquired through examination and testing
    b. data provided by the patient describing signs, symptoms, and feelings
    c. the provider's diagnosis
    d. the course of treatment
    e. patient referral

20. Gynecological instruments include
    a. pelvimeter
    b. uterine tenaculum
    c. vaginal speculum
    d. uterine curette
    e. all of the above

21. Antimicrobials include
    a. E-mycin
    b. Amoxil
    c. Veetids
    d. Tagamet
    e. (A), (B), and (C) only

22. Which of the following are precautions when using an AED?
    a. Do not touch the victim while the AED is analyzing.
    b. Do not touch the victim during defibrillation.
    c. Before shocking the victim, ensure no one is in contact with the victim or the equipment.
    d. Do not use alcohol to dry the victim's chest.
    e. All of the above

23. The media of choice for culturing *Neisseria gonorrhoeae* is
    a. tryptocase soy broth
    b. MacConkey
    c. Salmonella-shigella agar
    d. thioglycolate broth
    e. Thayer-Martin agar

24. A patient suffering from diabetic coma will require
    a. something sweet
    b. carbohydrates
    c. a dose of insulin
    d. immediate surgical care
    e. hospital admission

25. The right lateral position best describes which of the following?
    a. X-rays enter the left side and exit the right side of the body.
    b. X-rays enter the right side and exit the left side of the body.
    c. X-rays enter the front and exit the back side of the body.
    d. X-rays enter the back and exit the front side of the body.
    e. X-rays enter and exit the body at an acute angle.

26. An instrument used to perforate the injured area when a blood clot or infection makes drainage and pressure release necessary.
    a. Extractor
    b. Fingernail drill
    c. Alligator forceps
    d. Ear curette
    e. Retractor

27. Which of the following is the generic name for Diovan?
    a. losartan potassium
    b. valsartan
    c. amlodipine
    d. metoprolol
    e. benazepril hydrochloride

28. If you are alone and must leave the victim to call for help, the victim should be placed in which of the following positions?
    a. Prone
    b. Supine
    c. Recovery
    d. Trendelenberg
    e. Fowler's

29. A metabolic profile typically includes all of the following assays **EXCEPT**
    a. Na^+
    b. glucose
    c. BUN
    d. ketones
    e. K^+

30. The seven dietary guidelines include
    a. eating a variety of food
    b. maintaining an ideal weight
    c. eating foods low in fat and cholesterol
    d. reducing alcohol consumption
    e. all of the above

CMA PRE-TEST SCORE SHEET

Directions:

1. Comparing your answer sheet with the correct answers listed below for each section, circle the incorrect responses below.
2. Tally the number of incorrect responses in each column and record the total in the space provided.
3. Score each of the three sections as described in Chapter 1. Identify the section (general, administrative, or clinical) having the lowest score.
4. In the section having the lowest overall score, identify the column having the most incorrect responses and turn to the chapter indicated for further study.
5. Concentrate your study on the section with the lowest score by studying the next weakest area and the next, and so on.
6. After completing your study of the weakest content section, turn to the section having the next lowest score, concentrating your study on the column with the lowest score, and so on.

GENERAL: Percent correct: _____%

1=C	2=B	3=A	4=E	5=B	6=D
7=D	8=D	9=B	10=D	11=D	12=B
13=D	14=B	15=B	16=A	17=C	18=D
19=A	20=D	21=D	22=E	23=A	24=B
25=B	26=A	27=C	28=C	29=B	30=A
____	____	____	____	____	____
Ch. 4	Ch. 5	Ch. 6	Ch. 7	Ch. 8	Ch. 9

ADMINISTRATIVE: Percent correct: _____%

1=C	2=B	3=A	4=D	5=D	6=E
7=A	8=E	9=D	10=B	11=B	12=C
13=B	14=B	15=A	16=B	17=A	18=E
19=E	20=A	21=B	22=A	23=C	24=B
25=B	26=D	27=C	28=A	29=A	30=D
____	____	____	____	____	____
Ch. 10	Ch. 11	Ch. 12	Ch. 13	Ch. 14	Ch. 15

CLINICAL: Percent correct: _____%

1=A	2=B	3=D	4=A	5=E	6=A
7=C	8=A	9=C	10=C	11=D	12=B
13=C	14=E	15=D	16=A	17=D	18=B
19=B	20=E	21=E	22=E	23=E	24=C
25=A	26=B	27=B	28=C	29=D	30=E
____	____	____	____	____	____
Ch. 16	Ch. 17	Ch. 18	Ch. 19	Ch. 20	Ch. 21

General:

If you answered three or more questions incorrectly in any of the columns, turn to the appropriate chapter for further study.

Administrative:

If you answered three or more questions incorrectly in any of the columns, turn to the appropriate chapter for further study.

Clinical:

If you answered three or more questions incorrectly in any of the columns, turn to the appropriate chapter for further study.

Total percent correct (_____ /90 × 100): _____%

CMA standard score = (Raw score × 10) − 200
(Standard score ≥ 445 is passing)

CMA PRE-TEST ANSWERS AND RATIONALES

General:

1. C. Option A would be –emia; B would be –lysis; D would be ptosis; E would be –itis.

2. B. Blood returning to the heart from the body via the superior and inferior venae cavae enters the right atrium.

3. A. B is a behavioral aspect characterized by an increase in the complexity of function and skill; C is the outward expression of the inner self; D is the source of instinctive and unconscious urges that are chiefly sexual in nature; and E is formed through the realization that satisfying one's urges and impulses conflicts with reality and gratification must be delayed.

4. E. Of the options listed, jargon is not an element in the communication process.

5. B. Respondeat superior is Latin for "let the master answer."

6. D. A, B, and C are terms related to a beneficial nature or outcome and so relate to the concept of confidentiality.

7. D. Option A means rib; B means mouth; C means eye; E means nose.

8. D. Option A is the eighth; B is the fifth; C is the first; E is the seventh cranial nerve.

9. B. A represents physical changes with accompanying increase in size; C is the outward expression of the inner self; D is the source of instinctive and unconscious urges that are chiefly sexual in nature; and E is formed through the realization that satisfying one's urges and impulses conflicts with reality and gratification must be delayed.

10. D. Option A refers to the need for food and water; B refers to freedom from anxiety; C refers to love and belonging; E refers to meeting one's potential.

11. D. Generally, a consent form should be required for all patient treatments; however, when a person is unable to provide consent and an emergency exists, it is assumed that the patient would desire life and/or limb to be restored.

12. B. Option A is a custom; C is a positive spirit; D is a study of moral thought; E is a positive character trait.

13. D. Of the options listed, "o" is the most common vowel.

14. B. The epiglottis is a flap of tissue that covers the trachea during swallowing to prevent choking.

15. B. A is cephalocaudal growth and development, and the remaining options are nonsense distracters.

16. A. Option B means to unconsciously avoid the reality of a situation; C means to divert unacceptable thoughts or feelings into acceptable behaviors; D means to put unpleasant thoughts or feelings out of one's mind.

17. C. Patients should never be coerced or forced to accept treatment, nor should they be dismissed or their care terminated in such a case.

18. D. Option A means do good; B means do no harm; C means fairness; E means loyalty.

19. A. Option A is the definition for tachycardia.

20. D. Option A refers to the foot bones; B refers to the ankle bones; C refers to the hand bones; E refers to the finger bones.

21. D. A–C are the three levels of personality.

22. E. Option A means to adopt the feelings of others; B means to disconnect the emotional significance of an idea or event; C means to justify a feeling or thought; D means to ascribe to another person one's own feelings.

23. A. Option B means to perform an improper act; C means to perform a bad or illegal act; D is a general term meaning to act carelessly; E refers to the negligent acts of a professional person.

24. B. Option A means obligations; C means fairness; D means study of moral principles; E means legal claims.

25. B. Balanitis means inflammation of the penis, a reproductive organ.

26. A. The ureter is a tube that extends from the kidney to the bladder.

27. C. A is Sigmund Freud, B is Jean Piaget, D is Lawrence Kohlberg, and E is James Fowler.

28. C. Dr. Elisabeth Kübler-Ross formulated the five stages of dying.

29. B. Option A refers to unlawfully prying into another's private life; C refers to defamation using spoken words; D refers to unlawfully diverting organizational funds or resources for private use; E refers to deception.

30. A. Being truthful to the patient regardless of the unpleasantness involved is our duty and the patient's right.

Administrative:

1. C. Option E is elite pitch; the other options are nonsense distracters.

2. B. Option A refers to a specific time slot; C is a staggered wave system; D is scheduling more than one patient for the same time slot; E is scheduling patients having similar needs during a common time frame.

3. A. Option B is the depositor; C and E refer to the person receiving the funds; D is the person writing the check.

4. D. The remaining options are procedures and are assigned a CPT code.

5. D. A warranty covers the cost of repairs resulting from defects.

6. E. All are typical responsibilities of the chairperson.

7. A. Two lines separate the inside address and the salutation.

8. E. Day of the week is the least important factor to consider when scheduling appointments.

9. D. 4050 + 1025 − 700 = 4375

10. B. The other options are procedures and are assigned a CPT code.

11. B. An honorarium is a gratuitous payment for professional services.

12. C. Option A is a form used to monitor the handling of evidence; B is a chart identifying the positions with an organization; D is a charter; E is a nonsense distracter.

13. B. The tab key allows one to move the cursor a predetermined number of spaces to the right.

14. B. Option A means scheduling more than one patient for the same time slot; C means scheduling patients for individual time slots; D is a nonsense distracter; E means scheduling a number of patients at the beginning of an hour and seeing them in the order of arrival.

15. A. The remaining options are nonsense distracters.

16. B. Option A is for the elderly and disabled; C and D are conventional plans; E is for military personnel and their dependents.

17. A. Option B refers to stock that is depleted, C refers to stock that is replaced, D is stock on the shelf, and E refers to when stock delivery that is delayed.

18. E. Marital status is not a bona fide occupational qualification and is an illegal question to ask during an interview.

19. E. The alt and ctrl keys triple the tasks the function keys can perform.

20. C. Option A is full block; B is modified block; D is hanging identification; E is simplified.

20. A. Because the appointment book is a legal document, nonerasable ink should be used.

21. B. Option A is twice a month; C is every 2 months; D is twice a week; E is twice a year.

22. A. Option B is additional insurance to pay for expenses not covered by a policy; C refers to a provider who accepts the payment directly from the carrier; D is an uncovered peril; E is a nonsense distracter.

23. C. Options A and B refer to general, non-medical facilities; D is true for facilities that specifically service disabled persons.

24. B. One hour is the standard for domestic flights.

25. B. Six lines represent an inch.

26. D. There is a 1-hour difference between Minnesota and Georgia.

27. C. Option A is assets less liabilities; B is a debt obligation; D is business income; E is business cost.

28. A. HMO is a plan that emphasizes health promotion.

29. A. Generally, only one entrance must be made accessible.

30. D. A–C. Payroll guidelines are not part of the job description.

Clinical:

1. A. PERRLA means pupils are equal, round and reactive to light and accommodation—this is part of the head and neck examination.

2. B. Option A is used for cutting; C for visualizing body orifices and cavities; D and E for probing orifices and cavities.

3. D. Tylenol is the trade name for acetaminophen, its generic name.

4. D. The compression to ventilation ratio is 30:2; this ratio is the same for adults and children, per AHA guidelines.

5. E. Option A is a carbohydrate; B through D are noncardiac enzymes.

6. A. Option B yields 9 kilocalories, and the remaining options yield none.

7. C. The Fowler's or semi-sitting position is the best position for orthopnea (difficulty breathing if not upright).

8. A. Boiling water physically destroys bacteria, whereas the other options are chemical agents.

9. C. Under normal conditions, a 5/8-inch needle is optimal for subcutaneous injections.

10. C. Option A relates to infants; B relates to children; D and E are nonsense distracters.

11. D. Although blood may be present in all the options, urinary hemorrhage is the most obvious and common reason.

12. B. Proteins chemically are composed of carbon, hydrogen, oxygen, and nitrogen, not potassium.

13. C. The three-point gait refers to when two crutch tips and one foot are in contact with the ground.

14. E. All of the options are typical responsibilities of medical assistants.

15. D. 600 mg ÷ 200 mg × 0.5 mL = 3 × 0.5 mL = 1.5 mL.

16. A. Nothing is done until a person has been determined to be unconscious—she could merely be sleeping.

17. D. A normal hematocrit is approximately 35 to 45%, which is about three times the normal hemoglobin, 12 to 15 g/dL.

18. B. Unlike the other options, hydrogen, a gas, is not considered a mineral.

19. B. Option A refers to O—objective; C refers to A—assessment; D refers to P—plan; E is a nonsense distracter.

20. E. All are common gynecological instruments.

21. E. A through C are antimicrobials, whereas D is an articles agent

22. A. The most common streptococci are the gram-positive variety.

22. E. Precautions are necessary to prevent injury to the victum or rescuer

23. E. This bacteria requires a rich media, such as Thayer-Martin agar, to grow

24. C. Patients suffering from diabetic coma have abnormally high blood glucose levels. This condition requires insulin so that the body can metabolize the glucose for energy.

25. A. Option B describes the left lateral position; C describes the AP (anterior-posterior) position; D describes the PA (posterior-anterior) position; E describes the oblique position.

26. B. Option A is used to remove substances from the superficial layer of skin; C, forceps inserted through a speculum to remove foreign bodies; D, scrapes accumulated cerumen from the ear canal; and E, is used to pull back tissue to allow viewing of the operative site.

27. B. Option A is Cozaar, C and E is Lotrel, and D is Toprol.

28. C. The recovery position minimizes any further injury to the victim and helps to ensure that vomitus will not be aspirated and block the airway.

29. D. Ketones are typically not tested in a metabolic profile.

30. E. All are elements of the seven dietary guidelines.

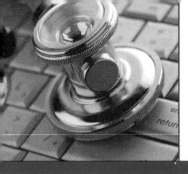
Pre-Test

90-question, 90 minute, timed diagnostic exam

PART 1: GENERAL

DIRECTIONS

Each of the questions or incomplete statements below is followed by four suggested answers or completions. Select the *one* answer or completion that is *best* in each case and fill in the circle containing the corresponding letter on the answer sheet. Perforated answer sheets are located at the back of the book.

1. Which of the following combining forms means "eyelid"?
   a. cost/o
   b. or/o
   c. ocul/o
   d. blephar/o

2. The most common connecting vowel found in combining forms is
   a. a
   b. i
   c. o
   d. u

3. The term tachycardia is synonymous with
   a. fast heart rate
   b. slow heart rate
   c. normal heart rate
   d. irregular heart rate

4. Balanitis refers to which body system?
   a. nervous system
   b. reproductive system
   c. digestive system
   d. circulatory system

5. Hematopoiesis means
   a. blood condition
   b. hemorrhage
   c. blood formation
   d. bloody discharge

6. The twelfth cranial nerve is
   a. acoustic
   b. trigeminal
   c. olfactory
   d. hypoglossal

7. The structure that prevents material from entering the windpipe is the
   a. trachea
   b. epiglottis
   c. bronchus
   d. alveolus

8. The wristbones are collectively known as
   a. metatarsals
   b. tarsals
   c. metacarpals
   d. carpals

9. The tube extending from the kidney to the bladder is the
   a. ureter
   b. urethra
   c. epididymis
   d. seminal vesicle

10. The aqueous humor is situated _____ to the lens.
    a. lateral
    b. distal
    c. medial
    d. anterior

11. Represents physical changes with accompanying increase in size.
    a. Growth
    b. Development
    c. Personality
    d. Id

12. A behavioral aspect that is characterized by an increase in the complexity of function and skill.
    a. Growth
    b. Development
    c. Personality
    d. Id

13. Proximodistal growth and development progresses from
    a. head to toe.
    b. the center outward.
    c. the front to the rear.
    d. the left to the right.

14. According to Sigmund Freud, which of the following is **NOT** a personality level.
    a. Id
    b. Ego
    c. Superego
    d. Libido

15. Erik Erikson is credited with formulating which of the following theories:
    a. Psychosexual development
    b. Cognitive development
    c. Psychosocial development
    d. Moral development

16. In Abraham Maslow's Hierarchy of Needs, the need to be respected describes the
    a. physiological need
    b. safety need
    c. social need
    d. self-esteem need

17. Exhibiting immature behavior as a result of stress or anxiety describes
    a. regression
    b. denial
    c. sublimation
    d. repression

18. An unconscious defense mechanism characterized by behavior that is the opposite of one's true feelings describes
    a. introjection
    b. dissociation
    c. rationalization
    d. reaction formation

19. Elisabeth Kübler-Ross is credited with establishing the
    a. elements of the communication process
    b. steps in dealing with the emotionally distressed client
    c. five stages of dying
    d. development of the unconscious defense mechanisms

20. A patient expresses fear about dying; the medical assistant should
    a. ask the patient to discuss something more cheerful
    b. indicate that fearing death is futile
    c. describe in detail the stages of dying
    d. attempt to be attentive and understanding

21. A consent form is not required if the patient is
    a. a minor
    b. elderly
    c. incompetent
    d. unconscious and critically injured

22. Failing to act when one has the duty to act describes the tort
    a. nonfeasance
    b. misfeasance
    c. malfeasance
    d. negligence

23. Defamation of character employing the written word describes
    a. invasion of privacy
    b. libel
    c. slander
    d. fraud

24. Negligence requires the following elements **EXCEPT**
    a. inconvenience
    b. duty
    c. causation
    d. damage

25. Defenses against negligence include which of the following?
    a. tolling of the statute of limitations
    b. contributory negligence
    c. assumption of the risk
    d. all of the above

26. Confidentiality is ethically supported by the concept of
    a. beneficence
    b. onmaleficence
    c. fidelity
    d. all of the above

27. A standard or principle that guides our behavior regarding what is right and what is wrong is a(n)
    a. norm
    b. moral
    c. morale
    d. ethic

28. Telling the truth best defines
    a. beneficence
    b. nonmaleficence
    c. justice
    d. veracity

29. Positive character traits are
    a. duties
    b. virtues
    c. justice
    d. ethics

30. Disclosing unpleasant information to a patient is best supported by the ethical concept of
    a. veracity
    b. right
    c. nonmaleficence
    d. justice

PART 2: ADMINISTRATIVE

DIRECTIONS

Each of the questions or incomplete statements below is followed by four suggested answers or completions. Select the *one* answer or completion that is *best* in each case and fill in the circle containing the corresponding letter on the answer sheet. Perforated answer sheets are located at the back of the book.

1. When using a typewriter to complete a pre-printed form, pica pitch consists of what number of characters per inch?
   a. 8
   b. 10
   c. 12
   d. 14

2. The tab key allows one to
   a. set the margins
   b. move the cursor a predetermined number of spaces to the right
   c. center the cursor
   d. return the cursor to the left margin

3. What number of lines of text represent 1 inch?
   a. 6
   b. 8
   c. 10
   d. 12

4. The keyboard keys most commonly used with function keys (F1–F12) are
   a. alt
   b. space bar
   c. ctrl
   d. (A) or (C)

5. In word processing, to remove a portion of text and transport it to another section of the document describes
   a. cut and paste
   b. concatenate
   c. copy and paste
   d. purging

6. Scheduling the number of patients who can be seen in 1 hour based on the average appointment describes the
   a. time specified
   b. wave system
   c. modified wave system
   d. double-booking system

7. All of the following should be considered when scheduling appointments **EXCEPT**
   a. patient need
   b. day of the week
   c. provider preference
   d. available facilities

8. Scheduling patients with similar diagnoses, treatments, or needs within a specified time frame describes
   a. double-booking
   b. grouping (clustering)
   c. time specified
   d. wave

9. To mitigate potential legal difficulties, appointments should be recorded in
   a. indelible ink
   b. erasable ink
   c. pencil
   d. any of the above

10. When it is 2 p.m. in Minnesota, it is _____ in Georgia.
    a. 1 p.m.
    b. 2 p.m.
    c. 3 p.m.
    d. 4 p.m.

11. The bank is also known as the
    a. drawee
    b. drawer
    c. payee
    d. payor

12. The bank statement shows a balance of $4,050.00. Outstanding deposits total $1,025.00, and outstanding checks total $700.00. The checkbook balance should be
    a. $2,325.00
    b. $3,725.00
    c. $4,375.00
    d. $5,775.00

13. Categorizing accounts according to the number of days the account is pastdue describes
    a. aging accounts receivable
    b. accounts receivable turnover
    c. accounts receivable analysis
    d. none of the above

14. A medical assistant who is compensated every other Friday is being paid
    a. semimonthly
    b. biweekly
    c. bimonthly
    d. semiannually

15. A property or right owned by a business defines
    a. capital
    b. liability
    c. asset
    d. revenue

16. Which of the following would require an ICD-9 (or 10) CM code?
    a. hysterosalpingo-oophorectomy
    b. cystopexy
    c. cleidorrhaphy
    d. glossitis

17. All of the following would require a CPT code **EXCEPT**
    a. myringotomy
    b. atherosclerosis
    c. herniorrhaphy
    d. rhinoplasty

18. A health care entitlement program for the indigent that is funded by both state and federal revenues but is administered by the state is
    a. Medicare
    b. Medicaid
    c. Blue Cross
    d. Tricare

19. An amount that is paid on an insurance contract before the payment of benefits is
    a. deductible
    b. coinsurance
    c. assignment
    d. exclusion

20. A prepaid health plan that emphasizes health prevention and promotion is a(n)
    a. HMO
    b. PPO
    c. IPA
    d. PID

21. A purchase agreement provision that covers the cost of repair resulting from faulty design or manufacturing is the
    a. service agreement
    b. garnishee
    c. guarantee
    d. warranty

22. The amount of supplies used as a buffer while awaiting receipt of additional supplies is called
    a. safety stock
    b. stock-out
    c. replenishment
    d. inventory

23. According to the Americans with Disabilities Act (ADA), outpatient facilities should provide how many accessible parking spaces?
    a. One for every 25 or fewer spaces.
    b. Two for every 26 to 50 spaces.
    c. Ten percent of available spaces.
    d. Twenty percent of available spaces.

24. Assuming a clinic has five entrances, how many must be accessible according to federal law?
    a. One
    b. Two
    c. Three
    d. Four

25. Which of the following represent good electrical safety?
    a. Never remove the third (grounding) prong from any three-prong piece of equipment.
    b. Floor-mounted outlets should be carefully placed to prevent tripping hazards.
    c. Cords should never be placed on radiators, steam pipes, walls, or windows.
    d. All of the above

26. The meeting chairperson is responsible for which of the following?
    a. developing the meeting agenda
    b. determining who should be present
    c. deciding on the meeting time, place, and duration
    d. all of the above

27. Protocol regarding who reports to whom within an organization's hierarchy is the
    a. chain of custody
    b. organizational chart
    c. chain of authority
    d. chain of infection

28. A gratuitous payment for professional services for which custom or propriety forbids a price to be set is a(n)
    a. professional fee
    b. honorarium
    c. gratuity
    d. tip

29. Integrating the various resources to meet organizational objectives is known as
    a. planning
    b. organizing
    c. coordinating
    d. directing

30. An employee's ability to perform a task is a function of all of the following **EXCEPT**
    a. knowledge
    b. skill
    c. experience
    d. commitment

PART 3: CLINICAL

DIRECTIONS

Each of the questions or incomplete statements below is followed by four suggested answers or completions. Select the *one* answer or completion that is *best* in each case and fill in the circle containing the corresponding letter on the answer sheet. Perforated answer sheets are located at the back of the book.

1. The acronym PERRLA is typically recorded in what part of the Review of Systems?
   a. head and neck
   b. cardiovascular
   c. respiratory
   d. urinary

2. The "S" of SOAP notes represents
   a. data acquired through examination and testing
   b. data provided by the patient describing signs, symptoms, and feelings
   c. the provider's diagnosis
   d. the course of treatment

3. Which of the following represents hypotension?
   a. 130/84
   b. 120/80
   c. 142/90
   d. 90/58

4. The typical pulse range for adults is
   a. 50 to 70
   b. 60 to 80
   c. 70 to 90
   d. 60 to 100

5. Which of the following factors affect body temperature?
   a. age
   b. environment
   c. activity
   d. all of the above

6. The position of choice for orthopnea is
   a. lithotomy
   b. dorsal recumbent
   c. Fowler's
   d. supine

7. Instruments designed to grasp objects are
   a. scissors
   b. forceps
   c. scopes
   d. sounds

8. Which of the following is a gynecological instrument?
   a. bayonette forceps
   b. hemostat
   c. tenaculum
   d. obturator

9. Which of the following is a physical disinfection agent?
   a. boiling water
   b. alcohol
   c. Betadine
   d. bleach

10. The medical assistant's responsibilities in surgical care and treatment include
    a. preparing the room
    b. preparing the patient
    c. assisting the health care provider
    d. all of the above

11. Gynecological instruments include
    a. pelvimeter
    b. vaginal speculum
    c. uterine curette
    d. all of the above

12. An instrument used to perforate the injured area when a blood clot or infection makes drainage and pressure release necessary.
    a. Extractor
    b. Fingernail drill
    c. Alligator forceps
    d. Ear curette

13. Tylenol is an example of a
    a. generic name
    b. chemical name
    c. synthetic name
    d. trade name

14. A subcutaneous injection typically employs a
    a. 1.5 inch needle
    b. 3/4 inch needle
    c. 5/8 inch needle
    d. 1/4 inch needle

15. OS means
    a. left eye
    b. right eye
    c. both eyes
    d. either eye

16. The healthcare provider orders 600 mg Augmentin; however, 200 mg per 0.5 mL is the available strength. The medical assistant should administer
    a. 0.5 mL
    b. 0.75 mL
    c. 1 mL
    d. 1.5 mL

17. Antimicrobials include
    a. E-mycin
    b. Amoxil
    c. Veetids
    d. all of the above

18. Which of the following is the generic name for Diovan?
    a. losartan potassium
    b. valsartan
    c. amlodipine
    d. metoprolol

19. During two-rescuer CPR, the compression to ventilation ratio for children is
    a. 15:1
    b. 15:2
    c. 30:1
    d. 30:2

20. In adult CPR, the depth of chest compressions is
    a. 0.5 to 1.0 inches
    b. 1.0 to 1.5 inches
    c. 1.5 to 2.0 inches
    d. 2.0 to 2.5 inches

21. When encountering an unconscious person, the medical assistant should *first*
    a. assess the person's responsiveness
    b. call for help
    c. administer artificial respirations
    d. control any bleeding

22. A patient suffering from diabetic coma will require
    a. something sweet
    b. carbohydrates
    c. a dose of insulin
    d. hospital admission

23. All of the following are common causes of breathing emergencies **EXCEPT**
    a. choking
    b. obstruction
    c. strains
    d. asthma

24. If you are alone and must leave the victim to call for help, the victim should be placed in which of the following positions?
    a. Prone
    b. Supine
    c. Recovery
    d. Trendelenberg

25. Which of the following is a cardiac enzyme?
    a. glucose
    b. coagulase
    c. lipase
    d. CPK

26. A metabolic profile typically includes all of the following **EXCEPT**
    a. Na^+
    b. K^+
    c. glucose
    d. ketones

27. All of the following are electrolytes **EXCEPT**
    a. sodium
    b. potassium
    c. nitrogen
    d. chloride

28. Which of the following assays is used to manage diabetic patients?
    a. BUN
    b. bilirubin
    c. potassium
    d. hemoglobin A_1C (glycated hemoglobin)

29. Which of the following illustrates an engineering control?
    a. sharps container
    b. handwashing
    c. lab coat
    d. none of the above

30. The presence of hemoglobin in the urine is most likely indicative of
    a. UTI
    b. glomerulonephritis
    c. hydronephrosis
    d. urinary hemorrhage

RMA PRE-TEST SCORE SHEET

Directions:

1. Comparing your answer sheet with the correct answers listed below for each section, circle the incorrect responses below.
2. Tally the number of incorrect responses in each column and record the total in the space provided.
3. Identify the column having the lowest score and turn to the chapters indicated for further study.
4. Focus your attention on the columns having the lowest scores.
5. After completing your study of the weakest content area, turn to the column having the next lowest score, concentrating on that area, and so on.

GENERAL: Percent correct: _____%

1=D	6=D	11=A	16=D	21=D	26=D
2=C	7=B	12=B	17=A	22=A	27=B
3=A	8=D	13=B	18=D	23=B	28=D
4=B	9=A	14=D	19=C	24=A	29=B
5=C	10=D	15=C	20=D	25=D	30=A
____	____	____	____	____	____
Ch. 4	Ch. 5	Ch. 6	Ch. 7	Ch. 8	Ch. 9

ADMINISTRATIVE: Percent correct: _____%

1=B	6=B	11=A	16=D	21=D	26=D
2=B	7=B	12=C	17=B	22=A	27=C
3=A	8=B	13=A	18=B	23=C	28=B
4=D	9=A	14=B	19=A	24=A	29=C
5=A	10=C	15=C	20=A	25=D	30=D
____	____	____	____	____	____
Ch. 10	Ch. 11	Ch. 12	Ch. 13	Ch. 14	Ch. 15

CLINICAL: Percent correct: _____%

1=A	7=B	13=D	19=A	25=D
2=B	8=C	14=C	20=C	26=D
3=D	9=A	15=A	21=A	27=C
4=D	10=D	16=D	22=C	28=D
5=D	11=D	17=D	23=C	29=A
6=C	12=B	18=B	24=C	30=D
____	____	____	____	____
Ch. 16	Ch. 17	Ch. 18	Ch. 19	Ch. 20

General, Administrative, and Clinical

If you answered three or more questions incorrectly in any of the columns, turn to the appropriate chapter for further study.

Total percent correct (____/90 × 100): _____%

RMA scaled score = (Raw score × 0.6) + 40
(Scaled score ≥ 70 is passing)

RMA PRE-TEST ANSWERS AND RATIONALES

General:

1. D. This is the combining form for eyelid. Cost/o means rib; or/o means mouth; ocul/o means eye.

2. C. "O" is the most common connecting vowel.

3. A. Tachy means fast and cardia means pertaining to heart.

4. B. Balanitis means inflammation of the glans penis, a reproductive organ.

5. C. Hemato refers to blood and poiesis to formation.

6. D. hypoglossal: This is the twelfth cranial nerve. Acoustic is the 8th; trigeminal is the 5th; olfactory is the 1st.

7. B. The structure that closes the trachea during swallowing.

8. D. Metatarsals are foot bones; tarsals are ankle bones; metacarpals are hand bones.

9. A. Urethra is the tube connecting the bladder to the meatus; epididymis is the tube that transports semen; the seminal vesicle is a bilateral pouch posterior to the bladder.

10. D. The aqueous humor is situated in front of the lens.

11. A. B is a behavioral aspect that is characterized by an increase in the complexity of function and skill; C is the outward expression of the inner self; D is the source of instinctive and unconscious urges that are chiefly sexual in nature.

12. B. A represents physical changes with accompanying increase in size; C is the outward expression of the inner self; D is the source of instinctive and unconscious urges that are chiefly sexual in nature.

13. B. A is cephalocaudal growth and development, and the remaining options are nonsense distracters.

14. D. Options A though C are the three levels of personality.

15. C. A is Sigmund Freud; B is Jean Piaget; D is Lawrence Kohlberg.

16. D. Physiological need relates to food and water; safety need relates to shelter and freedom from harm; social need relates to love and belonging.

17. A. Denial is avoiding reality; sublimation is diverting unacceptable thoughts and impulses into acceptable behaviors; repression is putting unpleasant thoughts and feelings out of one's mind.

18. D. Introjection is adopting the feelings of others; dissociation is disconnecting emotional significance from specific ideas or events; rationalization is justifying one's thoughts or feelings.

19. C. The others are nonsense distracters.

20. D. Options A through C do nothing to help the patient to deal with the fear of dying or the dying process.

21. D. A consent form is normally required for all patient care; however, when an emergency precludes obtaining one, it is assumed that the patient would want life or limb to be maintained.

22. A. Nonfeasance: Misfeasance means improper act; malfeasance means bad act; negligence means careless act.

23. B. Slander is defamation by the spoken word; invasion of privacy and fraud are unrelated distracters.

24. A. The elements of negligence include duty, causation, and damage.

25. D. Recovery for negligence is barred if the statute of limitations has expired, the plaintiff contributed in any way to the injury, or the patient assumed the risk for injury.

26. D. Options A though C are terms related to a beneficial nature or outcome and so relate to the concept of confidentiality.

27. B. A is a custom; C is a positive spirit; D is a study of moral thought.

28. D. A means to do good; B means to do no harm; C means fairness.

29. B. A means obligations; C means fairness; D means study of moral principles.

30. A. Being truthful to the patient regardless of the unpleasantness involved is our duty and the patient's right.

Administrative:

1. B. 10. 12 is elite; 8 and 14 are nonsense distracters.

2. B. The others are nonsense distracters.

3. A. 6: The others are nonsense distracters.

4. D. A or C: The alt and ctrl keys triple the number of tasks the function keys can perform.

5. A. Concatenate means to combine records; copy and paste moves text elsewhere while it remains in its original position; purging means to omit data or records.

6. B. A is a specific time allotted for each patient; C is a staggered wavelike method; D is booking more than one patient for the same time slot.

7. B. A, C, and D should always be considered when scheduling appointments. Although B is plausible, it is the least attractive of the four choices.

8. B. A, C, and D are wrong for the reasons identified in answer 11.

9. A. The appointment book is a legal record and should ideally be recorded using ink that cannot be erased.

10. C. There is a one-hour difference between Minnesota and Georgia.

11. A. B is the depositor; C is the recipient of funds; D is the one providing the funds.

12. C. $4050 + 1025 - 700 = 4375$.

13. A. B is how often accounts receivable are paid in a period; C and D are nonsense distracters.

14. B. A is twice a month; C is every two months; D is twice a year.

15. C. A is the difference between assets and liabilities; B is a debt obligation; D is money generated from operations.

16. D. The others are medical procedures and typically use CPT codes.

17. B. The others are medical procedures and typically use CPT codes.

18. B. A is for the elderly and disabled; C is commercial insurance; D is for military personnel and their dependents.

19. A. B is an insurance policy used to supplement another policy; C is transferring the payment of an insurance benefit to a provider; D is a peril that is not covered by a policy.

20. A. A is best even though B and C are plausible. D is a nonsense distracter.

21. D. The others are nonsense distracters.

22. A. B is inventory that has been depleted; C is the replacement of stock; D is the stock itself.

23. C. Options A and B refer to general, non-medical facilities; D is true for facilities that specifically service disabled persons.

24. A. Generally, only one entrance must be made accessible.

25. D. Options A through C are all good safety measures.

26. D. The chairperson is typically responsible for all of these tasks.

27. C. A is a means of maintaining legal control of physical evidence, e.g., blood specimens; B is a chart that illustrates the reporting relationships in an organization; D is a nonsense distracter.

28. B. This is a small payment of appreciation for providing a volunteer-like or professional service. A is not gratuitous. C and D, although synonymous, represent additional payments of appreciation over and above a regular payment.

29. C. Option A refers to developing objectives; B is assembling organizational resources; D is overseeing the use of the resources.

30. D. A person's commitment is not a function of ability.

Clinical:

1. A. Pupils are Equal, Round, and Reactive to Light and Accommodation—visual examination of the eye is part of head and neck section of the ROS.

2. B. S refers to subjective data; that is, information reported by the patient.

3. D. Hypotension is a systolic below 90 and/or a diastolic below 60.

4. D. Although all are plausible, D is the best choice.

5. D. Body temperature is affected by A, B, and C.

6. C. This is a reclining or semi-sitting position, best for orthopneic patients.

7. B. A is used to cut; C is used to visualize cavities; D is used to probe cavities.

8. C. It is used to grasp uterine tissue.

9. A. Boiling water physically destroys pathogens; the others are chemical agents.

10. D. The MA is typically responsible for all of these duties.

11. D. All are gynecological instruments.

12. B. Option A is used to remove substances from the superficial layer of skin; C, forceps inserted through a speculum to remove foreign bodies; D, scrapes accumulated cerumen from the ear canal; and E, is used to pull back tissue to allow viewing of the operative site.

13. D. Tylenol is the name given the drug by the manufacturer.

14. C. Usually this is the case unless the patient is emaciated or obese.

15. A. Oculus sinister, L. left eye.

16. D. 600 mg ÷ 200 mg × 0.5 mL = 1.5 mL.

17. D. A through C are all antimicrobials.

18. B. Option A is Cozaar, C is Lotrel, and D is Toprol.

19. D. The compression to ventilation ratio is 30:2; this ratio is the same for adults and children, per AHA guidelines.

20. C. A and B are too shallow; whereas D is too deep.

21. A. B and C would be inappropriate if the person were asleep; A would rule this out.

22. C. A and B will provide no benefit. C will likely occur in the field before the patient is transported to the hospital.

23. C. All can cause a breathing emergency **EXCEPT** a strain, which is a stretched muscle or tendon.

24. C. The recovery position minimizes further injury to the victim and ensures vomitus will not be aspirated, causing a blocked airway.

25. D. CPK is the only cardiac enzyme listed.

26. D. Ketones are not typically included in a metabolic profile.

27. C. All are electrolytes **EXCEPT** nitrogen.

28. D. The others have little to do with diabetes management.

29. A. B is a work practice control; C is personal protective equipment.

30. D. Although hemoglobin could possibly be present in all of these conditions, the obvious and most common cause is hemorrhage.

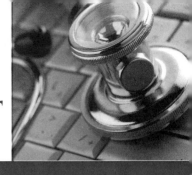

Pre-Test

100-question, 90 minute, timed diagnostic exam

Each of the questions or incomplete statements below is followed by four suggested answers or completions. Select the *one* answer or completion that is *best* in each case and fill in the circle containing the corresponding letter on the answer sheet. Perforated answer sheets are located at the back of the book.

1. Which of the following word parts is a suffix?
   a. ante
   b. post
   c. organ/o
   d. itis

2. Which of the following word parts is a prefix?
   a. pre
   b. cleid/o
   c. osis
   d. rrhea

3. Which of the following terms relates to a respiratory disorder?
   a. MI
   b. HBP
   c. COPD
   d. RIH

4. Which of the following terms relates to a gynecological disorder?
   a. epididymitis
   b. salpingitis
   c. stomatitis
   d. rhinitis

5. Which of the following terms is spelled incorrectly?
   a. sinusitis
   b. hysterectomy
   c. arteriosclerosis
   d. rabdomyoma

6. Unclear vision resulting from hardening of the crystalline lens, common among the elderly, is known as
   a. diplopia
   b. presbyopia
   c. amblyopia
   d. myopia

7. Inflammation of the gallbladder is known as
   a. cholelithiasis
   b. colitis
   c. cholecystitis
   d. cystitis

8. Radiographic study involving the urinary system is called
   a. intravenous pyelogram
   b. intravenous infusion
   c. intravenous cardiogram
   d. intravenous injection

9. The medical abbreviation meaning *by mouth* is
   a. ad lib
   b. p.o.
   c. n.p.o.
   d. b.i.d.

10. The medical abbreviation meaning *as desired* is
    a. stat
    b. p.r.n.
    c. ad lib
    d. q.o.d.

11. In the structural hierarchy of organisms, which of the following immediately precedes the organ level?
    a. organism
    b. systems
    c. tissues
    d. cells

12. Which of the following tissues consist of neurons?
    a. epithelial
    b. nervous
    c. connective
    d. muscle

13. Which of the following is considered an appendage of the skin?
    a. dermis
    b. epidermis
    c. subcutaneous
    d. sudoriferous glands

14. Which of the following best describes a bony projection?
    a. spine
    b. fissure
    c. process
    d. fossa

15. Turning a body part inward, especially the sole of the foot is
    a. flexion
    b. abduction
    c. circumduction
    d. inversion

16. The right atrioventricular valve is known as the
    a. bicuspid
    b. mitral
    c. semilunar
    d. tricuspid

17. The structure known as the voice box is the
    a. pharynx
    b. larynx
    c. epiglottis
    d. oropharynx

18. A fingerlike projection of the soft palate is the
    a. uvula
    b. frenulum
    c. epiglottis
    d. villi

19. The structure that houses the glomerulus is the
    a. Loop of Henle
    b. proximal convoluted tubule
    c. Bowman's capsule
    d. distal convoluted capsule

20. The innermost layer of the uterus is the
    a. epimetrium
    b. fimbria
    c. myometrium
    d. endometrium

21. All of the following are reasons for revocation or suspension of a healthcare provider's license **EXCEPT**
    a. conviction of a crime
    b. unprofessional conduct
    c. administering atypical treatments
    d. physical incapacity

22. Behavior or actions that can be reasonably presumed to be consensual is
    a. express consent
    b. self-determination
    c. informed consent
    d. implied consent

23. Which of the following may require notification of the appropriate health agency?
    a. auto accident
    b. roseola
    c. staph infection
    d. phenylketonuria

24. Confidentiality is legally supported by the
    a. Self-Determination Act
    b. Health Care Quality Improvement Act
    c. Americans with Disabilities Act
    d. Privacy Act

25. Confidentiality is ethically supported by the concept of
    a. beneficence
    b. nonmaleficence
    c. fidelity
    d. all of the above

26. A civil wrong committed against other persons or their property is
    a. a tort
    b. a breach of contract
    c. negligence
    d. malpractice

27. A provider who guarantees the outcome of a course of treatment may be in jeopardy of committing
    a. a tort
    b. a breach of contract
    c. negligence
    d. malpractice

28. Negligence of a professional person is known as
    a. nonfeasance
    b. misfeasance
    c. malfeasance
    d. malpractice

29. The least serious degree of negligence is
    a. minor
    b. ordinary
    c. inconsequential
    d. gross

30. The principle that the healthcare provider has a professional obligation to care for a patient is known as
    a. duty
    b. dereliction of duty
    c. direct causation
    d. damage

31. A facilitative communication technique that repeats what the patient has said to demonstrate understanding is
    a. accepting
    b. mirroring
    c. clarification
    d. focusing

32. All of the following are facilitative communication techniques **EXCEPT**
    a. exploring
    b. clarifying
    c. focusing
    d. advising

33. An unconscious defense mechanism characterized by behaving in the opposite way to one's actual feelings is called
    a. introjection
    b. projection
    c. reaction formation
    d. sublimation

34. Mimicking the behavior of another to cope with feelings of inadequacy is called
    a. dissociation
    b. rationalization
    c. substitution
    d. identification

35. The reason a patient may desire to continue the sick role is
    a. fear of reestablishing responsibility
    b. financial gain such as workers' compensation
    c. to generate sympathy and attention
    d. all of the above

36. All of the following may be considered losses associated with adopting the sick role **EXCEPT**
    a. autonomy
    b. privacy
    c. mobility or function
    d. none of the above

37. Methods of discovering what is important to a patient include
    a. asking the patient
    b. observing patient behavior
    c. asking family and friends
    d. all of the above

38. Adopting the view of other persons relative to their situation and experience is known as
    a. empathy
    b. sympathy
    c. reinforcement
    d. projection

39. Which of the following will most likely promote the perception of professional competence?
    a. shaking when performing a procedure
    b. behaving in a nonchalant manner
    c. poor enunciation
    d. appearing confident

40. Interacting with a health professional as one would interact with a parental figure is known as
    a. inference
    b. dependence
    c. transference
    d. countertransference

41. The smallest piece of information processed by a computer is the
    a. data
    b. bit
    c. byte
    d. ASCII

42. The process of activating the input of the operating system into main memory is known as
    a. start-up
    b. shutdown
    c. booting
    d. program installation

43. The process of organizing a blank disk into sectors so that it can store data is known as
    a. booting
    b. configuration
    c. WYSIWYG
    d. formatting

44. A key that moves the cursor to the left, right, top, or bottom margins when pressed is the
    a. Backspace key
    b. Tab key
    c. Delete key
    d. Home key

45. A blinking dash or small rectangle that identifies where on the computer screen data will be entered is the
   a. pausebreak
   b. icon
   c. cursor
   d. page-up

46. The number of characters contained within an inch is the
   a. macro
   b. font
   c. widow
   d. pitch

47. Which of the following permits the printing of identical information at the top of each page?
   a. pagination
   b. header
   c. justification
   d. orphans

48. The last paragraph line appearing alone at the top of a page is a
   a. block
   b. prompt
   c. word wrap
   d. widow

49. A predefined computer setting that is automatically loaded with each new document unless changed by the user is the
   a. default
   b. directory
   c. menu
   d. macro

50. An index of files on a disk is known as the
   a. macro
   b. block
   c. menu
   d. directory

51. Which of the following would be indexed first?
   a. Allison B. Wilson
   b. Alice A. Wilson
   c. Mrs. Anthony (Alma) Wilson
   d. Alice B. Wilson

52. Which of the following would be indexed last?
   a. John P. St. John
   b. John Q. St. George
   c. Paul M. St. Paul
   d. Alfred O. San Luis

53. Annual reports are best filed using a(n)
   a. alphabetical system
   b. subject system
   c. geographic system
   d. numerical system

54. The best method of controlling charts removed from the office is with a(n)
   a. out guide
   b. subpoena duces tecum
   c. borrowed charts log
   d. archival record

55. A simple method to check the accuracy of a postal scale is to see if 1 ounce is displayed when weighing
   a. 6 pennies
   b. 7 pennies
   c. 8 pennies
   d. 9 pennies

56. The computer command that organizes data alphabetically or numerically is
   a. sort
   b. presort
   c. macro
   d. function

57. A computer application that allows multiple applications to operate simultaneously is
   a. spreadsheet
   b. DOS
   c. Windows
   d. thesaurus

58. The software program that permits rapid calculations applied to a table of numerical data is
   a. Windows
   b. word processing
   c. telecommunications
   d. a spreadsheet

59. The data entered into a spreadsheet comprising alphanumeric characters primarily used as column and row headings is known as the
   a. value
   b. label
   c. formula
   d. cell

60. Cell A3 is located at
   a. column A, row 3
   b. row A, column 3
   c. columns 1 to 3, and row A
   d. rows 1 to 3, and column A

61. The person most likely to handle equipment purchases is the
    a. receptionist
    b. medical assistant
    c. office manager
    d. nurse

62. When a pharmaceutical representative arrives unannounced, it is best to
    a. request a business card and see if the provider is available for a visit
    b. immediately escort the representative to the provider's office
    c. ask the representative to wait until the provider is free
    d. refer the representative to the next available medical assistant

63. Ideally, the phone should be answered before the
    a. first ring
    b. second ring
    c. third ring
    d. fourth ring

64. When a second line rings, it is best to
    a. answer with "please hold"
    b. ask the first caller if she can hold
    c. indicate to the first caller, "my other line is ringing, I will place you on hold"
    d. ignore it until you have finished with the first caller

65. All of the following are typically recorded on a telephone message **EXCEPT**
    a. date and time of call
    b. person called
    c. message
    d. caller's demographic data

66. The assistant's telephone voice should convey all of the following **EXCEPT**
    a. confidence
    b. warmth
    c. disinterest
    d. concern

67. When dialing direct, the caller dials
    a. 0 + area code + seven-digit number
    b. 1 + area code + seven-digit number
    c. 1 + 800 + seven-digit number
    d. Caller ID number + seven-digit number

68. The time zone difference between California and New Jersey is
    a. 1 hour
    b. 2 hours
    c. 3 hours
    d. 4 hours

69. WATS stands for
    a. Washington Tax Service
    b. Western Area Transit System
    c. World Arena Telephone System
    d. Wide Area Telephone Service

70. An effective answering service is necessary to avoid
    a. liability
    b. malpractice
    c. negligence
    d. abandonment charges

71. A signature card must be completed to
    a. file medical practice income taxes
    b. authorize reconciliation of bank statements
    c. pay medical practice professional dues
    d. open a checking account

72. Special characters that simplify the sorting and routing of financial documents are
    a. FONT
    b. PITCH
    c. MICR
    d. OCR

73. A check that the bank refuses to pay is
    a. postdated
    b. debited
    c. honored
    d. dishonored

74. A personal record of relevant information regarding a check and checking account balance is a
    a. deposit ticket
    b. debit memo
    c. check register
    d. credit memo

75. Carbonless copies of checks use a special paper known as
    a. NCR paper
    b. OCR paper
    c. MICR paper
    d. DOD paper

76. A check that has been honored and appropriately stamped to prevent if from being reissued is a(n)
    a. NSF check
    b. postdated check
    c. dishonored check
    d. canceled check

77. The bank statement shows a balance of $4,250, deposits in transit that total $1,200, and outstanding checks that equal $300. The check register balance should be
    a. $2,750
    b. $3,350
    c. $4,550
    d. $5,150

78. An organization's ability to pay its debts is known as
    a. solvency
    b. profitability
    c. effectiveness
    d. efficiency

79. The property of value owned or controlled by an organization is known as
    a. capital
    b. liability
    c. asset
    d. revenue

80. All of the following are common users of a clinic's accounting information **EXCEPT**
    a. owners
    b. patients
    c. managers
    d. government agencies

81. A direction to consider additional codes is
    a. see condition
    b. NEC
    c. NOS
    d. see also

82. An organizational arrangement that provides medical service for a fixed, prepaid fee best describes
    a. PPO
    b. SEC
    c. HMO
    d. HRM

83. The underlined portion of: Hypertension (<u>orthostatic, benign, simple</u>) identifies a(n)
    a. main term
    b. subterm
    c. essential modifier
    d. nonessential modifier

84. An insurance policy designed to pay fees not covered by conventional plans is a
    a. commercial plan
    b. government plan
    c. private plan
    d. companion plan

85. AOB means
    a. actual observable behavior
    b. assignment of benefits
    c. average objective benefits
    d. archives of business records

86. The person or party designated by the policyholder to receive the value of a policy is the
    a. carrier
    b. beneficiary
    c. provider
    d. insured

87. Title 18 of the Social Security Act best describes
    a. Medicare
    b. Tricare
    c. Blue Cross/Blue Shield
    d. CHAMPVA

88. A CPT modifier that identifies bilateral procedures is
    a. -20
    b. -30
    c. -40
    d. -50

89. Who of the following is most likely eligible for Medicaid?
    a. persons age 65 and older
    b. dependents of retired military personnel
    c. workers afflicted with end-stage renal disease
    d. persons receiving Supplemental Security Income (SSI) for the aged and disabled

90. COBRA requires that government claim forms and attachments be maintained for at least
    a. 2 years
    b. 3 years
    c. 4 years
    d. 5 years

91. Details regarding the health status of the patient's parents and siblings are known as
    a. chief complaint
    b. social history
    c. past medical history
    d. family history

92. Which of the following identifies the action to be taken to solve a medical problem such as treatment, medication, surgery, referral, etc?
    a. subjective
    b. objective
    c. assessment
    d. plan

93. The patient's name, date of birth, marital status, education, occupation, etc., is known as
    a. social history
    b. demographics
    c. family history
    d. personal history

94. Questions regarding each of the major body systems and parts are known as
    a. CC
    b. PMH
    c. FH
    d. ROS

95. All of the following instruments are commonly used during a routine physical examination **EXCEPT**
    a. stethoscope
    b. otoscope
    c. percussion hammer
    d. thumb forceps

96. Initial examination of the breasts is usually performed when the patient is in which of the following positions?
    a. lithotomy
    b. Trendelenburg
    c. sitting
    d. dorsal recumbent

97. The Ishihara test is associated with which of the following examinations?
    a. otological
    b. ophthalmological
    c. gynecological
    d. orthopedic

98. Schedule II inventories must be made every
    a. year
    b. 2 years
    c. 3 years
    d. 4 years

99. The Rx symbol is classified as the
    a. prescription
    b. subscription
    c. signature
    d. superscription

100. Which of the following is not performed in the handwashing procedure?
    a. remove all jewelry except perhaps wedding rings
    b. allow the hands to become completely wet
    c. rinse so that the water flows from the fingertips to the wrist
    d. scrub for at least 30 seconds

CMAS PRE-TEST SCORE SHEET

Directions:

1. Comparing your answer sheet with the correct answers listed below for each section, circle the incorrect responses below.
2. Tally the number of incorrect responses in each column and record the total in the space provided.
3. Identify the column having the lowest score and turn to the chapters indicated for further study.
4. Focus your attention on the columns having the lowest scores.
5. After completing your study of the weakest content area, turn to the column having the next lowest score, concentrating on that area, and so on.

Percent correct: _____ %

1=D	11=C	21=C	31=B	41=B	51=B	61=C	71=D	81=D	91=D
2=A	12=B	22=D	32=D	42=C	52=D	62=A	72=C	82=C	92=D
3=C	13=D	23=D	33=C	43=D	53=B	63=C	73=D	83=D	93=D
4=B	14=C	24=D	34=D	44=D	54=A	64=B	74=C	84=D	94=D
5=D	15=D	25=D	35=D	45=C	55=D	65=D	75=A	85=B	95=D
6=B	16=D	26=A	36=D	46=D	56=A	66=C	76=D	86=B	96=C
7=C	17=B	27=B	37=D	47=B	57=C	67=B	77=D	87=A	97=B
8=A	18=A	28=D	38=A	48=D	58=D	68=C	78=A	88=D	98=B
9=B	19=C	29=B	39=D	49=A	59=B	69=D	79=C	89=D	99=D
10=C	20=D	30=A	40=C	50=D	60=A	70=D	80=B	90=D	100=C
___	___	___	___	___	___	___	___	___	___
Ch. 4	Ch. 5	Ch. 8–9	Ch. 6–7	Ch. 10	Ch. 10	Ch. 11	Ch. 12	Ch. 13–15	Ch. 16

CMAS:

If you answered five or more questions incorrectly in any of the columns, turn to the appropriate chapter for further study.

Total percent correct (____/100 × 100): ____%

CMAS scaled score = (Raw score × 0.6) + 40
(Scaled score ≥ 70 is passing)

CMAS PRE-TEST ANSWERS AND RATIONALES

1. D. A and B are prefixes; C is a combining form.
2. A. B is a combining form; C and D are suffices.
3. C. A is myocardial infarction; B is high blood pressure; C is chronic obstructive pulmonary disease; D is right inguinal hernia.
4. B. Salpingitis is inflammation of the fallopian tubes, a gynecological disorder. A is inflammation of the epididymis, a male reproductive disorder; C is inflammation of the mouth; D is inflammation of the nose.
5. D. It should be rhabdomyoma.
6. B. A is double vision; C is dull vision; D is nearsightedness.
7. C. A means gallstones; B means inflammation of the colon; D means inflammation of the bladder.
8. A. The others are distracters.
9. B. Per os, L. "by mouth." A means as desired; C means nothing by mouth; D means twice a day.
10. C. Ad libitum, L. "as desired." A means immediately; B means as needed; D means every other day.
11. C. A collection of cells forms tissues; a collection of tissues forms organs; a collection of organs forms a system; a collection of systems comprises an organism.
12. B. Neurons are made up of nervous tissue, the others are not.
13. D. An appendage is a structure that supplements the primary purpose of an organ. D is the only appendage listed.

14. C. A is a sharp projection; B is a groove; D is a depression.

15. D. A means bending upon itself; B is drawing a part away from the midline; C is a rotating motion.

16. D. A and B are synonymous for the left atrioventricular valve; C is a half-moon–shaped valve found in the great vessels.

17. B. The larynx contains the vocal cords (voice box).

18. A. B is the web of tissue under the tongue; C is a tissue flap that closes the trachea during swallowing; D is fingerlike projections of the small intestinal wall.

19. C. The glomerulus is housed by the Bowman's capsule.

20. D. A is the outermost layer of the uterus; B is part of the fallopian tube; C is the muscular layer of the uterus.

21. C. All the other reasons are grounds for forfeiture of licensure. A healthcare provider is free to choose the manner of patient treatment barring any acts of negligence.

22. D. A is spoken or recorded consent; B relates to self-rule; C is express consent for risky procedures.

23. D. Most states require that PKU be reported to the local health department.

24. D. Patient privacy is the main concern of confidentiality.

25. D. A through C support the idea of confidentiality.

26. A. B is failing to carry out the terms of an agreement; C is a tort due to carelessness; D is a tort due to carelessness of a professional person.

27. B. By failing to deliver a result that is guaranteed, the provider has committed a breach of contract.

28. D. The others are ways in which one can be negligent.

29. B. D is the most serious; A and C are nonsense distracters.

30. A. A professional obligation is a duty.

31. B. Mirroring means to repeat what the patient has said to demonstrate understanding.

32. D. Advising, unlike the other three, serves to steer the patient in a direction that may not be acceptable to the patient.

33. C. A means adopting the feelings of others; B means ascribing to another person one's own feelings; D means diverting unacceptable thoughts and feelings to acceptable behaviors.

34. D. A means disconnecting emotional significance from specific ideas or events; B means justifying one's thoughts or feelings; C means making up for a deficiency by concentrating on a more easily attainable goal.

35. D. All are reasons for continuing the sick role.

36. D. All are potential losses; therefore, none of the above are exceptions.

37. D. All may be effective in learning what is important to a patient.

38. A. B is feeling sorry for another; C is strengthening a behavior; D is an unconscious defense mechanism.

39. D. The others would most likely exhibit a lack of professional competence.

40. C. D is the opposite of C; A and B are nonsense distracters.

41. B. C is 8 bits; A and D are nonsense distracters.

42. C. Booting activates the operating system.

43. D. Formatting organizes a blank disk to facilitate data storage.

44. D. The Home key when pressed moves the cursor to the margins of a document or screen.

45. C. The cursor is the blinking dash on the computer screen.

46. D. The number of characters contained within an inch is the pitch.

47. B. The header allows the same information to be printed at the top of each page.

48. D. The last paragraph line appearing alone at the top of a page is a widow.

49. A. The default setting is automatically loaded with each new document unless changed by the user.

50. D. An index of files on a disk is known as a directory.

51. B. Then D, A, and C.

52. D. San Luis comes after any of the Sts, which would be spelled out Saint.

53. B. Filed by subject and then numerically by year.

54. A. The others are nonsense distracters.

55. D. Nine pennies will approximate an ounce.

56. A. The sort function will organize data numerically or alphabetically.

57. C. Windows operating system allows multiple applications to run simultaneously.

58. D. A spreadsheet permits rapid calculations of tables of data.

59. B. Alphanumeric entries are called labels because math functions cannot be applied to them.

60. A. A3 refers to column A, row 3.

61. C. Equipment represents capital expenditures, and typically only the practice owners or managers make such purchases.

62. A. B through D may cause the representative to wait for a lengthy time when the provider cannot or does not wish to see the person. MAs do not make drug selection decisions.

63. C. The phone should not be permitted to ring more than three times before it is answered.

64. B. The other options display discourteousness.

65. D. Demographic data such as marital status, age, and education are rarely included in a phone message.

66. C. Disinterest is the obvious response.

67. B. 1 + area code + seven-digit number.

68. C. There is a 3-hour difference between California and New Jersey.

69. D. Wide Area Telephone Service.

70. D. Although all are plausible, D is the best choice. A patient who is unable to reach the provider can be said to have been abandoned if reasonable steps have not been made for alternative means of communication.

71. D. A signature card is required when opening a checking account.

72. C. Magnetic ink character recognition.

73. D. A dishonored check is one that the bank refuses to pay usually because of insufficient funds.

74. C. The check register allows for recording the relevant information concerning a check.

75. A. No carbon required paper.

76. D. A canceled check has been stamped so that it cannot be reused.

77. D. 4250 + 1200 − 300 = 5150.

78. A. Solvency is the ability to pay one's debts on time.

79. C. Assets are property owned or controlled by a business.

80. B. Patients are not given access to a practice's financial records.

81. D. "See also" directs the user to consider additional codes that may be more appropriate.

82. C. Although A is plausible, C is the best choice. B and D are nonsense distracters.

83. D. Nonessential modifiers can be included or ignored when assigning a diagnosis code.

84. D. A companion plan is a policy designed to pay fees not covered by a conventional plan.

85. B. The others are nonsense distracters.

86. B. A is the insurance company; C is the health care professional providing services; D is the policyholder.

87. A. B is available for military personnel and their dependents; C is a conventional insurance plan; D is available for veterans.

88. D. −50 is a CPT modifier for bilateral procedures.

89. D. A and C are eligible for Medicare; B is eligible for Tricare.

90. D. COBRA requires that government insurance claim forms be maintained at least 5 years.

91. D. The family history details the health status of parents and siblings.

92. D. Plan identifies the action to be taken to resolve the medical problem.

93. D. Personal history data.

94. D. Review of systems. A is chief complaint; B is past medical history; C is family history.

95. D. A through C are commonly used, unlike the thumb forceps.

96. C. Breasts are also examined in the supine position; however, the patient is usually in the sitting position first.

97. B. The Ishihara test assesses color blindness—ophthalmological.

98. B. Schedule II drug inventories must be made every 2 years.

99. D. The Rx symbol is the superscription.

100. C. The water should flow in reverse direction, from the wrists to the fingertips.

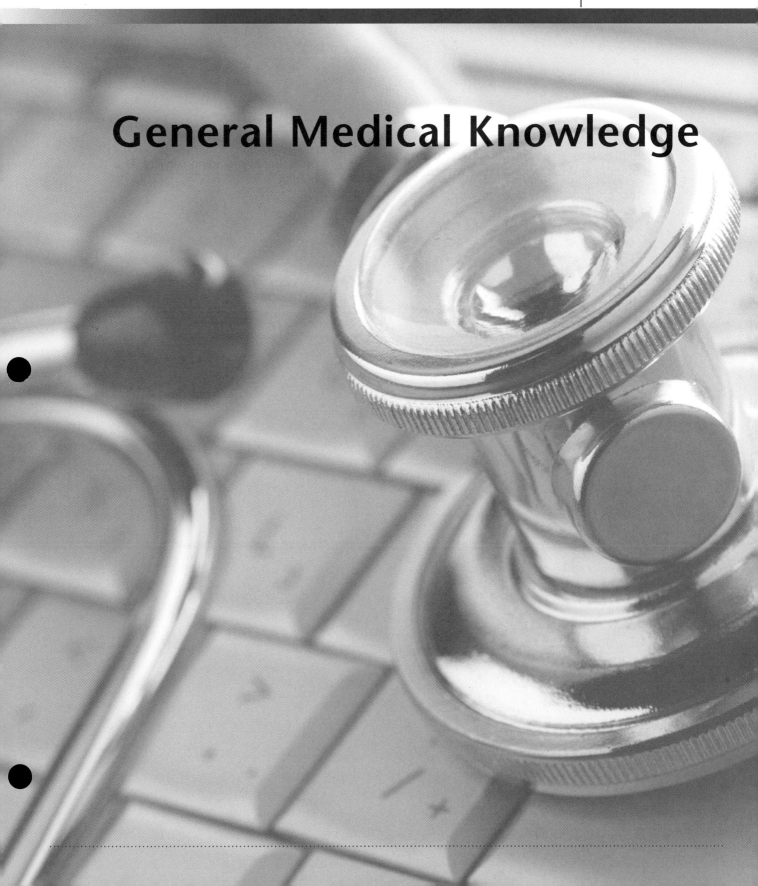

SECTION III

General Medical Knowledge

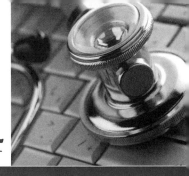

CHAPTER 4

Medical Terminology

I. WORD STRUCTURE

A. Derivation: Medical terminology is generally derived from Greek and Latin word roots.
  1. Latin (L) names are generally ascribed to anatomical structures.
  2. Greek (G) names are generally ascribed to the disease processes or medical procedures affecting these structures.
B. Root (R): A basic word element that identifies the central meaning of a word and serves as a foundation for developing more complex words through the addition of other word parts.
C. Combining form (CF): A root plus a vowel allowing for the addition of other word parts (suffixes or other roots) to form a word. The vowel "o" is most commonly used to construct combining forms.
D. Prefix (P): A word part that precedes other word parts to modify the meaning of a word.
E. Suffix (S): A word part that is terminally placed to modify the meaning of a word.
F. Word construction: Medical terms generally require at least a root or combining form and a suffix (see Figure 4–1); however, any of the following word part combinations are possible:

- P / S: Dia / gnosis
- R or CF / S: Arthr / itis
- P / R or CF / S: Anti / arthr / itic
- R or CF / R or CF / S: Oste / o / arthr / itis
- P / R or CF / R or CF / S: Anti / oste / o / arthr / itic

On occasion, there can be three or more roots or combining forms in a word (see Figure 4–2).
- CF / CF / R / S:
  Hyster / o / salping / o / oophor / ectomy.

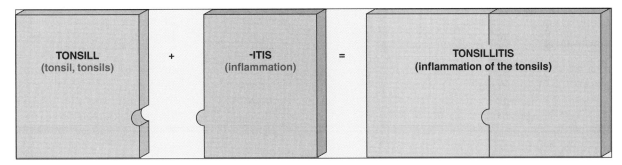

Figure 4-1

The term tonsillitis is created when the word root "tonsill" is added to the suffix "itis". Delmar/Cengage Learning.

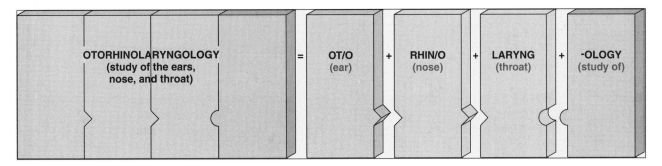

Figure 4-2

Words can have multiple word roots. Delmar/Cengage Learning.

1. Connecting a root ending with a consonant to a suffix beginning with a consonant requires a connecting vowel (the root is now a combining form).
   - Arth*r* + *pathy* = Arthr / o / pathy.
2. With a few exceptions*, word parts can be directly connected when a root ending with a consonant is combined with a suffix beginning with a vowel.
   - Arth*r* + *itis* = Arthritis
   - *Trach*e* + *itis* = Tracheitis
3. Regardless of their composition, connecting two or more roots usually requires a connecting vowel.
   - Salping / o / oophor / itis
4. Prefixes can generally be connected directly to other word parts without a connecting vowel.
5. When building a medical term from its definition, the beginning of the definition is usually the suffix of the term. Roots and combining forms representing anatomical structures are usually ordered from upper to lower, inner to outer, or in the order they are studied.
   - *Disease* of the colon:
     Colon / o / pathy
   - *Inflammation* of the ear:
     Ot / itis
   - *Pertaining to* the intestine and stomach:
     Gastr / o / intestin / al
   - *Bleeding* from the mouth and tongue:
     Gloss / o / stomat / o / rrhagia

II. PREFIXES

A. Common prefixes denoting color

Leuk/o-:	White
Erythr/o-:	Red
Xanth/o-:	Yellow
Melan/o-:	Black/dark
Chlor/o-:	Green
Cyan/o-:	Blue
Purpur/a-:	Purple

B. Common prefixes denoting number

Uni-:	(L) One
Mono-:	(G) One
Prim/i-:	First
Bi-:	(L) Two
Di-:	(G) Two
Diplo-:	Double
Tri-:	Three
Quad-:	Four
Hemi-:	Half
Semi-:	Partial
Multi-:	(L) Many, much
Poly-:	(G) Many, much
Nulli-:	None

C. Common prefixes denoting degree

Hypo-:	Below, under, decreased
Hyper-:	Above, excessive, increased

Olig/o-:	Few, deficient, scanty
Pan-:	Total, all

D. Common prefixes denoting size

Micro-:	Small
Macro-:	(G) Large
Mega(lo)-:	(G) Large

E. Common prefixes denoting relativism

Normo-:	Normal
Eu-:	Good, easy, normal, true
Pseudo-:	False
Iso-:	Equal, same
Aniso-:	Unequal, dissimilar
Homo-:	(L) Man
Homo-:	(G) Same
Homeo-:	Similar
Hetero-:	Different, unequal
Poikilo-:	Irregular, variable
Ortho-:	Straight, upright

F. Common prefixes denoting relative time

Ante-:	(L) Before
Pre-:	(L) Before
Pro-:	(L/G) Before
Post-:	After

G. Common prefixes denoting direction

Ab-:	Away from
Ad-:	Toward
Dia-:	(G) Through
Per-:	(L) Through
Trans-:	(L) Across, through

H. Common prefixes denoting position

Ambi-:	Both (sides)
Amphi-:	Both sides
Dextr/o-:	Right side
Sinistr/o-:	Left side
Epi-:	Upon
Retro-:	Backward, behind
Inter-:	Between
Sym(n)-:	Together
Infra-:	(L) Under, below
Sub-:	(L) Under, below
Mid-:	Middle
Meso-:	(G) Middle
Medi-:	(L) Middle
Ecto-:	(G) Outside
Exo-:	(G) Outside
Endo-:	Inside
Intra-:	Within
Ultra-:	(L) Beyond
Meta-:	(G) Beyond
Para-:	Beside, near
Super-:	(L) Above
Supra-:	(L) Above
Circum-:	(L) Around
Peri-:	(G) Around

I. Common prefixes denoting negation

A(n)-:	Without, lack of
Im(n)-:	Not

Anti-:   (G) Against
Contra-:   (L) Against

J. Common prefixes denoting pathology

Mal-:   (Fr) Bad, ill
Dys-:   (G) Bad, difficult, painful
Brady-:   Slow
Tachy-:   Fast
Neo-:   New, recent
Py/o-:   Pus
Pyr/o-:   Fire
Scler/o-:   Hard
Presby/o-:   Old

K. Common miscellaneous prefixes

Apo-:   Separate
Auto-:   Self
Astr/o-:   Star
Hydr/o-:   Water
Antr/o-:   Cavity
Idio-:   Own

III. SUFFIXES

A. Adjectival suffixes

-ac: Pertaining to
-al: Pertaining to
-ar(y):   Pertaining to
-(t)ic(al):   Pertaining to
-ile: Pertaining to
-ine: Pertaining to
-ory: Pertaining to
-ous: Pertaining to
-form: Resembling
-oid: Resembling
-age: Related to

B. Noun suffixes

-ia: Condition of
-ism: Condition of
-y: Condition of
-osis: Abnormal condition of
-iasis: Abnormal condition of
-(o)logy: Study of
-(iatr)ist: One who specializes in
-(ic)ian: One who specializes in
-iatr(y/ics):   Medical specialty

C. Diminutive suffixes

-ole: Small, minute
-icle: Small, minute
-ula: Small, minute
-ule: Small, minute

D. Condition and pathology suffixes

-algia: (G) Pain
-dynia: (G) Pain
-cele: Hernia
-emesis: Vomiting
-emia: Blood condition
-asthenia: Weakness
-cusis: Hearing

-cyesis: Pregnancy
-itis: Inflammation
-lysis: Destruction
-malacia: Softening
-mania: Madness
-oma: Tumor
-pathy: Disease
-penia: Deficiency, lack of
-phobia: Fear
-plegia: Paralysis
-ptosis: Prolapse, drooping
-rrhage: To burst forth
-rrhexis: Rupture
-rrhea: Discharge, flow

E. Verb (procedural) suffixes

-centesis: Surgical puncture
-cide: To kill
-clysis: Injection
-crit: To separate
-desis: Binding
-ectasis(y):   Dilation, distention
-ectomy: Excision
-gram: To record
-graph(y):   To record (recording)
-metry: To measure
-pexy: Fixation
-plasty: Surgical repair
-rrhaphy: Suture
-stasis: Control, stop
-stomy: New opening
-tomy: Incision
-tripsy: Crushing
-gnosis: To know

F. Miscellaneous suffixes

-ase: Enzyme
-blast: Immature cell
-cyte: Cell
-genesis: Formation
-plasm: Formation, plasma
-poiesis: Formation
-glia: Glue
-globin: Protein
-kinesis: Motion
-meter: Measuring instrument
-mnesia: Memory
-opia: Eye, vision
-orexia: Appetite
-pepsia: To digest
-phagia: To eat
-phasia: To speak
-pnea: Breathing
-ptysis: To spit
-scope: Viewing instrument
-tome: Cutting instrument
-tone: Tension
-trophy: Nourishment, development
-uria: Urine

G. Plural forms (suffixes)

Singular	Plural	Examples	
a	ae	bursa	bursae
ax	aces	thorax	thoraces
en	ina	lumen	lumina
ex	ices	index	indices
ix	"	appendix	appendices
is	es	diagnosis	diagnoses
"	a	femoris	femora
"	ides	iris	irides
nx	nges	phalanx	phalanges
on	a	ganglion	ganglia
um	"	ovum	ova
oon	oa	spermatozoon	spermatozoa
us	i	fungus	fungi
y	ies	artery	arteries

IV. ROOTS AND COMBINING FORMS

A. Anatomical orientation

Dors/o:	(L) Back
Poster/o:	(L) Back
Anter/o:	(L) Front
Ventr/o:	(L) Front
Later/o:	Side
Dist/o:	Distance, further from
Proxim/o:	Toward, nearer to
Viscer/o:	Organ
Caud/o:	Tail
Cephal/o:	Head
Cervic/o:	Neck
Thorac/o:	Chest
Abdomin/o:	Abdomen
Lumb/o:	Lower back, lumbar
Acr/o:	Extremity
Brachi/o:	Arm
Chir/o:	Hand
Ped/o:	Foot
Dactyl/o:	Finger
Pub/o:	Pubis
Cost/o:	Rib
Axill/o:	Axilla
inguin/o:	Groin

B. Cells and tissues

Cyt/o:	Cell
Kary/o:	Nucleus
Hist/o:	Tissue
Fibr/o:	Fiber
Aden/o:	Gland
Muc/o:	Mucus
Phag/o:	Ingest, eat
Lip/o:	(G) Fat, lipid
Adip/o:	(L) Fat

C. Integumentary

Cutane/o:	(L) Skin
Dermat/o:	(G) Skin
Hidr/o:	Sweat
Ichthy/o:	Scaly, dry
Kerat/o:	Horny layer
Onych/o:	(G) Nail
Ungu/o:	(L) Nail
Seb/o:	Sebum
Trich/o:	(G) Hair
Pil/o:	(L) Hair

D. Musculoskeletal:

Oste/o:	Bone
Myel/o:	Bone marrow
Chondr/o:	Cartilage
Arthr/o:	Joint
Synov/i:	Synovial fluid
Burs/o:	Bursa
Crani/o:	Cranium
Vertebr/o:	(L) Vertebra
Spondyl/o:	(G) Vertebra
Rachi/o:	Spine
Cost/o:	Rib
Sacr/o:	Sacrum
Coccyg/o:	Coccyx
Pelvi/o:	Pelvis
Ili/o:	Ilium
Stern/o:	Sternum
Humer/o:	Humerus
Carp/o:	Wrist
Ischi/o:	Ischium
Ten(d)/o:	Tendon
My/o:	Muscle
Leiomy/o:	Smooth muscle
Rhabdomy/o:	Striated muscle

E. Circulatory

Cardi/o:	Heart
Aort/o:	Aorta
Ventricul/o:	Ventricle
Atri/o:	Atria
Angi/o:	(G) Vessel
Vas/o:	(L) Vessel
Arteri/o:	Artery
Phleb/o:	(G) Vein
Ven/o:	(L) Vein
Sphygm/o:	Pulse
Varic/o:	Twisted, swollen vein
Lymph/o:	Lymph
Lymphaden/o:	Lymph node
Lymphangi/o:	Lymph vessel
Hem(at)/o:	Blood
Thromb/o:	Clot

F. Respiratory

Rhin/o:	(G) Nose
Nas/o:	(L) Nose
Pharyng/o:	Pharynx
Laryng/o:	Larynx
Trache/o:	Trachea
Epiglott/o:	Epiglottis
Bronchi/o:	Bronchus
Pneum(o/ato):	(G) Lung, air, breath

Pulmon/o: (L) Lung
Alveol/o: Avleolus
Pleur/o: Pleura
Phren/o: Diaphragm (mind)
Steth/o: Chest
Spir/o: Breathe
Ox/o: Oxygen

G. Urinary
Ren/o: (L) Kidney
Nephr/o: (G) Kidney
Pyel/o: Renal pelvis
Ur/o: Urine, urinary
Ureter/o: Ureter
Urethr/o: Urethra
Cyst/o: (G) Bladder
Vesic/o: (L) Bladder
Glomerul/o: Glomerulus

H. Reproductive
Balan/o: Glans penis
Orchi(d)/o: (G) Testes
Test/o: (L) Testes
Andr/o: Male
Osche/o: Scrotum
Epididym/o: Epididymis
Prostat/o: Prostate
Vas/o: Vas deferens (vessel)
Vesicul/o: Seminal vesicle
Spermat/o: Sperm
Gyn/o: Woman
Men/o: Month, menstruation
Oo: (G) Ovum
Ov/o: (L) Ovum
Oophor/o: (G) Ovary
Ovari/o: (L) Ovary
Salping/o: Fallopian tube
Uter/o: (L) Uterus
Hyster/o: (G) Uterus
Metr/o: (G) Uterus
Vagin/o: (L) Vagina
Colp/o: (G) Vagina
Vulv/o: (L) Vulva
Episi/o: (G) Vulva
Clitor(id)/o: Clitoris
Mamm/o: (L) Breast
Mast/o: (G) Breast
Labi/o: Labia, lip
Nat/a: Birth
Toc/o: Labor
Lact/o: Milk
Galact/o: Milk
Amni/o: Amnion, sac

I. Gastrointestinal
Or/o: (L) Mouth
Stomat/o: (G) Mouth
Gloss/o: (G) Tongue
Lingu/o: (L) Tongue
Bucc/o: Cheek

Cheil/o: Lip
Dent/o: Tooth
Sial/o: Saliva
Sialaden/o: Salivary gland
Gastr/o: Stomach
Esophag/o: Esophagus
Pylor/o: Pyloris
Enter/o: Intestine
Duoden/o: Duodenum
Jejun/o: Jejunum
Ile/o: Ileum
Cec/o: Cecum
Col(on)/o: Colon
Sigmoid/o: Sigmoid colon
Rect/o: (L) Rectum
Proct/o: (G) Rectum
An/o: Anus
Hepat/o: Liver
Bili/o: Bile
Chol(e)/o: Bile, gall
Cholecyst/o: Gallbladder
Cholangi/o: Bile duct
Pancreat/o: Pancreas
Splen/o: Spleen

J. Nervous
Neur/o: Nerve
Mening/o: Meninges
Radicul/o: Spinal nerve root
Encephal/o: Brain
Cerebr/o: Cerebrum
Cerebell/o: Cerebellum
Thalam/o: Thalamus
Medull/o: Medulla oblongata
Myel/o: Spinal cord (bone marrow)
Phren/o: Mind (diaphragm)

K. Sensory
Audi/o: Hearing
Ot/o: Ear
Tympan/o: (L) Tympanum
Myring/o: (G) Tympanum
Staped(i)/o: Stapes
Labyrinth/o: Labyrinth, inner ear
Vestibul/o: Vestibulet
Cochle/o: Cochlea
Blephar/o: (G) Eyelid
Palpebr/o: (L) Eyelid
Lacrim/o: Tear duct
Dacry/o: Tear
Opt/o: Eye, vision
Ocul/o: (L) Eye
Ophthalm/o: (G) Eye
Scler/o: Sclera (hard)
Corne/o: (L) Cornea
Kerat/o: (G) Cornea
Phak/o: Lens
Irid(t)/o: Iris
Pupill/o: (L) Pupil

Core/o:	(G) Pupil
Retin/o:	Retina
Ambly/o:	Dull, dim
Cycl/o:	Ciliary body

L. Pathology

Carcin/o:	Cancer
Onc/o:	Tumor
Path/o:	Disease
Lith/o:	Stone
Py/o:	Pus
Pyr/o:	Fire, fever
Scler/o:	Hard (sclera)
Scirrh/o:	Hard
Tox(ic)/o:	(G) Toxic, poison
Sept/o:	(G) Toxic, poison
Sarc/o:	Flesh (cancer of connective tissue)
Icter/o:	Jaundice (yellow)
Infarct/o:	Choke
Myc/o:	Fungus
Bacill/o:	Bacillus
Xer/o:	Dry
Strept/o:	Twisted chain (bacteria)
Staphyl/o:	Grapelike cluster (bacteria)
Bacteri/o:	Bacteria
Vir/o:	Virus
Cocc(i)/o:	Round bacteria
Immun/o:	Immune
Lys/o:	Destruction
Crypt/o:	Hidden

V. HEALTH CARE PERSONNEL

A. Independent Health Practitioners

1. **Physician:** A person who has successfully completed the requisite education and training to be licensed to practice medicine; that is, to diagnose and treat physical and psychological diseases and disorders in a particular locale.
   a. **Doctor of Medicine (M.D.):** Providers who diagnose and treat health problems by means of physical, medicinal, and surgical methods.
   b. **Doctor of Osteopathy (D.O.):** Providers who also diagnose and treat health problems using physical, medicinal, and surgical methods. Osteopaths, however, rely more on physical manipulation of the body and environment to achieve healing.

2. **Doctor of Chiropractic (D.C.):** Chiropractors rely primarily on the physical manipulation of the spinal column and related structures to restore health, as well as other therapies such as diet and selected holistic approaches.

3. **Doctor of Optometry (O.D.):** Optometrists primarily measure visual acuity and prescribe corrective lenses as well as selected medications and surgical interventions.

4. **Doctor of Podiatric Medicine (D.P.M.):** Podiatrists diagnose and treat diseases and disorders of the foot.

5. **Doctor of Dental Surgery (D.D.S. or D.M.D.):** Dentists diagnose and treat diseases and disorders of the teeth and gums.

6. **Psychologist (Ph.D., Psy.D., M.A., M.S.):** A practitioner who, holding either a master's or doctorate degree, is licensed to diagnose and treat behavior and personality disorders through counseling.

B. Primary Care Specialties: Primary care involves the initial diagnosis and treatment services patients receive for common injuries and illnesses. Primary care specialists are responsible for coordinating the total care of their patients and, as warranted, refer their patients to consultative care specialists.

1. **Family Practice (M.D./D.O.):** Family practitioners diagnose and treat the entire family for various health problems. Family practitioners are particularly interested in how the family social process affects health.

2. **Pediatrics (M.D./D.O.):** Pediatricians are primary care providers who diagnose and treat health problems of children, adolescents, and young adults.

3. **Internal Medicine (M.D./D.O.):** Internists diagnose and treat diseases and disorders of the internal organs, mainly confining their practice to adult patients.

4. **Gynecology (M.D./D.O.):** Gynecologists can be described as internists specializing in the diagnosis and treatment of female health problems, especially those associated with the female genitourinary system.

C. Consultative Care Specialties: Consultative care physicians (M.D. or D.O.) gain additional training in a medical specialty to diagnose, treat, and often perform surgical interventions. These providers generally require a referral from a primary care provider before seeing a patient.

1. **Allergy/Immunology:** An allergist/immunologist is concerned with the diagnosis and treatment of immune disorders as well as diseases associated with the allergic response.

2. **Anesthesiology:** An anesthesiologist administers agents to manage pain as well as to administer and maintain an anesthetic state during surgical operations.

3. **Aerospace Medicine:** Aerospace medicine specialists are concerned with the health problems associated with space travel.

4. **Dermatology:** Dermatologists diagnose and treat diseases and disorders of the integumentary system.

5. **Endocrinology:** Endocrinologists diagnose and treat diseases and disorders associated with the endocrine system.

6. Gastroenterology: Gastroenterologists diagnose and treat diseases and disorders of the digestive system, principally the stomach and intestines.
7. Geriatrics: Gerontologists diagnose and treat diseases and disorders associated with the aging process.
8. Hematology: Hematologists diagnose and treat diseases and disorders of the blood and hemopoietic system.
9. Infertility: An infertility specialist diagnoses and treats disorders associated with conception and pregnancy.
10. Nephrology: Nephrologists diagnose and treat diseases and disorders of the urinary system, principally the kidney.
11. Neurology: Neurologists diagnose and treat diseases and disorders of the nervous system.
12. Nuclear Medicine: Nuclear medicine specialists employ radioactive substances to diagnose and treat various diseases and disorders.
13. Obstetrics: Obstetricians care for women during and shortly after pregnancy, as well as diagnose and treat associated disorders.
14. Occupational Medicine: Occupational medicine specialists diagnose and treat job-related illnesses and injuries.
15. Oncology: Oncologists diagnose and treat tumors and cancerous growths.
16. Ophthalmology: Ophthalmologists diagnose and treat diseases and disorders of the eye as well as perform the tasks performed by optometrists.
17. Otorhinolaryngology: Otorhinolaryngologists diagnose and treat disorders of the ear, nose, and throat (ENT specialists).
18. Pathology: Pathologists study disease processes as well as perform autopsies and provide diagnostic services by examining cells and tissues.
19. Physical Medicine: Physical medicine specialists (physiatrist) diagnose and treat disorders by means of physical agents, especially through physical therapy.
20. Psychiatry: Psychiatrists diagnose and treat psychological disorders using psychotherapy and medication (psychologists, not being physicians, cannot prescribe medications).
21. Pulmonary Medicine: Pulmonary specialists diagnose and treat disorders of the respiratory system.
22. Radiology: Radiologists diagnose and treat diseases and disorders using imaging techniques and radiant energy such as X-rays, CAT scans, MRIs, etc.
23. Sports Medicine: Sports medicine specialists diagnose and treat disorders associated with athletic injuries.
24. Trauma Medicine: Trauma specialists diagnose and treat disorders requiring immediate, emergency intervention to restore life or limb.

25. Urology: Urologists diagnose and treat disorders of the urinary system in females and the genitourinary system in males.

D. Surgical Specialties: Surgeons diagnose and treat diseases and disorders through invasive operative means.
1. General Surgery: General surgeons are trained to perform a myriad of surgical interventions, but principally confine their surgical practice to the abdominal organs.
2. Colon and Rectal Surgery: Colorectal surgeons concentrate on surgically treating the colon and rectum.
3. Neurosurgery: Neurosurgeons diagnose and surgically treat the nervous system and surrounding tissues.
4. Orthopedic Surgery: Orthopedic surgeons diagnose and treat diseases and disorders of the musculoskeletal system.
5. Oral Surgery: Oral surgeons, a subspecialty of dentistry, extract teeth and surgically treat the jaw, oral tissues, and maxillofacial bones.
6. Plastic Surgery: Plastic (cosmetic) surgeons provide surgical treatments to restore function and aesthetics.
7. Cardiovascular Surgery: Cardiovascular (thoracic) surgeons diagnose and surgically treat diseases and disorders of the heart, vessels, lungs, and chest cavity.

E. Nursing Specialties: Nurses are health professionals who care for and administer prescribed treatments to patients by monitoring the patient's response to illness and medical interventions.
1. Registered Nurse (R.N.): Registered nurses are licensed nurse professionals who care for the ill and infirm.
2. Nurse Practitioner (N.P.): Nurse practitioners are R.N.s who have gained additional training to provide basic primary care.
3. Licensed Practical/Vocational Nurse (L.P.N./L.V.N.): Practical nurses provide nursing care under the supervision of a registered nurse or physician.
4. Nurse Anesthetist: Nurse anesthetists are R.N.s who have been trained to administer anesthetic agents.
5. Nurse-midwife: Nurse-midwives are R.N.s who have been trained to provide obstetrical care to include delivery and postpartum care.

F. Allied Health Specialties: Health professionals serve as support personnel for health care providers, nurses, and other allied health professions in the provision of health care services.
- Electrocardiography Technician
- Paramedic
  Emergency Medical Technician
- Histology Technician
- Medical Assistant
- Medical Technologist
  Medical Laboratory Technician

- Medical Record Administrator
  Medical Record Technician
- Medical Secretary (Administrative Assistant)
- Occupational Therapist
  Occupational Therapy Assistant
- Physical Therapist
  Physical Therapist Assistant
- Physician Assistant
  Surgeon Assistant
- Radiology Technologist
  Radiology Technician
- Respiratory Therapist
  Respiratory Therapy Technician
- Surgical Technologist
  Surgical Technician

NOTE:
- See also Section II, Chapter 5, for acronyms and abbreviations associated with diseases as they may also be part of this section of the exam.
- See also Section III, Chapter 10, for concepts associated with letters, memos, and transcription guidelines as they may also be part of this section of the exam.
- See also Section IV, Chapter 16, for common charting terminology, acronyms, and abbreviations, as well as Chapter 18 for pharmacological terminology, acronyms, and abbreviations as they may also be part of this section of the exam.

CHAPTER 5

Anatomy and Physiology

I. INTRODUCTION: ANATOMICAL ORIENTATION

A. Anatomy and Physiology defined: The scientific study of the structures and functions of the body.

B. Structural hierarchy

   1. Cells: Basic structural unit of all organisms. Cells take on a variety of morphological characteristics depending on the function it is intended to serve; e.g., cardiac cells.

   2. Tissues: A collection of cells having similar morphology to carry out a specific function; e.g., cardiac tissue.

   3. Organs: A collection of tissues serving a common function; e.g., heart.

   4. Systems: A collection of organs working concertedly to carry out a bodily function; e.g., cardiovascular system.

   5. Organism: A living entity comprising an integration of systems to carry out the necessary functions to maintain life.

C. Body system organization

   1. Outer protection: The integumentary system serves to protect, regulate temperature, and synthesize chemicals and hormones, as well as function as a sense organ. It is composed of the skin, hair, nails, and associated structures.

   2. Support and movement
      a. Skeletal: Comprises the bones, joints, ligaments, tendons, and associated structures.
      b. Muscular: Comprises muscles, tendons, and associated structures.

   3. Communication, control, and coordination
      a. Nervous: Comprises the brain, spinal cord, nerves, and associated structures.
      b. Sensory: Comprises the organs of sight, hearing, smell, taste, and touch.
      c. Endocrine: Comprises hormone-secreting glands.

   4. Transportation and defense: Circulatory system comprises the heart, blood and lymph vessels and tissues, and associated structures.

   5. Processing, regulating, and maintenance
      a. Respiratory: Comprises the lungs, trachea, bronchi, pharynx, and associated structures.
      b. Digestive: Comprises the stomach, intestines, liver, gallbladder, pancreas, and associated structures.
      c. Urinary: Comprises the kidneys, ureters, bladder, urethra, and associated structures.

   6. Reproduction and development: The reproductive system comprises sex glands and associated sex organs.

D. Body regions and locations

1.	Axilla:	Armpit
2.	Brachial:	Upper arm
3.	Buccal:	Cheek
4.	Oral:	Mouth
5.	Cervical:	Neck
6.	Cranial:	Head (skull)
7.	Deltoid:	Shoulder
8.	Femoral:	Thigh
9.	Gluteal:	Buttocks
10.	Iliac:	Hip
11.	Inguinal:	Groin
12.	Lumbar:	Small of back
13.	Mammary:	Breast
14.	Nasal:	Nose
15.	Orbital:	Eye
16.	Patellar:	Kneecap
17.	Popliteal:	Back of knee
18.	Pectoral:	Chest
19.	Plantar:	Sole of foot
20.	Sacral:	Lower spine
21.	Umbilical:	Navel
22.	Abdominal:	Abdomen
23.	Palmar:	Palm
24.	Pedal:	Foot
25.	Pelvic:	Pelvis
26.	Pubic:	Pubis
27.	Carpal:	Wrist
28.	Tarsal:	Ankle

E. Abdominal regions: The abdominal area is divided into nine regions (see Figure 5-1).
  1. Epigastric region: Upper middle sector overlying the stomach.
  2. Umbilical: Central middle sector just below the epigastric; includes the navel.
  3. Hypogastric: Lower middle sector below the umbilical.
  4. Hypochondriac (right and left): Upper side sectors.
  5. Lumbar (right and left): Middle side sectors.
  6. Iliac (right and left): Lower side sectors.
F. Abdominal quadrants: The abdominal area is divided into four regions (see Figure 5-2).
  1. Right Upper Quadrant (RUQ)
  2. Left Upper Quadrant (LUQ)
  3. Right Lower Quadrant (RLQ)
  4. Left Lower Quadrant (LLQ)
G. Anatomical planes: Cross-sectional imaginary surfaces that organize the body for anatomical reference (see Figure 5-3).
  1. Coronal (frontal): Imaginary plane dividing the body into front and back parts.
  2. Sagittal: Imaginary plane dividing the body into left and right parts.
  Midsagittal (median): Imaginary plane dividing the body into left and right halves (equal).
  3. Transverse (horizontal): Imaginary plane dividing the body into upper and lower parts.

H. Body cavities: Hollow body spaces that house internal organs (see Figure 5-4).
  1. Dorsal cavity: Comprises two cavities that house organs along the posterior (back) aspect of the body.
    a. Cranial cavity: Houses the brain.
    b. Spinal cavity: Houses the spinal cord.
  2. Ventral cavity: Comprises two cavities that house organs along the anterior (front) aspect of the body.
    a. Thoracic cavity: Chest cavity that contains organs located above the diaphragm.
    b. Abdominopelvic cavity: Contains organs located below the diaphragm.
I. Anatomical terms denoting position or direction
  1. Anatomical position: Used as a standard anatomical reference where the body is standing erect with arms extended at the sides with palms facing forward.
  2. Anterior (ventral)—Posterior (dorsal): Anterior indicates toward the front. Posterior indicates toward the back.
  3. Inferior—Superior: Inferior indicates downward or below. Superior indicates upward or above.
  4. Medial—Lateral: Medial indicates toward the middle or midline. Lateral indicates away from the middle or toward the side.

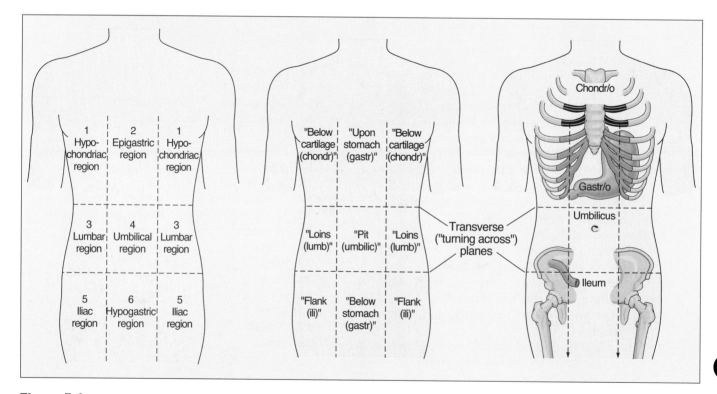

Figure 5-1

Abdominal regions. Delmar/Cengage Learning.

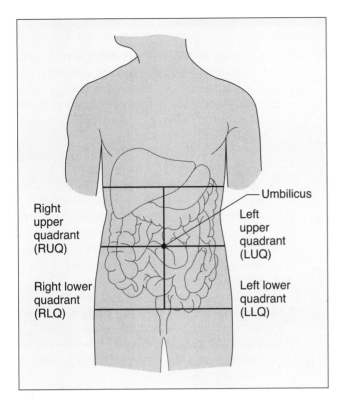

Figure 5-2
Abdominal quadrants. Delmar/Cengage Learning.

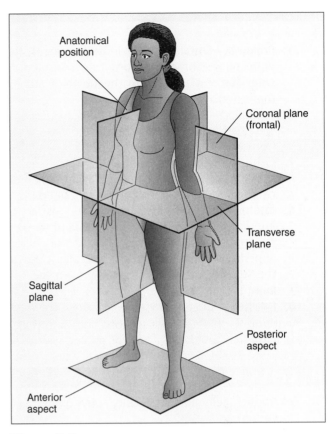

Figure 5-3
Anatomical planes. Delmar/Cengage Learning.

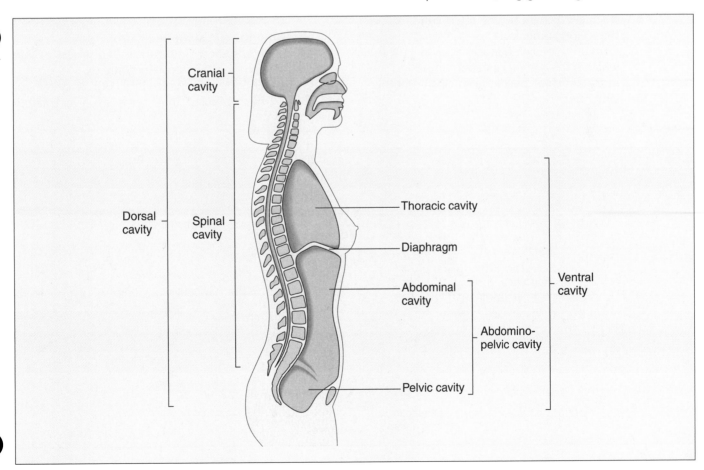

Figure 5-4
Major body cavities. Delmar/Cengage Learning.

5. Proximal—Distal: Proximal indicates nearest the point of attachment or body trunk. Distal indicates furthest away from the point of attachment or body trunk.

6. Cephalad—Caudal: Cephalad indicates toward the head as in superior. Caudal indicates away from the head as in inferior.

7. Central—Peripheral: Central indicates that a structure is part of a main part. Peripheral indicates a structure extends from the main part.

8. Internal—External: Internal indicates within or interior to. External indicates outside of or exterior to.

9. Superficial—Deep: Superficial indicates close to the surface. Deep indicates away from the surface.

10. Parietal—Visceral: Parietal indicates the cavity wall. Visceral indicates the organs within a cavity.

II. CELLS AND TISSUES

A. Eukaryotic cell anatomy and physiology (see Figure 5-5)

1. Nucleus: Serves as the control center of the cell.
   a. The largest organelle of the cell. The nucleus is usually spherical, but often conforms to the shape of the cell.
   b. Contains deoxyribonucleic acid (DNA) which is the genetic material comprising the instructions for building proteins and other structures.

2. Cell membrane: Flexible membrane that serves as a barrier by enclosing the cell contents, thus separating them from the environment.
   a. The membrane generally consists of a double layer of lipids known as phospholipids.
   b. Proteins float within the lipid membrane serving the function of enzymes and carriers that transport substances across the membrane or act as receptor sites for hormones.
   c. Certain cell membranes have a convoluted arrangement appearing similar to finger-like projections called microvilli that increase the surface area of the membrane, allowing absorption to occur more quickly and efficiently.

3. Cytoplasm: Consists of cellular material outside the nucleus and inside the cell membrane. The cytoplasm is the site of most cellular activity.
   a. The structural elements of the cell are suspended in a semitransparent fluid (mostly water) known as cytosol.
   b. The cytoplasm may also contain nutrients, fat, glycogen, pigments (melanin), mucus, and crystals.

4. Organelles: Compartmentalized microscopic structures that carry out specific cellular functions. Most have their own membrane to maintain an internal environment distinct from the surrounding cytosol.
   a. Ribosomes: Tiny, dark, round structures that are the site of protein synthesis.
   b. Endoplasmic Reticulum (ER): A system of microtubules that serve as a circulatory

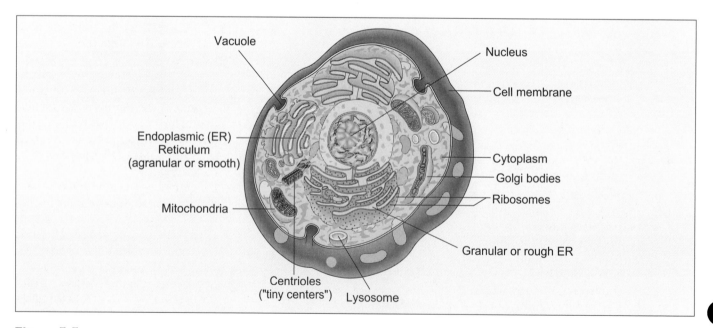

Figure 5-5

Anatomy of a cell. Delmar/Cengage Learning.

system for transporting substances through-out the cell.

    (1) Granular (rough) Endoplasmic Reticulum: ER that is studded with ribosomes. Serves to transport proteins.

    (2) Agranular (smooth) Endoplasmic Reticulum: Present in cells that produce steroid-based hormones. Also thought to be involved in fat metabolism and detoxification.

  c. Golgi bodies: Appear as flattened membranous sacs located close to the nucleus that modify and package proteins such as mucus and digestive enzymes.

  d. Lysosomes: Membranous sacs containing digestive enzymes.

  e. Peroxisomes: Membranous sacs containing oxidase to detoxify harmful substances.

  f. Mitochondria: Sausage-shaped structures that activate aerobic respiration and energy production.

  g. Centrioles: Pair of rod-shaped structures perpendicularly situated near the nucleus that are composed of microtubules that organize the spindle formation during cell division.

  h. Cilia/Flagella: Some cells have cilia, which are hairlike projections that serve to move substances along cellular surfaces. Some have flagella, which provide a whiplike action to propel a cell.

B. Tissues: Cell groups that are similar in structure and function form tissues. There are four primary tissues: epithelium, connective, nervous, and muscle tissue.

  1. Epithelial tissue: Lines, covers, and comprises glandular tissue.

    a. Functions include protection, absorption, filtration, and secretion.

    b. Epithelial cells fit closely together to form membranes or continuous sheets of cells.

  2. Connective tissue: Is the most common tissue type.

    a. Serves to protect, support, and bind together other body tissues.

    b. Includes bone, cartilage, adipose, and hemopoietic tissue.

  3. Nervous tissue: Consists of neurons that receive and conduct electrochemical impulses.

  4. Muscle tissue: Specialized tissue that contracts or shortens to produce movement.

    a. Skeletal (striated) muscle: Muscle tissue that is attached to bones causing voluntary movement of body parts.

    b. Cardiac muscle: Located solely in the heart causing involuntary, rhythmic contractions.

    c. Smooth muscle: Involuntary muscles found in the walls of hollow organs.

III. INTEGUMENTARY SYSTEM

A. General

  1. The integumentary system includes the skin and its appendages, the hair, nails, and glands.

  2. The integumentary system is the largest organ of the body, 1.5 to 2.0 square meters in the average adult.

B. Functions

  1. Protection: Provides an external barrier to harmful environmental forces.

  2. Sensation: Embodies receptors for pain, temperature, touch, and pressure.

  3. Secretion: Secretes sebum, which retards microbial growth.

  4. Thermoregulation: Sweat and the large surface area serve to dissipate heat.

  5. Vitamin D synthesis: A form of cholesterol in the skin is converted to vitamin D when exposed to ultraviolet radiation from the sun.

  6. Excretion: Although a minor function, the skin excretes small amounts of waste products such as urea.

C. Skin structure (see Figure 5-6)

  1. Epidermis: Surface layer of the skin lacking blood vessels comprising stratified squamous epithelium divided into five strata (sublayers).

  2. Dermis (corium): True skin

    a. Middle layer of the skin that is comprised of connective tissue, blood vessels, nerves, and appendages.

    b. Functions

      (1) Provides strength to the skin.

      (2) Stores water and electrolytes.

      (3) Blood vessels serve to regulate heat.

    c. Appendages: Supplementary or accessory structures that support the function of a system, in this case the integument.

      (1) Glands

        (a) Sudoriferous glands: Sweat glands comprising coiled, tube-like structures located in the dermis and subcutaneous layers that function by producing and transporting sweat to the skin surface for evaporation to cool the body.

        (b) Ceruminous glands: Modified sweat glands located in the ear canal that produce earwax.

        (c) Ciliary glands: Modified sweat glands located along the edge of the eyelid.

        (d) Sebaceous glands: Saclike structures opening into the hair follicle that produce sebum to lubricate and prevent drying of the skin and hair.

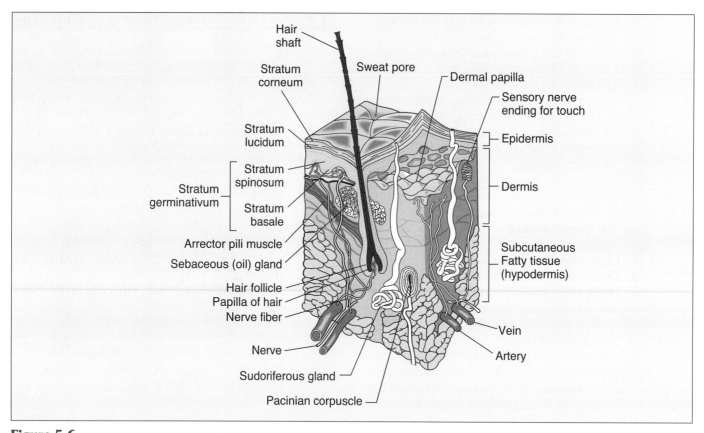

Figure 5-6

Anatomy of a cell. Delmar/Cengage Learning.

(2) Hair: Dead tissue comprised of keratin found over most of the body.

(3) Muscles: The arrector pili muscles cause the hair to become erect, producing "goosebumps."

(4) Nails: Hard, protective structures comprised of keratin located at the tips of fingers and toes.

3. Subcutaneous (hypodermis): Innermost layer of the skin that is comprised of elastic tissue, fibrous tissue, and adipose tissue.

  a. Known as the superficial fascia because it provides the means of connecting the dermis to the surface of muscles.

  b. The adipose tissue (fat) serves as insulation and a source of reserve energy.

D. Melanin provides skin, hair, and eye color (pigmentation). Darker skin contains a greater quantity of melanin.

E. Thermal regulation

  1. The skin plays a critical role in the balance between heat loss and heat gain.

  2. Approximately 80% of heat loss occurs through the skin. The remaining 20% is lost through the mucosa of the respiratory, digestive, and urinary systems.

  3. The hypothalamus monitors internal temperature. Increased body temperature causes the hypothalamus to send nervous impulses to the sudoriferous glands and blood vessels until temperature returns to normal.

F. Age-Related Changes

  1. Epidermal cells replaced less frequently.

  2. Less elasticity: Dermal fibers thicken, less collagen. Skin loosens and wrinkles.

  3. Decreased adipose tissue in face and hands. Increased sensitivity to cold.

  4. Fewer blood vessels and sweat glands. Maladjustment to temperature changes.

  5. Decreased melanocytes: Hair grays, increased skin pallor.

  6. Decreased number of hair follicles: allopecia.

G. Pathophysiology

  1. Discoloration

    a. Jaundice: Yellowing of the skin due to hyperbilirubinemia often caused by liver, gallbladder, or blood disorders.

    b. Carotinemia (or xanthemia): Yellowish color caused by excessive ingestion of carotene found in yellow/orange vegetables such as carrots. This can be distinguished from jaundice by lack of yellow discoloration of the sclera (white-of-the-eye).

    c. Poisoning: May cause a gray or brown tinge to the skin.

d. Addison's disease: An adrenal gland dysfunction that may cause a bronze skin color.

e. Albinism: Extreme whiteness of the integument resulting from lack of the pigment melanin.

f. Vitiligo: White patches on the skin caused by discontinuation of melanin production often caused by an autoimmune disorder.

g. Erythema: Redness of the skin often the result of local irritation or inflammation.

h. Cyanosis: Bluing of the skin caused by hypoxia (lack of oxygen).

2. Injuries and wounds

a. Excoriation: Scratch.

b. Abrasion: Scrape.

c. Laceration: Rough, irregular tear or cut.

d. Lesion: Spot or circumscribed irregularity.

e. Ulcer: Open sore often resulting from lack of circulation caused by pressure.

f. Keloid: Abnormal scar formation following surgery or trauma.

g. Avulsion: Torn away tissue.

h. Hematoma: A bruise caused by the collection of blood under tissue resulting from blood vessel damage.

i. Burns: Tissue injury resulting from thermal, chemical, electrical, or radioactive agents.

(1) First degree: Superficial involvement limited to the outer layer of the epidermis characterized by erythema, tenderness, and pain.

(2) Second degree: Involvement of the epidermis and superficial dermis characterized by vesicles.

(3) Third degree: Destruction of epidermis and dermis with injury to underlying tissues characterized by charring and tissue coagulation.

(4) Rule of Nines: Topographical method of determining the percentage of body surface area affected.

(a) Head and neck: 9%

(b) Torso: 36%

(c) Arms: 18%

(d) Legs: 36%

(e) Genitals: 1%

3. Eruptions

a. Macule: Flat lesion (e.g., freckle, measles).

b. Nevus: A pigmented flat lesion (e.g., mole).

c. Papule: Firm, raised lesion (e.g., pimple, chicken pox).

d. Comedo: A papule having a small dark central region (blackhead) or pallor region (whitehead).

e. Wheal: Circular, raised lesion having central pallor and circumscribed redness (e.g., insect bite).

f. Nodule: Raised lesion comprising a solid tissue mass.

g. Vesicle: Raised, fluid-filled lesion (e.g., blister).

h. Bulla (bleb): Large vesicle.

i. Pustule: Pus-filled vesicle.

j. Cyst: Raised or flat fluid-filled sac (may also contain solid tissue).

k. Polyp: Pediculated (having a stalk) growth of a mucous membrane.

l. Callus: Thickened area of stratum corneum due to friction or pressure.

m. Corn: Similar to a callus, but more distinct.

n. Fissure: A crack, crevice, or groove.

o. Eschar: Crust or scab.

4. Acne vulgaris: Inflammation of the sebaceous glands characterized by papules, pustules, or comedos.

5. Alopecia: Absence of hair, especially on the head (baldness).

6. Psoriasis: Chronic skin disease characterized by red lesions and silvery scaling thought to be caused by an autoimmune disorder.

7. Urticaria (hives): Acute condition characterized by the appearance of wheals usually resulting from an allergic reaction.

8. Impetigo: Infectious bacterial inflammation caused by staphylococcus or streptococcus bacteria characterized by vesicles, pustule, and bullae that develop a classic honey-colored crust, especially on the face and around the mouth.

9. Furuncle (boil): Abscess involving the hair follicle and adjacent tissue characterized by edema, erythema, and perhaps fever. Carbuncles are several localized furuncles.

10. Pediculoses: Infestation of parasitic insects of the genus *Pediculus* (lice) characterized by pruritus (itching) and inflammation.

a. Pediculosis capitis: Head lice caused by *Pediculus humanus capitis*.

b. Pediculosis corporis: Body lice caused by *Pediculus humanus corporis*.

c. Pediculosis palpebrarum: Lice infestation of eyebrows and lashes caused by *Pediculus humanus palpebrarum*.

d. Pediculosis pubis: Infestation of the body, especially the genital region by the crab louse, *Phthirius pubis*.

11. Dermatophytoses: Chronic superficial fungal infection called tinea caused by the *Dermatophyte* genus characterized by round, gray, scaly, or ring-shaped lesions.

a. Tinea capitis: Involving the scalp.

b. Tinea corporis (ringworm): Involving the exposed skin.

c. Tinea unguium: Involving the nails.

d. Tinea pedis: Athelete's foot.

e. Tinea cruris: Jock itch.

12. Verrucae (warts): Characterized by raised lesions caused by hypertrophy of the epidermis caused by the papilloma virus.

13. Scleroderma: Thick, densely fibrous skin thought to be caused by an autoimmune disorder.

14. Dermatitis: General inflammation of the skin characterized by pruritus, erythema, and various lesions.

    a. Seborrheic dermatitis: Chronic dermatitis caused by an increase and alteration of sebaceous secretions characterized by dry, moist, greasy scales, pruritus, and dandruff.

    b. Eczematous dermatitis (eczema): Idiopathic skin inflammation characterized by severe pruritus.

    c. Contact dermatitis: Acute inflammation caused by an irritant.

15. Herpes zoster (shingles): Acute inflammatory eruption of painful vesicles along the course of a peripheral nerve caused by the herpes zoster virus.

16. Herpes simplex (cold sore/fever blister): Small, pale, painful vesicles or ulcers around the mouth, lips, nose, or mucous membranes caused by herpes simplex type 1 virus.

17. Decubitus ulcer (bedsore): Localized open lesion often caused by poor blood flow to the region resulting from pressure against the skin surface.

18. Carcinomas: Basal cell and squamous cell carcinomas, as well as malignant melanomas, are cancerous skin lesions on the exposed skin often resulting from overexposure to ultraviolet rays and radiation.

IV. SKELETAL SYSTEM

A. General

    1. The adult skeleton is composed of 206 bones.

    2. Bone names provide the basis for names of other structures such as the muscular and vascular systems.

B. Function

    1. Support: Provides a framework to support bodily structures.

    2. Protection: Provides housing that protects the internal organs.

    3. Movement: Provides the points of attachment for muscles to create movement.

    4. Reservoir: Stores important minerals for release into peripheral circulation as required.

    5. Hematopoiesis: Blood production.

C. Bone anatomy (see Figure 5-7)

    1. Diaphysis: Bone shaft composed of both compact and spongy bone which functions to provide strong support without increased weight.

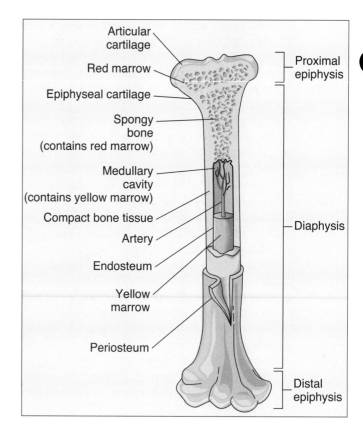

Figure 5-7

Anatomy of a cell. Delmar/Cengage Learning.

2. Epiphysis: The bulbous ends of long bones that provide attachment for muscles and stability to joints.

3. Epiphyseal cartilage: Layer of cartilage medial to the epiphysis and diaphysis where ossification (bone growth) occurs.

4. Articular cartilage: Sheet of cartilage that covers bones where they articulate to provide lubrication and cushioning to the joint.

5. Periosteum: Outer membrane of the bone excluding the epiphysis composed of fibrous connective tissue, to provide attachments for tendons, blood vessels, and ossification (growth) cells known as osteoblasts.

6. Endosteum: Thin epithelial lining of the internal cavity (medulla) that serves to balance bone growth at the periosteum by producing osteoclasts that enlarge the diameter of the medulla.

7. Medulla: Cavity within long bones that house bone marrow.

8. Bone marrow

    a. Soft, diffuse connective tissue known as myeloid tissue responsible for blood cell production.

    b. Red marrow: Produces red blood cells.

    c. Yellow marrow: As one ages, red marrow becomes saturated with fat and turns to yellow marrow, thereby ceasing to produce blood cells unless blood supply is seriously decreased.

D. Bone classifications
   1. Long bones: The bone length exceeds its width (e.g., extremities).
   2. Short bones: Cube-shaped bones (e.g., wrist, ankle).
   3. Flat bones: Thinner, sheetlike bone (e.g., skull, ribs, breastbone).
   4. Sesamoid bones: Nodular, rounded bones embedded in tendons (e.g., kneecap).
   5. Irregular bones: Morphological characteristics outside 1–4 (e.g., spine, hip).

E. Bone landmarks: Surface characteristics such as projections, ridges, and depressions.
   1. Process: A bony projection (e.g., mastoid process).
   2. Trochanter: A large, blunt, irregularly shaped process.
   3. Tubercle: Small bone nodule.
   4. Tuberosity: Large, rough bone nodule.
   5. Spine: Slender, pointed process.
   6. Crest: A ridge on a bone (e.g., iliac crest).
   7. Condyle: A rounded projection distal to the epiphysis that articulates with other bones to form joints.
   8. Epicondyle: A rounded projection of a condyle.
   9. Fissure: A groove in which typically a vessel or nerve lies.
   10. Fossa: A shallow depression on a bone (e.g., glenoid fossa).
   11. Foramen: An opening through a bone (e.g., foramen magnum).
   12. Head: Large, rounded end of a bone distal to a constricted neck.
   13. Sinus: Bony cavity.

F. Axial skeleton: Bones forming the skull, spine, and chest (see Figures 5-8A and B).

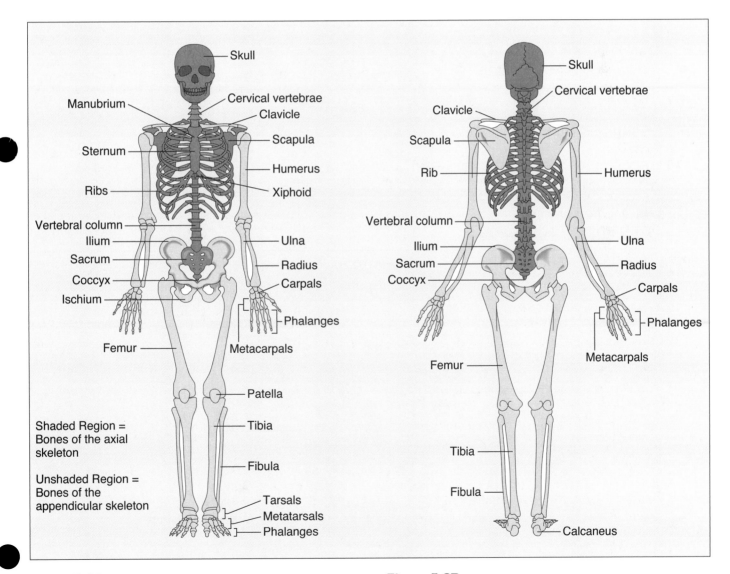

Figure 5-8A

Anterior view of the adult human skeleton. Delmar/Cengage Learning.

Figure 5-8B

Posterior view of the adult human skeleton. Delmar/Cengage Learning.

1. Cranium: Bones that house the brain (see Figures 5-9A, B and C).
    a. Frontal: Forms the forehead, frontal sinuses, and upper orbits of the eye.
    b. Parietal: Two bones joined at the top to form the roof.
    c. Temporal: Two bones forming the lower sides and floor of the cranium.
        (1) Auditory meatus: Ear canal of the temporal bone.
        (2) Ossicles: Bones of the middle ear:
            (a) Malleus: Hammer that articulates with the eardrum.
            (b) Incus: Anvil, which transmits energy from the malleus to the stapes.
            (c) Stapes: Stirrup, which transmits sound energy to the oval window.
        (3) Mastoid process: Projection located posterior to the auditory meatus.
        (4) Styloid process: Sharp projection inferior to the auditory meatus.
        (5) Zygomatic process: Bridge of thin bone forming the arch of the cheekbone.
    d. Occipital: Single bone forming the inferior, posterior wall of the cranium. Contains the foramen magnum where the spinal cord exits the skull.

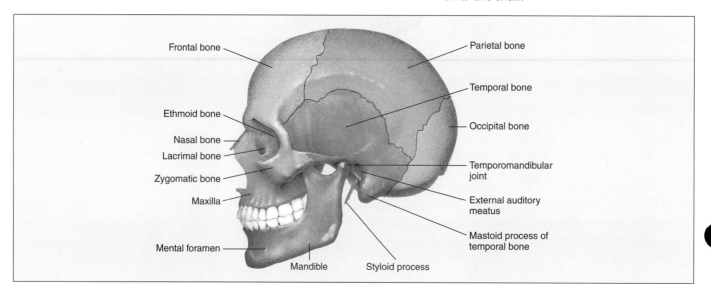

Figure 5-9A

Lateral view of the skull. Delmar/Cengage Learning.

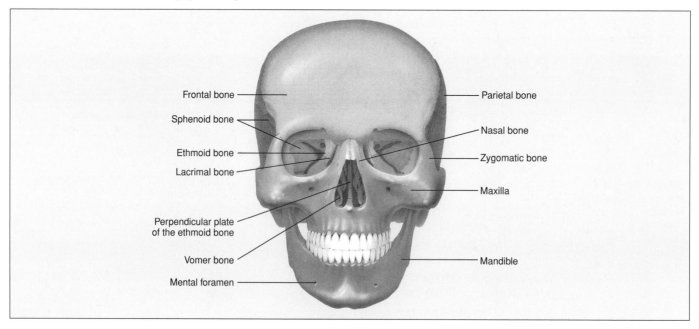

Figure 5-9B

Anterior view of the skull. Delmar/Cengage Learning.

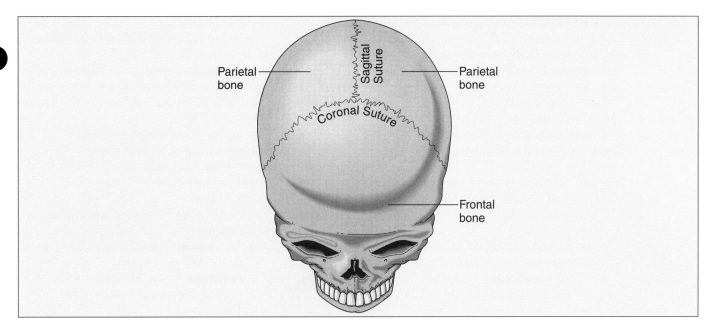

Figure 5-9C

Bones and structures of the skull. Delmar/Cengage Learning.

e. Sphenoid: Butterfly-shaped bone bridging the temporal bones to form the floor of the cranium. Contains the sella turcica, an indentation where the pituitary gland rests.

f. Ethmoid: Single bone forming the superior nasal cavity and posterior orbits.

2. Facial

a. Nasal: Two bones forming the superior nose bridge.

b. Vomer: Single bone forming the inferior portion of nasal septum.

c. Lacrimal: Two bones forming the medial orbits.

d. Zygomatic: Two bones forming the arch of the cheekbone and lateral orbits.

e. Palatine: Two bones forming the posterior hard palate and nasal floor.

f. Mandible: Lower jawbone.

g. Maxilla: Two fused bones forming the upper jaw, anterior hard palate, and orbital floors.

h. Hyoid: U-shaped bone suspended from the styloid process that supports the tongue. Only bone that does not articulate with another bone.

3. Spinal column: Comprised of vertebrae that house the spinal cord (see Figure 5-10).

a. Cervical vertebrae: First seven vertebrae, C1 to C7, forming the neck.

   (1) Atlas: First cervical vertebrae (C1) supporting the skull.

   (2) Axis: Second cervical vertebrae (C2) that allows rotation of the skull.

b. Thoracic vertebrae: Next 12 vertebrae, T1 to T12, that articulate with all 12 ribs.

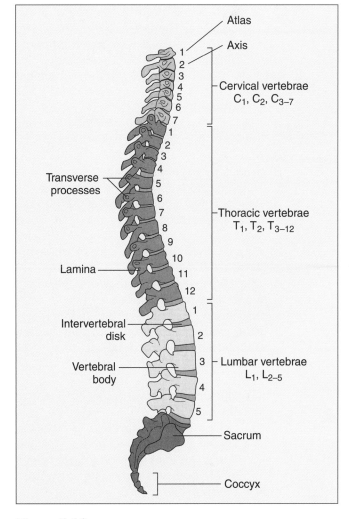

Figure 5-10

Spinal column. Delmar/Cengage Learning.

c. Lumbar vertebrae: Next five vertebrae, L1 to L5, forming the small of the back.

d. Sacrum: Single vertebrae comprised of five fused vertebrae forming the posterior pelvic wall.

e. Coccyx: Single vertebrae comprised of three to five fused vertebrae forming the tailbone.

f. Intervertebral disks: Cartilaginous material that provides cushions between vertebrae.

4. Thorax

a. Sternum: Breastbone forming the anterior articulation of the first seven ribs.

   (1) Manubrium: Superior portion of the sternum.

   (2) Body: Medial portion of the breastbone.

   (3) Xiphoid process: Slender, inferior terminal projection of the sternum.

b. Ribs: Curved flat bones that serve to house the thoracic cavity.

   (1) True ribs: Superior seven pair that articulate with both the sternum and vertebrae by means of costal cartilage.

   (2) False ribs: The next three pair articulate with the seventh rib by way of costal cartilage. The last two pair are known as floating ribs as they do not articulate anteriorly.

G. Appendicular skeleton: Bones of the extremities and pelvis.

1. Upper extremities

a. Clavicle: Two collarbones forming a bridge between the shoulder blade and breast-bone.

b. Scapula: Two shoulder blades.

c. Humerus: Bone forming the upper arms.

d. Radius: Lower armbone on the thumb side.

e. Ulna: Lower armbone on the little finger side.

f. Carpals: Two rows of four bones forming the wrist.

g. Metacarpals: Five bones that form the framework of the hand.

h. Phalanges: Three bones in each finger (proximal, medial, and distal) and two in each thumb (proximal and distal).

2. Lower extremities

a. Pelvis

   (1) Ilium: Superior, wing-shaped bones of the hip.

   (2) Ischium: Inferior portion of the hip known as the sit-down bone.

   (3) Pubis: Anterior portion of the pelvis where both sides articulate at the symphysis pubis.

b. Femur: Thighbone. Largest, heaviest bone of the body.

c. Patella: Kneecap.

d. Tibia: Shinbone.

e. Fibula: Smaller, lower legbone lateral to the tibia.

f. Tarsals: Seven ankle bones. Calcaneus, talus, navicular, cuboid, and three cuneiforms.

g. Metatarsals: Five bones forming the arch of the foot.

h. Phalanges: Three bones in each toe, except the great toe having only two.

H. Articulations: Point of attachment between bones, held together by ligaments, to form joints.

1. Joint classifications

a. Functional classification: Classified according to movement afforded.

   (1) Synarthroses: Immovable joints (e.g., cranial bones).

   (2) Amphiarthroses: Slightly movable joints (e.g., symphysis pubis).

   (3) Diarthroses: Freely movable joints (e.g., knee, elbow, etc.).

b. Structural classification: Classified according to the connective tissue comprising the joint.

   (1) Fibrous joints: Joints that fit tightly together and are generally synarthrotic.

   (2) Cartilaginous joints: Joints that are connected by cartilage and are generally amphiarthrotic.

   (3) Synovial joints: Joints that are filled with synovial fluid for continuous lubrication are generally diarthrotic.

2. Synovial (diarthrotic) joint types

a. Uniaxial: Movement around one axis or plane.

   (1) Hinge joints: Articulation that allows only flexion and extension (e.g., elbow, knee, fingers, toes).

   (2) Pivot joints: Rotation around the axis of a bone (e.g., atlas-axis vertebrae).

b. Biaxial: Movement around two perpendicular axes or planes.

   (1) Saddle joints: Convex-concave articulation (e.g., thumb).

   (2) Condyloid: Condyle fits into an elliptical socket (e.g., knee).

c. Multiaxial: Movement around three or more axes or planes:

   (1) Ball and socket: Ball-shaped head fits into concave socket (e.g., shoulder).

   (2) Gliding joints: Flat articulation allowing limited movement over most axes (e.g., carpals, tarsals).

I. Important bone landmarks

1. Cranial region

a. Frontal tuberosities: Ridges above the orbits.

b. Optic foramen. Opening in the orbit permitting passage of the optic nerve.

c. Mandibular fossa: Socket formed by the mandible articulating with the cranium.

d. Foramen magnum: Opening where spinal cord exits the cranium.

e. External occipital protuberance: Slight bump at the posterior base of the skull.

2. Upper extremities
   a. Acromion process: Tip of shoulder.
   b. Glenoid fossa: Shoulder socket.
   c. Olecranon process: Projection of the proximal ulna—the elbow.

3. Lower extremities:
   a. Acetabulum: Hip socket.
   b. Obturator foramen: Large openings of the ischium.
   c. Pelvic inlet: Large opening posterior to the symphysis pubis.
   d. Greater trochanter: Protuberance of the femur located laterally to the head.
   e. Lesser trochanter: Protuberance of the femur located medially to the head.
   f. Lateral condyle: Outer edge of the knee.
   g. Medial condyle: Inner edge of the knee.
   h. Lateral malleolus: Outer protuberance of ankle (fibula).
   i. Medial malleolus: inner protuberance of ankle (tibia).
   j. Calcaneus: Heel bone.

J. Age-Related Changes
   1. Cartilage calcifies: Bones become hard and brittle. Increased risk of osteoporosis.
   2. Bone resorption overcomes new bone creation. Requires greater healing time after fractures.

K. Pathophysiology
   1. Fractures: Break or crack in a bone.
      a. Simple (closed) fracture: A fracture with no external wound caused by the bone.
      b. Compound (open) fracture: A fracture in which the bone extrudes from the skin.
      c. Greenstick fracture: An incomplete break as when a soft twig is bent.
      d. Comminuted fracture: A fracture that shatters or creates bone fragments.
      e. Impacted fracture: A fracture in which one broken end is forced into the other.
      f. Transverse fracture: A straight break across the bone.
      g. Spiral fracture: A break caused by a twisting force creating an "S"-shaped fracture.
   2. Abnormal spinal curvatures (see Figures 5-11A to C)
      a. Kyphosis: Abnormal outward curvature of the spine creating a humpback appearance.
      b. Lordosis: Abnormal inward curvature of the spine creating a swayback appearance.
      c. Scoliosis: Abnormal sideward curvature of the spine creating an off-balanced appearance.
   3. Herniated nucleus pulposus (HNP): Displaced intervertebral disc that puts pressure on the spinal cord.
   4. Osteoporosis: Brittle, porous bones that are susceptible to fractures because of decreased calcium and phosphorus. Found especially among menopausal women.
   5. Osteomalacia: Softness of bones caused by poor mineralization or lack of vitamin D creating rickets in children.

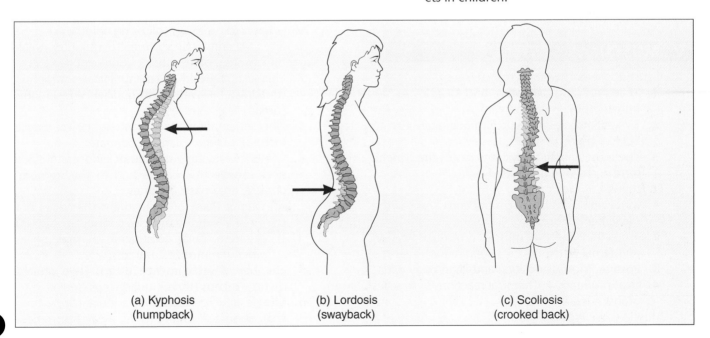

(a) Kyphosis (humpback)　　(b) Lordosis (swayback)　　(c) Scoliosis (crooked back)

Figure 5-11

(a) Kyphosis (humpback); (b) Lordosis (swayback); (c) Scoliosis (crooked back). Delmar/Cengage Learning.

6. Osteomyelitis: Infection of bone, usually following compound fractures or surgery.
7. Osteitis deformans (Paget's disease): Chronic metabolic skeletal disease causing bones to become thicker and softer.
8. Arthritis: Inflammation of a joint.
   a. Osteoarthritis: Chronic inflammatory joint disease resulting in degeneration of cartilage and subsequent hypertrophy of bone.
   b. Rheumatoid arthritis (RA): Chronic, systemic, inflammatory joint disease of the synovial joints that erode cartilage.
   c. Ankylosing spondylitis: Rheumatoid arthritis of the spine.
   d. Gout: Arthritis caused by the deposit of uric acid in synovial fluid.
9. Bursitis: Inflammation of bursae, a thin-walled sac that affords movement of tendons and muscles over bone.
10. Spina bifida: Congenital abnormality characterized by failure of the vertebrae to close around the spinal cord.
11. Talipes: Congenital deformity causing twisted or clubbed feet.
12. Pott's disease: Tuberculous osteitis of the vertebrae.
13. Neoplasms
    a. Osteosarcoma: Most common malignant tumor.
    b. Osteochondroma: Most common skeletal tumor.
    c. Chondrosarcoma: Malignant tumor of hyaline cartilage.
14. Subluxation: Joint dislocations.
15. Sprain: Stretching injury to ligaments of a joint.

V. MUSCULAR SYSTEM

A. General
   1. There are approximately 656 muscles in the human body.
   2. Skeletal muscle makes up approximately 40% to 50% of body weight.
   3. The musculoskeletal system creates the general form and shape of the body.
B. Functions
   1. Movement: Muscle contractions cause the movement of bones.
   2. Protection: Sheets of muscles provide protection to internal organs.
   3. Posture: Muscles position and align body parts.
   4. Heat production: Chemical reactions in muscles produce heat.
C. Muscle tissue types
   1. Smooth muscle tissue: Involuntary muscles not under conscious control operate automatically to carry out important metabolic functions.
   2. Cardiac muscle tissue: Striated involuntary muscles found only in the heart that is self-stimulating causing rhythmic contraction to maintain constant blood flow.
   3. Skeletal muscle tissue: Striated voluntary muscles under conscious control that serves to provide movement.
D. Skeletal muscle structure: Muscles are composed of bundles of muscle fibers held together by fibrous connective tissue.
   1. Fibers: Skeletal muscle cells are called fibers because of their threadlike appearance.
   2. Sarcolemma: Delicate plasma membrane covering each muscle fiber.
   3. Endomysium: Delicate connective tissue membrane that covers the muscle fiber.
   4. Fascicles: Group of skeletal muscle fibers.
   5. Perimysium: Tough connective tissue membrane that binds fascicles together.
   6. Epimysium: Tough connective tissue sheath that envelopes an entire muscle.
   7. Tendon: The three fibrous connective tissues endomysium, perimysium, and epimysium that form strong, cordlike structures for the attachment of muscles to the periosteum of bones.
   8. Aponeurosis: Sheetlike tendons which serve to attach muscles to muscles.
E. Muscle characteristics
   1. Irritability (excitability): Ability of the muscle to be stimulated or respond to nervous stimuli.
   2. Contractility: Ability to contract or shorten.
   3. Extensibility (elasticity): Ability to extend or stretch to return to resting length.
F. Morphology and nomenclature: Muscles may be named according to the following criteria:
   1. Size: Maximus (large), medius (middle), minimus (small), brevis (short), longus (long).
   2. Shape: Deltoid (triangular), trapezoid (quadrilateral with two parallel sides), latus (broad).
   3. Fiber orientation: Rectus (straight), transverse (across), oblique (slanted, pennate).
   4. Points of attachment: Sternocleidomastoid is a neck muscle that is attached to the sternum, clavicle, and mastoid bones.
      a. Origin: Point of attachment that does not move when the muscles contract.
      b. Insertion: Point of attachment that moves when the muscle contracts.
   5. Number of attachments: Biceps (two attachments), triceps (three), quadriceps (four).
   6. Muscle action: Adductors adduct (draw toward), abductor abduct (draw away from), flexors flex (bend upon itself), extensors extend (straighten), levators raise, and depressors lower.

G. Muscle actions
1. **Prime mover:** Muscles that produce movement.
2. **Antagonist:** Muscles that oppose prime movers to cause opposite movement or provide prime mover precision and control.
3. **Synergist:** Muscles that serve to make prime movers operate more efficiently and effectively.
4. **Fixator:** Muscles that stabilize the origin of prime movers or joints.

H. Body movement
1. **Flexion:** Movement that causes an extremity to bend upon itself thereby decreasing the angle of a joint.
2. **Extension:** Opposite of flexion; movement that causes an extremity to straighten thereby increasing the angle of a joint.
3. **Adduction:** Movement of a part toward the midline of the body.
4. **Abduction:** Opposite of adduction; movement of a part away from the midline of the body.

5. **Rotation:** Movement of a bone around its longitudinal axis thereby creating a twisting motion.
6. **Circumduction:** Movement of a part in a circular motion.
7. **Pronation:** Movement of a part to face downward, especially the hands.
8. **Supination:** Movement of a part to face upward, especially the hands.
9. **Inversion:** Turning a body part inward, especially the sole of the foot.
10. **Eversion:** Turning a body part outward, especially the sole of the foot.
11. **Dorsiflexion:** Movement of a part in the direction of its backside or dorsum, especially the feet.
12. **Plantarflexion:** Movement of the foot in the direction of its sole.
13. **Protraction:** Movement of a body part forward.
14. **Retraction:** Movement of a body part backward.

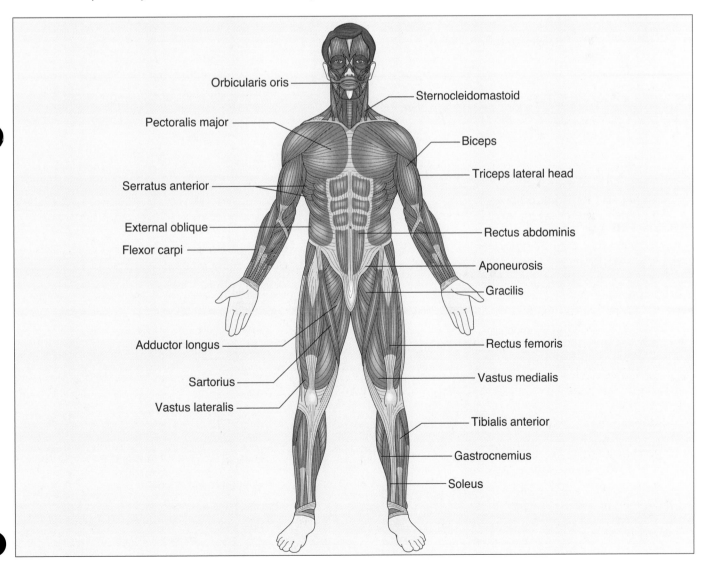

Figure 5-12A

Anterior surface muscles. Delmar/Cengage Learning.

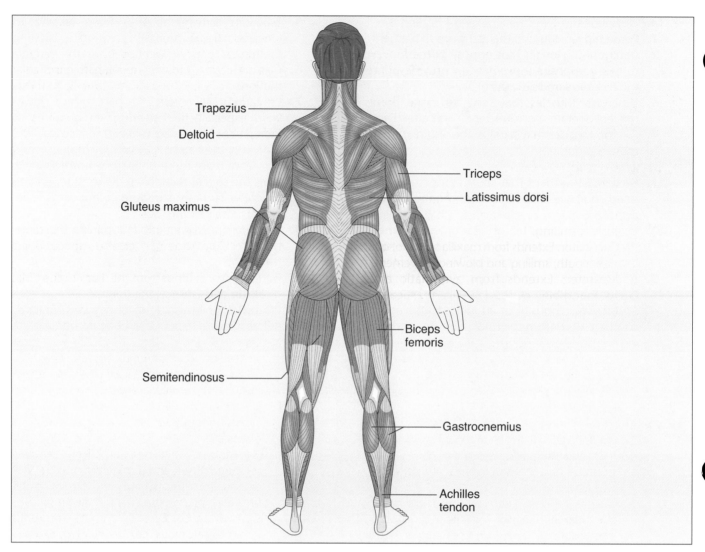

Figure 5-12B

Posterior surface muscles. Delmar/Cengage Learning.

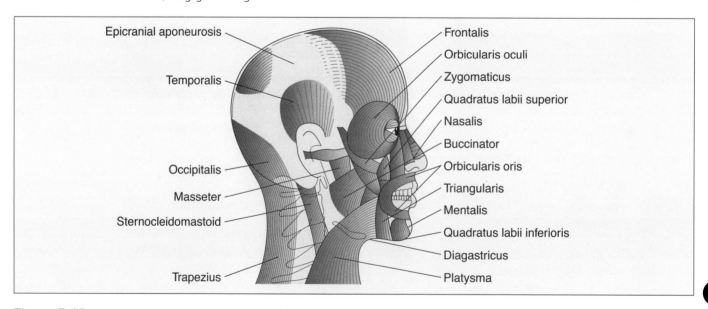

Figure 5-13

Cranial and facial muscles. Delmar/Cengage Learning.

I. Major skeletal muscles (see Figures 5-12A and B)
   1. Head and facial muscles (see Figure 5-13)
      a. Occipitofrontalis (epicranius): Extends from the frontal to occipital bone; raises eyebrows and wrinkles forehead.
      b. Temporalis: Lies over the temporal bone; closes jaw.
      c. Orbicularis oculi: Encircles the eyelids; closes eyes.
      d. Orbicularis oris: Encircles the mouth; draws lips together.
      e. Zygomaticus major: Extends from zygomatic to orbicularis oris; elevates angle of mouth during smiling.
      f. Buccinator: Extends from maxilla to skin of outside mouth; smiling and blowing movement.
      g. Masseter: Extends from zygomatic arch to mandible; closes jaw for mastication (chewing).
   2. Neck and thoracic muscles
      a. Sternocleidomastoid: Extends from the mastoid process to the sternum and clavicle; flexes the head in a bowing motion.
      b. Trapezius: Extends from the occipital to clavicle; raises and lowers shoulders, as in a shrug.
      c. Serratus anterior: Extends from the ribs to scapula; pulls shoulder up and forward.
      d. Pectoralis major: Extends from the clavicle, sternum, and ribs to humerus; flexes upper arm across chest.
      e. Latissimus dorsi: Extends from lower vertebrae to humerus; extends upper arm.
      f. Intercostals: Muscles situated between the ribs. External intercostals elevate the ribs; internal intercostals depress the ribs to aid in breathing.
      g. Diaphragm: Muscular sheet separating the thoracic and abdominal cavities; enlarges thorax for inspiration.
   3. Abdominopelvic muscles
      a. Obliques: Internal and external obliques extend from the ribs to the iliac crest and pubis; compresses abdomen, flattens lumbar curve of spine.
      b. Transversus abdominis: Extends from the ribs to the pubis; serves the same function as the obliques.
      c. Rectus abdominis: Extends from the ribs to the pubis; serves the same function as the obliques.
      d. Levator ani: Extends from pubis and ischium to the coccyx; forms floor of pelvic cavity to support pelvic organs.
   4. Upper extremity muscles
      a. Deltoid: Extends from the scapula and clavicle to humerus forming the shoulder cap; abducts upper arm.
      b. Biceps brachii: Extends from scapula to radius; flexes forearm.
      c. Triceps brachii: Extends from the scapula and humerus to ulna; extends forearm.
      d. Flexor carpi: Extends from humerus to metacarpals; flexes hand.
      e. Extensor carpi: Extends from humerus to metacarpals; extends hand.
      f. Flexor digitora: Extends from humerus and radius to finger tendons; flexes fingers.
      g. Extensor digitora: Extends from humerus to finger tendons; extends fingers.
   5. Lower extremity muscles
      a. Gluteus maximus, medius, minimus: Extends from ilium to femur; extends and abducts thigh.
      b. Sartorius: Extends from the ilium to the tibia; flexes and adducts the thigh.
      c. Adductor brevis, longus, magnus: Extends from pubis to femur; adducts thigh.
      d. Gracilis: Extends from pubis to tibia; adducts thigh, adducts and flexes leg.
      e. Quadriceps femoris: Four muscles, rectus femoris, vastus lateralis, vastus medialis, and vastus intermedius, that extend from the ilium and femur to the tibia; flexes thigh and extends leg.
      f. Hamstrings: Three muscles, biceps femoris, semitendinosus, and semimembranosus, that extend from the ischium and femur to the tibia and fibula; extends thigh, flexes leg.
      g. Gastrocnemius: Extends from the posterior femur to calcaneus; flexes lower leg, extends foot.
      h. Tibialis anterior: Extends from tibia to tarsals and metatarsals; flexes and inverts foot.
      i. Soleus: Extends from tibia and fibula to tarsals; extends and plantar flexes foot.
      j. Peroneus longus, brevis, tertius: Extends from the tibia and fibula to metatarsals; extends and everts foot.
      k. Extensor digitorum longus: Extends from tibia and fibula to phalanges; dorsiflexes foot, extends toes.
J. Age-Related Changes
   1. Decreased mass and strength.
   2. Deterioration is replaced by connective or adipose tissue.
   3. Fewer muscle cell mitochondria. Decreased endurance.
   4. Decreased function resulting from cardiovascular and nervous system changes.
K. Pathophysiology
   1. Sprain: Stretching or tearing injury of a ligament.
   2. Strain: Stretching or tearing injury of a muscle or tendon.

3. Tendonitis: Inflammation of a tendon.
4. Myasthenia gravis: Chronic, progressive neuromuscular disease thought to be caused by an autoimmune disorder characterized by muscle weakness, blepharoptosis, and dysphagia.
5. Polymyositis: Chronic, degenerative disease characterized by inflammation of muscle tissue coupled with weakness.
6. Muscular dystrophy: Congenital disorder characterized by progressive wasting of muscle tissue.

VI. CIRCULATORY SYSTEM

A. Function
 1. Transportation: The primary function of the circulatory system is to transport important physiological elements (such as cells, hormones, antibodies, oxygen, nutrients, etc.) throughout the body.
 2. Thermal regulation: Assists in the regulation of body temperature through blood vessel constriction and dilation.

3. Waste removal: With assistance from the lungs, kidneys, and liver, removes waste from the body.
4. Fluid balance: Maintains a balance between fluid retention and loss.
B. Heart anatomy and physiology (see Figure 5-14)
 1. The heart is a muscular, cone-shaped, hollow organ approximately the size of a fist situated slightly to the left of midline in the mediastinum, posterior to the sternum.
  a. Apex: The inferior, pointed portion of the heart that rests on the diaphragm.
  b. Base: The broader superior aspect.
 2. Heart walls: Composed of three distinct layers.
  a. Epicardium: Outer layer.
  b. Myocardium: Thick, muscular middle layer.
  c. Endocardium: Inner layer comprising delicate endothelial tissue.
 3. Pericardium: Double membranous sac that envelopes the heart to protect and reduce friction.
  a. Parietal pericardium: Outermost pericardial layer.
  b. Visceral pericardium: Innermost pericardial layer.

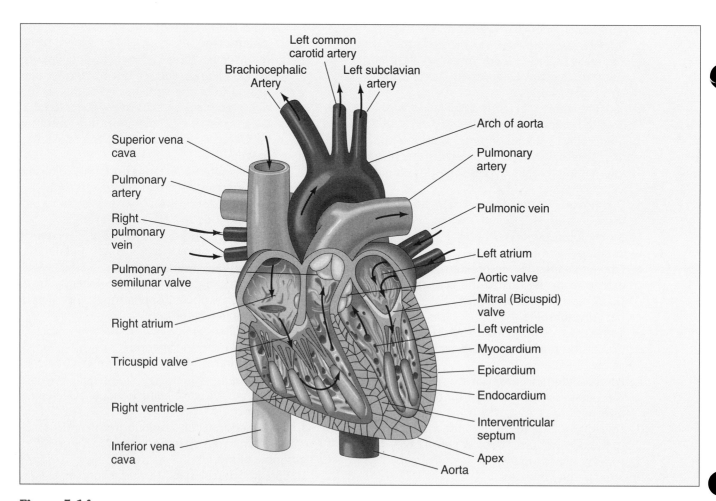

Figure 5-14

Coronal section of the heart. Delmar/Cengage Learning.

4. Chambers: Heart contains four chambers.
   a. Atria: Two superior chambers that receive blood transported through veins.
      (1) Atria relax to receive blood and contract to force blood into the ventricles.
      (2) Atrial walls are not as thick as ventricles because of the short distance the blood is pumped.
      (3) Atrial septum: Separates the left and right atria.
   b. Ventricles: Two inferior pumping chambers that receive blood from the atria and pump to body parts.
      (1) Ventricular walls are much thicker than atria because of the force needed to pump the blood throughout the body.
      (2) Left ventricular myocardium is thicker than the right due to the greater distance the blood must be pumped.
      (3) Ventricular septum: Continuous with the atrial septum, it separates the left and right ventricles.
5. Heart valves: Structures that ensure one-way bloodflow through the heart.
   a. Atrioventricular (AV) valves: Prevents the backflow of blood into the atria when the ventricles contract.
      (1) Tricuspid valve: Right AV valve composed of three flaps that permits flow of blood from the right atrium to the right ventricle.
      (2) Bicuspid (mitral) valve: Left AV valve composed of two flaps that permits flow of blood from the left atrium to the left ventricle.
      (3) Semilunar (SL) valves: Half-moon–shaped valves found in the major vessels arising from the ventricles.
         (a) Pulmonary valve: Valve at entrance of the pulmonary artery that prevents the backflow of blood into the right ventricle.
         (b) Aortic valve: Valve at entrance of the aorta that prevents backflow of blood into the left ventricle.
6. Electrical conduction system: Modified cardiac muscle that serves to initiate and maintain rhythmic heart contractions (see Figure 5-15).
   a. Sinoatrial (SA) node: Specialized cells located in the right atrial wall near the superior vena cava.
      (1) Initiates each heartbeat and sets its pace (pacemaker).
      (2) The impulse travels across both atria, causing them to contract.
      (3) Has an intrinsic rate of 60 to 80 impulses per minute.

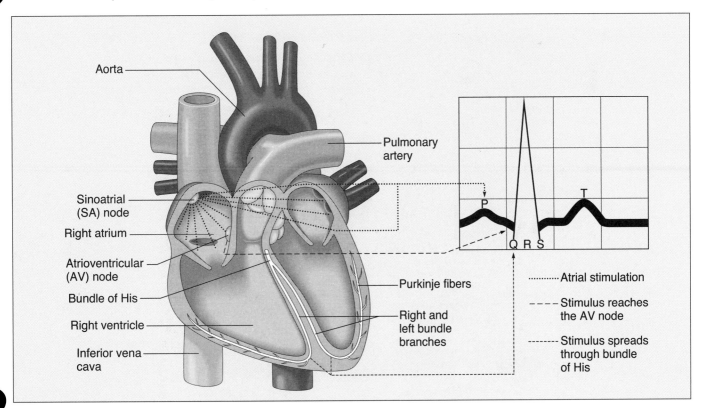

Figure 5-15

Electrical conduction system of the heart. Delmar/Cengage Learning.

b. Atrioventricular (AV) node: Specialized cardiac muscle located in the lower right atrial septum.

   (1) The impulse travels from the SA to the AV node at a reduced velocity to permit both atria to contract.

   (2) Should the SA node malfunction, the AV node has an intrinsic rate of 40 to 60 impulses per minute.

c. Bundle of His: Specialized cells located in the ventricular septum.

   (1) The impulse travels from the AV node to the bundle of His at an increased velocity.

   (2) Should the SA and AV node malfunction, the bundle of His has an intrinsic rate of 20 to 40 impulses per minute.

d. Bundle branches: Two branches, extending from the bundle of His, conduct impulses down the ventricular septum.

e. Purkinje fibers: Extend from the right and left bundle branches to the ventricular walls causing them to contract.

7. Nerve supply

a. Cardiac plexus: Cluster of nerves located near the aortic arch comprising sympathetic and parasympathetic nerve fibers.

b. Fibers from the cardiac plexus enter the heart by way of the coronary arteries.

c. Fibers end in the sinoatrial node, atrioventricular node, and atrial wall.

8. Cardiac cycle: Complete heartbeat consisting of contraction (systole) and relaxation (diastole) of both atria and ventricles.

a. Atrial systole: Contraction of the atria.

   (1) Atrial contraction empties the blood into the ventricles.

   (2) The AV valves open, and the SL valves close.

b. Ventricular diastole: The ventricles are relaxed and filling with blood from the atria.

c. Ventricular systole: Contraction of the ventricles.

   (1) Ventricular contraction forces the blood through the SL valves to the major vessels, aorta, and pulmonary artery.

   (2) The AV valves are now closed.

d. Atrial diastole: The atria are relaxed and filling with blood from the major veins, vena cavas and pulmonary veins, before the cycle is repeated with atrial systole.

C. Blood vessel anatomy and physiology (see Figure 5-16)

  1. Types and function

    a. Artery: Vessels that carry blood away from the heart. Small arteries are arterioles. Arterioles provide resistance important in blood pressure.

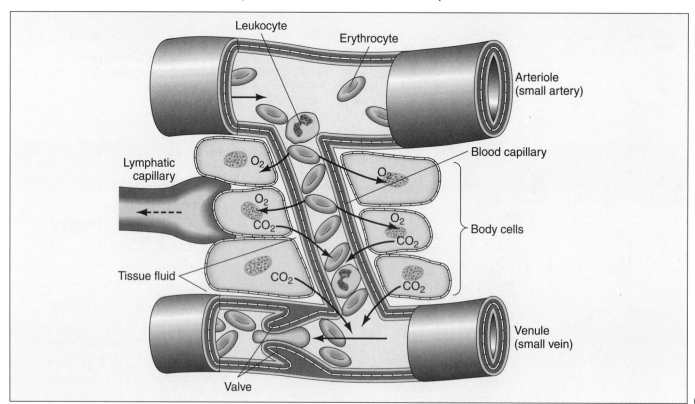

Figure 5-16

Blood vessel anatomy. Delmar/Cengage Learning.

b. Veins: Vessels that carry blood toward the heart. Small veins are venules. Serve as collectors and reservoir vessels.
c. Capillaries: Microscopic vessels that connect arterioles and venules. Permit the collection and delivery of important physiologic substances.

2. Structure
   a. Arteries/veins: Composed of three layers.
      (1) Tunica adventitia: Outermost layer comprising tough, fibrous connective tissue. Thickest layer in veins.
      (2) Tunica media: Middle layer comprising smooth muscle tissue. Allows vessels to contract and dilate.
      (3) Tunica intima: Innermost layer comprising endothelium. In veins forms semilunar valves to prevent backflow.
   b. Capillaries: Microscopic vessels composed of a single layer of endothelium to allow for the exchange of material between plasma and interstitial fluid.

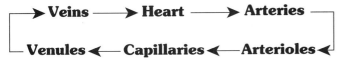

D. Circulation
   1. Deoxygenated (CO_2) blood returning to the heart from the body flows through the vena cavas.
      a. Blood returning from head, neck, and axilla flow through the superior vena cava.
      b. Blood returning from the torso and below flow through the inferior vena cava.
   2. From the vena cavae, the blood enters the right atrium.
   3. The right atrium contracts, forcing the blood through the tricuspid valve.
   4. The blood enters the right ventricle.
   5. The right ventricle contracts forcing the blood through the pulmonary valve.
   6. The blood enters the pulmonary artery to be transported to the lungs for oxygenation (O_2).
   7. Once oxygenated in the lungs, the blood enters the pulmonary veins for transport back to the heart.
   8. From the pulmonary veins, the blood enters the left atrium.
   9. The left atrium contracts forcing the blood through the bicuspid (mitral) valve.
   10. The blood enters the left ventricle.
   11. The left ventricle contracts forcing the blood through the aortic valve.
   12. The blood enters the aorta where it is transported to all body parts to deposit oxygenated (O_2)

blood and collect deoxygenated (CO_2) blood for return to the heart where the cycle is repeated.

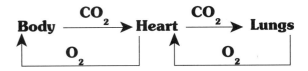

E. Major vessels (see Figures 5-17A and B)
   1. Major arteries (see Figure 5-17A)
      a. Pulmonary: Arising from the right ventricle, it transports deoxygenated blood to the lungs for oxygenation.
      b. Aorta: Largest artery arising from the heart where largest systemic arteries branch off from. The aorta is divided into the ascending, aortic arch, descending, and abdominal aorta.
      c. Coronary: Right and left arteries branch off from the ascending aorta to supply the heart with blood.
      d. Brachiocephalic: One of three major branches of the aortic arch. It branches off to supply blood to both the neck and head, and the axilla and upper arm.
      e. Subclavian: The left subclavian branches from the aortic arch; the right subclavian branches from the brachiocephalic to supply the arm and vertebrae.
      f. Carotid: The left carotid branches from the aortic arch; the right from the brachiocephalic to supply the neck and head.
      g. Facial: A branch of the carotid, it supplies the anterior face and cranium.
      h. Occipital: A branch of the carotid, it supplies the neck, mastoid, and lateral and posterior cranium.
      i. Axillary: An extension of the subclavian, it supplies the axilla.
      j. Brachial: An extension of the axillary, it supplies the upper arm.
      k. Radial: A branch of the brachial on the thumb side, it supplies the forearm, wrist, and hand.
      l. Ulnar: A branch of the brachial on the little finger side, it supplies the forearm, wrist, and hand.
      m. Celiac: A branch of the abdominal aorta, it supplies the upper abdominal organs.
      n. Splenic: Serves a similar function as the celiac.
      o. Renal: A branch of the abdominal aorta, it supplies the kidneys, suprarenal glands, and ureters.
      p. Mesenteric: A branch of the abdominal aorta, the inferior and superior mesenterics supply the intestine, colon, and rectum.

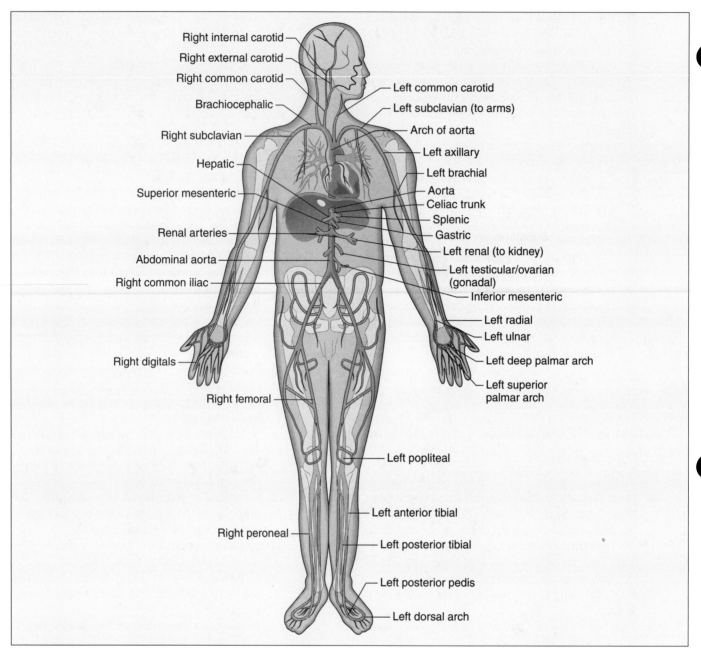

Figure 5-17A

Major arteries of the body. Delmar/Cengage Learning.

q. Iliac: A branching extension of the abdominal aorta, it supplies the abdominal, pelvic, and lower limb regions.

r. Femoral: An extension of the right and left iliac, it supplies the lower abdominal wall, genitalia, and upper leg.

s. Popliteal: An extension of the femoral, it supplies the knee and calf.

t. Tibial: An extension of the popliteal, the anterior tibial supplies the lower leg, ankle, and foot; the posterior tibial supplies the lower leg, foot, and heel.

u. Dorsalis pedis: An extension of the anterior tibial, it supplies the foot.

2. Major veins (see Figure 5-17B)

a. Pulmonary: Vein that transports oxygenated blood from the lungs to the left atrium.

b. Coronary: Leading into the coronary sinus of the right atrium, it drains blood from the heart.

c. Vena cava: Largest vein draining blood from the body into the right atrium. The superior vena cava drains the upper half of body; the inferior vena cava, the lower half.

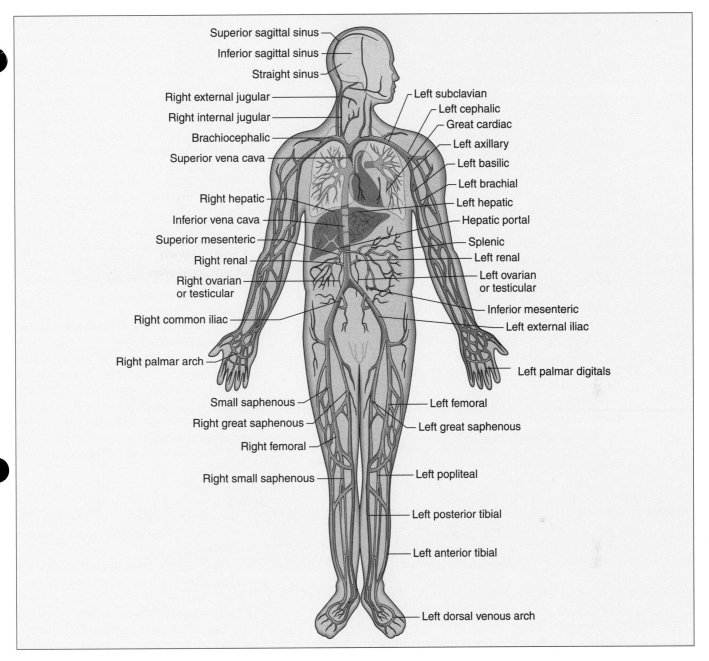

Figure 5-17B

Major veins of the body. Delmar/Cengage Learning.

d. Brachiocephalic: Left and right branches leading into the superior vena cava, it drains the head, neck, and upper extremities.

e. Jugular: Branches leading into the brachiocephalic, it drains the head and neck.

f. Facial: Branches leading into the jugular, it drains the face and anterior cranium.

g. Occipital: Branches leading into the jugular, it drains the posterior cranium.

h. Axillary: Branches leading into brachiocephalic, it drains the axillary and upper arm region.

i. Subclavian: Branches leading into the axillary, it drains the upper arms.

j. Cephalic: Superficial vein on the thumbside leading into the axillary, it drains the upper and lower arm.

k. Radial: Deep vein leading into the axillary that drains blood from the thumbside of the forearm and wrist.

l. Basilic: Superficial vein on the little-finger side leading into the axillary, it drains the upper and lower arm.

m. Ulnar: Deep vein leading into the axillary that drains blood from the little-finger side of forearm and wrist.

n. Splenic, gastric, cholecystic: Leading into the portal hepatic vein, it drains the spleen, stomach, and gallbladder, respectively.

o. Mesenteric: Leading into the hepatic portal vein, it drains blood from the intestines, colon, and rectum.

p. Hepatic: Leading into the inferior vena cava, it drains the liver.

q. Renal: Leading into the inferior vena cava, it drains the kidneys, suprarenal glands, and gonads.

r. Iliac: A branching extension of the inferior vena cava, it drains the abdominal, pelvic, and lower limb regions.

s. Femoral: An extension of the right and left iliac, it drains the upper leg.

t. Popliteal: An extension of the femoral, it drains the knee and calf.

u. Saphenous: The longest vein; the great saphenous leads into the femoral and drains the medial leg. The small saphenous leads into the popliteal and drains the lateral lower leg.

v. Tibial: Leading into the popliteal, the anterior and posterior tibial drains the lower leg.

w. Dorsal venous arch: Leading into the tibial veins, it drains the foot.

F. Lymphatics anatomy and physiology
1. General
a. Specialized component of the circulatory system comprising lymph fluid, lymphatic vessels, lymph nodes, tonsils, thymus, and spleen.
b. As part of the circulatory system, it functions to maintain fluid balance and provide immunity.
c. Lymph vessels serve to collect excess tissue fluid for transport into the veins before its return to the heart.
d. The lymphatic system transports tissue fluid, proteins, fats, and other elements to the general circulation.
e. Unlike the cardiovascular system, the lymphatic system is not a closed circuit.

2. Lymphatic fluid: Clear, watery, isotonic fluid resembling blood plasma.

3. Lymphatic vessels
a. Vessels similar to veins, but have thinner walls, more valves, and contain lymph nodes along the course of the vessels.
b. Lymphatic capillaries: Microscopic vessels composed of a single layer of endothelial cells.
c. Lacteals: Lymphatic capillaries that absorb fat in the villi of small intestine.

d. As lymphatic vessels increase in diameter, their walls become thicker and form three layers similar to blood vessels.
e. Semilunar valves: Are present every few millimeters and increase as the vessels get smaller.
f. Right lymphatic duct: Lymph from upper right quarter of the body drains into right lymphatic duct, which then drains into the right subclavian vein.
g. Thoracic duct: Lymph from the rest of the body drains into the thoracic duct, which then drains into the left subclavian vein.

4. Circulation
a. Lymph moves in a rightward direction because of the number of valves.
b. Breathing and skeletal muscle motion cause a pressure gradient, which moves the lymph fluid through the vessels.

5. Lymph nodes
a. Lymph nodes are oval-shaped filters enclosed by a fibrous capsule.
b. Lymph nodes generally occur in clusters the most significant of which include submental, submaxillary, cervical, cubital, axillary, and inguinal lymph nodes.
c. Lymph nodes filter and phagocytose toxins and microorganisms.
d. Site of final stages of maturation for some lymphocytes and monocytes.

6. Lymphatic tissues
a. Tonsils
(1) Located under the mucous membranes in the mouth and pharynx at the base of the tongue.
(2) Protect against bacteria invading the tissues between the nasal and oral cavities.
b. Thymus
(1) Pyramid-shaped organ located in the mediastinum; it is replaced by fat as one ages.
(2) Produces lymphocytes before birth.
(3) Shortly after birth, secretes thymosin which allows lymphocytes to develop into T-cells.
c. Spleen
(1) Oval-shaped organ located in the left hypochondriac region, below the diaphragm, above the left kidney, posterior to the stomach.
(2) Macrophages within the spleen phagocytose microorganisms from the blood.
(3) Site of final maturation of monocytes and lymphocytes.
(4) Macrophages phagocytize worn out RBCs and platelets and recycle iron and globin.
(5) Serves as a blood reservoir in case of sudden blood loss.

G. Age-Related Changes
   1. Heart increases in size. Increased risk for thrombosis and infarction.
   2. Adipose deposited in and around the heart. Varicosities develop.
   3. Valves thicken and stiffen.
   4. Resting and maximum cardiac rates decrease.
   5. Decreased pumping capacity.
   6. Decreased vascular elasticity and plaque build-up.
H. Pathophysiology
   1. Cardiopathies
      a. Rheumatic heart disease: Streptococcal infection resulting from rheumatic fever that causes inflammation of the heart and subsequent scarring of the heart valves.
      b. Carditis: Acute inflammation of the heart.
         (1) Pericarditis: Inflammation of the pericardium of the heart.
         (2) Myocarditis: Inflammation of the myocardium or muscular layer of the heart.
         (3) Endocarditis: Inflammation of the endocardium or inner layer of the heart including the valves.
      c. Mitral stenosis: Narrowing of the mitral valve preventing normal blood flow from the left atrium to ventricle often resulting from rheumatic fever, mitral valve prolapse, or infarction.
      d. Tricuspid stenosis: Narrowing of the tricuspid valve preventing normal blood flow from the right atrium to ventricle.
      e. Pulmonic stenosis: Narrowing of the pulmonary valve preventing normal blood flow from the right ventricle through the pulmonary artery to the lungs often causing right ventricular hypertrophy.
      f. Aortic stenosis: Narrowing of the aortic valve preventing normal blood flow from the left ventricle through the aorta to the body often causing left ventricular hypertrophy.
      g. Angina pectoris: Chest pain resulting from lack of blood nourishment to the heart.
      h. Myocardial infarction: Heart attack; usually the result of occlusion of a coronary artery that interrupts blood flow, causing necrosis of heart tissue.
      i. Congestive heart failure: Heart disease characterized by the inability of the heart to sufficiently keep the blood circulating, resulting in venous and pulmonary congestion and generalized edema.
      j. Tetralogy of Fallot: Heart condition characterized by four abnormalities: pulmonary stenosis, interventricular septal defect, dextraposed aorta, and right ventricular hypertrophy.
      k. Tachycardia: Rapid heart rate greater than 100 beats per minute.
      l. Bradycardia: Slow heart rate less than 60 beats per minute.
      m. Patent ductus arteriosus: Abnormal connection between the pulmonary artery and the aorta.
      n. Cardiac arrest: Sudden, unexpected interruption of heart function most often following myocardial infarction.
   2. Angiopathies
      a. Hypertension: High blood pressure usually greater than 140/90.
      b. Aneurysm: Dilation of an artery resulting from weakening of the vessel wall.
      c. Arteriosclerosis: Hardening of the arteries characterized by thickening of the arterial walls coupled with a loss of elasticity often contributing to hypertension.
      d. Atherosclerosis: A form of arteriosclerosis with the accumulation of fat, cholesterol, and cellular debris causing the vessels to narrow.
      e. Thrombophlebitis: Inflammation of a vein coupled with clot formations in the vessel.
      f. Embolism: Obstruction of a blood vessel by foreign substances or a blood clot.
      g. Varicosity: Large twisted superficial veins occurring especially in the lower legs.
   3. Lymphopathies
      a. Lymphedema: Abnormal accumulation of lymph especially in the extremities caused by obstruction of lymph vessels and resulting in swelling.
      b. Hodgkin's disease: Malignant neoplastic condition of the lymphatic system causing enlargement of lymphatic tissues (lymphadenopathy).
      c. Lymphosarcoma: Non-Hodgkin's lymphoma that is a malignant disease of the lymphatic system.
   4. Reye's syndrome: An acute illness found primarily among children, commonly following an upper respiratory infection, that results in the accumulation of ammonia in the blood, hypoglycemia, brain edema, and high intracranial pressure.

VII. RESPIRATORY SYSTEM

A. General: The respiratory system consists of three parts
   1. Upper respiratory tract: Organs outside the thoracic cavity include the nose, nasopharynx, oropharynx, laryngopharynx, and larynx.

2. Lower respiratory tract: Organs within the thorax such as the trachea, bronchial tree, and lungs.
3. Accessory organs: Organs that complement the respiratory system include the oral cavity, rib cage, and diaphragm.

B. Function
1. Air distribution and exchange: Allows for the distribution of oxygen and the elimination of carbon dioxide.
2. Filtration: The cilia in the nasal cavity traps dust and particles before air enters the trachea.
3. Humidification: Moistens air before entering the lungs.
4. Warming: Superficial blood vessels in the nasal cavity serve to warm the air before entering the lungs.
5. Sound production: Enhances sound production during speech.
6. Olfaction: Allows for the sense of smell.
7. Homeostasis: Aids in the regulation of pH.

C. Upper respiratory tract (see Figure 5-18)
1. Nose
   a. External nose: Consists of the nasal bone and cartilage which forms the tip and nostrils or nares.
   b. Nasal cavity (internal nose): Situated over the roof of the mouth.

(1) Divided into two halves by the nasal septum.
(2) Three subdivisions are created by lateral extensions called the superior, medial, and inferior turbinates.
   c. Paranasal sinuses: Four pairs of mucous-lined, air-filled spaces that drain into the nasal cavity: frontal, maxillary, ethmoid, and sphenoid sinuses.

2. Pharynx: Commonly known as the throat, it is a muscular passageway extending from the base of the skull to the esophagus consisting of three divisions:
   a. Nasopharynx: The proximal pharynx nearest the nasal cavity containing the adenoids.
   b. Oropharynx: The medial area posterior to the mouth containing the tonsils.
   c. Laryngopharynx: The distal pharynx leading to the trachea and esophagus.

3. Larynx: Commonly known as the voicebox.
   a. Located between the root of the tongue and the upper trachea.
   b. Consists of articulated cartilage structures and muscles lined with a ciliated mucous membrane.
   c. Houses the vocal cords.
   d. Serves as an air passageway from the pharynx to the trachea.

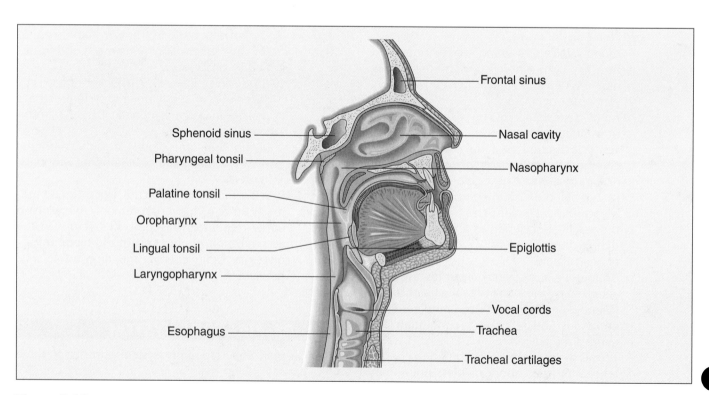

Figure 5-18

Sagittal section of the head and neck. Delmar/Cengage Learning.

D. Lower respiratory tract (see Figure 5-19)
  1. **Trachea:** Or windpipe is composed of 16 to 20 C-shaped rings of cartilage that extend from the larynx to the bronchi.
  2. **Bronchi:** The distal trachea divides into the right and left bronchus, which upon entering the lungs further divide into secondary bronchi that branch into bronchioles, and eventually branch into alveolar ducts.
  3. **Alveoli (air sacs)**
     a. Functional unit of respiration resembling a cluster of grapes.
     b. Formed at the terminal ends of the bronchioles, alveoli are composed of a single layer of epithelium to afford the exchange of gases with surrounding capillaries.
  4. **Lungs:** Cone-shaped organs responsible for air distribution and exchange.
     a. Located in the thoracic cavity extending from the diaphragm to above the clavicles.
     b. Contains approximately 300 million alveoli.
     c. Hilum: Slit or indentation where the bronchi and pulmonary vessels enter the lungs.
     d. Base: Interior surface resting on the diaphragm.
     e. Left lung: Divided into two lobes, the superior and inferior, which is further divided into eight segments.
     f. Right lung: Divided into three lobes, the superior, medial, and inferior, which is further divided into 10 segments.
     g. Pleura: Double-folded membrane containing pleural fluid that envelopes the lungs for lubrication to reduce friction during respiration.
        (1) Visceral pleura: Pleural membrane laying against the lungs.
        (2) Parietal pleura: Pleural membrane laying against the thoracic cavity wall.
  5. **Thorax:** Housing the lower respiratory organs, it permits inspiration and expiration.
E. Pulmonary Ventilation
  1. Carries out the breathing process by means of a pressure gradient
     a. Inspiration: Draws air into the lungs via contraction of the diaphragm making the thoracic cavity larger.
     b. Expiration: Expulsion of air from the lungs by way of relaxing the diaphragm.
  2. The air moving in and out, and remaining in the lungs is important to the process of proper gas exchange.
F. Gas exchange and transportation
  1. External exchange: The exchange of gases (O_2 and CO_2) between the alveoli and the surrounding capillaries.
  2. Internal exchange: The exchange of gases between the capillaries and the cells of the body.
     The common structure of internal and external respiration is the capillary.

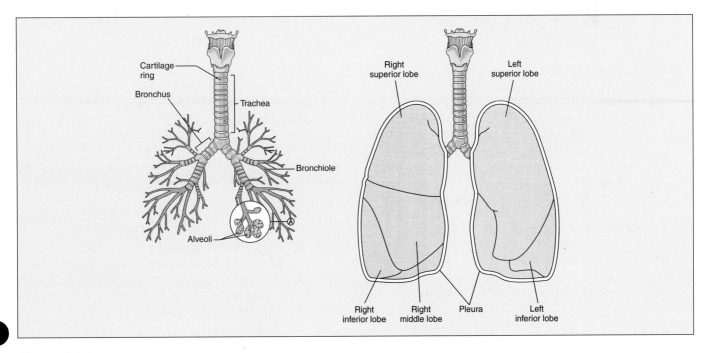

Figure 5-19

Structure of the lower respiratory track. Delmar/Cengage Learning.

G. Respiratory regulation: Is brought about by the respiratory control center of the medulla, which controls the rhythm and depth of inspiration and expiration by constantly monitoring the level of oxygen, carbon dioxide, and blood pH.

H. Age-Related Changes
1. Decline in respiratory capacity.
2. Increased risk of respiratory infections.
3. Decreased lung volume and gas exchange due to thickened capillaries and inelastic intercostal muscles.

I. Pathophysiology
1. Abnormal respirations
   a. Apnea: Lack of breathing.
   b. Hyperpnea: Increased volume of breathing.
   c. Hypopnea: Shallow breathing.
   d. Bradypnea: Slow breathing.
   e. Dyspnea: Difficulty or painful breathing.
   f. Tachypnea: Rapid breathing.
   g. Orthopnea: Difficult breathing unless positioned upright.
   h. Rales: Crackling or whistling sound during inspiration often as a result of accumulation of secretions in the bronchi.
   i. Rhoncus: Wheezing or squeaking sound.
   j. Stridor: High-pitched respiratory sounds resembling howling wind often the result of partial obstruction.
   k. Cheyne-Stokes: Alternating episodes of tachypnea and apnea.
2. Hypoxia: Oxygen deficiency.
3. Anoxia: Lack of oxygen.
4. Suffocation: External prevention of breathing such as drowning or choking.
5. Asphyxia: Insufficient oxygen intake.
6. Epistaxis: Nosebleeds.
7. Sinusitis: Inflammation of the paranasal sinus.
8. Pharyngitis: Inflammation of the throat.
9. Laryngitis: Inflammation of the larynx.
10. Bronchitis: Inflammation of the bronchi.
11. Infectious mononucleosis: Acute lymphatic viral infection caused by the Epstein Barr virus that often includes upper respiratory symptoms.
12. Pneumonia: Inflammation of the bronchioles and alveoli.
13. Pneumothorax: Collection of air in pleural space resulting in partial or complete lung collapse.
14. Hemotherax: Collection of blood in the pleural cavity.
15. Pleurisy: Inflammation of the pleural membranes.
16. Pleural effusion: Accumulation of fluid between the visceral and parietal pleura.
17. Chronic obstructive pulmonary disease (COPD): General term used to describe disease processes that decrease the lung's ability to perform its function.
18. Emphysema: Enlargement and loss of elasticity of the alveoli resulting from partial blockage of alveolar spaces.
19. Asthma: Bronchial spasms and edema resulting in dyspnea and wheezing.
20. Tuberculosis: Lung disease caused by *Mycobacterium tuberculosis* resulting in necrosis of lung tissue that may spread to other body regions.
21. Pneumoconiosis: Condition characterized by the collection of dust particles in the lungs.
    a. Silicosis: Caused by inhalation of silica (quartz) often seen in miners.
    b. Asbestosis: Caused by inhalation of asbestos fibers.
    c. Berylliosis: Caused by inhalation of beryllium often seen in metal and ceramics workers.
    d. Anthracosis: Caused by the inhalation of carbon particles or coal. Also called black lung disease.
    e. Byssinosis: Caused by inhalation of cotton, flax, or hemp particles. Also known as white lung disease.
22. Pulmonary edema: Accumulation of fluid in the pulmonary tissues.
23. Pulmonary embolism: A blood clot or undissolved matter located in the pulmonary artery or its branches.
24. Respiratory acidosis/alkalosis: Acidosis results in decreased pH levels of body fluids because of inadequate removal of carbon dioxide by the lungs. Alkalosis results in increased pH levels caused by excessive removal of carbon dioxide by the lungs.
25. Atelectasis: Partial or complete lung collapse.
26. Bronchiectasis: Permanent dilation of bronchial passageways as a result of pneumonia, obstruction, or poisonous gas.
27. Carcinoma: Malignant neoplasms of the respiratory system.
28. Croup: Acute viral infection characterized by dyspnea and a barklike cough.
29. Pertussis: Whooping cough; a bacterial lung disease caused by *Bordetella pertussis*.

VIII. DIGESTIVE SYSTEM

A. Function
1. Digestion: The physical and chemical breakdown of complex nutrients into simple nutrients.
2. Absorption: Transportation of nutrients from the gastrointestinal tract into the bloodstream.
3. Elimination: Excretion of waste material not absorbed.

B. Anatomy (see Figure 5-20)
1. Divisions
   a. Alimentary canal: Internal complex of tubal structures beginning with the oral cavity and ending with the anus.

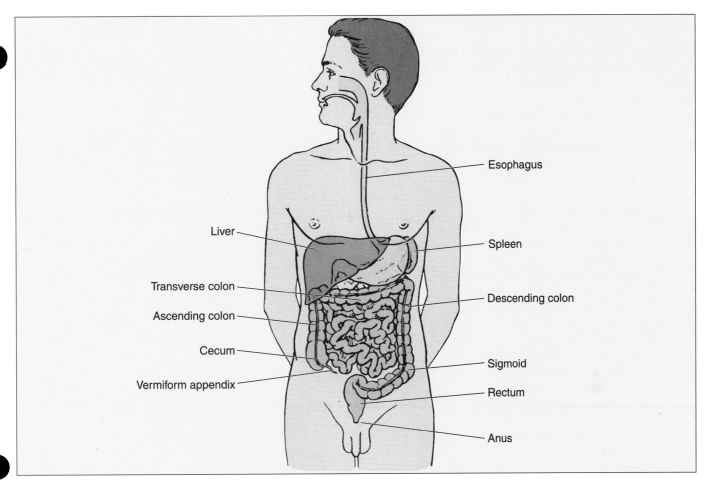

Esophagus

Liver

Spleen

Transverse colon

Descending colon

Ascending colon

Cecum

Sigmoid

Vermiform appendix

Rectum

Anus

Figure 5-20

The digestive system. Delmar/Cengage Learning.

b. Accessory structures: Organs that assist in the digestive process—salivary glands, liver, gallbladder, and pancreas.

2. Mouth
a. Oral cavity
  (1) Lips: Opening into the oral cavity.
  (2) Cheeks: Lateral walls of the oral cavity having a mucous membrane that secretes mucus.
  (3) Hard palate: Forms anterior roof of oral cavity.
  (4) Soft palate: Forms posterior roof of oral cavity.
  (5) Uvula: Fingerlike projection of the soft palate.
  (6) Tongue: Mass of skeletal muscle covered by a ridged mucous membrane.
  (7) Frenulum: Single web of tissue anchoring the tongue to the mouth floor.
b. Salivary glands: Three pairs of exocrine glands that secrete approximately 1 liter of saliva per day. Moistens food and begins chemical digestion (see Figure 5-21).
  (1) Parotid: Largest salivary glands located anterior to the ears.

  (2) Submandibular: Located in the lower jaw.
  (3) Sublingual: Smallest salivary glands located under the tongue.
c. Teeth: Organs of mastication.
  (1) Crown: Exposed portion of tooth covered with enamel.
  (2) Neck: Narrower portion covered by the gingivae.
  (3) Root: Terminal portion of the neck that fits into the alveolar socket of maxilla and mandible.
  (4) Dentin: Middle layer of tooth. At the crown it is covered by enamel, while at the neck and root, it is covered by cementum.
  (5) Pulp cavity: Innermost layer containing connective tissue, blood, and nerves.
  (6) Types.
    (a) Deciduous: Twenty baby teeth that eventually fall out.
    (b) Permanent: Thirty-two adult teeth, which replace deciduous teeth.
3. Pharynx: The throat region through which the bolus (chewed food) passes on to the esophagus.

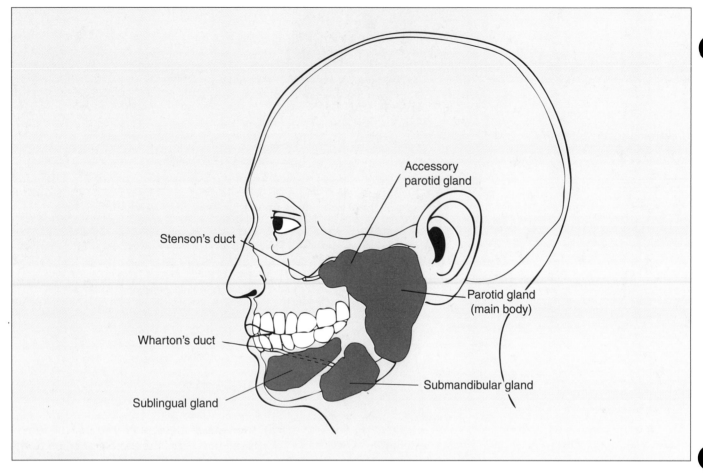

Figure 5-21

Salivary glands. Delmar/Cengage Learning.

4. Esophagus: Tube that extends from the oral cavity to the stomach.
5. Stomach
   a. Located in the upper abdominal cavity inferior to the liver and diaphragm, it is approximately the size of a large sausage when empty with an adult capacity of about 1 to 1.5 liters.
   b. Sphincters: Circular muscles that open and close to control the passage of materials.
      (1) Cardiac sphincters: Controls the opening of the esophagus into the stomach.
      (2) Pyloric sphincter: Controls the opening of the lower stomach into the small intestine.
   c. Stomach wall
      (1) Gastric mucosa: Epithelial lining having rugae that secrete gastric juice, enzymes, and acids.
      (2) Gastric muscularis: Muscular layer having three sublayers to allow for strong contractions.
   d. Functions
      (1) Reservoir: Temporarily stores and partially breaks down food before entering the small intestine.
      (2) Secretion: Secretes substances that aid in initial digestion.
      (3) Protection: Destroys bacteria ingested with food.
6. Small intestine
   a. A coiled tubular structure approximately 2 to 3 cm in diameter and 6 to 7 m in length that occupies most of the abdominal cavity.
   b. Divisions
      (1) Duodenum: First portion approximately 20 to 30 cm long.
      (2) Jejunum: Middle portion approximately 2 to 3 m long.
      (3) Ileum: Terminal portion approximately 3 to 4 m long.
   c. Villi: Microscopic to small fingerlike protrusions of the intestinal lining, containing capillaries and lacteals, which increase its surface area for efficient absorption of nutrients.
   d. Function: Completes chemical digestion and is the primary site of absorption of nutrients into the bloodstream.

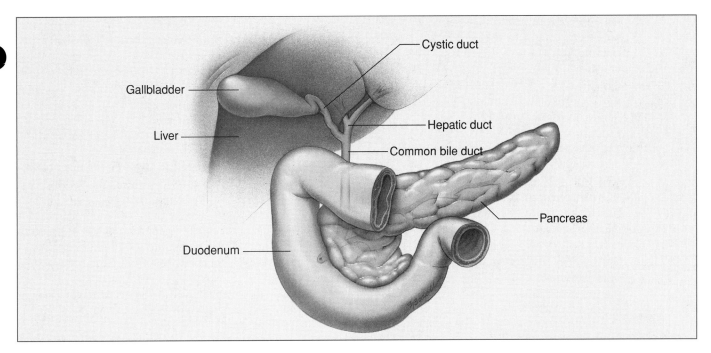

Figure 5-22

Accessory organs of the digestive system. Delmar/Cengage Learning.

7. Large intestine (colon)
    a. A folded tube approximately 6 cm in diameter and 1 to 2 m long.
    b. Divisions
        (1) Cecum: First 5 to 10 cm where the vermiform appendix is attached. Containing the ileocecal valve, it is connected to the ileum of the small intestine.
        (2) Ascending colon: Vertical length of colon along the right side of the abdomen.
        (3) Transverse colon: Length of colon passing horizontally across the abdomen from right to left.
        (4) Descending colon: Vertical length of colon along the left side of the abdomen.
        (5) Sigmoid colon: S-shaped length of colon connected to the rectum.
        (6) Rectum: Last 17 to 20 cm of the colon.
        (7) Anus: The terminal opening of the rectum.
    c. Functions
        (1) Receives and temporarily stores materials not absorbed in the small intestine, forming feces.
        (2) Absorbs residual fluids, causing the feces to become firm.
        (3) Produces vitamin K.
8. Peritoneum: Serous membrane covering most of the abdominal organs to hold them in place.
    a. Mesentery: Projection of the peritoneum that loosely holds the intestines in coils to prevent strangulation.
    b. Transverse mesocolon: Peritoneal membrane that binds the transverse colon to the posterior abdominal wall.
    c. Omentum: The greater and lesser omentum is a serosal sheet containing fat that lies over the abdominal organs to protect the organs in case of inflammation.
9. Liver (see Figure 5-22)
    a. The largest gland and internal organ of the body, it weighs approximately 1 to 2 kg and lies under the diaphragm in the right hypochondriac and epigastric regions.
    b. Functions
        (1) Detoxification: Filters and destroys toxic substances and waste such as urea.
        (2) Bile production: Bile salts are formed from cholesterol to emulsify fats for absorption in the small intestine.
        (3) Metabolism: Metabolizes proteins, fats and carbohydrates.
        (4) Storage: Stores iron, fat soluble vitamins, A, D, E, and K, and glycogen to regulate blood glucose levels.
        (5) Hemostasis: Produces heparin and fibrinogen to regulate blood clotting.
        (6) Recycle: Recycles iron and hemoglobin from old, worn-out RBCs.
10. Gallbladder
    a. Pear-shaped sac located along the inferior surface of the liver where it stores 30 to 50 mL of bile.

b. Functions: Stores, concentrates (5 to 10 fold), and ejects bile into the duodenum for fat metabolism.

11. Pancreas
a. Grayish-pink gland located along the posterior abdominal wall behind the stomach.
b. Serves both an exocrine and endocrine function:
(1) Acinar units (exocrine) secrete digestive enzymes.
(2) Beta cells (endocrine) secrete insulin for carbohydrate metabolism.
(3) Alpha cells (endocrine) secrete glucagon.

C. Physiological processes
1. Digestion
a. Mechanical digestion: Movements of the digestive tract causing the breakdown of complex nutrients.
(1) Mastication: Chewing action to reduce the size of food and mix with saliva to form a bolus for swallowing.
(2) Deglutition: Process of swallowing the bolus.
(3) Peristalsis: Wavelike motion of the alimentary canal to move food compounds along the digestive tract.
(4) Segmentation: Movements of the alimentary canal that cause food compounds to mix with digestive juices and brings digested food in contact with intestinal mucosa for absorption.
(5) Gastric motility
(a) Food is churned and mixed with gastric juices to form chyme.
(b) Chyme is then ejected every 20 seconds into the duodenum for about 2 to 6 hours until empty.
(6) Intestinal motility
(a) Segmentation in the duodenum and jejunum mixes chyme with the pancreatic, liver, and intestinal juices
(b) Peristalsis increases as chyme leaves the jejunum taking approximately 5 hours to exit the small intestine.
b. Chemical digestion: Chemically changes food as it travels through the digestive tract.
(1) Enzymes: Biological catalysts composed of proteins that speed up or retard certain chemical reactions to aid in digestion.
(2) Carbohydrate digestion
(a) Carbohydrates are initially broken down by enzymes known as amylases.
(b) Final breakdown is caused by sucrase, lactase, and maltase found in the villi.

(3) Protein digestion
(a) Proteases breakdown proteins into amino acids.
(b) Important proteases include pepsin (stomach), trypsin (pancreas), and peptidase (intestine).
(4) Fat digestion
(a) Fats are first emulsified by bile in the small intestine.
(b) Pancreatic lipase finally digests fat.
(5) Digestive residue: Material not digested is eliminated in the feces.

2. Absorption
a. The process of transporting nutrients from the intestinal mucosa into the blood or lymph.
b. Most absorption occurs in the small intestine.
c. After nutrients are absorbed, it travels through the portal system to the liver.

3. Elimination
a. The expulsion of waste matter in the form of feces is known as defecation.
b. As the rectum fills, receptors become stimulated causing the defecation reflex.

D. Age-Related Changes
1. Loss of teeth.
2. Peristalsis slows.
3. Increased risk of hiatal hernia, esophageal reflux, peptic ulcers, constipation, hemorrhoids, and cholelithiasis.
4. Diverticulosis.
5. Liver requires more time to metabolize drugs and alcohol.
6. Increased risk of colon and pancreatic cancer in elderly.

E. Pathophysiology
1. Gastritis: Inflammation of the stomach.
2. Gastroenteritis: Inflammation of the stomach and intestine.
3. Ulcer: Lesion of the mucosal lining of the stomach or intestine that may bleed.
4. Hernia: Protrusion of a stomach or intestinal part into an adjacent cavity.
5. Malabsorption syndrome: A collection of diseases of the small intestine that inhibit proper absorption of nutrients into the blood or lymph.
6. Celiac sprue: Malabsorption disease of the small intestine coupled with mucosal damage resulting from gluten (found in wheat products) intolerance.
7. Appendicitis: Inflammation of the vermiform appendix.
8. Intussusception: The slipping or telescoping of one part of the intestine into another part just below it. Occurs mainly in the ileocecal region of children.

9. Volvulus: Twisting of the bowel on itself, causing obstruction.
10. Irritable bowel syndrome (IBS): Collection of symptoms characterized by abdominal pain, constipation, and diarrhea having no organic cause.
11. Crohn's disease: Chronic, idiopathic inflammation of the intestine, usually the ileum.
12. Colitis: Acute inflammation of the colon.
13. Diverticulitis: Inflammation of the diverticula (small pouches) in the colon.
14. Hemorrhoids: Dilated, inflamed veins of the rectum and anus.
15. Pancreatitis: Inflammation of the pancreas.
16. Cholelithiasis: Gallstones. Hard deposits of cholesterol or calcium found in the gallbladder or bile duct.
17. Cholecystitis: Inflammation of the gallbladder.
18. Cirrhosis: Chronic degenerative disease of the liver.
19. Hepatitis: Inflammation of the liver.
20. Emesis: Vomiting.
21. Esophageal reflux: Backup of gastric juice into the esophagus as a result of poor cardiac sphincter function resulting in heartburn.
22. Jaundice: Yellowing of the skin caused by excess bilirubin in the blood caused by liver disorders.
23. Pyloric stenosis: Narrowing of the pyloric sphincter.
24. Mumps: Parotiditis or inflammation of the parotid salivary glands.
25. Gingivitis: Inflammation of the gums.
26. Stomatitis: Inflammation of the mouth.
27. Vincent's angina: Trench mouth. Painful ulcerations of the mucosa of the mouth.
28. Thrush: Infection of the mouth caused by the yeast *Candida albicans.*
29. Pyorrhea: General term used to describe infection or inflammatory diseases of the tissues surrounding the teeth.
30. Caries: Cavities caused by tooth decay.
31. Anorexia: Lack of appetite.
32. Diarrhea: Loose, watery stools.
33. Constipation: Hard, compacted stool making it difficult to defecate.
34. Carcinoma: Malignant neoplasms of the digestive system.

IX. URINARY SYSTEM

A. Function
1. Waste elimination: Excretes nitrogenous waste such as urea and uric acid.
2. Blood volume: Regulates blood volume and pressure by balancing water gain and loss.
3. pH balance: Regulates the gain and loss of hydrogen and bicarbonate ions to balance pH.

4. Mineral salts: Regulates mineral salt levels such as sodium, potassium, and chloride.
5. Detoxification: Assists the liver in neutralizing toxic substances.

B. Anatomy (see Figure 5-23)
1. Kidney (see Figure 5-24)
   a. Bean-shaped organs located in the retroperitoneal region surrounded by a cushion of fat.
   b. Cortex: Outer layer of the kidney.
   c. Medulla: Inner layer of the kidney.
   d. Renal pyramids: Triangular wedges distributed throughout the renal medulla that contain the nephrons.
   e. Calyces: The papilla (point) of the pyramids converge into a cuplike structure, the calyx.
   f. Renal pelvis: The calyces join together to form the renal pelvis where urine is collected.
2. Ureter
   a. Renal pelvis narrows as it exits the kidney to form the ureter.
   b. A tube that extends from the kidney to the urinary bladder.
3. Urinary bladder
   a. Flexible muscular sac located posterior to the symphysis pubis.
   b. Rugae: Folds in the inner lining that can distend to hold urine.
   c. Temporarily stores urine until its release through the urethra via voluntary relaxation of the sphincter.
4. Urethra: Small tube that permits passage of urine from the bladder to the urinary meatus to the outside.
5. Nephron: The microscopic functional unit of the kidney where blood is filtered and urine produced. Nephrons comprise the bulk of the kidney (see Figure 5-25).
   a. Bowman's capsule: Cup-shaped structure located in the renal cortex, which houses the glomerulus.
   b. Glomerulus: Tuft of capillaries within the Bowman's capsule. The Bowman's capsule and glomerulus are collectively known as the renal corpuscle.
   c. Proximal convoluted tubule: A winding extension of the Bowman's capsule, it is the first part of the renal tubule.
   d. Loop of Henle: Segment of the renal tubule extending from the proximal convoluted tubule. It comprises a thin descending tubule, a sharp turn, and an ascending tubular segment.
   e. Distal convoluted tubule: A winding extension of the loop of Henle.
   f. Collecting duct: Straight tubule formed by the union of other distal convoluted tubules.

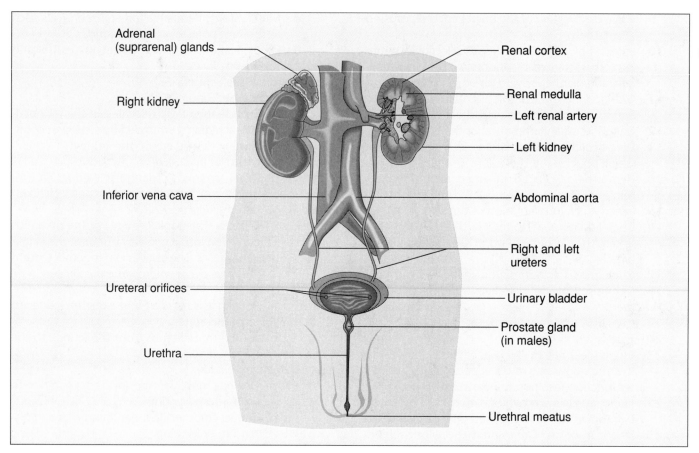

Figure 5-23

The urinary system. Delmar/Cengage Learning.

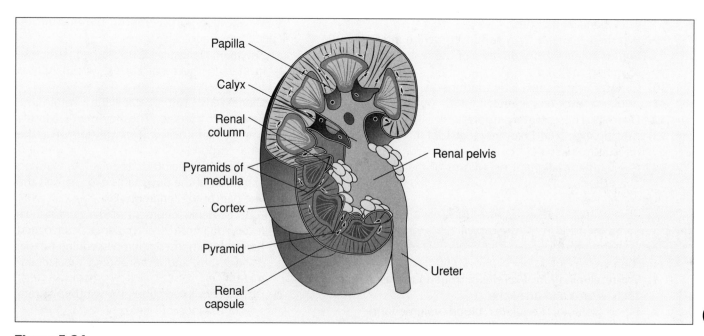

Figure 5-24

Cross section of the kidney. Delmar/Cengage Learning.

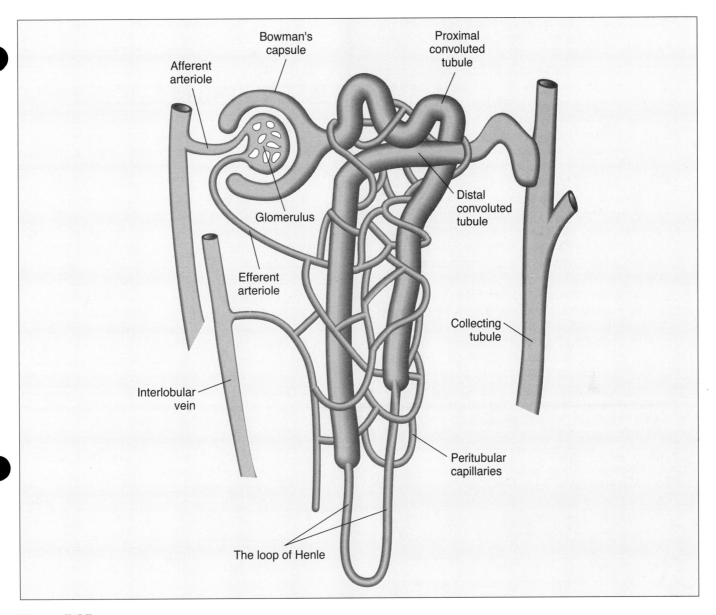

Figure 5-25

Anatomy of a nephron. Delmar/Cengage Learning.

(1) Larger ducts join together to form ducts of one renal pyramid.

(2) Ducts of renal pyramids join to form a calyx.

C. Renal blood flow

   1. Renal artery: A large branch of the abdominal aorta, it enters the kidney at the hilum.

   2. Afferent arteriole: The renal arteriole that enters the Bowman's capsule of the nephron.

   3. Glomerulus: The network of capillaries that form from the afferent arteriole.

   4. Efferent arteriole: The arteriole coming from the glomerulus that exits the Bowman's capsule.

   5. Peritubular capillaries: Extending from the efferent arteriole, the peritubular capillaries surround the renal tubule.

   6. Renal venule: Extending from the peritubular capillaries, the renal venule goes on to become the renal vein.

   7. Renal vein: Exits the kidney at the hilum and joins the inferior vena cava.

D. Urine formation

   1. Filtration: Transport of water and solutes from the blood in the glomerulus to be filtered through the Bowman's capsule.

   2. Reabsorption

a. Water and solutes, sodium, chloride, glucose, and urea enter the proximal convoluted tubule.
b. Most of the water and solutes are recovered by the blood via the peritubular capillaries in the proximal convoluted tubules, leaving only a small quantity to move through the loop of Henle.
c. Reabsorption continues in the loop of Henle and distal convoluted tubule, depending on the body's needs.
3. Secretion: Water and solutes not reabsorbed are transported to the collecting ducts, where they drain into the calyces and eventually through the renal pelvis, the ureters, the urinary bladder, the urethra, and out the urinary meatus.
4. Urine composition
a. Water: Water comprises 95% of urine.
b. Nitrogenous waste: Created through protein metabolism. Composed of urea, uric acid, ammonia, and creatinine.
c. Electrolytes: Mostly sodium, potassium, ammonium, chloride, bicarbonate, phosphate, and sulfate.
d. Toxins: Mostly bacterial poisons.
e. Pigments: Mostly urochrome.
f. Hormones.
E. Age-Related Changes
1. Decreased kidney size and function.
2. Increased risk of nephrolithiasis.
3. Decreased bladder capacity: Incontinence.
4. Enlarged prostate gland: Increased urge and frequency of urination.
5. Increase in UTIs.
F. Pathophysiology
1. Polycystic kidney disease: Groups of collecting tubules that are unable to empty into the renal pelvis swell into multiple, grapelike, fluid-filled sacs or cysts.
2. Nephrotic syndrome: A glomerular disease characterized by severe proteinuria.
3. Uremia: Accumulation of urea in the blood resulting from improper kidney function.
4. Renal failure: Gradual, progressive deterioration of kidney function.
5. Nephrolithiasis: Kidney stones caused by accumulation of mineral salts.
6. Acute tubular necrosis (ATN): Destruction of the tubules of the nephron.
7. Neurogenic bladder: Impairment of bladder function resulting from nervous system injury.
8. Urinary tract infections (UTI)
a. Pyelonephritis: Inflammation of the renal pelvis.
b. Glomerulonephritis: Inflammation of the glomerulus.
c. Cystitis: Inflammation of the urinary bladder.
d. Urethritis: Inflammation of the urethra.

X. REPRODUCTIVE SYSTEM

A. Function
1. Survival: Ensure survival of the species.
2. Female: Produce ova, receive sperm for fertilization. Provide nutrients and developmental elements to the fetus in preparation for birth.
3. Male: Produce, transfer, and introduce sperm into the female reproductive tract where fertilization can occur.
B. Female reproductive system (see Figure 5-26)
1. General
a. Essential organs: Ovaries—the female gonads, and ova—the female gamete.
b. Accessory organs: Uterus, tubes and ducts, vagina, vulva, and mammary glands.
2. Uterus (see Figure 5-27)
a. Pear-shaped organ located in the pelvic cavity between the urinary bladder and rectum.
b. Divisions
(1) Fundus: Upper region superior to entrance of fallopian tubes.
(2) Body: Larger medial region.
(3) Cervix: Lower neck region containing the cervical os.
c. Uterine layers
(1) Endometrium: Innermost layer where implantation of the fertilized cva occurs.
(2) Myometrium: Middle muscular layer.
(3) Epimetrium: Outer serosal layer.
d. Functions
(1) Allows for the passage of sperm to the fallopian tubes during fertilization.
(2) Site of fetal development.
(3) Contracts to deliver the offspring.
3. Fallopian tubes (oviducts)
a. Attached at the upper, outer angles of the uterus.
b. Function: Serve as the site of fertilization and as transport canals for the fertilized ovum to reach the uterus for implantation.
c. Fingerlike structures at the distal ends, fimbria, envelope the ovary to collect the ovum.
4. Ovaries
a. Nodular, almond-shaped glands located inferior and posterior to the fallopian tubes bilaterally.
b. Ovarian follicles contain the developing ova.
c. Function: Produce ova and the female sex hormones, estrogen, and progesterone.

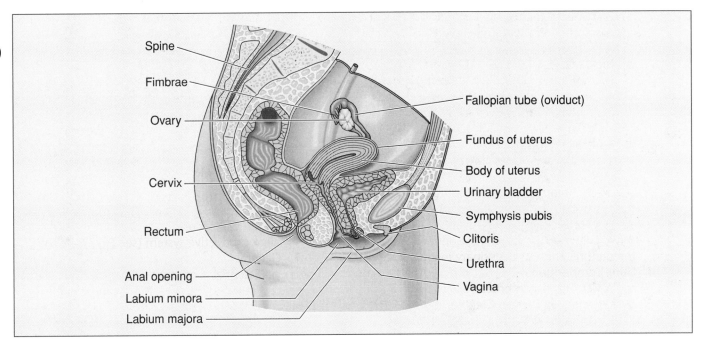

Figure 5-26

Sagittal section of the female reproductive organs. Delmar/Cengage Learning.

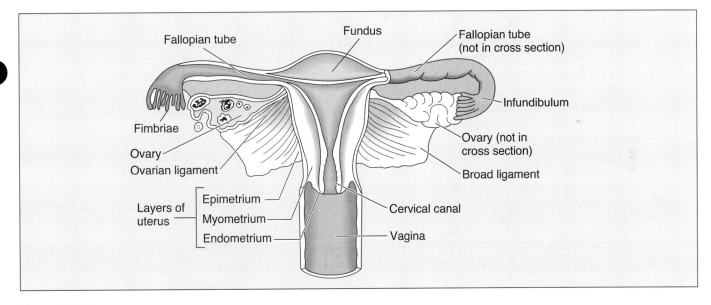

Figure 5-27

Anterior view of the female reproductive organs. Delmar/Cengage Learning.

5. Vagina
   a. Tubular structure located between the rectum and urinary bladder.
   b. Strong, muscular organ capable of great elasticity lined with a mucous membrane having rugae.
   c. Functions
      (1) Receives and stimulates the penis for delivery of sperm during intercourse.
      (2) Serves as a birth canal, and a means of shedding menstrual tissues.

6. Vulva: The external genitalia (see Figure 5-28).
   a. Mons pubis: Rounded fatty layer overlying the symphysis pubis.
   b. Labia majora: Two large longitudinal folds of skin extending from the mons pubis to the anus.
   c. Labia minora: Two smaller skin folds medial to the labia majora.
   d. Clitoris: Small, highly sensitive nodule of erectile tissue superior to the labia majora. It plays an important role in sexual arousal.

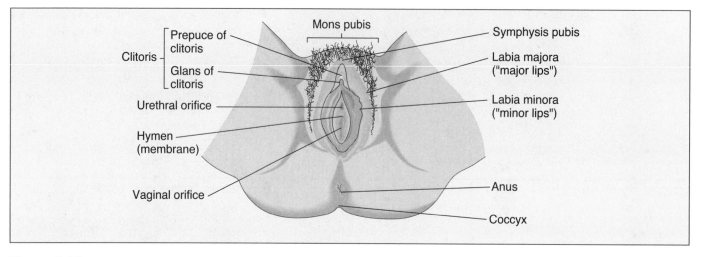

Figure 5-28

External female genitalia. Delmar/Cengage Learning.

e. Greater vestibular glands (Bartholin glands): Secrete lubricating fluid during intercourse.

7. Perineum: The region between the vaginal orifice and rectum. It may be torn during childbirth.

8. Breasts

a. Mammary glands surrounded by fatty tissue overlying the pectoral muscles.

b. Lactation: Produces milk for consumption by offspring.
   (1) Contains important nutrients.
   (2) Contains antibodies providing passive immunity.
   (3) Permits emotional bonding between parent and child.

c. Nipple: Protrusion serving to deliver milk from the mammary gland.

d. Areola: Dark pigmented region surrounding the nipple.

9. Reproductive cycle

a. Ovarian cycle: Development and maturation of the ovum in the ovary.

b. Menstrual (endometrial) cycle
   (1) Menses: Day 1 to Day 5 of the menstrual cycle. If the ovum is not fertilized, the blood-rich endometrium sloughs off causing menstrual bleeding.
   (2) Postmenstrual: Day 6 to Day 13. The endometrium thickens and the ovum matures in the ovarian follicle. Estrogen levels increase.
   (3) Ovulation: Day 14. The mature follicle ruptures releasing the ovum.
   (4) Premenstrual: Day 15 to Day 28. The corpus luteum secretes progesterone, which further thickens the endometrium in preparation for potential fertilization.

c. Myometrial phase: Uterine contractions occur during the 2 weeks before ovulation, but disappear between ovulation and the next menses in case the fertilized egg has implanted in the endometrium.

d. Gonadotropic phase: The anterior pituitary secretes two gonadotropic hormones, follicle-stimulating hormone (FSH) and luteinizing hormone (LH), which regulate the reproductive cycle.

10. Pregnancy

a. Ovulation and insemination
   (1) Ovulation: Release of a mature ovum into the fallopian tube.
   (2) Insemination: Expulsion of semen into the vagina where sperm travel through the cervix and uterus into the fallopian tube.

b. Conception: Sperm fertilizes the ovum.
   (1) Usually occurs in the outer third of the fallopian tube.
   (2) The entrance of sperm into ovum triggers a chemical reaction preventing other sperm from entering.
   (3) Zygote: The sperm cell contributes 23 chromosomes to the ovum's 23 chromosomes to create a genetically complete, 46-chromosome zygote.

c. Prenatal period: Time between conception and birth.

d. Placenta
   (1) Allows the exchange of nutrients between fetus and mother.
   (2) Performs excretory, respiratory, and endocrine functions.

(3) Secretes human chorionic gonadotropin (hCG) that maintains estrogen and progesterone secretions for continued pregnancy.
  e. Gestational periods: Pregnancy lasts approximately 39 weeks, divided into three 3-month segments called trimesters.
    (1) Embryonic phase: First 8 weeks of gestation.
    (2) Fetal phase: 9 to 39 weeks of gestation.
11. Parturition: Birth
  a. Stage one: Time between onset of uterine contractions and full cervical dilation (usually 10 cm).
  b. Stage two: Time between full cervical dilation to birth, also known as the transition stage.
  c. Stage three: Expulsion of placenta through the vagina.
12. Age-Related Changes
  a. Menopause occurs between 45 and 55 years of age. Cessation of ovarian and uterine cycles, with loss of ova and hormone production.
  b. Wrinkling of skin.
  c. Increased risk of osteoporosis and myocardial infarction.
13. Pathophysiology
  a. Premenstrual syndrome: Collection of symptoms that occur before menstruation such as irritability, fatigue, depression, headache, arthralgia, edema, swollen and tender breasts, abdominal pain.
  b. Amenorrhea: Absence or discontinuation of menstruation beyond age 16.
  c. Dysmenorrhea: Painful menstruation.
  d. Ovarian cyst: Solid or fluid-filled sacs found in the ovary.
  e. Endometriosis: Growth of endometrial tissue outside the endometrium within the pelvic cavity.
  f. Pelvic inflammatory disease (PID): Acute or chronic infection of the female reproductive organs.
    (1) Endometritis: Inflammation of the endometrium of the uterus.
    (2) Cervicitis: Inflammation of the cervix.
    (3) Salpingitis: Inflammation of the fallopian tubes.
    (4) Oophoritis: Inflammation of the ovary.
  g. Dyspareunia: Painful intercourse.
  h. Disorders of pregnancy
    (1) Spontaneous abortion: Miscarriage or premature expulsion of the embryo or fetus before viability.
    (2) Ectopic pregnancy: Implantation of the fertilized ovum outside the uterus, most often the fallopian tube.
    (3) Placenta previa: Placenta implants over the cervix.
    (4) Abruptio placentae: Premature separation of an implanted placenta from the uterine wall.
    (5) Premature labor: Early onset of uterine contractions.
    (6) Eclampsia: Toxemia is a collection of dangerous symptoms during pregnancy such as hypertension, edema, and proteinuria that, if untreated, may result in convulsions and coma.
    (7) Hyperemesis gravidarum: Excessive vomiting during pregnancy.
  i. Sexually transmitted diseases (STD): Venereal diseases (VD) that occur in both sexes.
    (1) Trichomoniasis: Parasitic infection caused by *Trichomonas vaginalis*.
    (2) Gonorrhea: Bacterial infection caused by *Neisseria gonorrhoeae*.
    (3) Syphilis: Bacterial infection caused by *Treponema pallidum*.
    (4) Genital herpes: Viral infection caused by herpes simplex 1 or 2 (HSVI or II).
    (5) Genital warts: Wart formations caused by the human papilloma virus (HPV).
    (6) Chlamydia: Bacterial infection caused by *Chlamydia trachomatis*.
C. Male reproductive system (see Figure 5-29)
  1. General
    a. Essential organs: Testes—the male gonad, and sperm—the male gamete.
    b. Accessory organs: Genital ducts, accessory glands, penis, and scrotum.
  2. Testes
    a. Glandular structures composed of seminiferous tubules and interstitial cells.
    b. Manufactures, stores, and releases sperm and testosterone.
  3. Epididymis
    a. A continuation of the seminiferous tubules of the testes, it lies on the superior surface of the testes.
    b. Function: Secretes part of seminal fluid in addition to serving as a duct for seminal fluid. Sperm become motile while passing through the epididymis.
  4. Vas deferens: An extension of the epididymis, it passes through the inguinal canal into the abdominal cavity arching over the urinary bladder to join the seminal vesicles posteriorly.
  5. Seminal vesicles: Bilateral pouches posterior to the urinary bladder which secrete a nutrient-rich fluid comprising 60% of seminal fluid.

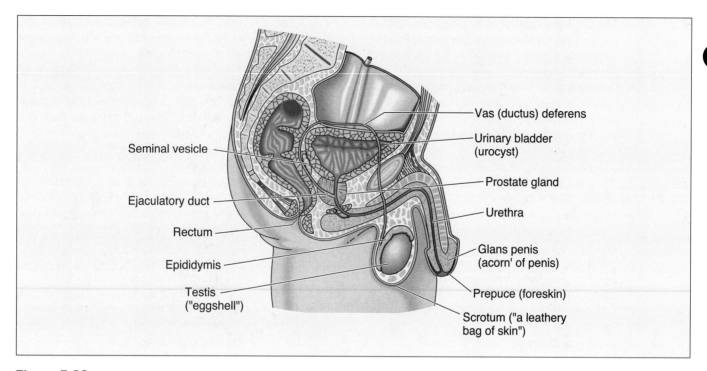

Figure 5-29

Sagittal section of the male reproductive organs. Delmar/Cengage Learning.

6. Ejaculatory duct: Formed by the union of the vas deferens and seminal vesicles.
   a. Passes through the prostate gland and enters the urethra.
   b. During orgasm, the ejaculatory duct contracts, propelling the sperm and seminal fluids into the urethra.
7. Prostate gland
   a. Doughnut-shaped gland encircling the base of urethra on the posterior surface of the urinary bladder.
   b. Secretes an alkaline fluid that protects the sperm when entering the acidic vaginal environment. It comprises 30% of seminal fluid.
8. Bulbourethral (Cowper's) gland
   a. Small, pea-shaped glands located on either side of the urethra.
   b. Secretes an alkaline fluid that provides lubrication during intercourse comprising 5% of seminal fluid.
9. Scrotum
   a. Pouch of skin suspended from the perineal region that houses the testes and epididymis.
   b. Suspended away from the body as sperm production requires temperatures below body temperature.
10. Penis
    a. External male genitalia composed of three cylindrical structures of erectile tissue.

    b. Contains the urethra. During sexual arousal, erectile tissues fill with blood and become erect to allow vaginal penetration.
    c. Prepuce: Foreskin of the penis; often removed by circumcision.
11. Age-Related Changes
    a. Decreased testosterone production after age 50.
    b. Prostatic hypertrophy.
    c. Decreased sperm production.
    d. Vascular and other diseases may cause erectile dysfunction.
12. Pathophysiology
    a. Prostatitis: Inflammation of the prostate.
    b. Epididymitis: Inflammation of the epididymis.
    c. Orchitis: Inflammation of the testes.
    d. Benign prostatic hypertrophy (BPH): Proliferation of cells within the prostate gland causing it to enlarge.
    e. Carcinoma: Malignant neoplasms of the reproductive system.
    f. Impotence: Inability to develop an erection.
    g. Premature ejaculation: Ejaculation very shortly after arousal or before orgasm.
    h. Cryptorchism: Failure of the testes to descend into the scrotum.
    i. Phimosis: Narrowing of the prepuce preventing its retraction.
    j. Hypospadias: Abnormal congenital opening of the urethra on the underside of the penis.

k. Priapism: Abnormal, painful, and continued erection resulting from a nervous system disorder.

l. Hydrocele: Accumulation of fluid in the scrotum.

XI. NERVOUS SYSTEM

A. General

1. Function: Serves to identify and evaluate internal and external environmental changes for appropriate response.

   a. Control: Regulates internal body processes and functions.

   b. Communication: Complementing the endocrine system, the nervous system directs communication processes among the body systems for effective integration of body function.

   c. Mental processes: Generates thought, feelings, emotions, perception, and sensations.

2. Organization

   a. Central nervous system (CNS)
      (1) Composed of the brain and spinal cord.
      (2) Integrates sensory information for responsive action.

   b. Peripheral nervous system (PNS)
      (1) Comprises nerves that lie in the outer region of the nervous system.
      (2) Includes the cranial nerves, originating from the brain, and the spinal nerves, originating from the spinal cord.
      (3) Divisions
         (a) Afferent (sensory) nervous system: Nerves that transmit sensory information to the brain.
         (b) Efferent (motor) nervous system: Nerves that transmit motor commands away from the brain to an organ or body part. Comprises two divisions:
            i) Somatic nervous system: Transmits impulses to skeletal (voluntary) muscles.
            ii) Autonomic nervous system: Transmits impulses to smooth and cardiac muscles (involuntary), and glands. Comprises two further divisions:
               a) Sympathetic nervous system: Prepares the body for stressful or threatening conditions.
               b) Parasympathetic nervous system: Coordinates normal resting activities.

3. Neuron: Nerve cell (see Figure 5-30).

   a. Excitable cells that initiate and conduct impulses essential to nervous system function.

   b. Components
      (1) Cell body: Contains the nucleus and organelles.
      (2) Dendrites: One or more branches that receive and conduct impulses toward the cell body of the neuron.

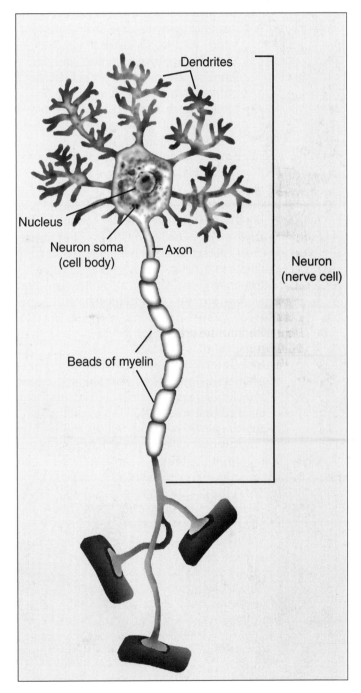

Figure 5-30

A neuron. Delmar/Cengage Learning.

(3) Axon: Processes extending from the neuron that conduct impulses away from the cell body.

(4) Synaptic knobs: Tiny enlargements of the distal axons that release neurotransmitters, chemical substances that transmit impulses across neurons.

(5) Synapse: Junction between the dendrite of one neuron and the axon of another to afford conduction of impulses from neuron to neuron via neurotransmitters.

(6) Myelin sheath: Inner membrane composed of Schwann cells that cover the axons of many neurons that act as insulators to speed electrical conduction. The presence of myelin gives structures a whitish appearance, whereas its absence demonstrates a grayish appearance.

(7) Neurilemma: Outer cellular membrane composed of Schwann cells that help regenerate injured neurons.

(8) Nodes of Ranvier: Gaps in the myelin sheath between successive Schwann cells.

4. Nerves

a. Collection of peripheral nerve fibers held together by several layers of connective tissue.

b. Tracts: Bundles of nerve fibers within the CNS.

5. Neurotransmitters: Chemical substances that allow neurons to communicate with each other.

B. Central nervous system

1. General

a. Includes the brain and spinal cord.

b. Meninges: Protective, membranous covering of the brain and spinal cord having three layers (see Figure 5-31).

(1) Dura mater: Strong, fibrous, white outer layer containing veins that drain blood from the brain.

(2) Arachnoid: Middle layer arranged in a cobweblike lattice for movement of cerebrospinal fluid (CSF).

(3) Pia mater: Inner, transparent layer containing vessels to supply blood to the brain.

c. Meningeal spaces

(1) Epidural space: Located between the dura mater and skull or vertebrae; contains fat for cushion.

(2) Subdural space: Located between the dura mater and arachnoid membrane; contains lubricating serous fluid.

(3) Subarachnoid space: Located between the arachnoid and pia mater; contains CSF.

d. Cerebrospinal fluid (CSF): A clear, colorless, thin, watery fluid found in the subarachnoid space and ventricle (cavities) of the brain. It serves two major purposes:

(1) Provides a supportive, protective cushion.

(2) As a circulating fluid, it is monitored by the brain to detect physiological changes in the body.

2. Cerebrum (see Figure 5-32A): Largest, superior portion of the brain divided into two hemispheres.

a. Right hemisphere: Controls the left side of the body and is responsible for auditory and tactile perception and interpreting spatial relationships.

b. Left hemisphere: Controls the right side of the body and is responsible for language and hand movements.

c. Cerebral lobes

(1) Frontal: Controls voluntary muscle movements and speech.

(2) Parietal: Receives and integrates sensory input.

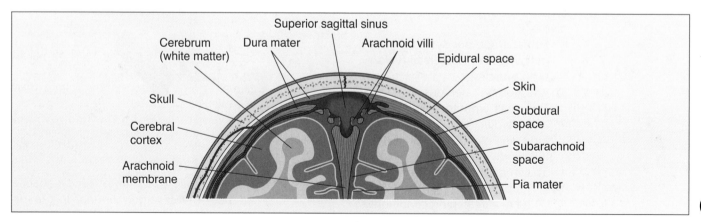

Figure 5-31

Structures of the meninges. Delmar/Cengage Learning.

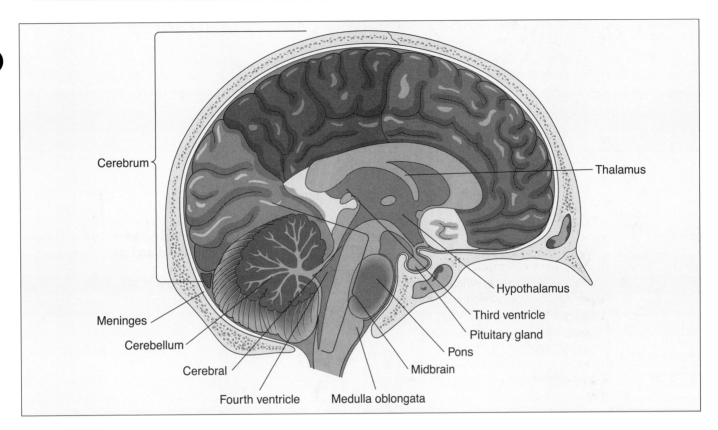

Figure 5-32A

Parts of the brain. Delmar/Cengage Learning.

(3) Temporal: Interprets sound as well as involved with emotion, personality, memory, and behavior.

(4) Occipital: Interprets sight.

d. Cortex: Outer surface of the brain comprised of gray matter.

(1) Gyri: Convolutions or folds of the brain.

(2) Sulci: Shallow grooves.

(3) Fissures: Deep grooves that divide the cerebrum.

3. Thalamus

a. Dumbbell-shaped mass of gray matter located between the cerebrum and midbrain.

b. Serves as a relay station for sensory impulses traveling to the brain.

c. Affords crude sensations associated with pain, temperature, and touch.

d. Affords complex reflex movements.

e. Affords certain emotions associated with pleasant and unpleasant sensations.

4. Hypothalamus

a. Collection of structures inferior to the thalamus.

b. Serves to link functions of the mind to that of the body.

c. Synthesizes hormones secreted by the posterior pituitary.

d. Assists in regulating appetite.

e. Assists in regulating body temperature.

5. Cerebellum

a. Second largest part located inferior to the posterior cerebrum.

b. Controls skeletal muscles by coordinating muscle groups for smooth, efficient movement and fine motor skills.

c. Controls equilibrium and posture.

6. Midbrain

a. Located below the central cerebrum at the base. Upper part of brain stem.

b. Serves as a relay center for certain eye and ear reflexes.

7. Pons: Located inferior to the midbrain links the cerebellum with the rest of the nervous system.

8. Medulla oblongata

a. Lowest part of the brain stem that is attached to the spinal cord just superior to the foramen magnum.

b. Controls respiration, cardiac and vascular activity.

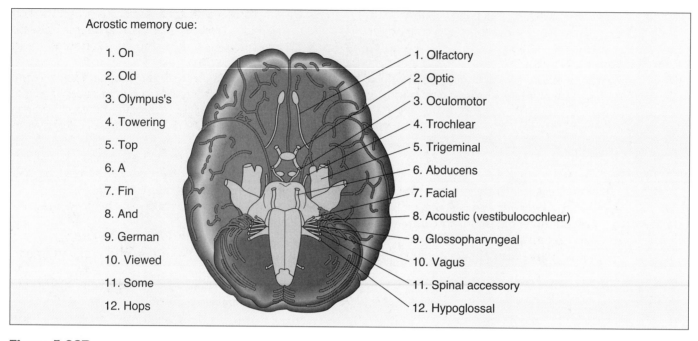

Acrostic memory cue:

1. On	1. Olfactory
2. Old	2. Optic
3. Olympus's	3. Oculomotor
4. Towering	4. Trochlear
5. Top	5. Trigeminal
6. A	6. Abducens
7. Fin	7. Facial
8. And	8. Acoustic (vestibulocochlear)
9. German	9. Glossopharyngeal
10. Viewed	10. Vagus
11. Some	11. Spinal accessory
12. Hops	12. Hypoglossal

Figure 5-32B

Cranial nerves. Delmar/Cengage Learning.

C. Peripheral Nervous System
1. Cranial nerves: Twelve pair of nerves arising from the brain, mostly the brain stem. Numbered according to order emerging anterior to posterior (see Figure 5-32B).
   a. I—Olfactory: Provides sense of smell.
   b. II—Optic: Transmits visual impulses from the eye to the brain.
   c. III—Oculomotor: Controls external eye muscles and iris.
   d. IV—Trochlear: Controls superior oblique eye muscles.
   e. V—Trigeminal: Three branches, ophthalmic, maxillary, and mandibular nerves. Provides sensation to head and teeth; controls chewing.
   f. VI—Abducens: Controls eye muscles.
   g. VII—Facial: Controls superficial muscles of face and scalp, salivary glands, and taste.
   h. VIII—Acoustic (vestibulocochlear): Provides sensation of balance and hearing.
   i. IX—Glossopharyngeal: Sensory, motor, and autonomic nerve involvement of the tongue and pharynx.
   j. X—Vagus: Nerve involvement of the pharynx, larynx, heart, lungs, bronchi, esophagus, stomach, small intestine, and gallbladder.
   k. XI—Spinal accessory: Assists the vagus by controlling the thoracic and abdominal viscera, pharynx, larynx, trapezius, and sternocleidomastoid.
   l. XII—Hypoglossal: Controls tongue muscle.

2. Spinal nerves
   a. Thirty-one pairs of nerves connected to the spinal cord.
   b. Numbered according to vertebrae emerging from the spinal cord.
      (1) Cervical nerves: Eight, C1 to C8.
      (2) Thoracic nerves: Twelve, T1 to T12.
      (3) Lumbar nerves: Five, L1 to L5.
      (4) Sacral nerves: Five, S1 to S5.
      (5) Coccygeal nerves: One pair.
   c. Cauda equina: Cluster of nerves emanating from the distal spinal cord resembling a horse's tail.
3. Somatic Nervous System
   a. Transmits impulses to the skeletal muscles outside the CNS.
   b. Somatic reflexes: Contraction of a muscle or glandular secretion resulting from an external stimuli.
      (1) Achilles reflex: Ankle jerk—extension of the foot in response to tapping the Achilles tendon.
      (2) Babinski reflex: Extension of great toe in response to tickling the lateral sole. Present to age 1.5 years.
      (3) Plantar reflex: Plantar flexion of all toes in response to tickling the lateral sole.
      (4) Corneal reflex: Blinking in response to touching the cornea.
      (5) Abdominal reflex: Drawing in the abdominal wall in response to stroking the lateral abdomen.

(6) Patellar reflex: Knee-jerk; extension of the lower leg in response to tapping the patellar tendon.

4. Autonomic Nervous System
   a. Regulate automatic functions such as heart activity, involuntary muscles, and glandular secretions.
   b. Divisions
      (1) Sympathetic nervous system: Serves to maintain normal tone of smooth muscles and to prepare the body for emergency conditions requiring immediate action.
      (2) Parasympathetic nervous system: Serves to promote digestion and elimination and return the body to a resting state after the emergency condition subsides.

D. Age-Related Changes
   1. Brain cells die and are not replaced. Learning, memory, and reasoning decrease.
   2. Cerebral cortex shrinks. Reflexes slow.
   3. Decreased production of neurotransmitters. Increased risk of Alzheimer's disease in the elderly.

E. Pathophysiology
   1. Paralysis: Loss of voluntary muscular control and sensation to a body part or region.
      a. Hemiplegia: Paralysis of one side of the body often resulting from stroke.
      b. Paraplegia: Paralysis of the trunk and lower extremities often caused by spinal cord injury.
      c. Quadriplegia: Paralysis of all four extremities and usually the trunk.
      d. Bell's palsy: Paralysis of muscles on one side of the face.
   2. Peripheral neuritis: Inflammation of terminal nerves.
   3. Cerebrovascular accident (CVA): Stroke caused by occlusion or hemorrhage of vessels supplying the brain resulting in impairment of consciousness and paralysis.
   4. Transient ischemic attack (TIA): Temporary, recurrent episodes of impaired neurological activity resulting from lack of blood flow to the brain often described as little strokes.
   5. Epilepsy: Abnormal electrical activity of the brain characterized by random, intense neuronal discharges that result in a seizure.
   6. Alzheimer's disease: Presenile dementia describes a chronic organic brain syndrome characterized by the degeneration of nervous tissue causing impaired intellectual function and ultimately death.
   7. Parkinson's disease: Chronic crippling disease characterized by muscle rigidity and tremors thought to be caused by a deficiency of dopamine.
   8. Amyotrophic lateral sclerosis (ALS): Lou Gehrig's disease is a motor neuron disease characterized by muscle atrophy and weakness.
   9. Hydrocephalus: Excess accumulation of cerebral spinal fluid characterized by macrocephaly.
   10. Multiple sclerosis: Chronic nervous disease caused by the degeneration of the myelin sheath.
   11. Cerebral palsy: Nonprogressive loss of sensation or control of movement resulting from congenital brain defects or injury at birth.
   12. Meningitis: Inflammation of the meningeal tissues.
   13. Encephalitis: Inflammation of the brain.
   14. Encephalocele: Protrusion of the brain through a cranial fissure.
   15. Trigeminal neuralgia: Sharp pain along the trigeminal nerve.
   16. Aphasia: Nervous impairment of the ability to communicate through speech, writing, or sign-making.

XII. SENSORY SYSTEM

A. General
   1. Sense organs: Work with the nervous system by acting as the medium through which external stimuli are transmitted to and interpreted by the brain.
   2. Sensory receptors: Allow the body to respond to stimuli by converting them to nerve impulses.
   3. Somatic senses: Senses that detect pain, temperature, pressure, touch, position, muscle tension, hunger, thirst, etc.
   4. Special senses: Receptor groups that coordinate the sense of smell, taste, hearing, equilibrium, and vision.

B. Smell
   1. Special sense known as olfaction.
   2. Olfactory receptors
      a. Located in the superior nasal cavity, they are chemoreceptors sensitive to gases and dissolved chemicals.
      b. Extremely sensitive and easily fatigued.

C. Taste (see Figure 5-33)
   1. Special sense known as gustation.
   2. Gustatory receptors
      a. Located within glossal papillae (tastebuds) on the tongue, they are chemoreceptors sensitive to dissolved chemicals in saliva.
      b. Primary taste sensations
         (1) Sweet: Tip of tongue.
         (2) Salty: Tip of tongue.
         (3) Sour: Sides of tongue.
         (4) Bitter: Back of tongue.

D. Ear: Sense of hearing and equilibrium (see Figure 5-34).
   1. External ear
      a. Auricle (pinna): The visible flap of the ear.
      b. External auditory meatus: Narrow canal extending from the auricle to the middle ear. Produces cerumen (earwax) to protect and lubricate the ear canal.

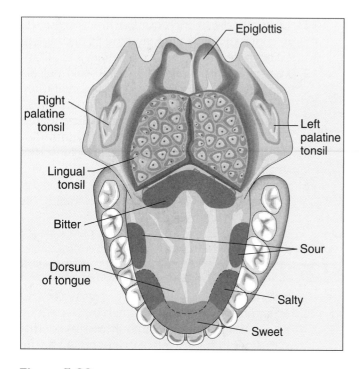

Figure 5-33

Sagittal section of the ear. Delmar/Cengage Learning.

2. Middle ear: Auditory structures within the temporal bone.
   a. Tympanic membrane: Eardrum.
   b. Ossicles: Three bones of the middle ear.
      (1) Malleus: Hammer—attached to the tympanic membrane.
      (2) Incus: Anvil—connects the malleus and stapes.
      (3) Stapes: Stirrup—attached to the incus and articulates with the oval window.
   c. Oval window: Oval membrane covering the opening into the vestibule into which the stapes fits.
   d. Round window: Opening in the cochlea of the inner ear covered with a membrane that allows the dissipation of fluid movement within the labyrinth.
   e. Eustachian tube: Tube extending from the middle ear to the pharynx that equalizes pressure internally.
3. Inner ear
   a. Labyrinth: Auditory structure of winding canals composed of the external bony labyrinth and internal membranous labyrinth.
   b. Vestibule: Middle part of the labyrinth involved with balance.
      (1) Utricle: Endolymph-filled tubes within the vestibule that responds to body position for balance.
      (2) Saccule: Smaller than the utricle, it serves a similar purpose.

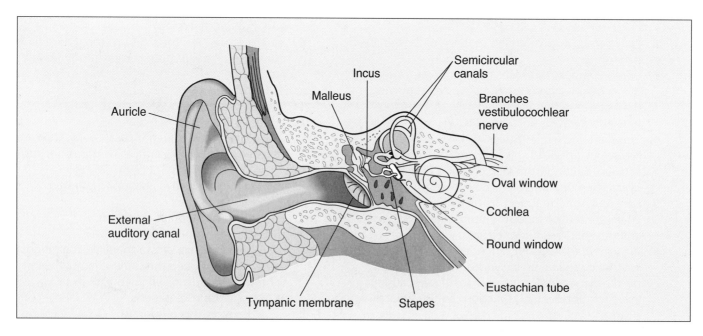

Figure 5-34

Sagittal section of the ear. Delmar/Cengage Learning.

c. Cochlea: Coiled, snail-shaped structure involved with hearing.
   (1) Cochlear duct: Triangular tube located inside the cochlea that contains endolymph.
   (2) Organ of Corti: Hearing sense organ within the cochlea.
d. Semicircular canals: Three superiorly situated ringlike canals arranged in right angles to each other that are involved in balance.
   (1) Membranous semicircular canals articulate with the utricle and saccule.
   (2) Able to sense the position of the head relative to gravity and to sense acceleration and deceleration.
e. Endolymph: Clear fluid that fills the labyrinth.
f. Perilymph: Fluid similar to CSF that fills the space between the bony and membranous labyrinth.

4. Vestibulocochlear (acoustic) nerve (cranial nerve X)
a. Vestibular nerve: Provides information regarding head and body position and the pull of gravity.
b. Cochlear nerve: Converts sound waves to nerve impulses.

5. Hearing process
a. Sound is the vibration of air. The ability to hear particular sounds depends on the volume, pitch, and frequency of sound waves.
b. Sound waves are collected by the auricles and enter the external auditory meatus.
c. Sound waves strike the tympanic membrane causing it to vibrate.
d. The vibration is transmitted from the tympanic membrane through all three ossicles.
e. The vibration picked up by the stapes causes it to move against the oval window.
f. The oval window, in turn, causes a ripplelike vibration within the endolymph and perilymph of the labyrinth.
g. As the ripple moves throughout the labyrinth, it stimulates the organ of Corti, where the cochlear nerve picks up the vibrations. Converting the vibrations into nerve impulses, the cochlear nerve transmits the impulses to the auditory region of the temporal lobe, where they are interpreted as sound.
h. The wave of fluid within the labyrinth dissipates at the round window.

E. Eye: Sense of vision (see Figure 5-35).
   1. Structural layers: Three layers.
   a. Sclera: Outer layer, mostly the white of the eye.
      (1) Composed of tough, white fibrous tissue.
      (2) Cornea: Transparent anterior portion positioned over the iris, the pigmented area of the eye.
   b. Choroid: Middle layer that is highly vascular and greatly pigmented.
      (1) Ciliary body: Anterior thickening of the choroid that serves as a point of attachment to suspend the lens.
      (2) Suspensory ligaments: Suspends the lens from the ciliary body.

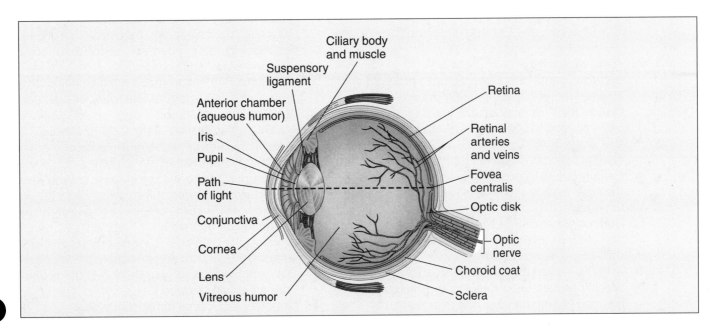

Figure 5-35

Sagittal section of the eye. Delmar/Cengage Learning.

(3) Iris: Pigmented part of the eye composed of smooth muscle fibers that dilate and contract causing the pupil (dark opening in the eye) to increase and decrease in diameter to control the amount of light entering the eye.

c. Retina: Innermost layer.
   (1) Photoreceptors: Receptors sensitive to light energy.
      (a) Rods: Photoreceptors sensitive to shades of gray.
      (b) Cones: Photoreceptors sensitive to color.
   (2) Fovea centralis: Pit in the macula lutea (yellow spot in center of retina) containing closely packed cones functioning as the area of sharpest vision.
   (3) Optic disk: Area in retina where the optic nerve exits the eye. Having no cones or rods, this is known as the blind spot.

2. Aqueous humor
   a. Clear watery fluid produced by vessels in the ciliary body.
   b. Located in the anterior cavity between the lens and cornea.
   c. Maintains the curvature shape of the cornea.
3. Vitreous humor: Semisolid, gelatinous fluid that fills the posterior chamber behind the lens to maintain the spherical shape of the eyeball.
4. Muscles: Two types.
   a. Extrinsic muscles: Skeletal muscles attached to the outer eye and orbital bones to afford eye movement.
   b. Intrinsic muscles: Smooth muscles located within the eye.
      (1) Iris: Regulates the size of the pupil.
      (2) Ciliary muscle: Controls the shape of the lens for focusing.
5. Accessory structures
   a. Eyebrows and eyelashes: Helps protect against foreign objects entering the eye.
   b. Eyelids: Blinking moistens the eye.
   c. Lacrimal apparatus: Structures such as glands and ducts that secrete and drain tears to maintain proper moisture levels.
   d. Conjunctiva: Mucous membrane that lines the inner eyelids and anterior eyeball.
6. Visual process
   a. Light rays from objects being observed strike the anterior eye where, initial refraction (bending of light) occurs.
   b. As the light enters the eye, structures of differing optical densities, i.e, cornea, aqueous humor, lens, and vitreous humor, cause refraction.
   c. Complementing these refractive structures, the iris adjusts the diameter of the pupil to prevent the entrance of stray light rays.

d. As the light passes through the lens, the lens automatically adjusts its curvature to refine the refraction; this is known as accommodation.
e. In conjunction with these processes, the eyes converge (move inward) to develop a single image. The closer the object, the more the eyes converge and vice-versa.
f. Once the light rays strike the retina, the photoreceptors, rods and cones, undergo structural changes that generate nerve impulses.
g. These impulses travel through the optic nerve to the occipital lobe of the brain where they are interpreted as vision.

F. Age-Related Changes
   1. Decline in visual acuity.
   2. Decline in taste acuity.
   3. Decline in auditory acuity.
   4. Decline in olfactory acuity.
   5. Increased risk for vertigo.
G. Pathophysiology
   1. Nystagmus: Repetitive, involuntary movements of the eye.
   2. Hordeolum (stye): Inflammatory, purulent infection of the sebaceous glands of the eyelid.
   3. Pterygium: Triangular thickening of the conjunctiva.
   4. Cataract: Opaque formation or cloudiness of the lens and surrounding tissues of the eye.
   5. Glaucoma: Accumulation of fluid pressure resulting from poor drainage of aqueous humor that damages the retina and optic nerve.
   6. Retinal detachment: Partial or complete separation of the retina from the choroid often caused by infiltration of vitreous humor behind the retina ultimately resulting in blindness.
   7. Macular degeneration: Degenerative disease changes in the pigmented cells of the macula causing a loss of fine vision.
   8. Conjunctivitis: Inflammation of the conjunctiva resulting from irritation, allergies, or infection (pinkeye).
   9. Uveitis: Inflammation of the uvea or choroid.
   10. Blepharitis: Inflammation of the eyelids.
   11. Keratitis: Inflammation of the cornea.
   12. Strabismus: Lazy eye is the inability of both eyes to focus on the same object.
   13. Astigmatism: Inability of the eye to sharply focus an image on the retina.
   14. Presbyopia: With age, the lens loses its elasticity making it unable to accommodate the visualization of objects at varying distances; bi- or trifocals are usually required.
   15. Amblyopia: General dimness of vision.
   16. Diplopia: Double vision.
   17. Nyctalopia: Inability to see at night or in dim light.

18. Exophthalmia: Protrusion of the eyeballs most often the result of endocrine dysfunction.
19. Myopia: Nearsightedness; the ability to clearly see objects near but not far.
20. Hyperopia: Farsightedness; the ability to clearly see objects far but not near.
21. Impacted cerumen: Compacted earwax within the auditory canal.
22. Otitis media: Inflammation of the middle ear.
23. Otosclerosis: Partial deafness caused by bone formation around the oval window and stapes.
24. Ménière's disease: Progressive deafness thought to be due to edema of the membranous labyrinth.
25. Presbycusis: Impairment in hearing caused by old age, otosclerosis, or nerve degeneration.
26. Deafness: Inability to hear.
27. Tinnitus: Ringing in the ears.
28. Vertigo: Dizziness.

XIII. ENDOCRINE SYSTEM

A. General (see Figure 5-36)
  1. Function
     a. Serves to identify and evaluate internal and external environmental changes for appropriate response.
     b. Control: Regulates internal body processes and functions.
     c. Communication: Complementing the nervous system, the endocrine system directs communication processes among the body systems for effective integration of body function.
  2. Endocrine glands: Specialized tissues that secrete hormones via the bloodstream to specific target cells within selected tissues or organs.

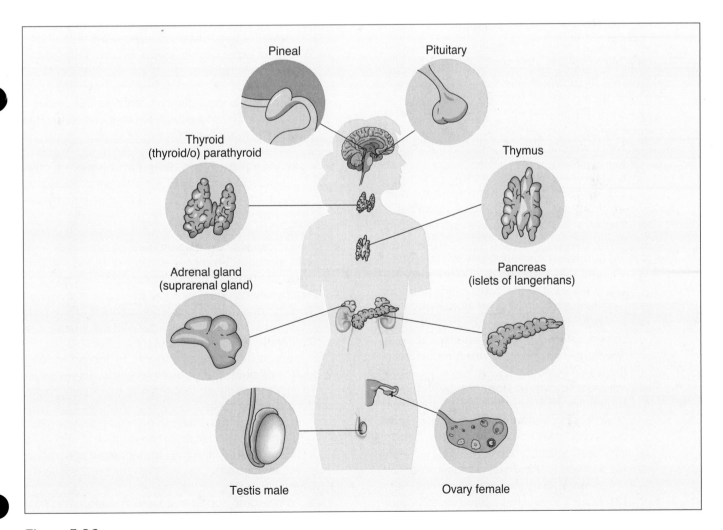

Figure 5-36

The endocrine system. Delmar/Cengage Learning.

B. Hormone: Chemical substance that stimulates other cells and tissues to increase functional activity or secrete their own hormones.
   1. Tropic hormones: Hormones that target other endocrine glands to stimulate their growth and secretion.
   2. Sex hormones: Hormones that target reproductive tissue to stimulate growth and development.
   3. Anabolic hormones: Hormones that target cells to stimulate growth and repair.
C. Prostaglandins
   1. Tissue hormones that are secreted to neighboring cells within the same tissue to integrate cellular activity.
   2. Secreted by a variety of tissues such as kidneys, lungs, brain, etc.
   3. Involved in blood pressure regulation, hydrochloric acid secretion in the stomach, and intestinal motility.
D. Pituitary gland
   1. General
      a. Commonly described as the "master gland". Also known as the hypophysis.
      b. Located on the inferior surface of the brain.
      c. Infundibulum: Stalk that connects the pituitary to the hypothalamus.
   2. Adenohypophysis (anterior pituitary)
      a. Somatotropic hormone (STH): Also known as growth hormone (GH).
         (1) Promotes the growth of tissue, especially bones and muscles.
         (2) Stimulates fat metabolism.
         (3) Is antagonistic with insulin to maintain homeostasis of blood glucose levels.
      b. Prolactin (PRL): Also known as lactogenic hormone.
         (1) Promotes development of the breast and milk secretion during pregnancy.
         (2) Works with the luteinizing hormone during the final phase of menstruation.
      c. Thyroid-stimulating hormone (TSH): Also known as thyrotropin. Stimulates growth, development, and hormone production of the thyroid gland.
      d. Adrenocorticotropic hormone (ACTH): Also known as adrenocorticotropin. Stimulates growth, development, and hormone production of the adrenal cortex.
      e. Follicle-stimulating hormone (FSH)
         (1) Female: Stimulates graafian follicle development and estrogen secretion.
         (2) Male: Stimulates seminiferous tube development and sperm production.

f. Luteinizing hormone (LH): Also known as gonadotropin.
   (1) Female: Stimulates secretion of estrogen and progesterone and follicle maturation in conjunction with FSH.
   (2) Male: Stimulates interstitial cell secretion of testosterone.
g. Melanocyte-stimulating hormone (MSH): Helps regulate normal pigmentation of skin and the adrenal gland's sensitivity to ACTH.
   3. Neurohypophysis (posterior pituitary)
      a. The posterior pituitary itself does not manufacture hormones but stores and releases hormones manufactured by the hypothalamus.
      b. Antidiuretic hormone (ADH): Prevents excess formation of urine, thereby conserving water.
      c. Oxytocin
         (1) In conjunction with PRL, causes milk ejection during lactation.
         (2) Stimulates contraction of uterus during childbirth.
E. Pineal gland
   1. Small, pinecone-shaped gland located in the posterior hypothalamus region.
   2. Produces melatonin, which regulates the body's biological clock.
F. Thyroid gland
   1. Butterfly-shaped gland located in the neck on the anterior and lateral surfaces of the trachea inferior to the larynx.
   2. Thyroxine
      a. Comprises two different hormones, tetraiodothyronine (T_4) which is a precursor to triiodothyronine (T_3) the principal thyroid hormone.
      b. Helps regulate metabolism including cell growth and differentiation.
   3. Calcitonin: Promotes transfer of blood calcium to the bone to reduce blood calcium levels.
G. Parathyroid glands
   1. Four pea-shaped glands embedded in the posterior surface of the thyroid's lateral lobes.
   2. Parathyroid hormone (PTH)
      a. Causes bone to dissolve to increase blood calcium and phosphate levels. Serves as an antagonist to calcitonin to maintain calcium homeostasis.
      b. Causes phosphate to be secreted by the kidney for excretion in the urine.
      c. Activates vitamin D for increased absorption of calcium.
H. Adrenal glands
   1. Located on top of the kidneys comprising two regions, the hormone-producing adrenal cortex and the neurosecretory medulla.

2. Adrenal cortex: Produce corticosteroids.
   a. Aldosterone: Mineralocorticoid hormone that regulates mineral salts.
      (1) Sodium regulation: Stimulates sodium reabsorption by the kidney to control blood sodium levels.
      (2) Potassium regulation: Increases water retention and promotes the loss of potassium.
   b. Cortisol: Principal glucocorticoid along with cortisone, and corticosterone.
      (1) Causes a shift from carbohydrate metabolism to fat metabolism as an energy source.
      (2) Maintains normal blood pressure with the aid of epinephrine and norepinephrine.
   c. Androgen and estrogen: gonadocorticoidal sex hormones.
3. Adrenal medulla: Comprises neurosecretory tissue that secretes epinephrine and norepinephrine, important to the sympathetic and parasympathetic nervous systems.

I. Pancreas
1. Elongated gland extending across the posterior stomach near the duodenum and spleen.
2. Glucagon: Produced by alpha cells to stimulate the conversion of glycogen in the liver to glucose to increase blood glucose levels.
3. Insulin: Produced by beta cells to metabolize glucose thereby reducing blood glucose levels.
4. Somatostatin: Produced by delta cells to regulate the endocrine functions of the other pancreatic cells.

J. Gonads
1. Testes: Testosterone produced by the interstitial cells stimulates development of male sex characteristics.
2. Ovaries
   a. Estrogen: Secreted by ovarian follicles to stimulate development of female sex characteristics.
   b. Progesterone: Secreted by corpus luteum to maintain the uterine lining during pregnancy.

K. Thymus
1. Located in the mediastinum below the sternum. Large in children but atrophies during adolescence.
2. Thymosin: Stimulates development of T-cells important in immunity.

L. Secondary endocrine organs
1. Placenta: Temporarily produces human chorionic gonadotropin (hCG).
2. Gastric and intestinal mucosa: Secretes gastrin, secretin, and cholecystokininpan-creozymin (CCK) responsible for coordinating digestion.

3. Heart: Secretes atrial natriuretic hormone (ANH) that acts as an antagonist to ADH and aldosterone, as well as opposes increases in blood volume or blood pressure.

M. Age-Related Changes
1. Glands shrink.
2. Increased risk for diabetes and thyroid disorders.

N. Pathophysiology: Principally involves the hyper- or hyposecretion of hormones.
1. Pituitary disorders
   a. Diabetes insipidus: Hyposecretion of ADH characterized by polyuria and polydipsia.
   b. Giantism: Hypersecretion of STH during infancy or youth characterized by abnormally large size.
   c. Acromegaly: Hypersecretion of STH after puberty characterized by enlarged head and extremities.
   d. Dwarfism: Hyposecretion of STH resulting in abnormally small size.
2. Thyroid disorders
   a. Grave's disease: Hyperthyroidism is due to the hypersecretion of thyroxine characterized by exophthalmia, nervousness, amnesia, diaphoresis, weight loss, and heat intolerance.
   b. Cretinism: Hypothyroidism is due to the hyposecretion of thyroxine during infancy characterized by retarded growth, impaired intelligence, and delayed development of secondary sex characteristics.
   c. Myxedema: Hyposecretion of thyroxine later in life characterized by fatigue, weight gain, and cold intolerance.
   d. Goiter: Enlargement of the thyroid gland resulting from iodine deficiency.
3. Parathyroid disorders
   a. Hypoparathyroidism: Hyposecretion of PTH causing hypocalcemia characterized by numbness of extremities and cramps.
   b. Hyperparathyroidism: Hypersecretion of PTH causing hypercalcemia characterized by weak, brittle bones, joint pain, and kidney stones.
4. Adrenal disorders
   a. Addison's disease: Hyposecretion of cortisol characterized by increased skin pigmentation, vitiligo patches, and hypotension.
   b. Cushing's disease: Hypersecretion of cortisol characterized by a round "moon" face with acne and "buffalo humps," fatty deposits on upper back.
5. Pancreatic disorders
   a. Diabetes mellitus: Hyposecretion of insulin causing impaired carbohydrate metabolism

characterized by hyperglycemia, polyuria, polyphagia, and polydipsia.

b. Hyperinsulinism: Hypersecretion of insulin characterized by hypoglycemia, weakness, polyphagia, diaphoresis, and diplopia.

> **NOTE:**
> - See also Section IV, Chapter 20 for information concerning the immune and hemopoietic systems as they may also be part of this section of the exam.

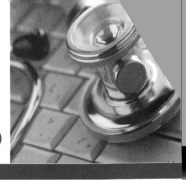

CHAPTER 6

Human Development

I. INTRODUCTION

A. Growth: Physical change with accompanying increase in size. Generally encompasses the first 20 years of life.

B. Development: Behavioral aspect of growth characterized by an increase in the complexity of function and skill. Progresses beyond the first 20 years of life.

C. Factors influencing growth and development
   1. Genetic: Established at conception and remains unchanged (e.g., gender and race).
   2. Environmental: Family, religion, culture, school, community, etc.

D. Principles
   1. Growth and development are continuous, orderly, sequential processes.
   2. All humans follow the same pattern of growth and development.
   3. The sequence of each stage is predictable. Time of onset, length, and effects of each stage are individual.
   4. Learning can either promote or hinder the maturational process.
   5. Each developmental stage has its own characteristics.
   6. Growth and development occur in a cephalocaudal (from head to toe) direction.
   7. Growth and development occur in a proximodistal (from the center outward) fashion.
   8. Development proceeds from simple to complex.
   9. Development becomes increasingly differentiated—from a general to a specific response.
   10. Certain stages of growth and development are more critical than others (e.g., 10 to 12 weeks after conception).
   11. The pace of growth and development is uneven—faster during infancy.

E. Personality development: The outward expression of the inner self (e.g., temperament, character traits, independence, etc.).

F. Theories attempt to explain the development of personality and the causes of behavior.

G. Theoretical Categories of Personality Development:
   1. Psychosexual Development.
   2. Psychosocial Development.
   3. Cognitive Development.
   4. Moral Development.
   5. Spiritual Development.
   6. Biophysical Development.

II. PSYCHOSEXUAL DEVELOPMENT (SIGMUND FREUD, 1923)

A. Unconscious: The part of the mind of which one is unaware.

B. Defense (adaptive) mechanisms: Behavioral responses resulting from the conflicts of inner impulses and the anxiety they create (discussed later).

C. Three levels of personality
   1. Id: Source of instinctive and unconscious urges that are chiefly sexual in nature, i.e., sources of pleasure and gratification.
   2. Ego: Formed through the realization that satisfying one's urges and impulses conflicts with reality and gratification must be delayed. Through the ego, id urges are satisfied.
   3. Superego: Refers to the moral aspects of personality, which include the source of guilt, shame, and inhibition.

D. Libido: The source of energy for satisfying the sexual urges that influence the three levels of personality.

E. Accordingly, the personality develops in five overlapping stages with corresponding change in the libido's location of emphasis.
   1. Oral: Mouth is center of pleasure (birth to 1 year).
      a. Feeding provides pleasure and comfort.
      b. Fixation may create mistrust along with nail-biting, drug abuse, smoking, overeating, etc.
   2. Anal: Anus and rectum are centers for pleasure (2 to 3 years).
      a. Toilet training provides pleasure and control.
      b. Fixation may result in obsessive-compulsive traits.

3. Phallic: Genitals are center of pleasure (4 to 5 years)
  a. Masturbation is pleasurable; child identifies with parent of opposite gender.
  b. Oedipus complex: Male child attracted to mother and hostile toward father.
  c. Electra complex: Female child attracted to father and hostile toward mother.
  d. Fixation may result in sexual identity and authority figure problems.
4. Latency: Focus on physical and intellectual activity—sexual impulses are repressed (6 to 12 years). Fixation may result in obsessiveness and lack of motivation.
5. Genital: Focus on attaining a mature sexual relationship (13+ years). Fixation may result in sexual problems.

III. PSYCHOSOCIAL DEVELOPMENT (ERIK ERIKSON, 1963)

A. Emphasizes the role environment plays in a person's development.
B. Each of Erikson's eight stages involves a conflict brought about by a person's need to adapt to the social environment.
C. Development is described in terms of a series of crises through which individuals progress. Each stage involves a conflict between new abilities or attitudes and inclinations that oppose them. Resolution of conflicts leads to a sense of competence.
D. Eight stages
  1. Trust versus Mistrust
    a. Infancy: Birth to 18 months.
    b. Positive resolution: Learns to trust others.
    c. Negative resolution: Mistrust, withdrawal, estrangement.
  2. Autonomy versus Shame and Doubt
    a. Early childhood: 18 months to 3 years.
    b. Positive resolution: Self-control without loss of self-esteem. Ability to cooperate and express oneself.
    c. Negative resolution: Compulsive self-restraint or compliance. Willfulness and defiance.
  3. Initiative versus Guilt
    a. Late childhood: 3 to 5 years.
    b. Positive resolution: Learns the degree to which assertiveness and purpose influence the environment. Onset of ability to evaluate one's own behavior.
    c. Negative resolution: Lack of self-confidence, pessimism, fear of wrongdoing, overcontrol and overrestriction of own activity.
  4. Industry versus Inferiority
    a. School age: 6 to 12 years.
    b. Positive resolution: Beginning to create, develop, and manipulate. Developing sense of competence and perseverance.
    c. Negative resolution: Loss of hope, sense of being mediocre, withdrawal from school and peers.
  5. Identity versus Role Confusion
    a. Adolescence: 12 to 20 years.
    b. Positive resolution: Coherent sense of self. Plans to actualize one's activities.
    c. Negative resolution: Confusion, indecisiveness, possible antisocial behavior.
  6. Intimacy versus Isolation
    a. Young adult: 18 to 25 years.
    b. Positive resolution: Intimate relationship with another person. Commitment to work and relationships.
    c. Negative resolution: Impersonal relationships; avoidance of relationships, career, or lifestyle commitments.
  7. Generativity versus Stagnation
    a. Adulthood: 25 to 65 years.
    b. Positive resolution: Creativity, productivity, concern for others.
    c. Negative resolution: Self-indulgence, self-concern, lack of interests and commitments.
  8. Integrity versus Despair
    a. Maturity: 65 years to death.
    b. Positive resolution: Acceptance of worth and uniqueness; acceptance of death.
    c. Negative resolution: Sense of loss, contempt for others.

IV. COGNITIVE DEVELOPMENT (JEAN PIAGET, 1966)

A. Manner in which one learns to think, reason, and communicate.
B. Mental abilities associated with intelligence, perception, and information processing.
C. Represents a progression of mental abilities from illogical to logical thinking, simple to complex problem solving, and from understanding concrete to abstract concepts.
D. Encompasses an orderly, sequential process in which new experiences must exist before intellectual abilities can develop.
E. Four stages
  1. Sensorimotor
    a. Infancy: Birth to 2 years.
    b. Focuses on motor and reflex action. Child learns through sensation and movement. Keen interest in faces and voices.
  2. Preoperational
    a. Toddler/early childhood: 2 to 7 years.

b. Focuses on language and symbols; has active imagination and vivid fantasies; personifies objects.

3. Concrete operational
   a. Elementary/early adolescence: 7 to 11 years.
   b. Begins to process abstract concepts such as numbers and relationships but needs concrete examples for comprehension. Can manipulate objects mentally.

4. Formal operational
   a. Adolescence/adulthood: 11 to 15+ years.
   b. Learns to reason logically and analytically without reference to concrete applications. Capable of hypothetical and deductive reasoning.

V. MORAL DEVELOPMENT (LAWRENCE KOHLBERG, 1971)

A. Pattern of change in behavior as it relates to determining what is right and wrong.
B. Rather than a concern for the morality of a decision, Kohlberg focuses on the reasons surrounding a moral decision.
C. Moral development progresses through three levels consisting of a total of six stages.
D. Levels and stages are not necessarily linked to a particular developmental stage because some can progress beyond others.
E. Levels and stages
   1. Level I—Preconventional: Focuses on cultural rules defining good, bad, right, and wrong.
      1. Stage 1—Punishment and obedience orientation: An activity is wrong if one is punished—not wrong if not punished.
      b. Stage 2—Instrumental-relativist orientation: Action is taken to satisfy one's desires.
   2. Level II—Conventional: Focuses on maintaining the expectations of referent groups.
      a. Stage 3—Interpersonal concordance: Good boy, nice girl. Action is taken to please another and gain approval.
      b. Stage 4—Law and order orientation: It is right to obey the law and follow rules.
   3. Level III—Postconventional: Focuses on developing values and principles without regard to outside authority or expectations.
      a. Stage 5—Social contract, legalistic orientation: Adheres to laws that protect the welfare and rights of others. Personal values and opinions are respected and not violated.
      b. Stage 6—Universal-ethical principles: Universal moral principles are internalized. Relationships are based on respect and mutual trust.

VI. SPIRITUAL DEVELOPMENT (JAMES FOWLER, 1985)

A. Deals with understanding one's relationship with the universe and one's notions concerning the direction and meaning of life.
B. Faith: According to Fowler, it is relational—the way we invest commitment, belief, love, risk, and hope in others.
C. Seven stages
   1. Undifferentiated
      a. Birth to 3 years.
      b. Infant is unable to develop concepts about the self or the environment.
   2. Intuitive-protective
      a. 4 to 6 years.
      b. Combination of images and beliefs are furnished by others, along with the child's own experience and imagination.
   3. Mythic-literal
      a. 7 to 12 years.
      b. Fantasy and wonder—dramatic stories and myths used to communicate spiritual meaning.
   4. Synthetic-conventional
      a. Adolescent to adult.
      b. Interpersonal focus—world and environment structured by the expectations and judgment of others.
   5. Individuating-reflexive
      a. After 18 years.
      b. Constructing one's own explicit system—high self-consciousness.
   6. Paradoxical-consolidative
      a. After 30 years.
      b. Awareness of truth from a variety of viewpoints.
   7. Universalizing
      a. May never develop.
      b. Becoming an incarnation of the principles of love and justice.

VII. BIOPHYSICAL DEVELOPMENT

A. Infant growth and development
   1. Reflexes: Automatic response to stimuli that govern the newborn's movements and serve a survival function. For example, the newborn has no fear of water. It will naturally hold its breath and contract its throat to keep water from rushing in.
      a. Moro reflex: When infants become startled, they arch their backs, throw their heads back, fling out their arms and legs then rapidly close them to the center of their bodies, and then flex as if they were falling.

b. Rooting reflex: Stroking the infant's cheek causes the head to turn in the direction of the stimulus.

c. Sucking reflex: An important means of obtaining nutrition and also an enjoyable, soothing activity.

d. Palmar grasp reflex: Up to age 6 months, infants will initiate a grasping movement when the palm is stimulated.

e. Stepping reflex: If the infant is held in a standing position and tilted forward, the infant will draw up each leg successively as if walking.

f. China doll reflex: Pulling the infant to a sitting position causes the eyes to open, the shoulders to tense, and the infant to try unsuccessfully to right its head.

2. Newborns spend 6% to 7% of their day crying. An infant's earliest cries are reflexive reactions to discomfort.

3. Newborns sleep for 16 to 17 hours a day. The patterns of sleep during the day do not always follow a rhythmic pattern.

4. By about 1 month of age, most infants have begun to sleep longer at night, and by about 4 months of age, they have usually moved closer to adultlike sleep patterns.

5. Physical growth and motor development

a. Newborns are about 20 inches long and weigh 7 pounds. Their hearts beat twice as fast as an adult's—120 beats a minute—and they breathe twice as fast as an adult, about 33 times a minute.

b. They urinate as many as 18 times and move their bowels from four to six times in 24 hours.

c. On the average, they are alert and comfortable for only about 30 minutes in a 4-hour period. At birth, the neonate has a gigantic head relative to the rest of the body that flops around in uncontrollable fashion.

d. In the span of 12 months, thin infants become capable of sitting anywhere, standing, stooping, climbing, and probably walking.

e. During the second year, growth decelerates, but rapid increases in such activities as running and climbing take place.

f. Cephalocaudal growth: The cephalocaudal pattern means that the greatest growth always occurs at the top of the individual—the head—with physical growth in size, weight, and feature differentiation gradually working its way down from top to bottom (e.g., neck, shoulders, middle trunk, and so on).

g. Proximodistal growth: Growth starts at the center of the body and moves toward the extremities. An example of this is the early maturation of muscular control of the trunk and arms as compared with that of the hands and fingers.

h. Gross motor skills: Include large muscle activities such as moving one's arms and walking.

i. Fine motor skills: Include more fine-grained movements like finger dexterity.

j. Rhythmic motor behavior: During the first year, repetitious movement of the limbs, torso, and head is common. Kicking, rocking, waving, bouncing, banging, rubbing, scratching, and swaying occur frequently and are pleasurable. It is an important transition between uncoordinated activity and complex, coordinated motor behavior.

k. Brain development
   (1) At birth, the infant probably has all of the nerve cells it is going to have in its entire life. However, at birth and in early infancy, nerve cells connectedness is impoverished.
   (2) As the infant moves from birth to 2 years of age, the interconnections of neurons increase dramatically as the dendrites of neurons branch out.

6. Sensory and perceptual development

a. Vision
   (1) The newborn's vision is about 20/600. But by 6 months of age, vision is 20/100 or better.
   (2) At about 3½ weeks, the infant is fascinated with the eyes, perhaps because the infant notices simple perceptual features such as dots, angles, and circles.
   (3) At 1 to 2 months of age, the infant notices and perceives contour. At 2 months and older, the infant begins to differentiate facial features.
   (4) By 5 months of age, the infant has detected other facial features—the face's plasticity, its solid, three-dimensional surface, the oval shape of the head, the orientation of the eyes and the mouth.
   (5) Beyond 6 months of age, the infant distinguishes familiar faces from unfamiliar faces.

b. Hearing: Immediately after birth, infants can hear, although a stimulus must be louder to be heard by a newborn than by an adult.

c. Smell: Infants can smell soon after birth.

d. Taste: Sensitivity to sweetness is clearly present in the newborn.

e. Touch: Infants also respond to touch. The main perceptual abilities—visual, auditory, and tactile—are completely uncoordinated at birth.

B. Childhood growth and development

1. The growth rate continues to slow down in early childhood following cephalocaudal development. At this time, the brain is closer to full growth than the rest of the child's body, attaining 75% of its adult weight by the age of 3.

2. The average child grows 2 ½ inches in height and gains 5 to 7 pounds per year during early childhood. As the preschool child grows older, the rate of growth decreases.

3. Girls are only slightly smaller and lighter than boys during this age period, a difference that continues until puberty. In early childhood, both boys and girls slim down as the trunks of their bodies become longer. Although their heads are still somewhat large for their bodies, by the end of early childhood most children have lost their top-heavy look.

4. The large muscles of preschool children develop extensively, especially those in the arms and legs.

5. Denver Developmental Screening Test: Devised to be a simple, inexpensive, and fast way to diagnose developmental delay in children from birth through 6 years of age.
   a. Gross motor skills: The child's ability to sit, walk, broad jump, pedal a tricycle, throw a ball overhand, catch a bounced ball, hop on one foot, and balance on one foot.
   b. Fine motor skills: Ability to stack cubes, reach for objects, and draw a person. Three-year-old children have deficiencies in mapping large-scale spaces.

6. Early childhood development: The following tasks are reasonable to expect in 75% to 80% of the children in the indicated ages.
   a. 2 to 3 years
      (1) Displays a variety of scribbling behavior.
      (2) Can walk rhythmically at an even pace.
      (3) Can step off low object, one foot ahead of the other.
      (4) Can name hands, feet, head, and some face parts.
      (5) Opposes thumb to fingers when grasping objects; releases objects smoothly from finger-thumb grasp.
      (6) Can walk a 2-inch wide line placed on the ground, for 10 feet.
   b. 4 years
      (1) Forward broad jump, both feet together and clear of ground at same time.
      (2) Can hop two or three times on one foot without precision or rhythm.
      (3) Walks and runs with arm action coordinated with leg action.
      (4) Can walk a circular line a short distance.
      (5) Can draw a crude circle.
      (6) Can imitate a simple line cross using a vertical and horizontal line.
   c. 5 years
      (1) Runs 30 yards in just over 8 seconds.
      (2) Balances on one foot (girls 6 to 8 seconds) (boys 4 to 6 seconds).
      (3) Child catches large playground ball bounced to him or her chest-high from 15 feet away, four to five times out of five.
      (4) Rectangle and square drawn differently (one side at a time).
      (5) Can high-jump 8 inches or higher over a bar with simultaneous 2-foot takeoff.
      (6) Bounces playground ball, using one or two hands, a distance of 3 to 4 feet.
   d. 6 years
      (1) Can block-print first name.
      (2) Can gallop, if it is demonstrated.
      (3) Can exert 6 pounds or more of pressure in grip strength measure.
      (4) Can walk balance beam 2 inches wide, 6 inches high, and 10 to 12 feet long.
      (5) Can run 60 feet in about 5 seconds.
      (6) Can arise from ground from back lying position, when asked to do so as fast as he or she can, in 2 seconds or under.

7. Middle to late childhood
   a. At about the age of 11, the average child is 58 inches tall and 85 to 88 pounds.
   b. Children's legs become longer and their trunks slimmer, and they are steadier on their feet. Fat tissue develops more rapidly than muscle tissue (which increases substantially in adolescence).
   c. Children's motor development becomes much smoother and more coordinated than in early childhood.
   d. There are marked sex differences in gross motor skills, with boys outperforming girls; however, girls outperform boys in fine motor skills like drawing and penmanship.
   e. Sensory mechanisms continue to mature. Early farsightedness is overcome, binocular vision becomes well developed, and hearing acuity increases. Children of this age also have fewer illnesses than younger children, especially fewer respiratory and gastrointestinal problems.

8. Growth chart
   a. A chart to plot the growth patterns of children's weight, height, and head circumference.
   b. The chart identifies statistically what percentile a child's growth falls in.
   c. Percentile increments are usually 10th, 25th, 50th, 75th, and 90th percentiles. The average is the 50th percentile.
   d. A 24-month child's weight falling in the 75th percentile means the child weighs more than does 75% of population at 24 months.

C. Puberty: Rapid physical maturation involving hormonal and bodily changes that take place primarily during early adolescence.
   1. A body weight approximating 106 pounds ±3 pounds signals menarche and the end of the adolescent growth spurt. For menarche to begin and continue, fat must make up 17% of the girl's body weight.
   2. Hormonal concentrations increase dramatically during adolescence.
   3. Noticeable pubescent changes include increased height and weight, and sexual maturation. The growth spurt for girls occurs around age 10, two years earlier than boys, lasting about 2 years. During this time, girls increase in height by about 3½ inches per year. Boys usually grow about 4 inches per year during this time frame.
   4. Male pubertal characteristics develop in this order: Increase in penis and testicle size, appearance of straight public hair, minor voice change, first ejaculation, appearance of kinky pubic hair, onset of maximum growth, growth of hair in armpits, more detectable voice changes, and growth of facial hair.
   5. Female pubertal characteristics develop in this order: First either the breasts enlarge or pubic hair appears. Later hair will appear in the armpits. As these changes occur, females grow in height and their hips become wider than their shoulders. The first menstruation comes rather late in the pubertal cycle.
   6. Adolescents are preoccupied with their bodies and develop individual images of what their bodies are like. General appearance, the face, facial complexion, and body build are thought to be the most important characteristics in physical attractiveness.

D. Young adults (20 to 40 years)
   1. Body systems are fully developed. Physically, in peak condition. Physiological efficiency begins to decline late in this phase.
   2. Physical changes are minimal, however, weight and muscle mass may change due to diet and exercise.
   3. Psychosocial development continues.
   4. Extensive physical and psychosocial changes occur in pregnant and lactating women.
   5. Developmental tasks
      a. Completing education and selecting a career.
      b. Selecting a partner.
      c. Raising a family.
      d. Developing a satisfactory sex life.

E. Middle-aged adults (40 to 65 years)
   1. This stage is more stable and comfortable.
   2. Metabolism, energy, and endurance tend to wane.
   3. Increase in weight.
   4. Skin elasticity decreases causing wrinkles; gray hair appears.
   5. Sense acuity is lessened, often necessitating the use of corrective devices.
   6. Menopause develops in women.
   7. Increased chance of chronic illness.
   8. Desire to provide volunteer service.
   9. Developmental tasks
      a. Adjusting to physical changes.
      b. Having grown children.
      c. Developing leisure-time activities.
      d. Adjusting to aging parents.

F. Older adults (65 and older)
   1. Activities of daily living (ADL) become increasingly challenging.
   2. Memory loss.
   3. Gross and fine motor skills become less coordinated; movement slows.
   4. Shortened stature.
   5. Loss of relationships because of illness and death.
   6. Developmental tasks
      a. Adjusting to decreased strength and loss of health.
      b. Retirement and reduced income.
      c. Coping with the death of a partner.
      d. Developing new friends and relationships.
      e. Preparing for one's own death.

CHAPTER 7

Professional Relations

I. PROFESSIONALISM

A. Professional: One who has acquired and applies a specialized body of knowledge, skills, and abilities.

B. Attributes of a professional
1. Empathy: Ability to understand another's perspective, feelings, and experience.
2. Attitude: To communicate and interact with others using a positive outlook.
3. Dependability: MA can be counted on to carry out one's responsibilities.
4. Initiative: Ability to anticipate the needs of others and to carry out responsibilities without direction.
5. Flexibility: Ability to adapt to changing circumstances.
6. Curiosity: To actively remain current on new information and developments—the desire to pursue lifelong learning.
7. Health: Adopting a healthful lifestyle and projecting a healthful role model.
8. Appearance: To project a desirable image by appropriate personal hygiene and attire.
9. Communicability: Ability to effectively convey meaning orally and in written form with both medical colleagues, patients, and the lay public.
10. Ethical: Adhering to moral standards, i.e. a code of ethics; conduct that is right and good and avoids what is wrong or bad.
11. Detailed: Appropriate attention to the specific elements that affect a process, procedure, or circumstance.
12. Prudence: To act with caution and careful consideration—to avoid waste.
13. Courteousness: To be polite and to have good manners.
14. Enthusiasm: To demonstrate interest in one's role and responsibilities.
15. Veracity: To be honest and truthful.
16. Patience: To calmly wait for events to unfold and to function within the constraints of various circumstances.
17. Perseverance: To exert the necessary effort to achieve a result.
18. Respectful: To demonstrate personal regard for another's feelings or perspective regardless of one's personal opinion.
19. Self-control: To show restraint and to avoid exhibiting inappropriate behavior.
20. Tactfulness: Ability to communicate information in a delicate fashion to avoid offense.
21. Punctuality: To arrive where and when expected.
22. Congeniality: To have a friendly disposition.

C. Professional organizations: Membership in one or more professional organizations provides myriad benefits.
1. Symbolizes professionalism.
2. Offer continuing education units to maintain professional credentials.
3. Provides newsworthy information that impacts the profession, the industry, and related institutions.
4. Provides opportunities to hold office, e.g., president, treasurer, etc., to develop leadership and other skills.
5. Affords opportunities to communicate and interact with colleagues for professional benefit.

D. Code of Ethics: Review Chapter 9, Health Care Ethics.
1. Represents standards of behavior and practice embodied by a profession.
2. Professionals are expected to adhere to applicable laws, regulation, and prescribed codes of ethics.
3. The AAMA, AMT, and AMA codes of ethics are most relevant to medical assistants and medical administrative specialists.

E. Promotion and protection of the profession
1. Promote the traditions, values, honor, and principles of the profession.
2. Mentorship: Provide opportunities to those in training to develop the skills, knowledge, and abilities of the profession, e.g. externships.
3. Behave in a fashion that sheds favorably on the profession.
4. Expose those who violate the laws and ethical code of the profession.

F. Competence
   1. Strive to maintain and develop professional skills, knowledge and abilities within one's scope of practice.
   2. Maintain professional credentials, e.g. CMA, RMA, CMAS.
G. Community service: Serve to advance the health, wellbeing, and good of society.

II. SEEKING EMPLOYMENT

A. Resumes
   1. A resume is merely a means to an interview.
   2. Resume types
      a. Historical resume: Arranged in reverse chronological order.
      b. Functional resume: Organizes duties, responsibilities, and accomplishments without regard to their historical perspective.
         (1) Functional resumes are very infrequently used.
         (2) Thought to be used when applicants attempt to hide something like a significant break in employment.
      c. Narrative resume: Reads like a letter. Usually, the candidate will highlight the different experiences that pertain to the position for which he or she wants to be considered.
   3. General content
      a. Full name, home address, home and business phone numbers, and email address.
      b. Education.
      c. Experience–responsibilities and accomplishments.
      d. Professional affiliations.
      e. Personal information (optional).
      f. Outside interests (optional).
      g. References.
   4. Begin each new page with your name in case the pages become separated during review or copying.
   5. Place the appropriate credentials after your name.
   6. Always place your home address on the resume, not your current employer's.
   7. Include the phrase "(to be used with discretion)" immediately below the business phone number.
   8. Be sure to use an answering service or have an answering machine to take your calls at home.
   9. Do not use an email address that is "cutesy" such as hireme@yahoo.com, or one that is especially long or difficult to type.
   10. Do not include a job objective.
   11. Education
      a. Put it first, because health care is a very education-oriented industry
      b. Begin with the highest degree earned.
      c. Indicate the year in which the degree was conferred.
      d. If you graduated with honors, include this information in the description of the degree.
      e. Omit your grade point average.
   12. Experience
      a. It is imperative that your resume be concise, easy to read, and easy to understand.
      b. Information needs to "jump off the page," so the reviewer can quickly decide if you meet the qualifications necessary for the job.
      c. Describe specific responsibilities and accomplishment.
      d. Whenever you complete an accomplishment, make a note, to yourself about the specifics and keep it in your personal career file; include your role in the project.
      e. Indicate the dates of continuous employment with one organization on the left side and note the dates corresponding to each position within the organization immediately after the job title.
      f. Listing the dates of different positions within one organization separately on the left-hand side of the resume confuses the reader.
      g. Try to abbreviate the responsibilities and accomplishments for earlier positions.
      h. The further you go back in time the more important it is to condense your responsibilities and accomplishments.
      i. Condense heavily the descriptions of jobs held prior to the 10-year mark.
      j. Focus on the truly exceptional projects and tasks you have successfully handled.
      k. Responsibilities tell the reader about the scope and breadth of the job.
      l. The number of full-time employees (FTEs) supervised, the number of departments reporting to you, amount of the budget you directed, and the names of committees on which you served.
      m. Describe what you did on the job to "make a difference."
      n. Quantify your accomplishments.
      o. Specificity allows the reader of your resume to understand your impact on the organization.
   13. Professional affiliations
      a. Professional affiliations demonstrate your active involvement in the healthcare profession.
      b. Do not overload this section.
      c. Show that you are active professionally, without causing the reader to question your credibility or your priorities.

14. Outside interests
    a. List active sports as outside interests.
    b. Healthcare professionals commonly golf, fish, or play tennis recreationally.
    c. Also, active hobbies, such as sports, will be looked at more favorably than passive hobbies, such as reading or watching films.
    d. Be careful if your outside interests might be considered outside the norm.
    e. Refrain from listing really offbeat outside interests.
    f. Omit mentioning membership in organizations whose agendas are primarily religious or political.
15. References
    a. State "References available upon request."
    b. Your actual list of references should be supplied only after the potential employer asks for it.
    c. The resume and the reference list alike should be printed on good-quality paper.
    d. Print your cover letter, resume, and reference list on the same kind of paper, using the same typeface.
    e. Use white paper only.
16. Avoid the inclination to be creative on your resume.
17. Do not use gimmicks or attention grabbers to make your resume stand out.
18. Ask two other people whose intelligence you respect to proofread it for you.
19. Check for correct spelling.
20. Do not exceed three pages—about 10 years of experience per page.
21. Use action verbs in your writing.
22. Cut out extra words by using verbs instead of nominalizations.
23. Avoid using the verbs "utilize" and "facilitate."
24. Make it "scannable" for the human resources department so that your name and your experience will be entered into their candidate pool as soon as possible.
    a. Use a chronological resume.
    b. Place your name at the top of the page on its own line.
    c. Use standard address format below your name.
    d. List each phone number on its own line.
    e. Use white or very light-colored 8½ × 11 paper, printed on one side only.
    f. Avoid colored paper.
    g. Avoid vertical and horizontal lines, graphics, and boxes.
    h. Avoid unusual fonts—san serif fonts work best.
    i. Don't condense spacing between letters (i.e. rn could be misinterpreted as m).
    j. Use key words to define your skills, education, experience, and professional affiliations.
B. Cover letters
    1. The cover letter should compel the reader to view the attached resume.
    2. The cover letter complements your resume.
    3. First paragraph
        a. Should explain why you are writing.
        b. Mention where you read the ad and specify the position that was advertised.
        c. The opening sentence allows the reader to easily determine where to route your letter.
    4. Second paragraph: Should detail your accomplishments, experience, or abilities and relate them to the job as you understand it.
    5. Third paragraph
        a. Should ask specifically for further consideration for the position and an interview.
        b. You should indicate your intent to follow up on your resume at a later date—and actually do it.
    6. Proofreading
        a. Proofread it for content.
        b. Does it include the most relevant information for that particular position?
        c. Have you carefully considered and explained why you are a qualified candidate?
        d. Have you expressed your interest in further discussing, i.e., interviewing for, the position?
        e. Correct all grammatical mistakes, misspelled words, and typographical errors.
        f. Your business correspondence reflects your standards of professionalism.
        g. Double check the spelling of the name, title, and address of the person to whom you are writing.
        h. Research the position and find out the name of the correct person to whom you are addressing your letter.
    7. Cover letter to search consultants
        a. Include your current salary and your salary expectations, as well as your geographic preferences.
        b. Include the types of positions in which you are interested and any special considerations.
C. References
    1. Should be separate from your resume.
    2. Have your reference list ready before you start your job search so you will not be caught off guard when an interested party requests it.
    3. References provide an interviewer with the opportunity to obtain independent verification of the information that you have supplied.

4. They provide the person listed as a reference with the opportunity to sell you to your potential employer with a glowing report.
5. Most thoughtful and cautious employers will require a list of references and will conduct reference checks.
6. Usually, the references are checked before an offer of employment.
7. Occasionally, an offer is made contingent on a satisfactory reference check.
8. Use your references sparingly and judiciously.
9. Wait until a prospective employer asks for your list of references before submitting it. This practice saves not only paper but, far more importantly, the time of your references.
10. Do not attach letters of reference to your resume.
    a. A letter of reference is an anachronism; you do not need to get one from an employer when you leave a job.
    b. Letters of reference are noted more for what they omit than for what they actually say.
11. Reference priority
    a. Supervisors
    b. Peers
    c. Subordinates
    d. Others
12. List supervisors from up to 10 years ago as references.
13. Prospective employers will look very favorably on someone who pleased former supervisors.
14. References from peers are a useful alternative if you are unable to obtain a positive reference from a supervisor because of a personality conflict or if a supervisor has died or cannot be located.
    a. They are especially good references when the search committee includes potential subordinates, or when the hiring committee wants to determine an individual's management style.
    b. References from subordinates are particularly important when the organization values participatory management.
15. Others who can supply references to your character and work ethic are people who were not part of the management team at your former position, but are familiar with your work.
16. Consultants and fellow professionals with whom you served on a committee can provide a reference.
17. Physicians are especially important "other" references.
18. Refrain from listing references simply because they have a national reputation when they have very little personal knowledge of your own situation.

19. List only those references with whom you have had active and direct professional contact.
20. Obtain permission from references
    a. Clear your references in advance.
    b. By asking, you may discern what kind of recommendation that person is likely to give.
    c. Being a reference can require a great deal of time and some inconvenience.
21. Check your own references.
    a. You need to have a feel for what your references say about you so that you can address any issues brought up by the reference with your potential employer.
    b. You can check your own references by asking directly of people who have called the reference what the reference had to say.
    c. You may enlist the aid of a friendly search consultant to make inquiries.
    d. If you are fair and nonconfrontational, the reference themselves will often tell you what they intend to say when people call.
22. Composing the reference list
    a. The actual list should include five or six people from the hierarchy of references.
    b. If you cannot use your current supervisor for any reason, try to find someone within your organization who fits into one of the other three categories to serve as one of your references.
    c. List the correct name, title, office address, and business phone number.
    d. Note in what capacity you know the reference.
    e. The more enthusiastic, the better.
    f. Some references "damn with faint praise." Therefore, when picking your references, concentrate on finding spirited, enthusiastic ones.
23. Personal references: References from a member of the clergy who knows you or personal references from your friends are neither necessary nor encouraged.
24. Involving your current employer: Weigh the decision to involve your current employer based on your knowledge of the organization and your relationship with your supervisor.

D. Interviewing
1. You must know two equally important things before the interview.
   a. Know the organization and the hiring manager.
   b. Know yourself.
2. Learn as much as you can about the job opportunity, the organization, and the hiring manager before the interview. Allows you to ask intelligent, forceful questions.

3. Obtain information on an organization
   a. Have the human resources department send information after the interview is scheduled.
   b. Call the public relations department and ask for some brochures.
   c. Call the local chamber of commerce and request a newcomer's package.
   d. Call the state association and find out what information is available.
   e. Read back copies of the local newspaper for information.
4. Obtain information about the hiring manager
   a. If he or she is a member of a professional organization, look up the individual's profile in the membership directory.
   b. Network with people who may have left the organization.
   c. Network with mutual acquaintances, such as vendors, consultants, and auditors.
   d. Make discreet inquiries with centers of influence such as association executives.
5. Anticipate what questions the interviewers will ask.
6. Frequently asked interview questions:
   a. Tell me about yourself. You don't need to be overly specific. Stick with accomplishments, both personal and business. Your answer should take less than 10 minutes.
   b. How would you describe your work, management or leadership style? Give a straightforward reply.
   c. Tell me about your experience. Include duties and specific accomplishments. Relate your experience to the opening.
   d. Why did you leave that job? Do not provide any negative information.
   e. Tell me about your strengths. Here is your opportunity to sell yourself. What is it that you do especially well? Try to give three to five strengths.
   f. What do you consider to be your weaknesses? "I work too hard." "I am too impatient for results." "I am too intent on accomplishing my goals." "I don't take enough time off." "I am too persistent."
      (1) This is one question for which you really do want to frame an answer in advance.
      (2) Don't give an answer if it does not actually fit your character.
      (3) Be ready to offer an example.
      (4) You can also mention a bona fide weakness and add that you are working on it, or better yet, have totally neutralized it.
      (5) Do not explore a weakness in any depth.
      (6) Avoid using the pronoun "I" as much as possible.
7. "We" is the appropriate word to use when noting accomplishments.
8. Illegal questions
   a. Rehearse firm, diplomatic responses.
   b. "You know, my mother told me that you wouldn't have the nerve to ask me that question!"
   c. "One of my friends told me she was asked a similar question, and she just chuckled and asked if it were a mock interview."
   d. "I know you are kidding, so I'll go ahead to your next question."
   e. "Is Mike Wallace in the next room?"
   f. To interview well, practice, practice, practice, especially on the tricky questions.
9. Preparation for the interview
   a. Arrive on time.
   b. Look your best.
      (1) Wear conservative clothes.
      (2) Men should wear a navy blue solid or pinstripe suit, white or pale blue shirt, and a conservative tie. Have neatly trimmed hair and mustache.
      (3) Women should choose a suit in the classic colors of navy blue, taupe, or black. Hairstyles should also be classic.
      (4) Polished shoes.
   c. Be especially nice to secretaries.
      (1) Secretaries are often confidants of the boss.
      (2) The secretary may cast the deciding vote.
   d. Do not smoke on an interview.
   e. Refrain from alcohol consumption.
   f. Check your handshake.
   g. Do not be glib.
10. Your contribution to the interview: Ask important questions.
    a. Tell me about this organization.
    b. Why is this position vacant?
    c. How many people have held the position in the last five years?
    d. If this is a new position, how will my success or failure be judged?
    e. What method of performance appraisal do you use?
    f. How is my supervisor viewed in the organization?
    g. What is my supervisor's management role?
    h. Whom do I supervise? What are their backgrounds, responsibilities, and so forth? What are they like?
    i. Ask for an organizational chart if one has not been provided.
    j. What is the organization's competitive position?

k. What is the greatest challenge facing this organization?
l. Direct the same questions to different people in the organization. Inconsistent answers or hedging should serve as red flags for you, indicating potential trouble.
m. You should direct questions about salary to one person and one person only—the hiring manager.
n. Maintain objectivity and some skepticism about the organization to balance your eagerness to get the job.
o. Asking questions of the different people with whom you interview will equip you with valuable, sometimes off-the-record, information you need if you want to work in the organization.
p. Even if you uncover a negative from your investigative questioning, or you think you do not want the job after all, conduct yourself during the entire interview as though you do.
q. Keep a poker face and an open mind.
r. At the end of the interview, be sure to state your interest in the position and a desire to pursue further discussions.
s. Ask what the next step will be and when they will plan to follow up with you on the results of your interview.
t. Even if the interview has not gone well, maintain your zeal and energy until you are out of the building.
u. Close the conversation with a strong handshake and a gracious acknowledgment for the interview.
v. Never accept a job on the spot. Sleep on it for at least 24 hours.
w. Get an offer in writing before you resign your current position.

11. Thank-you notes
a. Write a brief thank-you note and mail it within 24 hours of the interview.
b. Do the following three things in your note:
   (1) Express thanks for the interview and the interviewer's time.
   (2) Restate your interest in the position.
   (3) Refer to future communication.
c. It is also perfectly acceptable to send an e-mail note.
d. It is important to prepare a separate note for each individual you see because eventually all of your "thank you" notes will gravitate to the hiring manager.
e. It is much more favorable if each one of your notes is unique and not merely a copy of a form letter.

12. Second interview
a. The process typically proceeds in this order: You must let the process take its course.
   (1) Lead
   (2) Cover letter and resume
   (3) Reference request
   (4) First interview
   (5) Second interview
   (6) Offer
   (7) Acceptance
   (8) Transition
b. Just as the resume focuses on getting the first interview, the first interview focuses on getting the second interview.
c. Your goals for the first interview are the following:
   (1) Make a good impression.
   (2) Learn as much as you can.
   (3) Get the second interview.
d. Your goals for the second interview are slightly different:
   (1) Make a good impression.
   (2) Clarify as much as you can.
   (3) Involve your spouse.
   (4) Get the offer.
e. When you make it to the second interview, you are in the homestretch to obtaining an offer.
f. List all your questions in writing so that you can raise them in the second interview. No more than 20 questions.
g. Benefits
   (1) Ask for the benefits handbook or any written form of the organization's benefits policy.
   (2) What is written in the benefits handbook takes precedence over anything that the hiring manager may promise in good faith.
   (3) If there is any ambiguity, ask to meet with the appropriate human resources representative to get a more detailed explanation.
h. Find out about the organizational structure and authority issues in depth.
i. If a current job description is available, go over it with the hiring manager.
j. Has your contact at the hiring organization mentioned relocation costs? Will your prospective employer help out? Think about all these questions because you may be offered the job on the spot.
k. If you are, you need to be ready to discuss these important real estate issues, which may bear directly on whether the offer is an attractive one.

l. Request the itinerary for the visit in advance, with the names, titles, and employers of the people whom you will be meeting.

m. Interviewing at the senior level generally involves meeting with board members and, in some cases, prominent members of the community.

n. Second interviews include more social activities, so be ready to shift from business-related conversation to social conversation.

o. Avoid the topics of religion, controversial current events, and politics.

p. Ask lots of questions and listen attentively.

q. Find out about the social events ahead of time and the appropriate dress, and let your spouse know so you are both prepared.

r. At this part of the process, it is not your qualifications that are being scrutinized, but rather your personality.

13. Psychological testing
   a. Can help identify the optimal person for that particular position.
   b. The incidence of testing increases with annual salary.
   c. The objective is simple—to avoid turnover and to avoid selecting the wrong person for the job.
   d. The complete assessment, interview, and tests usually last about four hours.
   e. Approximately one-third of the time is taken up by the interview, with the balance devoted to the written tests.
   f. The client may specify some desirable characteristic that is a good indicator of success in the position or, conversely, may want to be alerted to any negative characteristic that would impede the candidate's performance.
   g. May include aptitude tests, interest inventories, personality tests, and honesty tests

14. Drug testing
   a. Because employment is a contractual relationship, prospective employers have the right to ask you to take a drug test as a condition of employment.
   b. Because you might jeopardize your chances of being considered for the position if you were to take offense, just take it in stride.

E. Follow-up
   1. You need to balance your presentation of yourself with your wish to find out whether you have the position.
   2. Healthcare organizations tend to make hiring decisions slowly.
   3. Try to be as patient as you can.
   4. If the decision to hire takes longer than 4 weeks, you may want to rethink whether you really want to work in a place that takes this long to make a decision.
   5. When you telephone the interviewer or company contact, you must strike the right balance.
   6. Try to sound enthusiastic, not desperate; confident, not arrogant; persistent, not pushy.
   7. A phone call every 2 weeks after the interviews is appropriate.
   8. The following questions are permissible points you might raise during a telephone call after the interviews:
      a. Do they need to schedule another interview?
      b. What is going on with the company in general?
      c. Is downsizing, expansion, or reorganization occurring?
      d. How do hiring decisions dovetail with the calendar?
      e. Are they going to hold off on an offer until after the fiscal year begins?
      f. How is the process coming?
      g. Have they been able to contact your references?
      h. What is the time frame?
      i. What in-house hurdles remain to be cleared before a decision is reached?
   9. Use a low-key plan to maintain contact and visibility
      a. Send an article on a topic that could prove useful to that person
      b. When you telephone to check on the status of the decision making, state your availability and willingness to provide more information.
   10. If at all possible, after you have interviewed, make an inside contact within the organization—perhaps someone you know professionally—who will be able to give you some helpful information.
   11. By knowing who makes the decisions about hiring for the position you want, you can make some reasonable assumptions about what kind of person the organization hopes to hire.
      a. In most cases, people hire people with whom they believe they can work well.
      b. Knowing who makes the hiring decisions does not give you license to contact them directly, especially if you are working with an intermediary.
   12. Do not go around people.
      a. You risk insulting the hiring manager.
      b. You risk offending the board members, or whomever else you contact.
      c. You risk seeming oblivious to how the game is played.

F. The job offer
1. Money
    a. "Money" really means total compensation: salary, bonus, benefits, deferred compensation.
    b. Check on state and local income and property taxes at the new location. Try the salary calculator at www.homefair.com
    c. Most compensation offers are negotiable.
    d. Negotiate a higher salary, perhaps by producing salary surveys indicating the earnings of individuals with your level of experience.
    e. Negotiate for a signing bonus or a moving expense allowance considerably higher than your actual moving expenses.
    f. Or you could accept the position with the provision that you will be guaranteed the salary you seek after a six-month review.
    g. If all else fails, accept the position like this:
        (1) "John [the boss], I am ready to go to work for Memorial Hospital. I accept the position right now if you can get the salary to $_____."
        (2) This approach gives John the chance to push for the salary change.
        (3) You have taken away the uncertainty of turning down his offer and given him the ammunition to clear the path for your contract and signing.
2. Opportunity
    a. The chance to expand the scope of your responsibilities, duties, or span of control.
    b. A chance to get away from a repressive management style, or a chance to run things your own way.
    c. If you are eager to pursue a new professional challenge that you deem an opportunity, be deliberate and thorough.
    d. Get the facts. Talk to people other than the ones to whom you have been introduced in the organization.
    e. Outsiders who have dealings with the facility or company can be helpful in characterizing its strengths, weaknesses, management organization; they are excellent sources of scuttlebutt.
    f. Ask about your career path.
3. Location
    a. Not only for recreational purposes after the workday ends, but also for the well-being of your family.
    b. A common mistake when evaluating location is to reject a position out-of-hand without ever making a site visit.
    c. You should remain flexible within a general region (such as the Southeast) and

population size (such as 100,000) and fill in the particulars after the site visit.
    d. In evaluating location, consider the general economic conditions of an area, demographic trends, quality of the school system, how you fit into the community, and the types of cultural activities.
    e. Location is also the factor on which a spouse exerts the greatest influence.
    f. Involve your spouse in the job change decision from the very beginning.
    g. If you are part of a dual-career marriage, one of you will have to compromise.
    h. When it comes to location, the whole family's opinion should be weighed heavily.
4. Verify the information with others who have had the job.
5. If you find that two of the three factors are very positive, then accepting the position will probably be a good move.
6. If only one factor is positive, pass and work toward getting a different, presumably better, offer.
7. If all three factors are positive, jump at the opportunity.
G. Employment transition
1. Beginning your new position is a continuation of your job search.
2. If you don't fit into the organization, you may lose the job you worked so hard to win.
3. Hold off on implementing changes too soon.
4. Assess the organization
    a. How do they do things?
    b. Who really runs the show?
    c. Adjust to the organization's culture
    d. View your new colleagues as allies.
    e. A positive and professional attitude.
5. Listen to what others say.
6. Pay attention to what the problems are.
7. New employees usually have a honeymoon period—use this time wisely.
8. Read in your spare time to find out all you can about your new organization and your particular function within in.
9. Resist getting involved in any political intrigue or gossip. Avoid this without seeming self-righteous. Get both sides of the story before making a decision.
10. Be courteous and friendly to everyone
11. When in doubt, cut it out.
12. Be businesslike and conduct yourself ethically.
13. Be visible: Meet with people in their office, let people know who you are, learn their names.
14. Focus on the work at hand: Solving problems and getting things done.
15. Resist importing too many ideas from your past organization. By constantly referring to your

past experience, you indirectly put down your current organization.

16. Unofficial rules can have the same weight as official rules.

H. Ending the job search
1. As a courtesy to your network and references, you should let them know that you have succeeded in finding the right job.
2. Notify all the members of your network once you have accepted a position.
3. Deactivate your candidacy with other organizations, and celebrate your success.
4. You should also use this opportunity to thank them for their contribution to your success.
5. Show your family your appreciation for their moral support and cooperation during the job search.

I. The student as job seeker
1. Experience is extremely important.
2. As a student, your objective is to get more experience relative to your peer group so that you can be more competitive.
3. You have to get as much experience as you can relative to your peer group to have the advantage in the job market.
4. The traditional road to experience in health care has been through internships.
5. Students are advised to treat the internship search as if it were a job search using all of the above techniques and advice.
6. Get the experience regardless of where the job is located.
7. Networking
   a. Obtain the alumni directory and call, write, or email all of the alumni currently in organizations or who have previously worked in those organizations where you would like to work.
   b. Look for things that you have in common.
   c. Seek help from your professors.
   d. Go to state, national, and local meetings.
   e. Seek out your elected leaders, chairman of the state hospital association, or any officer of a myriad of other organizations.
   f. Call them and engage them to help you, and let them know how much you appreciate their help.
   g. Tap into other people's networks.
8. You must have a degree of aggression to make networking effective.
9. Imagine yourself as an actor on stage. You have been given a role to play.
10. This role is not your normal self but merely a role, which will be temporary until you find a job.
11. Remember, lots of people have been where you are now in your career. They will be sympathetic and helpful.

12. But they can be neither of these unless you make contact with them.

III. WORKPLACE ETIQUETTE

A. General
1. Business etiquette puts social skills to work in business.
2. Benefits of etiquette
   a. Good manners allow one to make a positive impression.
   b. Being perceived as a professional enhances one's credibility.
   c. Allows one to feel relaxed and confident so the focus is on business.
   d. Polite protocol facilitates being a team player.
   e. Promotes comfortable interaction with others.

B. Meeting and greeting
1. How people are greeted influence how we are perceived.
2. Introductions
   a. When someone is not introduced, people feel uncomfortable or distracted.
   b. A = Authority.
      1. Say the name of the person who holds the position of most authority or importance first, regardless of gender and age.
      2. E.g. "Ms. Manager, I'd like you to meet Mr. New Employee."
   c. B = Basic.
      1. Keep it basic.
      2. You have to say each person's name only once.
      3. Avoid introducing everyone to each other.
   d. C = Clarify.
      1. If you can, provide some information about the people you are introducing.
      2. E.g. "Ms. Manager, I'd like you to meet Mr. New Employee. He comes to us from Good Samaritan Hospital, where he worked for 5 years. Ms. Manager has been our practice manager since last February."
3. Avoiding common faux pas
   a. When in doubt, don't use first names.
   b. If you don't know or if you forget the name of the person you are introducing, admit it.
   c. If someone neglects to introduce you, introduce yourself.
   d. When you are unsure which person has the position of most authority or importance, or if everyone's position is equal, introduce the person you wish to compliment first.
   e. Traditionally, you might introduce the elder person or woman.

f. When introduced, stand up and shake hands. Women should do this too.
   1. Move toward the person you are meeting, establish eye contact, look pleasant, and smile.
   2. Repeat the name of the person you've just met.
4. Introducing yourself: Have a planned and practiced way of describing who you are or what you do that is clear, interesting, positive, and well delivered.
5. Handshake
   a. Represents a traditional sign of trust.
   b. In the past, extending your hand in friendship demonstrated that you were unarmed.
   c. How to Shake Hands
      1. Say your name and extend your hand at a slight angle, with your thumb up.
      2. Touch thumb joint to thumb joint.
      3. Provide a firm handshake but not a bone-breaking one.
      4. About two or three pumps are enough.
      5. Greet disabled people in the same polite fashion that you would anyone else.
      6. You might ask a blind person, "Shall we shake hands?"
      7. You might extend your left hand if the person has an artificial right hand.
      8. If you get caught holding something, transfer the item and then shake hands.
6. The business card
   a. Your card represents you and should provide a professional image.
   b. It should be well designed and printed on quality paper.
   c. It's should not be too busy with extra information and graphics.
   d. Most important information: Name, title, address, phone number.
   e. Ensure the card is in good shape, not tattered, folded or flimsy.
   f. Ensure the card is readily available.
   g. Present your card at the appropriate time:
      1. Just before parting company.
      2. At the beginning of a meeting.
      3. Not during a meal.
   h. Personalizing the card by adding your home phone number in pen is a nice touch.
C. Small talk
   1. Contributes to one's credibility and ability to establish rapport; helps set clients at ease.
   2. Tuning-In (SOFTEN approach)
      a. S = Smile: a sign of friendliness and receptivity.
      b. O = Open posture: Appear attentive and face the speaker. Do not cross your arms or legs.

c. F = Forward lean: Leaning forward shows that you're alert. Don't invade the other person's space. Stay about an arm's distance away.
   d. T = Tone: Make your tone of voice show interest. Do not mumble, shout, or whisper.
   e. E = Eye Contact: Look directly at the speaker without staring.
   f. N = Nod: Indicates agreement or understanding of what is said. Avoid nodding too much.
3. Posture, eye contact, and gestures tell people that you are receptive to what they have to say.
4. Listening
   a. Create a setting in which you can listen.
   b. Tune out internal distractions—interfering thoughts and feelings.
   c. Monitor your body language.
   d. Reflect (mirror) back the person's words.
   e. Repeat or paraphrase what was stated, ask questions that clarify the comments, and offer words of encouragement or acknowledgment.
5. Topics to avoid
   a. Your health or someone else's health.
   b. Personal misfortunes.
   c. Income.
   d. Stories of questionable taste, dirty jokes, or gossip.
   e. Religion and highly controversial issues such as abortion.
   f. Intimate details about your personal life.
6. Temporal considerations
   a. Be punctual.
   b. Begin and end meetings on time.
   c. If events beyond your control make you late, inform the affected people and adjust the schedule.
   d. Give the person the option of canceling or rescheduling the meeting.
   e. Apologize for your delay when you arrive.
   f. Don't overstay your welcome.
   g. Don't stay longer than the business requires.
   h. Leaving on time is just as important as arriving on time.
D. Spatial diplomacy
   1. Doorway etiquette
      a. Generally, whoever gets to the door first opens it.
      b. Escorting a visitor: The host should try to get to the door first and hold it for the guest.
      c. It's polite to help anyone who needs help, e.g., someone carrying something.
      d. Tradition may be followed: A man holds the door for a woman or a young person opens the door for an elder person.

e. It's gracious to allow people to save face: If an older man would become upset if a woman doesn't allow him to hold a door, the woman should permit him to do so. The reverse is equally true.

f. Never allow a door to slam in someone's face.

g. Always thank someone who holds a door for you.

2. Revolving doors
   a. The host should lead the way by going first when entering or leaving.
   b. Once you have exited, wait for your party to join you.
   c. If more than one person is following you, wait until everyone has come through the revolving door.
   d. A slow walker should wait until most of the other traffic has cleared.
   e. If you happen to arrive immediately after a slow walker has entered the door, it's polite to either wait until she has exited or to slow your speed.

3. Elevator etiquette
   a. A host should walk a departing visitor to the elevator and wait with him until it arrives.
   b. A host who is accompanying the visitor to another floor should hold the elevator door and allow the guest to enter the elevator first.
   c. When leaving, the host should exit and hold the door for the guest while directing him where to go next.

4. Seating etiquette
   a. The host should indicate where the visitor should sit, and the visitor should wait for the host to do so before sitting down.
   b. The visitor should put a briefcase or purse on the floor, not on the host's desk.
   c. Sit up straight, don't slouch.
   d. Don't fidget, shift in your seat, or tap your feet.
   e. The host should sit next to the visitor if possible.

5. Proximity etiquette: A comfortable distance for people communicating in the workplace is approximately 3 feet, or about an arm's length away.

6. Taxi etiquette
   a. In some locations, you must call ahead rather than hail a cab on the street.
   b. To hail a cab, lean toward the street (do not step into it) and raise your hand.
   c. If a hotel doorman is present, allow him to perform this service.
   d. Doorman tip: $1; more if he helps you load luggage.

e. The one who arrived first gets the first cab.

f. Taxi fares: A flat rate, per person rate, or calculated by meter.

g. Taxi tip: 15 percent of the fare.

E. Office equipment etiquette
   1. Telephone
      a. Sound professional, pleased to hear from the caller, and ready to deal with the caller's concerns.
      b. Promptly and courteously answer: After the first ring but no later than the third.
      c. In a clear, pleasant voice, identify both yourself and your company.
      d. You're either in or out, available or not. Don't base your availability to talk on the identity of the caller.
      e. Callers are not favorably impressed if they are put through the third degree before they are allowed to talk with you.
      f. You should return telephone calls within 24 hours. If the person is not there, make sure you leave a message.
      g. Speak slowly and distinctly.
      h. Do not shout or raise your voice.
      i. Pay attention to your diction and grammar.
      j. Do not chew gum or eat while talking or listening on the phone.
      k. Be enthusiastic: Smile, or sound as if you're smiling.
      l. If you must sneeze or cough, turn your head, cover your mouth or the mouthpiece, and say, "Excuse me."
      m. Reduce distracting background noise, including interference on the line. If need be, switch to another location or call back.
      n. Holds and transfers
         1. Give the person a choice before putting the person on hold.
         2. When you return to the call, thank the caller for holding.
         3. If you put someone on hold, get back every 20 to 30 seconds or so to check if the person is still there. Let the person know what is happening.
         4. Before transferring a call, provide the extension in case of disconnection.
      o. Courtesy tips
         1. Apologize if you dial a wrong number.
         2. Identify yourself clearly.
         3. Ask if this is a good time to talk.
         4. When leaving a message, provide your phone number even if the person already has it.
         5. If using speaker phone or allowing a third person to listen in, let the person on the phone know at the beginning.
         6. Be organized.

7. Remember that the first call takes priority.
8. Deal with distractions.
9. Pay attention to your language.
10. Close the conversation with a thank you.
  p. Voice messages
    1. Don't use an answering machine to screen calls.
    2. It is much more polite to wait 10 minutes and call the person back than to pick up the phone after listening to the message.
    3. Identify yourself with your full name.
    4. Ensure the message is short and to the point.
  q. Leaving messages
    1. Listen to make sure you reached the person you dialed.
    2. Speak slowly and clearly, stating with your name and phone number.
    3. Make sure the messages you leave are intended for semipublic consumption.
    4. Repeat your name and phone number at the end.
2. Shared equipment
  a. Learn how to use the equipment properly. If you guess wrong, you may inconvenience others.
  b. Take turns.
  c. Clean up your mess before leaving the area.
  d. If it is empty, fill it.
  e. If it breaks, fix it or get it fixed.
  f. Do not take, borrow, or snoop through what isn't yours.
  g. Leave equipment ready for the next user.
3. Do not send unsolicited faxes.
4. Copier courtesy
  a. The person with the fewest number of copies to make gets priority.
  b. Check the paper supply after completing a job, and refill the copier if necessary.
  c. Do any necessary maintenance.
  d. Do not leave problems for the next person.
  e. Always remember to reset the machine after using it.
  f. Make sure that you take your original with you.
5. Computer access
  a. Try to coordinate projects on the computer so everyone knows in advance when the equipment is available.
    1. Be realistic about how much time you need.
    2. Respect office guidelines and timelines, and defer to projects with higher priority.
  b. Refill the paper supply in the printer, add toner, replenish the available supply of blank disks, and call the appropriate person when repairs are needed.
  c. Do not change the programming to suit your individual needs.
  d. Do not use someone else's disks or sign-on password without receiving permission.
  e. Do not read confidential plans, reports, or files.
  f. Remember to keep the area clean and to take all your papers with you when you leave.
6. Coffee machines
  a. If you drink from the coffee pot, help maintain it throughout the day.
  b. If you empty the pot, start a new one.
  c. Wipe up any spills.
  d. If you use the last of any supplies, get out refills or alert the appropriate person.
  e. If the system is pay as you go, make sure that you do.
F. Grooming
  1. The way you come across to others—created by dress and grooming.
  2. Appropriate, attractive packaging affects how one is perceived.
  3. Inappropriate or poor grooming is distracting and detracts from one's professional reputation.
  4. Grooming considerations:
    a. Hair is trimmed and well styled.
    b. Hair is clean and free of dandruff.
    c. Makeup is well designed and appropriately applied.
    d. Face is clean-shaven.
    e. Nose and ear hairs are trimmed.
    f. Fingernails are clean or polished.
    g. Amount of perfume or cologne is restrained.
    h. Teeth are polished.
    i. Breath is fresh.
    j. Glasses fit well and are clean.
    k. Posture is good–shoulders back, head up.
    l. Check the mirror periodically.
G. Attire
  1. Attire that calls attention to your body, positive or not, detracts from your skills, accomplishments, and contributions.
  2. Selection criteria
    a. Attire represents a nonverbal statement of your willingness to be a team player.
    b. Ensure it is appropriate for the job and the position.
    c. Consistent with what other people in the region, country, or organization wear.
    d. Appropriate for the season.
    e. Permits physical tasks to be performed comfortably.
    f. Suitable for the situation intended to be worn.

g. Fits suitably and looks good.

h. Able to sit down without the buttons pulling in front.

i. Attractive color.

j. Able to be worn often.

k. Communicates a professional message.

l. Buy the most expensive clothing that one can reasonably afford.

3. Wardrobe considerations

a. Differences in fabric, color, and styling all have an impact on the appropriateness of an outfit.

b. Woman's hosiery color: Nude, taupe, pale gray, bone, or one shade darker than skin tone.

c. Women should not wear sexy outfits to a company cocktail party.

d. Power colors: Navy, gray, charcoal, and black; brown should be avoided. Black can be intimidating.

e. Woman's shoes: Should be the color of her dress or skirt hemline or darker.

f. Man's tie: should extend to the belt. Contrast with color of jacket.

g. Man's suit jacket: Long enough to cover the buttocks.

h. Man's belt: Should match his shoes.

i. Man's shoes: Black shoes with gray, navy, or black suits.

4. Women's basic wardrobe

a. Suits: Black or gray, and navy.

b. Skirts: Three coordinating with jackets.

c. Dresses: One two-piece dress, one or more single-piece dress.

d. Blouses: Five solid-color blouses, two pastel or print blouses.

e. Scarf: Those that pick up colors from a suit.

f. Shoes: Pair of black, and navy or taupe pumps.

g. Black leather bag.

h. Belts: Black and navy.

i. Jewelry: Gold, silver, and good costume earrings, necklace, bracelet, pin, and good-quality watch.

j. Briefcase: Black, brown, or burgundy.

k. All-weather coat

5. Men's basic wardrobe

a. Suits: One navy, one charcoal gray, and one medium blue or gray. Two or three pin-striped or other subtle pattern suits.

b. Shirts: Six white cotton shirts, long-sleeved, and a blue or pin-striped shirt.

c. Ties: Five to eight solid, striped, or patterned silk ties.

d. Belts: Two black leather, and a brown or burgundy.

e. Shoes: One-two pair black, and a pair of brown or burgundy.

f. Jewelry: Tie tacks, tie clasps, and tie bars as appropriate; a good-quality watch.

g. Leather briefcase.

h. All-weather coat.

H. Gifts

1. Ability to handle gifts and other social niceties with finesse can improve one's professional image.

2. When professionally competent, social niceties are the polish on one's performance.

3. Ensure gift-giving is within organizational policy.

4. Ensure the situation conforms to organizational traditions.

5. Appropriate timing.

6. The gift should acknowledge the likes and dislikes of the recipient.

7. Cost of the gift is appropriate.

8. The gift itself is appropriate.

9. The main consideration is your own relationship with the recipient.

10. If the situation does not lend itself to a gift, a card may be appropriate.

11. A congratulations, thank-you, or a condolence card should include a handwritten note.

12. Occasions: Familial events—births, weddings, showers, and funerals—involving employees and their families.

13. You can observe a colleague's special birthday, e.g. 40th, even if you have ignored the day in other years.

14. A hostess gift is required every time you are treated to dinner at a co-worker's home. Boxed chocolates, packages of teas, party napkins, or flowers that are sent ahead of time or the following day.

15. Holiday cards are always appropriate, but they should have a general message, since not everyone celebrates religious holidays.

16. Give something of quality without excessive expense.

17. Should reflect the taste and desires of the recipient.

18. Avoid gifts with romantic connotations (such as long-stemmed roses) and highly personal gifts (such as clothing), and be careful about gag gifts.

19. Food: A generally appreciated gift that can be personalized to the recipient's taste.

20. Professional presents: Items such as a pocket calendar, a letter opener, a book, or bookends.

21. Presentation: Wrap the gift with appropriate paper. Write a short note and sign the card enclosed in an envelope. Present the gift in person, if possible.

22. Refusing a gift
  a. Be gracious while indicating the problem with the gift.
  b. E.g., "What a nice thought! However, since company policy prohibits my acceptance of this gift, I need to return it to you."
  c. If someone has deliberately sent an inappropriate gift, e.g. sexual overtones or implied business obligation—you want your refusal to tactfully communicate your displeasure at the situation.
  d. E.g., "I don't consider this gift appropriate. I am returning it to you," or "This gift is really not appropriate. Please don't send me any more presents."

23. Accepting a gift
  a. Remember to say thank you.
  b. Handle the gift with respect: Unwrap it carefully, admire the gift, if possible, and appear genuinely pleased.
  c. Find something positive—or at least pleasantly noncommittal—to say about the gift, such as "How nice of you to think of me."
  d. Write a thank-you note.

I. Entertaining clients
  1. Taking a client to a symphony concert or a baseball game is not the same as attending an official business meeting, but there is, nonetheless, a hidden agenda.
  2. Purpose: To get to know each other a little better outside the formal office environment, not to discuss business.
  3. You want the impression you make to be favorable, so that the next time you sit down to negotiate a contract or to place an order, the positive impact of your social time together may provide business dividends.
  4. Dress appropriately for the situation while maintaining a professional appearance.
  5. Attempt to ensure that the client has a good time.
  6. Make transportation and seating arrangements as required.
  7. Provide food and drinks.
  8. Be knowledgeable about the event you are attending and competent in performing any special skills it requires.
  9. React appropriately to performances by artists or players.
  10. Use the time to find out a little more about the client, interests, family, and personality.

J. Office parties
  1. Attend and be on time.
  2. Treat your managers with respectful friendliness.
  3. Look as if you are having fun.
  4. Limit talk about business.

  5. Don't flirt.
  6. Don't get drunk.
  7. Don't gossip or tell off-color jokes or stories.
  8. Send a thank-you note.

K. Dining
  1. The way applicants conduct themselves at a lunch shows how they will act in similar situations with the firm's important clients.
  2. The business lunch is much more than a meal; it's a test of manners.
  3. Lunch is the meal at which business is most likely to be transacted.
  4. You may encounter a slightly more formal setting at a business dinner.
  5. Making arrangements:
    a. Check out the food and the service beforehand.
    b. Ensure the atmosphere/ambiance is suitable and professional.
    c. Ensure you will not be rushed through the meal.
    d. Ensure enough time to discuss business.
    e. Call the guest a week or two in advance, offering a choice of possible locations, dates, and times.
    f. Ensure the restaurant knows the number in the party and the time of arrival.
    g. Provide clear directions to the restaurant, and explain where to wait for each other.
  6. Avoiding social faux pas
    a. The host pays for the lunch. When issuing the invitation, you can say, "Good Samaritan Clinic would like to take you out to lunch to celebrate the signing of the contract."
    b. It's polite to provide a reason for the lunch when inviting the guest.
    c. Let the guest know if anyone else is invited or if there are any materials you'd like the guest to bring along.
    d. The host should call the day before the luncheon to confirm the lunch with the guest or the guest's secretary.
    e. The host should plan to arrive at the restaurant before the guest. Ensures the reservations are in order and that the host can greet the guest on arrival.
    f. Call the guest's office if the guest is more than 15 minutes late.
    g. The host should wait to check his or her coat until the guest arrives.
    h. The maitre d' or hostess leads the way to the table, followed by the guest and then the host. When there is no hostess or maitre d', the host leads the way for the guest.
    i. The best seat goes to the guest, and the host sits to the left of that seat.
    j. The seat of honor is to the right of the host.

7. Server relations
   a. Pay attention to what your waiter or waitress looks like so you can recognize him or her later.
   b. Catch his or her eye or use a discreet wave of the fingers to request service. Do not snap your fingers to get his or her attention.
   c. Address the person by name if asked to do so, otherwise, use waiter, waitress, or server.
   d. Do not call someone Sweetie, Garçon, Boy, Dear, or Honey.
   e. As a guest, do not drink alcohol.

8. Ordering food
   a. As the host, suggest the restaurant's specialties and discuss what you might order to give your guest an idea of the price range of what you're eating.
   b. As a host, order in the higher price range.
   c. As a guest, order in the middle price range.
   d. Let the guest order first, and follow the guest's lead.
   e. If the guest orders soup or salad, the host should do the same. The same is true for dessert.
   f. Do not order foods that are too messy, e.g., lobster tail, French onion soup, or most forms of pasta.
   g. Do not share food.
   h. Do not be fastidious.

9. Utensils
   a. The more courses, the more utensils.
   b. Work your way through the utensils, from the outermost one to the innermost one on both sides.
   c. When you pause for bites or conversation breaks, put the utensils back on the entrée plate.
   d. Never rest the utensils half-on, half-off the plate.
   e. Forks on the left and knife and spoon on the right.
   f. On the left, from the outside in, may be a salad fork and then the entrée fork.
   g. On the right, from the outside in, are the dessert spoon and the knife.
   h. If you are still in doubt as to how to proceed, observe others.
   i. If you eat just slightly more slowly than they do, you might be able to follow their lead.
   j. If you happen to use the wrong utensil, do not panic or draw attention to your mistake.
   k. You can often substitute with the utensil you should have used, or you can quietly ask for a replacement.
   l. Do not become flustered or overwhelmed and ruin the meal by losing your perspective.

10. Place-setting
   a. Food dishes, including your bread and butter plate, are to your left. Remember this by the fact that "food" and "left" both have four letters.
   b. Your drink containers, including your coffee cup, are to the right. Both "drink" and "right" have five letters.
   c. Look to the left (four letters) for your fork (four letters) and to the right (five letters) for your knife and spoon (five letters).

11. Dining manners
   a. Any behavior that is unappetizing is automatically discourteous.
   b. Wait for everyone to be served before eating.
   c. Don't chew with your mouth open.
   d. Chew and swallow before speaking.
   e. Take small bites.
   f. Do not play with your food or wave it on your utensils.
   g. Keep your elbows off the table.
   h. Do not comb your hair (or do other grooming chores, including applying lipstick) at the table.
   i. Do not talk about gross things at the table.
   j. Do not criticize the food.
   k. Say please and thank you when passing food.
   l. Do not break crackers into your soup or hold a cracker in one hand and the soup spoon in the other.
   m. Do not blow on your coffee or soup; just give hot food or beverages time to cool.
   n. Do not chew ice cubes.
   o. Cup a lemon wedge in your hand before squeezing it to avoid squirting anyone.
   p. Discuss business after ordering.
   q. Keep papers off the table until after the entrée plates have been cleared.
   r. Do not push your plate away from you or stack dishes when you've completed your meal.

12. Gratuities
   a. Use a credit card: Makes paying quick, easy, and discreet; you also have a receipt for business purposes.
   b. A guest should not argue about who pays the bill.
   c. The guest should remember to say thank-you. Within two days send a handwritten note.
   d. Examine the bill to make sure the tip isn't already included, since this is the practice at some restaurants.
   e. For good service, a tip of 15 to 20 percent is appropriate.
   f. Pay the coatroom attendant $1 per coat and the garage attendant $1 to $2.

L. Gratitude
  1. Praise provides a good return on a minimal investment.
  2. Accept thanks and appreciation graciously to show respect for the person giving the praise; never take issue with the content of the remark.
  3. When in doubt, people should err slightly on the side of excess.
  4. Communicating praise
    a. Be consistent: Compliment everyone who deserves it; be nonsexist in your reasons for compliments.
    b. Be specific: Praise a specific action to make clear what you approve of, rather than issuing a blanket endorsement.
    c. Be direct and eliminate qualifiers: Qualifying a compliment detracts from it.
    d. Don't confuse praise with feedback: You generally don't want to give a compliment with one hand and take it away with the other.
      1. E.g. "You did a fine job on the briefing for the managers. It would have been even better if you had incorporated graphics."
      2. Don't attribute motives to the person you are complimenting. E.g. "Nice suit. Do you have a funeral or a job interview after work?"
    e. When appropriate, give praise in public or in writing. The impact increases dramatically. Putting praise in writing provides a permanent record.
    f. Be timely: No real reason to delay praise. It's a basic principle of behavior modification that immediate praise helps someone understand the connection between two events and encourages a repeat performance.
  5. Accepting praise
    a. Acknowledge the compliment. It should be the first step you take after receiving praise.
    b. Don't argue with or attempt to qualify the compliment. You're not only putting yourself down but also insulting the person giving the compliment by implying that he doesn't have sufficiently high standards.
    c. Even when you genuinely disagree with the reason for the compliment, don't insult the speaker.
    d. When possible, anticipate praise and prepare your response.
    e. Acknowledge the contributions of others.
  6. Power of gratitude
    a. Thank yous can help to personalize the business relationship.
    b. Can make you stand out from the crowd.
    c. Casts you in the role of a gracious and thoughtful individual.
    d. Thank yous can help you to demonstrate your attention to detail.
    e. It shows that you did not overlook the little things.
    f. Thank-yous can help further good public relations.
    g. You can use a thank-you note as a follow-up to establishing a business contact.
  7. Thank-you notes
    a. Timing is crucial as they lose their effectiveness rapidly.
    b. Ideally, you should send the note within 24 hours of the event that prompted it.
    c. If you have legible handwriting, a thank-you note should be handwritten.
    d. Use good quality note paper.
    e. Use the recipient's correct name and title.
    f. Keep your note short: Three to five sentences.
    g. Thank everyone who deserves it.
      1. Leaving someone out of the loop can cause more harm than not thanking anyone.
      2. If more than one person needs to be thanked, you can ask the recipient to convey your thanks to others.
      3. If everyone has equal status, send separate notes and make sure they all arrive on the same day.
      4. For a dinner thank-you, also thank the spouse.
    h. Use an appropriate closing.
    i. Read over the note to check for misspellings, grammatical errors, and omitted words.
    j. Sign your note, and send it promptly.
    k. Do not send a thank-you for a thank-you.
    l. Establish a file in which you save all the thank-you notes that you receive. It can help you when you are "stuck" while trying to write a thank-you of your own.

IV. COMMUNICATION

Communication is the process that involves the sharing of meaning.
  A. Elements of the communication process (see Figure 7-1)
    1. Source: The sender, originator of the communication message.
      a. The source may be a person, a group of people, a committee, a company, or a government.
      b. What the source chooses to communicate depends on the field of experience that affects the thoughts and feelings of the source.

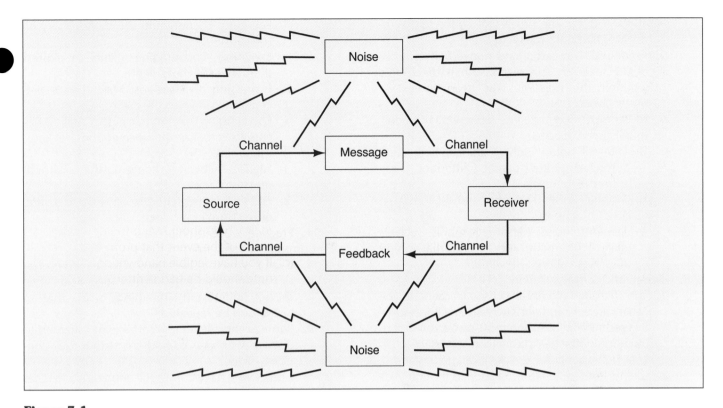

Figure 7-1

The communication process. Delmar/Cengage Learning.

c. The source is affected by past and present experiences: Mood, feelings, attitudes, beliefs, values, upbringing, sex, occupation, religion, as well as the environment.

d. One is best able to understand another's perspective by analyzing the person's field of experience; hence, the need for a complete physical, psychological, and social history.

2. Message: The communication process is initiated by the source sending some form of message. The message is the content that the source communicates. Messages have three components:

a. Meaning: Ideas or feelings. We have ideas such as how much to study for an exam. We have feelings such as hunger, anger, love, etc.

b. Symbols: Words or actions that represent meaning. To communicate meaning you must express ideas and feelings in the form of symbols.

(1) Encoding: The process of turning ideas and feelings into symbols.

(2) Intentional symbols: Consciously conveyed symbols serving a deliberate purpose.

(3) Unintentional symbols: Symbols conveyed, but not consciously selected.

(4) Receivers are more likely to pay attention to unintentional symbols as they may reflect the true feelings of the source.

(5) Approximately 70% of communication is nonverbal, 23% depends on tone of voice, and 7% comprises what is actually said.

c. Form/organization: This reflects the syntax and grammar of the message. One must put the symbols in an order that will facilitate comprehension.

3. Channel: The means by which symbols are conveyed.

a. Symbols are conveyed to one another via air waves, electromagnetic waves (light), and by touch.

b. Video: Television and cinema.

c. Audio: Radio, records, cassette, TV, and CDs.

d. Print: Periodicals, newspapers, and monographs.

e. Usually the more channels that are used to carry a message, the more likely the communication will be successful.

4. Receiver: The destination of the message. The purpose for which the message is conveyed.

a. The receiver, like the source, is affected by the receiver's field of experience.

b. Decoding: The process of converting symbols back into meaning.

5. Feedback: The verbal and nonverbal response of the receiver. This response tells the source whether the message was heard, seen, or understood.

6. Noise: Anything that interferes with the communication process.
   a. External noise: Sights, sounds, and other stimuli that draw people's attention away from the message.
   b. Internal noise: Thoughts and feelings that are distractions.
   c. Semantic noise: Message symbols, such as dialect, grammar, and accents that inhibit or prevent shared meaning.

B. Therapeutic communication
   1. The challenge of effective communication in the healthcare environment is twofold: Precise, descriptive technical information must be transmitted to members of the health care team as well as to clients, but in a manner the client can understand.
   2. Clients look to health professionals for comforting communication.
   3. The MA must always convey the message: "You are important. Your concerns are worthwhile and you can trust in my willingness and ability to help you."
   4. Provide immediate attention to the client; use the client's name and always indicate what the client can expect and offer explanations as needed.
   5. A way to communicate empathy is through verbal disclosure, a touch, or a gesture.
   6. Touching can be a powerful mode of therapeutic communication; however, it must be done tactfully and appropriately.
   7. Sensitivity and privacy are required when communicating with clients.
   8. Unpleasant information is typically delivered by the provider; however, the MA may be consulted regarding the best approach.
   9. Provide the opportunity for negative expression without retaliation.
   10. Facilitative communication techniques
       a. Accepting: Affirming the client's perceptions, feelings, and comments through eye contact and nodding.
       b. Reflecting: Encouraging clients to think through and answer their own questions.
       c. Mirroring: Repeating what the client has said to demonstrate that you understand.
       d. Clarification: Encouraging the client to explain ideas and feelings more clearly.
       e. Recognize: Demonstrating awareness of the client, especially positive, healthy behaviors.
       f. Focusing: Encouraging the client to stay on topic.
       g. Exploring: Encouraging clients to express themselves in more depth.
       h. Expressing observations: Making your perceptions known to the client.
       i. Encouraging communication: Asking clients to verbalize their perceptions, feelings, thoughts.
       j. Silence: Allowing clients to think without pressure to speak.
       k. Offering self: Offering to be with, to assure, or to console the client.
   11. Practice active listening

C. Communication barriers
   1. Clients, who may be in awe of the health professional, are often embarrassed to indicate they do not understand something, or ask that an instruction be repeated.
   2. Some clients feel uncomfortable or ashamed to discuss symptoms or body parts that they consider private.
   3. Clients who have communication disabilities are easily seen as intellectually inferior. The health professional, therefore, must guard against insulting the client's intelligence.
   4. The MA should observe for nonverbal cues that suggest that a client has been overwhelmed by information. Bad news is especially distressing and overwhelming.
   5. Withdrawal may occur. When the client does not respond to communication, the provider should be notified.
   6. Ineffective communication techniques
      a. Advising: Telling the client what you believe should be done.
      b. Minimizing feelings: Making light of the client's distress or discomfort.
      c. Defending: Protecting self, others, and the institution from criticisms.
      d. Responding stereotypically: Using clichés when responding to clients.
      e. Approval/disapproval: Overtly approving or disapproving client behaviors.
      f. Agree/disagree: Overtly agreeing or disagreeing with a client's thoughts, feelings, or perceptions.
      g. Reassuring: Indicating to the client that there is no need to worry or be anxious.
      h. Requesting rationales: Asking clients to provide reasons for their behavior.
      i. Probing: Discussing a topic the client has no desire to discuss.
      j. Changing topic: Demonstrating your desire not to discuss a topic by changing the subject.

V. PSYCHOSOCIAL ASPECTS OF THE PATIENT-PROVIDER RELATIONSHIP

A. The patient and sick role behavior
1. Patient needs: To interact effectively with clients, it is important to understand basic human needs.
   a. Abraham Maslow's Hierarchy of Needs: Lower level needs must generally be satisfied before higher level needs are pursued (see Figure 7-2).
      (1) Physiological need: Oxygen, food, water, sleep, and sex.
      (2) Safety need: Security, protection, shelter, freedom from anxiety.
      (3) Social need: Love, belonging, freedom from loneliness, alienation.
      (4) Self-esteem need: Self-worth, recognition, respect.
      (5) Self-actualization need: Meeting one's potential, self-fulfillment, creativity, spirituality.
   b. Needs, in part, are conditioned by one's social, cultural, and environmental background.
   c. Personality development is, to some degree, determined by the importance one places for each need.

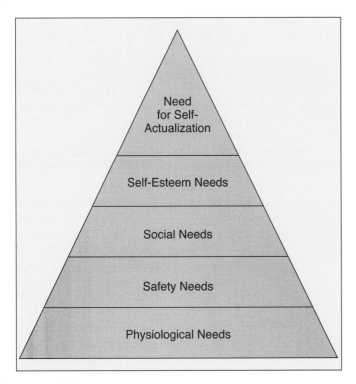

Figure 7-2

Maslow's Hierarchy of Needs (Adaptation based on Maslow's Hierarchy of Needs.) Delmar/Cengage Learning.

   d. It is possible to better understand and interact with the client if the needs that motivate the person's behavior can be determined, because behaviors are motivated by a desire to satisfy these needs.
   e. Assuming the patient role may interfere with any or all of these needs, especially safety, social, and self-esteem needs.
      (1) Adopting the sick role often results in the loss of self-assuredness, autonomy, and privacy.
      (2) The loss of autonomy is common as the patient role involves giving up control over time, circumstances, and outcome.
      (3) During the visit the client will disclose personal information, be prodded and poked, thus potentially causing the client to feel uncomfortable and vulnerable. The client may, therefore, experience the loss of privacy.
   f. Client's perception of welfare is determined by the level of experience of both social values and natural goods. Illness or disability may interfere with either or both.
      (1) Primary social values include rights, liberties, powers, opportunities, income, wealth, and dignity.
      (2) Primary natural goods include health, vigor, intelligence, and imagination.
   g. The MA must come to understand the needs, concerns and common reactions of clients in order to develop a professional, nonjudgmental attitude.
2. Anxiety and stress are common responses to illness, which may be characterized by feelings of uneasiness, fearfulness, worry, and nervousness.
3. Unconscious defense mechanisms: Defense mechanisms serve to protect the mind from anxiety, guilt, or shame.
   a. Introjection—Adopting the feelings of others.
   b. Projection—Ascribing to another, one's own feelings as if they had originated in the other person.
   c. Reaction formation—Behaving in the opposite to one's actual feelings to overcome undesirable impulses.
   d. Sublimation—Diverting unacceptable thoughts, feelings, and impulses into acceptable behaviors.
   e. Denial—Unconsciously avoiding the reality of an unpleasant or disturbing feeling, thought, or situation.
   f. Regression—Returning to former behavior or more immature behavior as the result of, and to escape stress or anxiety.

g. Repression—Putting unpleasant thoughts, feelings, or events out of one's mind.
h. Dissociation—Disconnecting emotional significance from specific ideas or events.
i. Rationalization—Justifying one's thoughts, feelings, or behavior to avoid admission of ulterior motives.
j. Substitution—Making up for an area of deficiency by concentrating on a more easily attainable goal.
k. Displacement—Shifting an impulse from a threatening object to a nonthreatening one.
l. Compensation—Overemphasizing a trait to make up for a perceived or actual failing.
m. Identification—Mimicking the behavior of another to cope with feelings of inadequacy.
n. Suppression—Deliberately forget or avoid dealing with an unpleasant situation.

4. One's capacity to deal with stress will determine whether the effects of illness are overcome or exacerbated.

5. Becoming a patient and the ability to return to society is influenced by gender, age, education, and income, as well as the following:
   a. Ability to redefine one's value system affected by the illness.
   b. Ability to interact effectively in a dependency relationship.
   c. Ability to interact with health professionals as a group.
   d. Ability to cope with the reactions of societal members. This is often based on:
      (1) Societal concepts of health.
      (2) Preconceived notions of the client's problems.
      (3) The visibility of signs and symptoms.
      (4) Societal knowledge of the prognosis.

6. Sustaining an illness or injury forces the client to adopt the sick role, which according to Parsons (1951), a medical sociologist, involves two rights and two duties:
   a. Right 1: Exemption from responsibility for the incapacity.
   b. Right 2: Exemption from normal social obligations.
   c. Duty 1: Obligation to make every effort to get well.
   d. Duty 2: Seek professional help and cooperate to achieve wellness.

7. Continuing the sick role may, however, generate certain benefits:
   a. Escape from fear of reestablishing responsibility.
   b. Financial gain: Workers' compensation or disability insurance.
   c. Social gain: Manipulating family and friends for sympathy and personal attention.

8. Losses associated with adopting the sick role
   a. An illness or injury entails some form of loss. The loss may be physical, psychological, or social.
   b. The significance of a loss is often determined by the pathology of the condition, the change in one's social role resulting from the condition, and one's ability to cope.
   c. Disorders that affect appearance can be quite disabling because of the close association among appearance, body image, and selfworth, as well as the social sanctions imposed by society for appearance that deviates from the norm.
   d. Hospitalization disrupts one's personal life, especially regarding family, friends, and work associates, as well as the loss of income and increased medical expenses.
   e. Hospitalization also signals to clients that they may be losing the battle imposed by the illness, which can be psychologically defeating.
   f. The sense of privacy is often lost; therefore, MAs must honor the client's privacy.
   g. Clients also lose their sense of independence.
   h. The client's condition may create social stigmas. The feeling associated with stigma can exacerbate the client's condition and make it difficult to find others with whom they can share their feelings.
   i. The outpatient experiences the difficulty of being ill, but not necessarily appearing ill, and can be stigmatized by both ill and healthy people.
   j. Illness and injury creates uncertainty about the future. This often results in anxiety causing some clients to become extremely rigid or conservative in their outlook.

9. Terminally ill and dying clients experience more profound stresses and exhibit behaviors that can be especially challenging.
   a. These behaviors have been described by Dr. Elisabeth Kúbler-Ross as the Stages of Dying:
      (1) Denial—Direct denial or periods of disbelief. This is generally a temporary defense. MAs should listen and not force clients to acknowledge or accept their circumstances.
      (2) Anger—Clients may suddenly realize what is really happening. At this stage they may become "problem patients" and are resentful. Rage and temper tantrums may occur.
      (3) Bargaining—Clients attempt to make deals with providers, God, or family. Clients may become more cooperative

and congenial. MAs should not be a party to bargaining.

    (4) Depression—The client may show signs of depression such as withdrawn behavior, sobbing, and lethargy. These are normal behaviors considering that the client's body is deteriorating, financial burdens may be increasing, pain is unbearable, and relationships will soon be severed.

    (5) Acceptance—Clients accept their fate. Again the client may withdraw and wish to be left alone. At this stage the client's family usually requires more support than the client.

  b. There is no standard time period, sequence, or pattern associated with the dying process because each person, as an individual, progresses uniquely.

  c. Although these stages relate to the dying process, many experts have generalized them to the grieving process as well.

B. The provider role

  1. Health professionals must be conscious of the unequal status posed by the provider-patient relationship. Clients should not be undermined by your helping role, but empowered by it to increase their likelihood of participating in their care.

  2. Elements of a caring relationship

    a. Concern for the client's well-being

      (1) Attend to client's personal hygiene needs.

      (2) Personal comfort needs.

      (3) Personal interest/preference needs.

      (4) Expanding awareness needs.

    b. Responsibly carrying out one's ethical duties.

    c. Respect for each person's individuality: The client should not be viewed as just a person with a disease, but as an individual whose mental, emotional, and social status has been affected by illness.

    d. Knowledge regarding what is important to that person: Avoid using your own values as a standard for others. This information can be obtained from four sources:

      (1) The client (by asking and observing behavior).

      (2) Family and friends.

      (3) The medical record.

      (4) Other health professionals.

    e. Positively interacting with the client

      (1) Get away from distractions.

      (2) Sit down and give the client your undivided attention; use eye contact.

      (3) Refrain from comments regarding how busy you are.

      (4) Do not permit interruptions unless warranted.

    f. Assisting the client to adapt to the experience of being a patient.

    g. Demonstrate empathy—Attempt to adopt the view of another person relative to their situation and experience.

      (1) To help develop an attitude of empathy, try to remember an experience similar to the client's that you experienced.

      (2) The more we see ourselves as similar to one another, the more likely we are to accept potential differences.

  3. Assume that the client will be cooperative.

  4. Sounding confident promotes the perception of competence.

  5. Encourage and positively reinforce proper client behavior where appropriate.

  6. The health professional must never imply that all will be well. The challenge is to help the client develop his or her old body image and value system or discover one that is realistically satisfactory.

  7. The MA significantly influences the client's perception of the medical office. Perception drives attitudes, and attitudes drive behavior. Research demonstrates that the manner in which health professionals interact with clients can, in itself, promote wellness or aggravate illness.

  8. Professional relationship difficulties

    a. Dependence: Emotional distance must always be great enough to facilitate the client's independence and autonomy.

      (1) Transference (detrimental dependence): Overdependence often based on excessive insecurities which can develop into a neurotic need to cling to another to the point at which the professional is no longer helpful to the client.

      (2) Constructive dependence: Dependence based on mutual respect to come together to achieve a desired outcome and who can sever the relationship if it becomes non-beneficial.

    b. Countertransference: The health professional responds to the client in a personal manner similar to that of a sibling or son or daughter.

    c. Overidentification: Difficulty seeing the client as an individual can arise, often creating the "I-know-how-you-feel" reaction that can be helpful or just as easily detrimental.

      (1) Client strongly personifies a stereotype.

      (2) Client strongly reminds the provider of someone else.

      (3) The client's experience is so similar to the provider's it is considered identical.

d. Personal biases
   (1) Personal bias describes one's feelings concerning a person or thing that influences the interpretation of it.
   (2) Prejudice is an adverse attitude toward a person by virtue of belonging to a particular group having objectionable characteristics.
e. Referrals: Clients should be referred under the following circumstances:
   (1) When required treatment is beyond the scope of the provider's training or experience.
   (2) When there are personality conflicts between the client and provider.
   (3) When there is a detrimental level of dependency between the client and provider.
9. Cultural influences
   a. Everyone brings different cultural, social, and ethnic biases. MAs must be aware of their biases and how those biases may interfere with objectivity and acceptance of clients.
   b. Distance awareness: Culturally defined distances between people during communicating and interaction. Providing medical care will almost invariably interfere with some person's social distance or personal space parameters, especially within the intimate and personal domains where most of health care is conducted.
      (1) Intimate distance: Physical contact
      (2) Personal distance: 1.5 to 4 feet
      (3) Social distance: 4 to 12 feet
      (4) Public distance: 12 to 25 feet
   c. Time awareness: The right time and the amount of time is relative according to cultural norms.
C. Therapeutic interaction
   1. The therapeutic relationship serves to assist the client to grow and resolve problems associated with an illness or injury. This is in contrast to a social relationship which serves to provide mutual benefits to both parties.
   2. A client is confronted with a new language, new technology, and new people and places that can bring about feelings of insecurity and inferiority or "culture shock."
   3. Maximizing client comfort will enhance the client's ability to direct individual energies toward healing.
   4. The MA must be cognizant of the client's physical safety as a result of emotional instability.
   5. The terminally ill client
      a. Most terminal illnesses are accompanied by gradual losses in strength, endurance, mobility, and sensation. Helping the client and family adjust to these losses is important.
      b. Support for the client and family are the major objectives of care in dealing with the terminally ill client.
      c. The health professional may need emotional support as well, the provider will lose a valued client relationship too.
      d. Communicating with the terminally ill client may be difficult because the process of dying is psychologically and physically stressful for the client and loved ones.
      e. Common fears include the fear of isolation, pain, dependence, and death itself.
      f. The MA should be willing to listen if the client expresses the need for discussion.
      g. The terminally ill client will likely experience some or all of the stages of dying.
   6. The angry client
      a. Anger and hostility are often caused by the medical condition. The goal of the MA is to calm the client and to contain the situation.
      b. Clients who lose much autonomy are prone to anger. Anger that is poorly managed may result in aggression.
      c. The MA should not get caught in the circle of anger, but should remain calm, objective, firm, and direct.
      d. The MA should never give in to unreasonable demands; however, public displays of anger in front of other clients should be extinguished without further inciting the client. The following is recommended:
         (1) Do not get upset. Do not take the client's anger personally.
         (2) Do not interrupt an irrational line of reasoning; just listen.
         (3) Keep your tone calm and in control.
         (4) If the client is loud and disruptive, lead the client to a quiet and private area to discuss the problem.
         (5) Mirror the client's statements of anger to exhibit your understanding of the problem.
         (6) If the client refuses to calm down, ask him or her to wait a few moments alone in an exam room. This may have a calming effect; however, allowing the patient to wait too long may have the opposite effect.
         (7) A psychiatric consult may be indicated.
   7. The sensory–impaired client
      a. For hearing–impaired and foreign language speaking clients, an interpreter my be necessary; otherwise, position yourself directly in front of the client and speak slowly (see Figure 7-3).

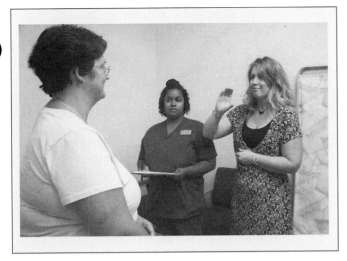

Figure 7-3

When working with an interpreter, the hearing impaired patient should be able to see both the medical assistant and the interpreter. Delmar/Cengage Learning.

b. For the sight impaired, the MA should ask the client, "How can I be of assistance?" rather than taking the client's hand or arm and directing her.

c. When communicating with sensory impaired clients, the MA should be open, flexible, and supportive.

8. Children: Most people must make an effort to adjust to being ill, but this can be more problematic for children, who may not understand their situation and may even feel that illness is a means of punishment.

a. Be aware of your feelings toward children. They can sense how you feel.

b. The MA should establish a friendly relationship with children.

c. Speak to children in quiet, pleasant tones while kneeling down to meet their level.

d. Use language (without clichés) that is appropriate to the child's age.

e. Allow children to choose in situations in which any choice will be correct.

f. Allow children to assist in their treatment without losing control.

g. The longer children have to wait, the more irritable they become.

h. Children tend to regress when ill.

i. Be truthful to children and help them deal with their fears and feelings. Explain what you are going to do and why; do so as close to the time of the procedure as possible.

j. Never shame a child and do not use labels such as baby or sissy.

k. Offer rewards such as stickers, inexpensive toys, and the like.

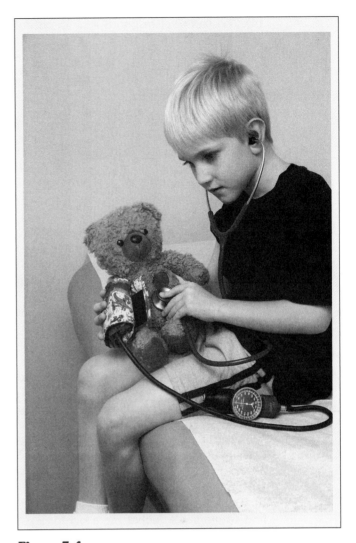

Figure 7-4

Allowing the child to play with equipment is a way to gain the child's cooperation. Delmar/Cengage Learning.

l. If safe, allow child to play with equipment to be used (see Figure 7-4).

m. Demonstrate the procedure on a doll.

n. Describe sensations the child may feel during or after the procedure.

o. Do not provide more information than is necessary.

p. Infants should be comforted by being held at each visit and after painful procedures.

q. Developing trust in infants: Three C's—*consistency* of approach, *constancy* of presence, and *continuity* of care.

(1) An infant expresses need through generalized behavior.

(2) The caregiver responds, satisfying the infant's need.

(3) The infant predicts the caregiver's response and repeats the behavior.

(4) The caregiver responds in a consistent manner, satisfying the infant's need.

(5) The infant develops trust and when the need recurs is confident that the caregiver will respond appropriately.

r. Temperaments of babies

(1) Difficult: Fussy, easily upset, finicky.

(2) Slow to warm up: Interacts cautiously, responds slowly to others.

(3) Easy: Cheerful, is easily occupied, outgoing.

9. The adolescent client: Adolescents are caught between childhood and adulthood; as a result, they often demand independence, yet require the comfort and consoling frequently afforded children.

a. Permit privacy and the right to be examined in the parent's absence.

b. Be prepared that adolescent clients may not have accurate information regarding sex.

c. Treat adolescents with respect and dignity.

d. Set limits that are fair and consistent.

10. The elderly client: The elderly are presented with myriad problems and challenges associated with aging ranging from physical disability to social isolation.

a. Allow additional time for tasks we complete easily and quickly.

b. Afford the elderly physical and environmental comforts.

c. As humans are creatures of habit, the elderly find comfort in a routine, so allow for a set schedule.

d. Do not be overattentive or overprotective.

e. Afford the elderly as much independence as possible.

11. The frightened client

a. Denial of fear is a common defense mechanism.

b. Frightened clients are often uncooperative, because to accept help is to acknowledge that the fear exists. This is especially true among male clients.

c. Recognize, accept, and help the client deal with the fear.

d. Afford as much control over the situation as possible.

e. Intense fear can bring about a panic response causing the person to withdraw. Act for the person.

12. Depressed clients

a. The client experiences feelings of dread, gloom, hopelessness, and negative self-worth.

b. Reactive depression: Depressive response to the loss of anything having significant meaning.

(1) Symptoms include weight loss, increased depression later in the day, insomnia, and decreases in activity and metabolic processes.

(2) Therapeutic interactions include sympathy and support, attentive listening, and demonstrating interest in the client's needs.

c. Endogenous depression: Depression that originates from within, without any recognizable source. It tends to be cyclical as with the seasons and holidays. Symptoms include weight loss and decreased activity as the day progresses.

d. Involutional depression (melancholia): Depressive episodes that typically occur during middle-age or later. Personality changes include behavioral rigidity, over-conscientiousness, and emotional instability. Symptoms include depression, feelings of guilt, obsession with death, and general irritability.

e. Manic depression (bipolar affective disorder): Characterized by alternating periods of severe depression and excessive well-being and hyperactivity. Symptoms include difficulty in maintaining a coherent conversation, extremely short attention span, mispronouncing words, hyperactivity, and insomnia.

f. A nonthreatening environment that provides security to freely express feelings is often therapeutic.

13. Suicidal clients

a. Suicide is often the final response to depression.

b. Clients often verbally test or disclose their intentions.

c. Four stages to contemplating suicide:

(1) Frustration, anger, and hostility are directed inwardly when needs are not being met.

(2) The situation becomes so stressful, panic manifests itself causing the client to seek escape.

(3) The client makes efforts to communicate the situation or sense of helplessness.

(4) If no one intervenes, feelings of unworthiness are perceived to be confirmed, and the client begins the suicidal process and prepares a plan to commit suicide.

d. Common behaviors include past suicide attempts, arranging one's affairs, giving away important possessions, attempting to right wrongs, or even saying good-bye to loved ones.

e. Threats or attempts should be taken seriously: Listen, avoid minimizing problems, demonstrate empathy, and avoid arguments. Seek professional advice or action.

14. Sexually suggestive clients
    a. Sexual suggestiveness usually indicates insecurities over one's sexuality and is a way of seeking reassurance.
    b. Maintain a positive and professional demeanor regarding sexuality. Address the behavior, but do not attack the person.
    c. Express the normalcy of sexual needs and desires, but emphasize that certain behaviors are unacceptable.
    d. Clients who have adopted altered sexual images (often resulting from surgery) are in need of assurances regarding their attractiveness.
    e. Never become sexually involved with clients.

15. Drug-dependent clients
    a. Drug dependency generally can be ascribed to biological, psychological, and cultural forces creating a myriad of causal factors such as lack of self-esteem, inability to deal with life stressors, lack of responsibility, and perhaps emotional problems.
    b. Do not belittle or rebuke clients for their behavior; attempt to exhibit compassion, empathy, and patience,
    c. Attempt to involve their family in their treatment.

16. Mentally impaired clients
    a. Are often in a state of confusion and disorientation.
    b. Gently correct the confusion unless doing so makes the client more agitated, violent, or disoriented.
    c. Correcting the confusion often makes the client less frightened.
    d. Such clients should be treated kindly but not condescendingly. Exercise gentle authority to instill a sense of security.

17. Abusive and abused clients
    a. Phases of violence
       (1) Triggering: A stressor precipitates verbal aggression or threats.
       (2) Escalation: The threat of aggression heightens as the perpetrator becomes more enraged.
       (3) Crisis: The perpetrator loses control over anger and resorts to physical aggression.
       (4) Recovery: The perpetrator calms down and returns to the pretriggering state.
       (5) Postcrisis: The perpetrator will either rationalize the behavior and/or attempt to make amends and promise not to be abusive again.
    b. Physical injuries should be treated promptly.
    c. Resource material should be available to refer clients to agencies skilled in handling such problems.
    d. Focus on the victim and provide assurances of self-worth.
    e. Observe the abuser's personal space to avoid being perceived as a threat; accept the abuser's feelings, but not the violent behavior.

18. Illiterate clients
    a. Communicate orally using simple, direct language.
    b. Ask patients to repeat the information you communicated to them.
    c. Demonstrate procedures for the patient; have the patient demonstrate the procedure.
    d. Use visual models to illustrate a procedure or condition. There is a growing body of patient education material that uses pictures effectively, e.g., medication instructions.
    e. Provide literature that includes pictures with simply written captions, i.e., at second grade reading level.
    f. Pictures should be closely linked to the text they represent so that readers or listeners connect the two in their minds.
    g. They should be simple, with a minimum of distracting details.
    h. People with low literacy skills are especially vulnerable to being distracted by details that do not relate to the picture's purpose.
    i. The MA can make drawings while talking to patients. These can be very simple, even crude. If the patient takes the drawings home, they will be reminders of what the MA said.

19. Interacting with significant others
    a. Family and friends form an emotional support group for the client and should not be discounted. The MA should administer to the needs and questions of the client's loved ones.
    b. In most cases, the wishes of the client should be addressed regarding loved ones.
    c. Young children need to be accompanied by an adult; however, as children approach adolescence, they require more autonomy and privacy.
    d. Waiting friends and relatives should be periodically notified of the progress of the client and informed of any delays.
    e. Family and friends are an important factor in the client's healing; their concerns can be as important to successful treatment as the client's.

VI. PATIENT EDUCATION

A. Learning needs assessment: Identify the patient's learning needs. Things to consider include the following:
  1. Patient knowledge of the American healthcare system and its workings.
  2. Current knowledge of the disorder.
  3. Desire to learn more about the disorder.
  4. Specific information needs required for informed consent.
  5. Benefits of a treatment regimen.
  6. Side effects of a medication.
  7. Demonstration of a procedure.
  8. Ethnic and cultural aspects.
  9. The patient's readiness to learn: Is the person motivated to learn? Does the person want to understand how the treatment will help? Is the person too anxious, exhausted, or in too much pain to concentrate on learning?
  10. Limitations that could interfere with learning or treatment (e.g., language, financial resources, time constraints, etc.). Attempt to resolve any limitations before beginning an education program.

B. Teaching plan
  1. Develop a teaching plan that is a well organized, written presentation identifying what the patient is to learn and how you will present the information.
  2. Invite the patient's family to the teaching sessions to help ensure the program is followed.
  3. The teaching method should be based on the patient's preferred learning style, e.g., written material (verbal), video (visual), or practice (kinesthetic).
  4. Demonstrate and have the patient demonstrate the best method when teaching procedures.
  5. Use analogies: Using the familiar to explain the new.
  6. Prepare learning objectives.

C. Implementation and evaluation
  1. Schedule learning sessions with the patient and family.
  2. Invite specialists to assist in the teaching as appropriate (e.g., dietitian, physical therapist, pharmacist, etc.).
  3. Follow up as needed with phone calls, home visits, questionnaires, and the like.
  4. Determine the extent to which the patient has achieved the learning objectives.
  5. If the patient experiences a setback (e.g., discontinues a diet), reassess the patient, evaluate the teaching plan, update it, and reimplement it.

D. Cultural considerations
  1. Treat patients as individuals while respecting their culture.
  2. Establish rapport: Patients are more likely to learn from you if they like and trust you.
  3. Use the patient's primary language if possible—use an interpreter when necessary.
  4. Discuss the patient's cultural perspectives on illness and treatment.
  5. Rather than shout, speak softly and clearly when providing instructions.
  6. Reduce any noise that may interfere with the communication process.
  7. Avoid rushing.
  8. Use simple, brief, and direct sentences and questions.
  9. Repeat instructions using different words.
  10. Use more literal expressions, such as *swallow* rather than *take.*
  11. Avoid idioms (e.g., why rather than how come, better than nothing, start from scratch, etc.).
  12. Attempt to explain the reason for the symptom before discussing a treatment regimen.
  13. Consider the patient's explanation of why the illness developed and how it might be treated.
  14. When providing explanations, use gestures and simple lay terms rather than technical medical terminology: Repeat key words.
  15. Explain the steps in a procedure in sequence.
  16. Use props and diagrams to explain procedures.
  17. Observe how the patient responds to your instructions.
  18. Make it easy for the patient and family to contact you for additional information.
  19. Recognize that patients from diverse cultures may have legitimate reasons for noncompliance that are consistent with their cultural values.

E. Documentation: Make a chart entry noting the relevant details of the assessment, plan, implementation, and evaluation of the patient education episode.

CHAPTER 8

Health Care Law

I. INTRODUCTION

A. Law defined: General rules of conduct that are enforced by government through a system of penalties.

B. Functions
   1. Remedy: To right wrongs that have been committed.
   2. Punish: To enforce penalties as a means of preventing or discouraging wrongs.
   3. Regulate: To control or direct according to rules, principles, methods, or standards.
   4. Benefit: To benefit society, e.g., Social Security payments.
   5. Contractual enforcement: To enforce legal agreements.

C. Sources of law
   1. Common law: Derived from custom, biblical law (Ten Commandments), English law (Law of the King), and judicial decisions emanating from court trials.
   2. Statutory law: Derived from federal and state legislation.
   3. Administrative law: Public law issued by administrative agencies serving to administer the enacted laws of the state and federal government.
   4. Constitutional law: Derived from the U.S. Constitution, which defines the structure and function of federal, state, and local government.

D. Classifications of law
   1. Civil law: Wrong committed against a person or property.
   2. Criminal law: Wrong committed against the state whereby the welfare and safety of the public are at stake.
   3. Crimes are acts forbidden by law or omission of acts required by law.
      a. Misdemeanor: A crime that is punishable by imprisonment in a house of correction or jail for less than one year.
      b. Felony: A crime that is punishable by death or imprisonment in a state penitentiary.

II. LICENSURE AND ACCREDITATION

A. Licensure, certification, and registration
   1. Licensure: This is the strongest form of professional regulation and a mandatory process whereby the state has verified that the incumbent has met the minimum standards required by law. A license authorizes and protects the use of a recognized professional job title such as MD, RN, etc.
   2. Certification: This is a voluntary process that identifies a health professional as having achieved minimum standards (usually through examination) established by a professional organization.
   3. Registration: Generally this is a voluntary process that identifies a health professional as listed on a registry, but may also involve a process similar to certification or licensure. A person may be permitted to perform the same or similar functions as a licensed practitioner; however, the registered person may not use the title afforded and protected under licensure.

B. Medical Practice Act: State statute found in all 50 states that defines the practice of medicine, licensing requirements, and guidelines for license revocation or suspension. All practicing physician providers must be licensed.
   1. Common requirements for licensure
      a. Graduation from an accredited medical school.
      b. Successful completion of an internship.
      c. Passing a recognized licensing exam.
      d. Demonstration of good moral character.
   2. Methods of gaining licensure
      a. Written examination: Passing a state's written examination.
      b. Endorsement: A state's acceptance of a delineated national examination score.
      c. Reciprocity: A state's acceptance of another state's licensing requirements.
   3. Reasons for license revocation or suspension
      a. Conviction of a crime.
      b. Unprofessional conduct.
      c. Incapacity.

C. Nurse Practice Act: Similar in nature to the Medical Practice Act although specific to nursing.

D. Regulatory issues
1. CON (Certificate of Need): A process whereby certain healthcare organizations seek approval, based on need, to add or expand services, or acquire capital in excess of a specified threshold.
2. Clinical Laboratory Improvement Act of 1988 (CLIA): Any facility performing quantitative, qualitative, or screening assays on materials derived from the human body are subject to CLIA, which identifies the standards of laboratory testing.
3. The Joint Commission, formerly JCAHO: An organization that offers voluntary accreditation of healthcare institutions.
4. Physician Office Laboratory (POL): Laboratory assays performed in a clinic or healthcare provider's office.
5. Ambulatory Surgical Centers (ASC): Healthcare facilities designed to perform minor surgical procedures or sameday surgeries on an outpatient basis.

III. CONSENT

A. Consent defined: Permission voluntarily granted by one, legally capable to do so, to receive medical treatment.
1. Express: Verbal expression (oral or in writing) of consent.
2. Implied: Behavior or actions that can be reasonably presumed to be consent.

B. Patient Self-Determination Act of 1990: Protects the rights of patients to make decisions regarding their own healthcare, including the right to accept or refuse medical care.

C. Doctrine of Informed Consent: A provider's duty to explain and make comprehensible to the patient information that enables the patient to evaluate a proposed medical procedure before submitting to it.
1. Necessary for procedures involving risk.
2. Elements of informed consent
   a. The nature of the patient's condition.
   b. Description of the nature and purpose of the proposed treatment or procedure.
   c. The risks, consequences, and benefits of the proposed treatment.
   d. Alternative treatments with associated risks, consequences, and benefits.
   e. The consequences, assuming no treatment is rendered.
   f. A means of assessing the patient's comprehension of the above issues.
   g. Dated signatures of the patient, provider and potential witnesses.

3. Successful lawsuits under the theory of informed consent must meet the following criteria:
   a. The healthcare provider failed to adequately inform the patient of a material risk.
   b. If the patient had been informed of the risk, the patient would not have consented to the treatment (subjective test). An objective test would be that of a hypothetical reasonably prudent person refusing consent in light of the risk.
   c. The risk that was unknown to the patient did in fact occur.
   d. The patient was harmed as a result of submitting to treatment.
4. Possible defenses barring recovery
   a. The undisclosed risk is too commonly known to warrant disclosure.
   b. The patient assured the provider that consent would be given regardless of the risks.
   c. The patient requested not to be informed of the risks.
   d. Acquiring consent was not reasonably possible.
   e. The provider, in her or his best medical judgment, determined that full disclosure would adversely affect the patient's condition.

D. Consensual powers: Generally persons who are mentally competent and of the age of majority have the power to grant, refuse, or rescind consent on their behalf.
1. Minors require the consent of a parent, legal guardian, someone acting *in loco parentis* (someone charged with standing in the parent's stead), or a guardian *ad litem* (representation by someone for litigation purposes only) except in the following cases:
   a. Minors serving on active duty in the armed forces.
   b. Emancipated minors: Minors who have been granted independent status by a court of law.
   c. Mature minors: Minors who are recognized as being of the age, intellect, and maturity to make certain decisions on their own.
   d. Minors who have communicable or sexually transmitted diseases.
   e. Minors involved in an unwed pregnancy, or seeking abortion or contraception counseling.
2. Persons who are *non compos mentis* (not of sound mind, insane) or *non sui juris* (incompetent) do not have consensual power and require some form of guardianship to represent their interests in granting consent.
3. In emergency situations whereupon the patient is unconscious or does not have consensual power and consent cannot be obtained in light of the circumstances, it is assumed that a reasonably

prudent person would want his or her life or limb restored, therefore implying consent.

E. Refused consent: Persons who are mentally competent and of the age of majority have the right to refuse medical care.
  1. Procedure to avoid litigation for failure to provide medical care if consent is refused:
     a. Do not render the care.
     b. Ask the patient to sign a release protecting the practitioner from liability for not rendering the care.
     c. Document the refused consent in the patient's chart. If the patient refuses to sign the release, document this as well with, perhaps, a witness's signature.
  2. Patients who initially grant consent can change their minds and rescind consent at their discretion. If possible, the procedure should be aborted.
  3. In circumstances in which there is a compelling state interest, a patient's refusal to consent can be legally overruled.

F. Fraudulently obtained consent: Consent obtained through fraud or misrepresentation is not binding and is considered as if the patient had given no consent.

G. Assault and battery
  1. Assault: The deliberate threat and perceived ability of one to make bodily contact with another without that person's consent.
  2. Battery: An intentional physical contact with another without that person's consent.
  3. Rendering care to a patient without consent may result in a charge of assault, battery, or both.

H. Living will: An advance directive authorizing the withholding or withdrawal of artificial life support in the event of terminal illness or injury. The Patient Self-Determination Act of 1990 encourages the use of advance directives before life-sustaining measures become necessary.

I. Uniform Anatomical Gift Act of 1968: Allows for competent adults to dispose of their own bodies or body parts by will or other recognized written document for medical or dental education, research, or transplantation.

IV. PUBLIC HEALTH DUTIES

A. Police power of the state: State government authority to protect the public health is based on "police power," which affords the power to provide for the health, safety, and welfare of the people. Police power, when exercised, generally preempts patient consent provisions.

B. Reporting obligations: For the state to satisfy its duty to provide for the public's health, safety, and welfare, the state requires certain information about its citizenry.

1. Births: All states require documentation of births. Generally the healthcare provider or birth attendant completes a birth certificate.
2. Deaths: All states require documentation of deaths. Providers in attendance or someone having greater authority, such as a coroner, medical examiner, or county health officer (especially regarding suspicious or violent deaths) generally must complete a death certificate citing the cause of death. A medical examiner must be consulted in the following cases:
   a. Death caused by criminal activity or violence.
   b. Death without a healthcare provider present.
   c. Death from an undetermined cause.
   d. Death within a predetermined time of hospital or licensed healthcare facility admission (usually 24 hours).
   e. Death without prior medical care for a predetermined period of time.
3. Communicable diseases: Reports of communicable diseases are usually made to the county health department.
   a. Communicable diseases include smallpox, scarlet fever, measles, rubella, tuberculosis, cholera, plague, sexually transmitted diseases, etc.
   b. National Childhood Vaccine Injury Act: This Act requires that providers who administer vaccines and toxoids such as diphtheria, tetanus, pertussis, measles, mumps, rubella, and polio that have injurious outcomes are required to report the following information to the appropriate public health agency:
      (1) Date of vaccine administration.
      (2) Manufacturer and lot number.
      (3) Adverse reactions.
      (4) Name, title, and address of person administering the vaccine.
4. Diseases in newborns
   a. Inborn errors of metabolism such as phenylketonuria (PKU).
   b. Certain instances of diarrhea, staphylococcal infections, ophthalmia neonatorum, etc.
5. Abuse: In circumstances where abuse is suspected, providers have a legal duty to make a report consistent with each state's statutes. If a report is made in good faith, the provider is generally protected from liability.
   a. Child abuse.
   b. Elder abuse: Abuse of persons age 60 and older.
   c. Spouse abuse.
   d. Patient abuse in hospitals and nursing homes.
   e. Drug abuse: The Drug Enforcement Agency (DEA) is responsible for the enforcement of the Comprehensive Drug Abuse Prevention

and Control Act of 1970. Loss of controlled substances is to be reported to the DEA and local authorities.

6. Criminal acts
   a. Injuries caused by lethal weapons.
   b. Rape victims: Unless there is a statutory reporting requirement, the provider, in guarding a patient's confidence, may require a release to divulge such information.
   c. Assault.
   d. Attempted suicide.

C. Professional misconduct: The Health Care Quality Improvement Act of 1986 requires that hospitals and healthcare entities that take adverse licensure or professional review actions lasting more than 30 days make report of such actions to the National Practitioner Data Bank.

V. HEALTH INFORMATION

A. Purpose
   1. Provide a chronological record of a patient's medical care.
   2. Provide a means of intra- and interoffice communication regarding a patient's care.
   3. Provide data for education and research.
   4. Provide legal protection to patients and evidentiary documentation for litigation.

B. Ownership
   1. Generally, ownership of the medical record resides with the person or organization generating the entries.
   2. There are competing claims upon the contents of a medical record. Although the provider may exercise property rights for the medical record, patients have an interest protected by law. Providers may own the records but patients own the information and are generally given access to that information.
   3. Records requested by patients or third parties can be released if (1) the provider grants approval, and (2) the patient grants consent, usually via a release form.
   4. Doctrine of professional discretion: Records can be withheld from patients if the information can be reasonably expected to cause harm to the patient, such as those associated with psychiatric, drug, and alcohol treatment.

VI. CONFIDENTIALITY AND DISCLOSURE

A. To help ensure effective treatment and care, information regarding a patient is privileged (special, protected communication between the patient and provider) and considered confidential.

B. This confidentiality is conditional and can be waived by the patient or overruled through court order or subpoena depending on the circumstances.

C. Privacy Act of 1974: Safeguards individual privacy from misuse of federal records and provides personal access to records maintained by federal agencies such as medical records maintained by VA hospitals.

D. Releasing patient information without acquiring the patient's consent could lead to a charge of invasion of privacy.

E. Redisclosure Prohibition: If disclosure occurs electronically (e.g., fax), a redisclosure prohibition statement is required to notify the recipient that the patient's information can be used only for the purpose specifie, cannot be redisclosed to other third parties without proper patient consent, and must be properly destroyed after its purpose has been achieved.

F. The federal government requires such a notice for information associated with alcohol or drug abuse, regardless of the manner or medium of disclosure.

G. The drug Abuse, Prevention, Treatment, and Rehabilitation Act; and the Comprehensive Alcohol Abuse and Alcoholism Prevention, Treatment, and Rehabilitation Act of 1970: Providers and organizations are generally prohibited from confirming that a patient is, has been, or ever was a patient at a substance abuse treatment facility.

H. Patient must be given notice of federal confidentiality requirements upon admission to a substance abuse treatment program.

I. HIV/AIDS: In many states, the release of information cannot be a general open-ended form, but must be specific to the release of HIV information to include a redisclosure prohibition statement.

J. Medical Devices: The Safe Medical Devices Act of 1990 requires the disclosure of any death resulting from the use of a medical device to the Department of Health and Human Services within 10 days of the episode or its discovery. If a device causes illness or injury, the manufacturer must be notified.

VII. HIPAA

A. Health Insurance Portability and Accountability Act of 1996.

B. Title II—Administrative Simplification: Requires standardized electronic data interchange when protected health information is involved. Includes standards concerning the protection and security of personal health data.

C. Electronic transactions standards
   1. Electronic transactions include health claims, health eligibility and enrollment determinations, premium and care payments, claim status, first

injury reports, coordination of benefits, and related transactions.

2. Virtually all health plans must adopt standard electronic formats when transacting medical claims and related business.
3. Providers using nonelectronic transactions are not required to adopt these standards for use with commercial third-party payers.
4. Electronic transactions are required for Medicare and Medicaid claims.
5. Health organizations must adopt standard coding systems (e.g., ICD and CPT) related to diagnosis and treatment services.

D. Unique identifier standards: Healthcare providers, employers, and health plans must use a standard identification code (e.g., employer identification number) when communicating with each other.

E. Security rule
1. Providers are required to ensure the confidentiality, integrity, and availability of all electronic protected health information (PHI) that is created, received, maintained, or transmitted.
2. Providers must protect against any reasonably anticipated threats or hazards to the security or integrity of such information.
3. Required safeguards include enforcement of appropriate policies and procedures, safeguarding physical access, and ensuring technical security measures are in place to protect networks, computers, and other electronic devices.

F. Privacy rule
1. Patients have the right to access their PHI, restrict access by others, request changes, and to learn how their PHI has been accessed.
2. Restrict disclosure of PHI to the minimum needed for medical care and business operations.
3. Patients must be formally notified of a provider's privacy practices.

VIII. RETENTION AND INTEGRITY

A. The medical record must be a complete, accurate, up-to-date report of the patient's medical history and care.

B. The length of time to retain a medical record is controversial. Generally, it depends on state statutes; however, some are of the opinion that records should be retained permanently or at least equal to the statute of limitations beyond a patient's death or age of majority.

C. Records to be destroyed should either be shredded or burned.

D. All records should be typed or written using permanent ink.

E. Falsification of medical records is a criminal offense potentially resulting in civil liability.

F. Errors should not be erased, whited out, blotted out, or scribbled over. The proper method of correcting errors is to cast a single line through the erroneous entry so that it is still legible, write out the correction, include the corrector's initials or signature, and date.

G. Entries unrelated to the patient's medical status and care should be avoided. Defensive, derogatory, critical, emotional, and extraneous remarks can precipitate a malpractice claim.

H. Information absent from the record is equally as important as what is contained in the record. Legally, undocumented medical care is presumed to have never occurred.

IX. TORTS

A. Tort defined: Civil wrong, other than a breach of contract, committed against another person or property. Torts are classified as negligence (unintentional) or intentional.

B. Negligence: Generally an unintentional tort that is characterized by an omission or commission of an act that a reasonably prudent person would or would not do in a given circumstance.
1. Tort versus contract theory: Generally, negligence associated with malpractice has its basis in tort law (discussed later); however, if the provider guarantees the outcome of a course of treatment, any breach can be litigated on the basis of contract law.
2. Forms of negligence
   a. Nonfeasance: Failure to act when there was a duty to act; e.g., failure to order an X-ray film for a joint injury.
   b. Misfeasance: Improper performance of an act resulting in harm; e.g., prolonged exposure to heat therapy causing a burn.
   c. Malfeasance: Performance of an unlawful or improper act; e.g., administering a contraindicated medication.
   d. Malpractice: Negligence (nonfeasance, misfeasance, or malfeasance) of a professional person such as a provider, nurse, medical assistant, pharmacist, attorney, accountant, etc.
   e. Criminal negligence: Gross carelessness characterized by wanton disregard for a person's safety.
3. Degrees of negligence
   a. Ordinary: Omission or commission of an act that a reasonably prudent person would or would not do in a given circumstance.
   b. Gross: Intentional or wanton omission or commission of an act that would be proper in a given circumstance.

X. MALPRACTICE

A. Duty: There must exist a provider-patient relationship whereby the provider has a professional obligation to care for the patient.

   1. Standard of care: The standard of care to which a provider or other professional is held is generally determined by the profession and affiliated associations. This standard may also be based on the degree of care that is expected, customary, acceptable, and reasonable; the current state of scientific knowledge; and one's training and philosophical frame of reference (i.e., MD versus DO, or general versus specialty training).

   2. Rescuers: In emergency situations, there exists no general duty to rescue.

      a. Except for family members, or if the victim was imperiled by the rescuer.

      b. With exceptions, rescuers can generally abandon the victim if the victim is not imperiled any further.

      c. Some states by statute require their citizens to render emergency aid to the best of their ability or suffer potential misdemeanor charges.

      d. Good Samaritan Act: Statutes protecting providers and certain others from liability when rendering emergency aid.

B. Dereliction of duty: The practitioner breached his or her duty by failing to meet or departing from the accepted standard of care owed to the patient.

   1. *Res Ipsa Loquitur:* Circumstantial evidence doctrine (Latin for "the thing speaks for itself") that describes a situation in which the nature of the injury strongly or obviously implicates negligence. Res ipsa must meet the following criteria:

      a. Inference of negligence: Injury to the patient would not have normally occurred in the absence of negligence.

      b. Exclusive control: Instrumentality that caused the injury was in the sole control of the health professional.

      c. Patient conduct: The patient must not have contributed to the injury.

   2. *Ybarra v. Spangard:* A California case that supports the application of res ipsa loquitur in situations implicating multiple health professionals in which no one person is clearly liable. All persons implicated are considered guilty until proven innocent.

C. Direct causation: There must be a reasonable, close, and causal connection between the health professional's negligent act and the harm suffered by the patient.

   1. Causation in fact: But for *(sine qua non)* the actions of the health professional, the injury would not have occurred.

   2. Proximate cause: The action or inaction that set off the chain of events that resulted in the injury must have been close enough in proximity to the injury to warrant liability.

D. Damages: The patient must have suffered some injury or harm as a result of the negligence.

   1. General (compensatory): Money awards assessed according to the injuries that naturally flowed from the negligence that are difficult to assess, such as pain and suffering, mental anguish, etc.

   2. Special: Compensatory money awards for assessable costs incurred that naturally flowed from the negligence such as medical bills, etc.

   3. Punitive: Additional money awards resulting from negligence caused by wanton disregard or gross negligence.

E. Defenses: Situations that defend against malpractice claims either by barring recovery of damages or limiting the award of damages.

   1. Tolling of the statute of limitations: The statute of limitations determines the maximum amount of time that can elapse before a malpractice claim can be made.

      a. The statute of limitations can begin when the incident occurs, or when the patient discovers the injury or should have discovered the injury.

      b. With minors, the statute of limitations may not begin until the patient reaches the age of majority.

      c. Depending on state statute, a medical assistant may be viewed as either a layperson or a professional. If viewed as a layperson, the statute of limitations for negligence is used, which, in some states, is longer than that for malpractice. If the medical assistant is viewed as a professional, the statute of limitations for malpractice is used.

   2. Contributory negligence: Patients, through their own actions or inactions, contributed to the cause of injury, thus barring recovery for that injury.

   3. Comparative negligence: Patients are allowed to recover damages for that portion of the negligence that was caused by the health professional, but not their own.

   4. Assumption of the risk: Voluntarily accepting a known risk or consequence of treatment.

   5. Good Samaritan Act: In rendering emergency aid outside one's place of employment, health professionals may be protected from ordinary negligence.

   6. Intervening cause: An act of an independent agent that compromises the causal connection between the negligence and the injury.

XI. INTENTIONAL TORTS

A. Assault and battery
   1. Assault: The deliberate threat and perceived ability of one to make bodily contact with another without that person's consent.
   2. Battery: An intentional physical contact with another without that person's consent.
B. Abandonment: Unilateral termination of the provider-patient relationship by the provider without proper notice to the patient.
   1. Elements
      a. A provider-patient relationship exists.
      b. Discontinuance of care by the provider.
      c. Failure to arrange substitute care.
      d. Foresight that discontinued care may cause harm to the patient.
      e. Actual harm suffered by the patient.
   2. Steps to avoid abandonment charges
      a. Provide adequate notification of intent to terminate care in writing using certified mail.
      b. Remain available during the notification period.
      c. Provide competent substitute care if needed.
      d. Cooperate with the patient's new provider.
C. Invasion of privacy: Divulging patient information acquired though privileged communications without the patient's consent.
D. Defamation: Injury to a person's reputation or character caused by the false statements of another made to a third person.
      a. Libel: False or malicious writing that is intended to defame or dishonor another person.
      b. Slander: False oral statements made in the presence of third persons that injure the character or reputation of another.
E. Infliction of mental distress: Outrageous conduct that causes mental suffering from painful emotions such as grief, public humiliation, despair, shame, and wounded pride.
F. False imprisonment: Unlawful restraint of an individual's personal liberty.
G. Fraud: Willful and intentional misrepresentation that could cause harm or loss to a person or property.

XII. PRODUCT AND VICARIOUS LIABILITY

A. Liability of a manufacturer, seller, or supplier, of products for injuries sustained because of defect.
B. Lawsuits are based on three legal theories:
   1. Negligence: Negligence requires the establishment of duty, dereliction of duty, direct causation, and damage.
      a. Liability will not be incurred if the patient negligently uses the product.
      b. Liability will be incurred for unsafe designs.
   2. Breach of warranty: Nonconformity to specific promises or affirmations made about a product.
C. Strict liability: A breach of duty to make safe any product that is used in the prescribed manner.
D. Defenses
   1. Contributory negligence, assumption of the risk, and intervening causes (discussed earlier).
   2. Disclaimers: Warnings regarding usage, safety, and contraindications.
E. Vicarious liability: Liability endured on another person's behalf.
   1. *Respondeat Superior:* Latin for "Let the master answer." Employers such as providers and healthcare organizations are liable for the conduct of employees while serving within the scope of their employment.
   2. Borrowed Servant Rule: If "A" borrows the services of "B" from employer "C," "A" may be vicariously liable for the conduct of "B" if "A" has the requisite degree of control over "B."

XIII. LABOR LAW

A. NLRA (National Labor Relations Act of 1935): Identifies and defines unfair employer and employee labor practices and provides for the hearing and remediation of complaints.
B. FLSA (Fair Labor Standards Act of 1938): Also known as the Federal Wage and Hour Law. Concerns minimum wage, overtime, equal pay for equal work, record-keeping requirements, and child labor restrictions.
C. EPA (Equal Pay Act of 1963): An amendment to the FLSA that addresses wage disparities based on gender.
D. EEOA (Equal Employment Opportunity Act of 1972): An amendment of Title VII of the Civil Rights Act of 1964 prohibiting employment discrimination based on age, race, color, religion, gender, or national origin.
E. ADEA (Age Discrimination in Employment Act of 1967): Prohibits employment discrimination based on age for citizens 40 years or older.
F. ADA (Americans with Disabilities Act of 1990): Prohibits employment discrimination against qualified individuals with disabilities.
G. OSHA (Occupational Safety and Health Act of 1970): Ensures safe and healthy working conditions.
H. Workers' Compensation Laws: State mandated programs to provide wage benefits in the case of work-related illnesses and injuries.
I. Pregnancy Discrimination Act (1978): Discrimination on the basis of pregnancy, childbirth, or related medical condition is unlawful gender discrimination under Title VII.

J. Drug-Free Workplace Act (1988): Requires organizations having $25,000 or more in federal contracts or grants to certify that they will make good-faith efforts to maintain a drug-free workplace and to establish employee drug education and awareness programs.

K. Employee Retirement Income Security Act (ERISA, 1974): Does not require that employers provide retirement benefits for employees, but protects the benefits to which they are entitled. Adequate funds must be reserved to provide the promised benefits.

L. Family Medical Leave Act (FMLA, 1993): Eligible employees are permitted to take up to 12 weeks of unpaid leave during any 12 month period when unable to work because of a serious health condition; or to care for a child upon birth, adoption, or foster care; or to care for a spouse, parent, or child with a serious health condition.

XIV. SEXUAL HARASSMENT

A. Elements of sexual harassment
   1. The behavior in question must be sexual in nature.
   2. The behavior must be unwelcome.
   3. The behavior must affect a condition of employment.
B. Forms of sexual harassment
   1. *Quid pro quo* (Latin for "something for something"): A situation in which the conditions of employment, positive or not, are based on an individual's acceptance or rejection of unwelcome sexual conduct.
   2. Hostile work environment: Unwelcome sexual behavior that creates an intimidating, hostile or offensive work environment, or unreasonably interferes with a person's job performance.

XV. CONSUMER CREDIT LAW

A. Truth in Lending Act (Regulation Z of the Consumer Protection Act of 1969): Requires written disclosure regarding fee payments in more than four installments.
B. Fair Credit Reporting Act of 1971: Covers guidelines for reporting and acquiring credit information.
C. Equal Credit Opportunity Act of 1975: Prohibits discrimination in the extension of credit.
D. Fair Collection Practices Act of 1978: Identifies fair collection guidelines.

XVI. PAYROLL LAW

A. FLSA (Fair Labor Standards Act) requires that records of employee hours must be maintained.
B. Employment designations

   1. Employer: One who employs one or more persons for performance of services in the United States.
   2. Employee: One who performs services in a covered employment.
      a. The employee is under the control and direction of an employer. An employee may be told what to do and how to do it and receives a wage or salary.
      b. Employees must be assessed payroll deductions consistent with federal and state payroll laws.
   3. Independent contractor: One who provides a professional service for a fee.
      a. Independent contractors are told what needs to be done, i.e., the desired end result, but not how it should be done.
      b. Independent contractors are not employees and therefore require no payroll deductions. It is unlawful for an employee as described above to be treated as an independent contractor.

C. FICA (Federal Insurance Contributions Act): Social Security tax that is applied toward old age survivor's insurance, Medicare and hospital insurance, and disability insurance.
D. FUTA (Federal Unemployment Tax Act): Tax to provide economic security during periods of temporary unemployment.
E. Forms and reports
   1. SS-5: Social Security number application.
   2. Form 941 (Employer's Quarterly Federal Tax Return): Filed every three months with payment of quarterly federal income tax.
   3. Form 8109 (Federal Tax Deposit Coupon Book): Used to pay FICA and federal income tax.
   4. Form W-2 (Wage and Tax Statement): Given to employees itemizing annual wages and taxes withheld.
   5. W-3 (Transmittal of Income and Tax Statement): Submitted to the Social Security Administration comparing the tax withheld on form W-2 to that stated on Form 941.
   6. Form W-4 (Employee's Withholding Allowance Certificate): Allows the employee to determine the number of withholding allowances based on number of dependents.
   7. Form 940 (Employer's Annual Federal Unemployment Tax Return): A quarterly unemployment tax return.

XVII. CONTRACT LAW

A. Defined: Mutual agreement between two or more parties to perform or refrain from performing certain duties usually for the benefit of those contracting.

Contracts can be oral or in writing, express or implied.

B. Elements of a contract: If any of the following elements are missing, a contract does not legally exist.
1. Offer: There must be an offer where one party offers to enter into a legal agreement with another. The offer should include the parties, the subject, the quantity, price, and time.
2. Acceptance: Another party must accept the terms of the offer such that the acceptance is a mirror image of the offer.
3. Consideration: There must be a detriment to each party such that it is reasonably balanced and fair.
4. Contractual capacity: Each party must be legally capable of contracting, which generally includes being of the age of majority and mentally competent.
5. Legality: The contract must be legal in nature and not against public policy.

C. Statute of frauds: Prevents fraud by requiring certain contracts to be in writing.
1. Sale of land.
2. Prenuptial agreements.
3. Contracts incapable of being performed within a year.
4. Sale of goods over $500.
5. Collateral contracts: A contract that allows a third party to carry out any contractual obligations not satisfied by the primary party as in a cosigner arrangement.

D. Breach of contract: Without legal excuse, failing to perform the obligations of a contract.

E. Defenses against breaches
1. Impossibility of performance: For example, destruction of the subject matter, or the terms of the agreement become illegal after the contract was formed.
2. Frustration of purpose: Possible to perform, but value has been significantly altered or destroyed.
3. Impracticability: Impractical to perform because of extreme or unreasonable economies.
4. Waiver: Waiving a contractual term.

F. Damages are awarded according to the benefit of the bargain.

CHAPTER 9

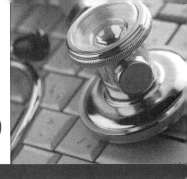

Health Care Ethics

I. INTRODUCTION

A. Morality: Standards and principles that guide our behavior relative to that of others and to that of society. Morals generally provide rules regarding right and wrong.

B. Ethics: A branch of philosophy, typically called moral philosophy, that describes the systematic study and analysis of morality.

C. Normative ethics: Addresses concrete moral questions in determining what is morally right or wrong.
  1. Deontology: (fr. Gk, *deos* "duty")—Means or duty theories supporting the notion that the means justifies the ends. Some actions are intrinsically moral or immoral regardless of the consequences. One's duty takes priority over associated consequences (or ends).
  2. Teleology: (fr. Gk, *telos* "end")—Ends or consequentialist theories supporting the notion that the ends justify the means. An act (duty or means) is right if the associated consequences create overall good (utilitarianism).

D. Situation ethics: Six guidelines developed by Joseph Fletcher (1966)—Human need determines what is or is not ethical.
  1. Compassion for people as human beings.
  2. Consideration of consequences.
  3. Proportionate good.
  4. Priority of actual needs over ideal or potential needs.
  5. A desire to enlarge choice and reduce chance.
  6. Acceptance of the need to make decisions having certain consequences.

II. ETHICAL PRINCIPLES

A. A norm is the basic unit of morality. A norm is a pattern of behavior or conduct that is valued by a society.

B. Duties: Obligations or commitments to act in certain ways.
  1. Nonmaleficence: Not committing any harm—*primum non nocere* (fr. L "first, do no harm"). As human beings we have the general duty not to harm others.

  2. Beneficence: Acting to create benefit or good. Often, nonmaleficence and beneficence are viewed as varying degrees of the concept of good.
  Do no harm → Prevent harm → Remove harm → Create good
  3. Fidelity: (fr. L *fides* "faithful")—Meeting the patient's reasonable expectations.
    a. Respect.
    b. Competence.
    c. Adhering to professional codes of ethics.
    d. Adhering to laws, rules, regulations, and policies.
    e. Honoring agreements.
  4. Veracity: Telling the truth.
  5. Justice: Ensuring that individuals in like circumstances receive their fair share of benefits and burdens—an equitable distribution of benefits and burdens.
    a. Distributive justice: Comparative treatment of individuals in the allotment of benefits and burdens.
    b. Compensatory justice: Restitution for wrongs that have been committed.
    c. Procedural justice: Impartial processes that serve to administer justice in a fair manner.

C. Rights: Stringent claims made on a person, group, or society. Rights are correlated to duties; if a right exists, there is usually a corollary duty to see that the right is satisfied or protected.
  1. According to Feinberg (1982), in order to bear rights one must meet the following criteria of personhood:
    a. Possess interests, wants, desires, needs.
    b. Possess cognitive awareness.
    c. Be capable of relationships.
    d. Possess a sense of futurity.
  2. Right to life.
  3. Right to self-determination (autonomy).
  4. Right to privacy.

D. Virtues: Character traits or behavioral dispositions to act in certain ways. Moral character has great significance in health care because of the unequal status within most patient-health professional relationships.

Taken together, the basic principles of ethics encompass duties, rights, and virtues.

E. Almost all ethical problems in health care arise from conflicts among two or more duties, two or more competing rights, or duties competing with rights.

F. Codes of Ethics: Most ethical codes subscribe to the following principles (see Figures 9-1 and 9-2)
   1. Respect for persons affording patient dignity.
   2. Communicate honestly and keep patient communications confidential.
   3. Promote the traditions, honor, and high principles of the profession.
   4. Strive to maintain professional competence within one's scope of practice by improving skills, knowledge, and abilities.
   5. Expose those who violate applicable laws and ethical codes.
   6. Promote the health, well-being, and good of society.

G. Principles of ethical decisions
   1. Ethics Check: Model proposed by Blanchard and Peale (1988) to help sort out ethical dilemmas by answering three questions:
      a. Is it legal? Generally if one answers "no" to this question, the other two need not be considered. This question can encompass organizational policies, rules, and regulations, as well as organizational or professional codes of ethics. This question considers existing standards of conduct.
      b. Is it balanced? Will the decision be fair or will it significantly favor one over the other—a clear winner and loser. This question considers the issue of justice.
      c. How will it make me feel about myself? This question considers issues of moral character, conscience, and emotions. Consider how you would feel if your decision were made public.
   2. Core principles of ethical decision making: The Five P's of Ethical Power (Blanchard & Peale, 1988):
      a. Purpose: Decide what your purpose in life is and use it along with ethics as guiding principles.
      b. Pride: Develop self-esteem by believing in yourself and having faith in your abilities so that you have the strength to do what is right.
      c. Patience: Once a decision is made, do not expect immediate results or reassurances that the decision was right. Impatience can undo morally sound decisions.
      d. Persistence: Adhere to one's purpose and behave ethically all of the time, not just when it is convenient.
      e. Perspective: The capacity to see the big picture, the important issues, the right path.

III. DUTY TO SELF

A. Duty to maintain personal integrity: "To thine own self be true."
   1. When presented with a moral dilemma, one must call upon one's own personal value system.
   2. Two major forces threaten personal integrity
      a. Bad laws, policies, or regulations.
      b. Self-deception: Protecting self-esteem by evading what one knows to be true.
   3. Integrity safeguards
      a. Integrity of the profession: Society knows that the professions have values that must be protected, e.g., codes of ethics.
      b. Moral repugnance: Means of protecting those who refrain from activities believed to be morally wrong, e.g., conscientious objection.

B. Duty to improve oneself: Because of the nature of the work, health professionals have a duty to maintain their professional credentials and competence.
   1. Continuing education.
   2. Maintaining or developing competence.
   3. Exemplifying a healthy lifestyle and being a role model.

IV. ROLE FIDELITY

To practice your professional role with faithfulness.

A. Gatekeeping: Looking out for the interests of the profession or of others practicing the profession to maintain the genuine honor and high principles of the profession, and to protect and serve the best interests of patients.

B. A profession's code of ethics provides guiding principles to maintain role fidelity.

C. Scope of practice: It is expected that health professionals will provide professional services within the constraints of their skills, knowledge, and abilities, and of the law. Services needed beyond one's scope of practice require appropriate referrals.

D. Disparagement: Constructive criticism of colleagues and the profession is often appropriate, but professionals should reserve their criticisms for the proper forum. It is generally unprofessional to criticize or disparage colleagues in the presence of patients.

E. Conflicts of interest: When the interests of the professional and of the patient collide, the patient must generally be given priority (e.g., self-referral and fee-splitting).

F. Impaired colleagues: Colleagues who engage in substance abuse, or who are incompetent put patients at risk. It is one's professional duty to address this issue.

G. Sexual misconduct: The health professional-patient relationship is an unequal one. Patients rely on the professional expertise of the health practitioner and are, therefore, vulnerable. Sexual misconduct by the practitioner directed toward the patient takes

AAMA CODE OF ETHICS

The Code of Ethics of AAMA shall set forth principles of ethical and moral conduct as they relate to the medical profession and the particular practice of medical assisting.

Members of AAMA dedicated to the conscientious pursuit of their profession, and thus desiring to merit the high regard of the entire medical profession and the respect of the general public which they serve, do pledge themselves to strive always to:

A. render service with full respect for the dignity of humanity;
B. respect confidential information obtained through employment unless legally authorized or required by responsible performance of duty to divulge such information;
C. uphold the honor and high principles of the profession and accept its disciplines;
D. seek to continually improve the knowledge and skills of medical assistants for the benefit of patients and professional colleagues;
E. participate in additional service activities aimed toward improving the health and well-being of the community.

CREED

I believe in the principles and purposes of the Profession of Medical Assisting.
I endeavor to be more effective.
I aspire to render greater service.
I protect the confidence entrusted to me.
I am dedicated to the care and well-being of all people.
I am loyal to my employer.
I am true to the ethics of my profession.
I am strengthened by compassion, courage, and faith.

Figure 9-1

AAMA Code of Ethics and Creed. Reprinted with permission of the American Association of Medical Assistants.

advantage of the patient's vulnerable state and is morally indefensible.
H. Whistle-blowing: Impaired colleagues and episodes of sexual misconduct justify whistle-blowing—reporting the perpetrators to the appropriate professional body for disciplinary action. The following criteria, as suggested by Haddad and Dougherty (1991), justifies whistle-blowing:
  1. The wrongdoing is egregious and could potentially create serious harm.

AMT STANDARDS OF PRACTICE

AMT seeks to encourage, establish, and maintain the highest standards, traditions and principles of the practices which constitute the profession of the Registry. Members of the AMT Registry must recognize their responsibilities, not only to their patients, but also to society, to other health care professionals, and to themselves. The following standards of practice are principles adopted by the AMT Board of Directors, which define the essence of honorable and ethical behavior for a health care professional:

1. While engaged in the Arts and Sciences, which constitute the practice of their profession, AMT professionals shall be dedicated to the provision of competent service.
2. The AMT professional shall place the welfare of the patient above all else.
3. The AMT professional understands the importance of thoroughness in the performance of duty, compassion with patients, and the importance of the tasks, which may be performed.
4. The AMT professional shall always seek to respect the rights of patients and of health care providers, and shall safeguard patient confidences.
5. The AMT professional will strive to increase his/her technical knowledge, shall continue to study, and apply scientific advanced in his/her specialty.
6. The AMT professional shall respect the law and will pledge to avoid dishonest, unethical or illegal practices.
7. The AMT professional understands that he/she is not to make or offer a diagnosis or interpretation unless he/she is a duly licensed physician/dentist or unless asked by the attending physician/dentist.
8. The AMT professional shall protect and value the judgment of the attending physician or dentist, providing this does not conflict with the behavior necessary to carry out Standard Number 2 above.
9. The AMT professional recognizes that any personal wrongdoing is his/her responsibility. It is also the professional health care provider's obligation to report to the proper authorities any knowledge of professional abuse.
10. The AMT professional pledges personal honor and integrity to cooperate in the advancement and expansion, by every lawful means, of American Medical Technologists.

Figure 9-2

AMT Standards of Practice. Reprinted with permission of the American Medical Technologists.

2. The whistle-blower has the proper information and is competent to judge the wrongdoing as such.

3. The whistle-blower has consulted colleagues to solicit their judgment.

4. All other internal resources to resolve the issue have been exhausted.

5. It is likely that the whistle-blowing will serve the greater good.

V. BENEVOLENT HEALTH CARE

A. Benevolent health care requires a balance between technical competence and emotional sensitivity.

B. Components of benevolent health care
  1. People are inherently worthy of concern.
  2. People should be treated as unique.
  3. People are irreplaceable.
  4. People should be allowed autonomy.
  5. People deserve warmth and compassion.

C. Individualized care: The manner in which your personal integrity manifests itself in your professional role.
  1. Think about how you should address a patient: Ask patients their preference; otherwise, initially, err on the side of formality. Eventually, however, with the patient's permission, informal address may be acceptable.
  2. Recognize efficiency as a trait expressing care when it does not constrain patient interaction.
  3. Demonstrate interest without fostering dependence or interference.
  4. Be a careful listener.
  5. Maintain a balance between sound service and compassion.
  6. Communicate to learn about patients and their lives.

D. Mistakes must be dealt with using the same or greater degree of humanizing principles.

VI. HEALTH INFORMATION

A. Confidentiality
  1. Ethics argument
    a. Deontological perspective: Upholds the duties of beneficence, nonmaleficence, and fidelity.
    b. Teleological perspective: Breached confidentiality will potentially compromise the patient-provider relationship.
  2. Rights argument: Upholds the right to self-determination (autonomy) and privacy.
  3. Virtues (moral character) argument: Upholds the fiduciary responsibility of a special and privileged relationship.
  4. Confidentiality is not valued as an end but rather as a means to serve trust and afford dignity. *Keeping confidences → Builds trust → Maintains patient dignity*

  5. Medical records
    a. Untrue information should not be recorded.
    b. Questionable information should be labeled as such.
    c. True information not relevant should not be recorded.
    d. Handle information to maintain patient privacy and dignity.
  6. The patient with AIDS poses a special problem because of the added risk for harm should confidentiality be breached. This harm may be in the form of discrimination or even physical threats.

B. Disclosure
  1. Disclosure to the patient is related to the duty of veracity.
  2. Arguments against disclosure
    a. Benevolent deception: The health professional's role is to maintain the patient's hope, and hope may be destroyed by bad news.
    b. The basis for this argument is paternalism.
  3. Arguments favoring disclosure
    a. Veracity is as important as, and not in conflict with, beneficence.
    b. Patients have a right to information about their condition, if wanted; therefore, there is a corollary duty for someone to provide it.
  4. If information is withheld, it must be on the basis of other more compelling moral considerations than the patient's rights and accompanying professional duties.
  5. A lie is an intent to deceive.

C. Informed Consent
  1. Related to the right of autonomy and duty of beneficence.
  2. Raises issues of competence: Ideally, four levels should be present.
    a. Ability to communicate choices.
    b. Ability to understand information upon which the choice is based.
    c. Ability to appreciate the situation according to one's own values.
    d. Ability to weigh various values to make a decision.
  3. Persons with diminished autonomy stand in need of protection, thus allowing for a range of justified paternalism.
  4. A guardian must be appointed for those who have never been competent: The "best interest" standard helps identify who can speak for the best interest of the patient, usually next of kin.
  5. For patients who have in the past been competent, a "substituted judgement" standard is used. This is usually based on the patient's personality, opinions, feelings, and communications as described by friends and relatives.

6. A "reasonable person" standard is sometimes used as well. This is based on what one believes a reasonably prudent person would do in similar circumstances.

VII. SPECIAL PATIENT CONSIDERATIONS

A. The difficult patient

1. The difficult patient raises concerns regarding respect, compassion, and social justice.
2. Derogatory labels
   a. GOMER: Get Out of My Emergency Room. Typically a dirty, debilitated person who abuses alcohol. Often subsists on public funds and has a history of multiple emergency room visits and hospitalizations. Experiences organic disease often resulting from poor hygiene, malnutrition, and self-destructive behaviors.
   b. GORK (vegetable): Often starts out as a Gomer but becomes sicker, is often unresponsive, and suffers from irreversible brain damage.
   c. CROCK: Hypochondriac or malingerer.
3. Most health professionals come from middle-class backgrounds. Patients coming from different social classes challenge materialistic and associated values and are thus psychologically threatening.
4. Physical disfigurement has a similar effect.
5. Uncooperative patients are frustrating because their attitudes and behavior appear to reject professional advice. Moreover, health professionals cannot feel gratification from curing people when patients are noncompliant.
6. Patients with mental/emotional disorders threaten our self-image. Psychological diseases are often seen as evidence of a weak or deficient character. When emotional problems manifest themselves physically, health professionals may react with impatience and contempt.
7. Working with difficult patients
   a. Noncompliant and self-destructive behavior can often be attributed to psychosocial stresses.
   b. Stressful work such as this can lead to burnout causing one to either react outwardly with anger or inwardly with depression/hopelessness.
   c. Health professionals have a duty to take care of themselves.
   d. Guidelines
      (1) Do not use derogatory labels.
      (2) The caring function is as important as the cure.
      (3) Be realistic about your powers as a health professional.
      (4) Do not blame the victim.
      (5) Take care of your own emotional well-being.

B. The suicidal patient

1. Some view suicide as resulting from mental derangement, psychological maladjustment, or social maladjustment.
   a. May be seen as the ultimate act of despair.
   b. Persons may attempt to communicate feelings of hopelessness to gain assurances—if none are forthcoming, their feelings are confirmed.
2. Some view suicide as an act against God.
   a. Jewish traditions view suicide as an act of shedding blood and is therefore murder.
   b. Christian traditions view suicide as an act against the God-given sense of self-preservation. Suicide is taking control over something only God should have control over.
   c. Hindu traditions view suicide as violating one's Karma.
   d. Islamic traditions view suicide as taking the destiny of one's life from the rightful control of God.
3. Some view suicide as an ignominious act
   a. If not insane, one is socially irresponsible.
   b. Causes emotional harm to loved ones.
   c. Giving up on life sets a bad example.
   d. Demonstrates cowardice and moral unworthiness.
4. Some view suicide as the person exercising self-determination: Ending one's life that no longer has meaning or utility, especially in terminal illnesses.
5. Responding to suicidal patients
   a. Err on the side of life.
   b. A person's suicidal comments may be a sign of testing.
   c. Be prepared for the possibility of its occurrence—comfort and help each other.

C. The terminally ill patient

1. Creates issues regarding quality of life. The one most qualified to judge quality of life is the person whose life it is.
2. Biological life versus biographical life: Death may be seen as a process of withdrawal: *Social life → Intellectual life → Biological life.* First, as a terminal illness progresses, one's social connections tend to diminish. In time, one's mental faculties fail, and ultimately physical death occurs, concluding the process of withdrawal.
3. Terminally ill patients make health professionals susceptible to committing psychological abandonment (distancing).
4. Paradoxically, for most health professionals, it is difficult to know when to stop treatment.
5. Heroic treatments may inflict undue physical, psychological, or spiritual harm.

6. Advance directives: Documents that allow patients to express their wishes when they no longer can do so themselves.

    a. Living will: A document that directs health professionals, in advance, regarding the patient's wishes concerning medical care while the patient is still able to communicate them.

    b. Durable power of attorney: A document serving to appoint an individual, chosen by the patient, to represent the patient's interests.

7. Father Gerald Kelly's (1957) Determinants of Extraordinary Care: Whether extraordinary care is provided or withheld depends on such factors as cost, pain, inconvenience, and potential benefit.

    a. CPR may be considered a heroic medical intervention (extraordinary) in circumstances in which extending the patient's life prolongs suffering or has no achievable purpose.

    b. Do Not Resuscitate orders (DNR) or other advance directives may be indicated.

8. The patient's family requires emotional support as well: Do not alienate them, because family support is important during the dying process.

9. Patients will often hesitate to express desires for fear they will seem irrelevant or silly.

10. Be sensitive to the patient's remaining time frame.

11. Discontinuing curative efforts indicates the beginning of efforts to control pain and provide comfort.

12. Euthanasia: from Greek for "good or easy death."

    a. Types

        (1) Passive versus active: Passive euthanasia generally describes allowing a person to die by discontinuing treatment. Active euthanasia, however, describes engaging in actions that will assist or hasten the dying process.

        (2) Voluntary versus involuntary: Voluntary euthanasia describes assisting a patient, at the patient's request, in the dying process, actively or passively. Involuntary euthanasia, on the other hand, describes assisting a patient, without the patient's request, in the dying process, actively or passively.

    b. Pro: According to duty and utilitarian terms, euthanasia is an extension of personal autonomy.

    c. Con: Our lives are not ours but a gift from God. Slippery slope—Where do we draw the line regarding those allowed or not allowed euthanasia?

VIII. ABORTION

A. Background

1. Abortion is the termination of a pregnancy through one of five methods:

    a. Uterine aspiration: Suctioning out the uterus.

    b. Dilatation and curettage (D&C): The cervix is dilated and the uterine lining is scraped away.

    c. Saline injection: To cause a miscarriage in late pregnancy.

    d. Cesarean section.

    e. Medication: RU 486—"morning after pill."

2. *Roe v. Wade:* The 1973 Supreme Court decision legalizing abortion based on the right to privacy. The Court constrained abortion rights by providing restrictions based on the length of pregnancy.

    a. First trimester: Abortions can be secured at the woman's discretion.

    b. Second trimester: The state may restrict abortions according to compelling state interests in maternal health.

    c. Third trimester: The state may regulate or prohibit abortions, except in cases in which the woman's life or health is in danger.

3. Pro-life versus pro-choice

    a. Pro-life: Anti-abortion—abortion is murder and should be outlawed.

    b. Pro-choice: The decision to abort is one of personal choice and should be legal.

        (1) Some pro-choice advocates believe abortion is wrong, but should be decided upon individually, without governmental interference.

        (2) Others believe whether abortion is right or wrong, there are more compelling consequences to consider.

4. Fetal development

    a. Conceptus: The initial union of the spermatozoon and ovum.

    b. Zygote: The state of the fertilized cell after 24 hours.

    c. Embryo: Approximately 2 to 8 weeks after fertilization.

        (1) Pro-choice advocates: Argue that up to this point the embryo does not remotely resemble anything human.

        (2) Pro-life advocates: Argue that such judgments should not be made on appearance, resorting to the example of how racism developed.

    d. Fetus: From 8 weeks to birth.

    e. After approximately the first trimester (third month), the fetus begins to move and can generally be felt by the fourth month.

f. By the fifth month the fetus can feel pain. Does this present any duties?

g. Viability is possible at the sixth month.

h. By the seventh month neuronal development creates minimal consciousness.

B. Moral issues, arguments, and questions

1. If the right to life begins at birth, what is the argument for allowing abortions 5 minutes before birth, assuming there is no medical change up until birth?

2. Killing

a. Generally killing another is wrong except in self-defense.

b. Some believe that abortion is morally defensible if the mother's life is in danger.

c. Others believe that the self-defense rule holds true only for murderous intent; therefore, because the fetus is innocent, abortion is wrong.

d. The doctrine of double effect distinguishes the intended effect of an action from unintended ones. This is a common argument for aborting a fetus to save the mother. Saving the mother is the intended effect; whereas, aborting the fetus is not intended, but rather a consequence of saving the mother.

3. Personhood: The right to life is embedded in the notion of personhood. The argument may be based on Mary Ann Warren's (1984) model of traits central to personhood.

a. Consciousness of objects and events.

b. Ability to feel pain.

c. Reasoning.

d. Self-motivated activity.

e. Communicability.

f. Self-awareness.

4. Viability: Biological independence

a. Once viability is achieved, the mother no longer has exclusive rights. Compelling state rights may come into force.

b. Viability varies over time and place depending on available technology.

5. Women's liberty

a. In order for women to be free, control over reproduction must be in place, especially with regard to the immense responsibility of raising children.

b. Women should have the same control of their life plan as men. If men could become pregnant, would there be an abortion controversy?

6. Justice

a. If you consent to sex and get pregnant, it is only just that you should raise the child.

b. Should we, then, regard children as a form of punishment?

c. The task of raising children is too difficult and demanding to turn it over to someone who is regarded as irresponsible in the first place.

IX. GENETIC SCIENCE

A. Eugenics: Manipulating the genes of offspring through either breeding or alteration.

B. Genetic testing—moral questions

1. Should parents be allowed to prevent the birth of a child with defects?

2. Should parents carrying genetic abnormalities be prevented from producing offspring?

3. Should parents be allowed to select the gender of their children?

4. Is it beneficial to eliminate all genetic disease?

5. Should genetic test data be confidential?

C. Genetic research and technology—moral questions

1. Should genetic research be used for military purposes?

2. As new research and technology becomes more commonplace and accessible, what problems might this pose regarding its use?

X. AIDS AND MEDICINE

A. Background

1. Acquired immune deficiency syndrome (AIDS) is caused by the human immunodeficiency virus (HIV).

2. HIV has been isolated from blood, vaginal secretions, semen, breast milk, saliva, tears, and CSF; however, HIV is generally transmitted via sex, blood, or breast milk.

3. Seems to have originated from mutant genes transmitted by the bite of a species of African monkey before spreading to Haiti and the United States.

B. Treatment duties

1. Minuscule risk to providers does not provide a suitable rationale to refuse treatment.

2. American Nurses Association Committee on Ethics (ANA, 1985) developed the criteria for identifying the duty to treat as either a moral option or a moral duty:

a. Risk or harm to the patient is significant in the absence of treatment.

b. Professional intervention is required to prevent such harm.

c. Benefits to the patient far outweigh risks to the provider.

Affirmation of all three criteria establishes a duty or moral obligation to treat. Negation of one or more, however, poses a moral option; i.e., based on personal principles and values, one is free to choose.

3. HIV-positive patients and patients with AIDS are protected under Section 504 of the Rehabilitation Act of 1973 as a handicapped condition, thus affording protection against discriminatory practices.

XI. RESOURCE ALLOCATION

A. United States healthcare issues
1. According to various polls, many Americans believe in the right to high-quality health care, but few are willing to contribute additional tax dollars to support a national health insurance program.
2. The United States has more healthcare providers per capita than most industrialized nations.
3. Although the current generation of Americans is the healthiest ever, the apparent improvement in health has not been subjectively experienced proportionately.
4. Americans live longer and better, yet we report more frequent and longer episodes of serious acute illness than in the past.
5. The United States healthcare system is expected to spend over 3 trillion dollars (18% of GDP) by 2013.
6. We rank twentieth in the world in infant mortality and eighteenth in longevity.
7. Forty to forty-five million Americans (15%) are without any form of health insurance.
8. Disparities between the rich and poor, black and white have widened: Infant mortality among the African American population is twice that of the white population. Early death from cancer, heart disease, and other chronic illnesses is more common among the poor than the United States population overall.

B. Microallocation and macroallocation
1. Macroallocation is the distribution of scarce resources as determined by society usually through the mechanism of government.
2. Microallocation is the distribution of scarce resources on a more personal level.

C. Distributive justice
1. Formal distributive justice: According to Aristotle in distributing scarce resources, equals are treated equally, and unequals treated unequally.
2. Material distributive justice: Principles that specify the relevant criteria in distributing scarce resources.
   a. To each an equal share.
   b. To each according to need.
   c. To each according to merit.
   d. To each according to probability to benefit.
   e. To each according to effort.
   f. To each according to past or future contribution.
   g. To each according to ability to pay.
3. Triage: Common ordering system, developed by the military, to prioritize the allocation of treatment regimens according to need and urgency.
   a. Walking wounded: Those who have sustained superficial injuries requiring minimal care. Patients either wait or are immediately "patched up" to return to battle.
   b. Fatally wounded: Are treated for pain, but not their injuries.
   c. Seriously wounded: Are treated immediately, because their care will have the best outcome.
4. Fairness issues
   a. Fair opportunity rule: No person should be granted social benefits on the basis of undeserved advantage, and no person denied social benefits on the basis of undeserved disadvantage. Gender, race, IQ, nationality, affectional preference, and social status, therefore, are not relevant criteria.
   b. Because resources may be used by someone else for the same purpose, the issue of fairness must be carefully weighed.
   c. Resources may be channeled in a different direction to solve other, perhaps more far-reaching problems.
5. Theories
   a. Egalitarian: Equal access to resources.
   b. Utilitarian: The greatest good for the greatest number.
   c. Libertarian: Emphasizes personal rights to social and economic liberty—the choice of an allocation system should be freely chosen.
6. The function of medicine is to respond to human need.
7. We often value a single life more highly than probabilities of saving multiple others, especially because we are not convinced such resources will be used to achieve such ends.
8. Rescher's (1969) Proposed Method: Once patients have been selected as equal regarding need, likelihood of successful outcome to treatment, and projected life expectancy post-treatment, the following selective criteria may be used:
   a. Likelihood of future service to society.
   b. The extent of past service to society.
   c. The extent of familial obligations.

D. Compensatory justice
1. Those who are marked for special treatment because of past wrongs are often stigmatized.
2. How do we address the question: Who will bear the costs?

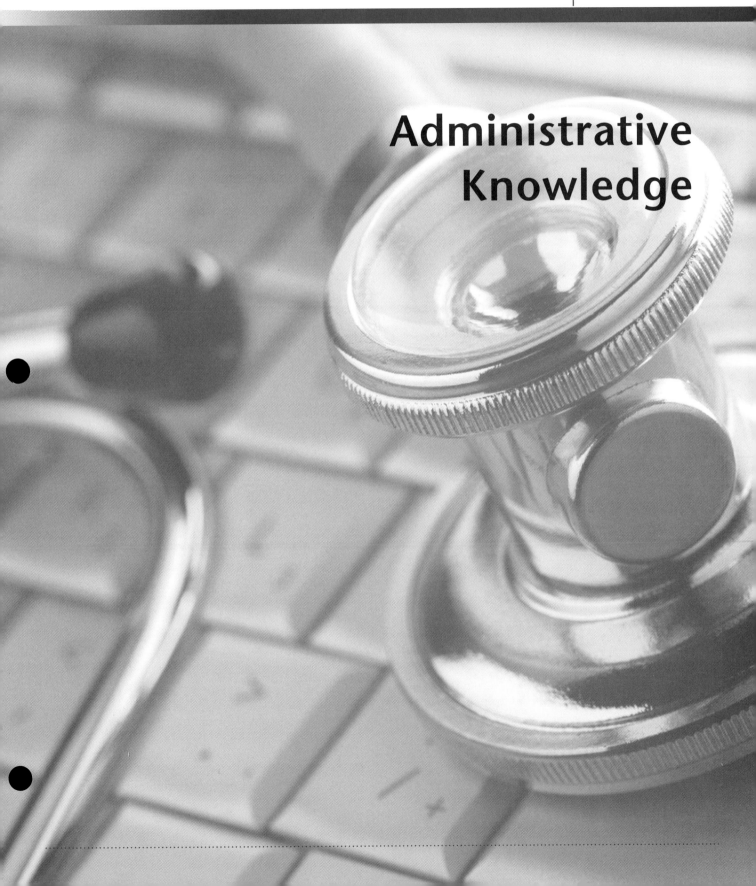

SECTION IV

Administrative Knowledge

CHAPTER 10

Information Management

I. COMPUTER CONCEPTS

A. General

1. **Computer:** Electronic device that receives, manipulates, and stores data.
2. **Computer classifications**
   a. According to size: Generally, larger computers have greater storage capacity and faster processing times.
      (1) Supercomputer: Large, complex computer system capable of performing rapid, complex functions, such as national defense and weather forecasting and research.
      (2) Mainframe: Large computer capable of handling hundreds of users.
      (3) Minicomputer: Medium-sized computer that can handle multiple users.
      (4) Microcomputer: Desktop personal computer (PC).
   b. According to type of data processed
      (1) Analog: Computers that process continuous or measurement data such as sound waves.
      (2) Digital: Computers that process discrete or binary numerical data.
      (3) Hybrid: Computers that perform the functions of both analog and digital computers.

B. Computer system elements
   1. **Hardware:** Physical computer equipment (see Figure 10-1).
      a. Central processing unit (CPU): Collection of three components that process data (see Figure 10-2).
         (1) Control unit (CU): Although it does not perform the actual data processing, it supervises the data processing operations. The CU performs the following functions called the *machine cycle:*
            (a) Retrieving: Obtains instructions from the primary storage unit.
            (b) Decoding: Translates the instructions into language the computer understands.
            (c) Executing: Carries out the instructions.
            (d) Storing: Results of the instructions are stored in the primary storage unit (PSU).
         (2) Arithmetic logic unit (ALU): Processes the data in two ways.
            (a) Arithmetic operations: Mathematical calculations involving addition, subtraction, multiplication, and division.
            (b) Logic operations: Compares data to determine whether two or more values are greater than, less than, or equal to each other.
         (3) Primary storage unit (PSU): Main computer memory that stores data and program instructions.
            (a) Random access memory (RAM): Temporary memory within the CPU that is lost once power is discontinued.
            (b) Read only memory (ROM): Permanent memory within the CPU installed by the manufacturer that allows the computer to carry out its operations.
      b. Peripherals: Input/output devices that communicate between the user and hardware (see Figure 10-3).
         (1) Input devices: Allows for input of data into a computer.
            (a) Keyboard: Allows for the input of alphanumeric data.
            (b) Mouse: Handheld device that, when moved across a flat surface, moves the cursor to any spot on the monitor screen.
            (c) Trackball: A ball embedded in a base that when rolled, moves the cursor on the screen.
            (d) Joystick: A vertical stick embedded in a base that moves the cursor in the direction the stick is moved.

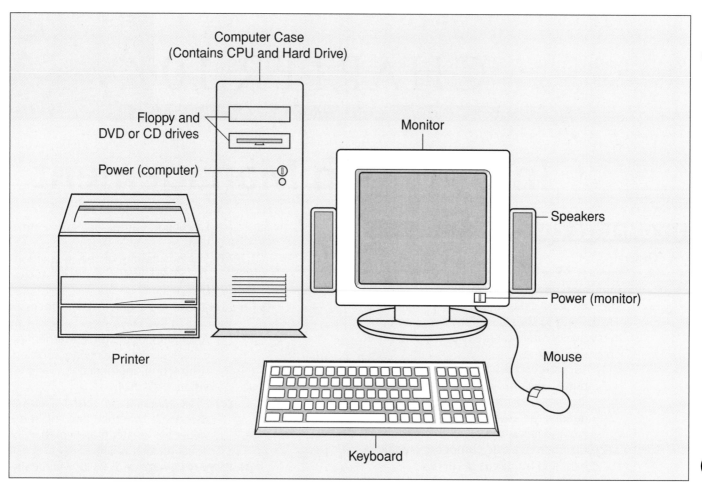

Figure 10-1

Components of the personal computer (PC). Delmar/Cengage Learning.

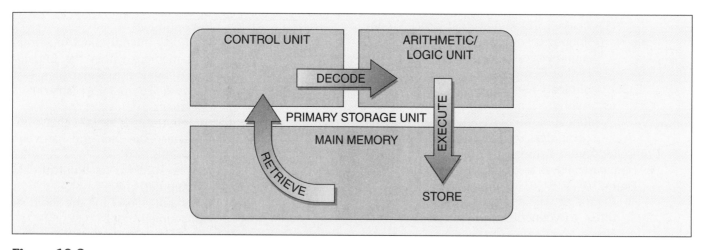

Figure 10-2

Basic computer components and functions. Delmar/Cengage Learning.

(e) Digitized tablet: A pressure sensitive pad that produces on the screen any outline drawn on the pad.

(f) Light pen (wand): A pen that is sensitive to the light emanating from the screen. When placed close to the screen, it can control the cursor and activate various functions.

(g) Scanners: A device such as a wand that bounces a beam of light off an

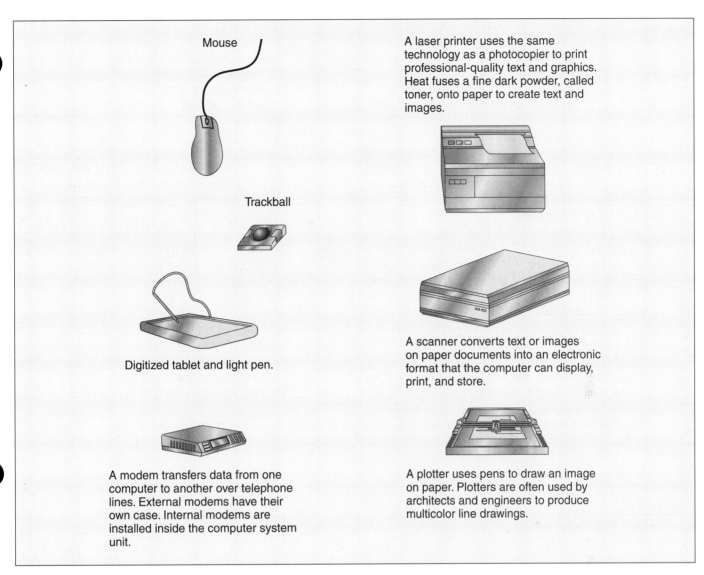

Figure 10-3

Peripheral devices. Delmar/Cengage Learning.

image such as a bar code that receives the reflected light as input.

(2) Output devices: Allows for data to be displayed or recorded.
    (a) Monitor: Cathode ray tube (CRT) or screen that visually displays data.
    (b) Printer: A device that records data on hard copy (paper).
    (c) Plotter: Device that converts computer-generated graphs, charts, and drawings into high-quality hard copy.

(3) Ports: Means of connecting peripherals to the CPU.
    (a) Serial port: Sequentially transfers data one piece at a time.
    (b) Parallel port: Transfers groups of data at a time.

c. Secondary storage: Due to the temporary nature of RAM in the primary storage unit, it is necessary to use secondary storage components to store data and programs (see Figure 10-4).
    (1) Hard disk: Internally contained magnetic disk for data and program storage.
    (2) Floppy disk: External magnetic disk that, when inserted into a disk drive, can store and load data and programs.
    (3) Disk drive: Electronic device that retrieves and stores data on a diskette.
    (4) Magnetic tape: Magnetic cassette tape or reel used to store data and programs.

(5) Optical disks: DVDs (digital video disks) and CDs (compact disks). Data is stored on a metal surface that can be read by a laser.

(6) Solid-state devices: Small (size of thumb or car key), removable storage/memory cards that have no moving parts. They plug into a USB port on the computer, and have various names depending on the manufacturer (e.g., flash drive, flash pen, thumb drive, key drive, and mini-USB drive).

2. Software: A computer program that provides processing instructions to the computer.

a. Systems software: Programming instructions that manage the overall operations of a computer system. Operating systems: Programming instructions that control, interface, and communicate between the applications software and computer hardware; e.g., MS-DOS, Unix, OS/2, Windows 95.

b. Applications software: Prepared programs, often commercially developed, that perform a specific data processing function such as word processing, spreadsheets, database management, and telecommunications.

C. Data processing
1. Transforming data into useful information.
   a. Data: Raw information such as numbers and letters that the computer processes.
   b. Information: Processed data that can be used in a meaningful way.
2. Memory
   a. Bit: Binary digit. Smallest piece of information processed by a computer.
      (1) When an electrical charge is present, the bit is on and takes the binary value 1.
      (2) When an electrical charge is absent, the bit is off and takes the binary value 0.
   b. Byte: An 8-bit unit. One byte of memory is required to represent a character.
   c. Kilobyte (K): Represents 1024 bytes.
   d. Megabyte (M): Represents 1000 kilobytes.
3. Machine language: Binary computer coding system that represents each data character.
   a. ASCII: American Standard Code for Information Interchange. A machine language used in many microcomputers.
   b. EBCDIC: Extended binary coded decimal interchange code. A machine language used by larger computers.

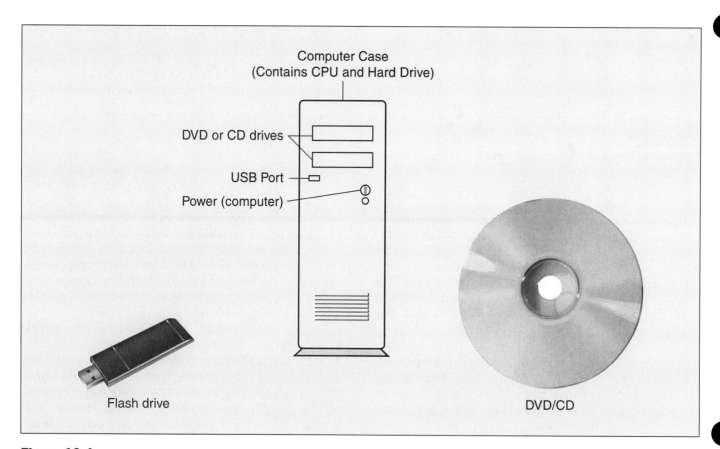

Computer Case
(Contains CPU and Hard Drive)

DVD or CD drives

USB Port

Power (computer)

Flash drive

DVD/CD

Figure 10-4

Secondary storage devices. Delmar/Cengage Learning.

4. Data processing cycle
   a. Input: Data is entered into the computer via an input device.
   b. Processing: Manipulation of the data that has been inputted.
   c. Output: After the data is processed, the resulting information can be accessed via an output device.
   d. Storage: Input or output data or information is stored on a storage medium such as a floppy disk.
D. Miscellaneous computer terms and concepts
   1. Computer care and maintenance
      a. Screen wipes: Thin paper sheets that keep monitors free of dust while providing anti-static protection.
      b. Compressed air: Cans of compressed air with strawlike nozzles used to blow out dust and particles from inside the keyboard.
      c. Cotton-tipped applicators: Used to clean the keyboard surfaces.
      d. Dust covers: Placed over hardware components to protect them from airborne particles.
   2. Computer start-up
      a. If the operating system is stored on the hard disk (C drive) simply turn on the computer, ensuring that no floppy disks are in the A or B drive.
      b. If, however, you must boot the system, that is, load the operating system, simply place the CD containing the operating system into the default drive (usually drive D or CD/DVD), and then turn on the computer.
      c. Turn on monitor and printer.
   3. Computer shutdown
      a. Ensure that you save whatever you are working on before turning off the computer.
      b. Escape out of the current application being used until you see the C:\> prompt.
      c. Remove all diskettes; turn off the computer.
   4. Diskette care
      a. Do not bend or fold diskettes.
      b. Do not expose to extreme heat or cold.
      c. Do not place near magnets or materials having a magnetic field.
      d. Keep away from dust, food, liquid, etc.
      e. Remove from the disk drive when not in use.
      f. Store in protective jacket when not in use.
   5. Booting: Process of activating the input of the operating system into main memory.
   6. Program installation: Process of loading the software instructions onto the hard disk of the computer. Specific installation instructions are included with the software package.
   7. Disk formatting: Process of organizing a blank disk into sectors so that it can store data.
   8. Disk copy: Process of copying a file on a diskette or copying the contents of an entire diskette onto a second diskette, especially backup copies.
   9. Configuration: Disk drive arrangement.
      a. Computer with a hard (C drive) and one or more diskette drives (A and B drive).
      b. Computer with no hard drive and one or more diskette drives.
      c. A computer connected with other computers with one of them designated the server (F drive), which has a high-capacity hard disk that contains files that can be accessed by the other computers.
   10. Cursor: A blinking dash shown on a screen that identifies where on the screen data will be entered.
   11. WYSIWYG: What you see is what you get. A document can be designed on the screen exactly as it will appear on paper.
   12. Site license: A license granted to software purchasers to make multiple copies for use at a particular location without violating copyright laws.
   13. Icon: A graphical interface that performs basic functions when clicked on by the mouse; e.g., clicking on the printer icon will cause the document to be printed.
   14. Buffer: Location for temporary data storage during computer processing.
   15. Bus: Any path that data travels inside the computer.
   16. CD-R: Recordable compact disk. Cannot be erased to be written on again.
   17. CD-ROM: Compact Disk-Read Only Memory. A laser is used to read bumps on the disk as 0 or 1 for digital data. Data can only be read, not written.
   18. CD-RW: Rewritable compact disk. Data can be saved, erased, and resaved.
   19. Clipboard: A section of computer memory used to temporarily hold data that has been cut or copied for transfer to another document or location within a document.
   20. Data compression: Program that forces data into less space on the storage medium.
   21. Digitizer: Device that converts drawings, photos, etc., to digital signals.
   22. Glidepad: Touch-sensitive pad for controlling cursor motion. Click by tapping the pad. The cursor follows the path of one's finger upon the pad. Common on laptop computers.
   23. Instant messaging (IM): Application that allows the user to write messages that can be exchanged instantly.

24. Kilobyte (K or KB): Represents 1024 bytes, historically. New standards will use kilobyte for 1000 bytes and kibibyte for the binary 1024.
25. Laptop: Portable personal computer with a screen in the cover.
26. Machine cycle: One round of steps from getting an instruction back to getting the next instruction. The four steps are retrieve, decode, execute, store.
27. Megabyte (MB): Represents 1024 kilobytes, historically. Approximately 1 million bytes.
28. Megahertz (MHz): 1 million cycles per second.
29. Nesting: Placing directories or folders inside other directories or folders.
30. Network: A set of computers that are permanently linked together.
31. Node: Each device connected to a network.
32. OCR software: Software that changes a scanned document from an image to editable text—commonly used for insurance claims.
33. PDA: Personal Digital Assistant. Small personal computer with limited capabilities.
34. Pocket PC: Handheld device similar to a PDA but more powerful—can use Microsoft Office applications, access the Internet, etc.
35. Point size: Measures the height of letters where 1 point is 1/72 inch.
36. Query: A way to arrange records in a particular kind of order or to show only the records that match certain criteria.
37. Queue: The set of print jobs waiting to be done.
38. Server: A computer that handles network tasks and data.
39. Suite: A set of separate applications that are packaged together usually at a lower price than they would cost separately, e.g., Microsoft Office Suite.
40. Touchscreen: Monitor screen that reacts to being touched by one's finger.
41. Tower: Vertical case for a personal computer.
42. Wizard: An automatic set of steps that lead you through a process, e.g., to create a letter.

II. WORD PROCESSING

Document production tool.
  A. Software programs that permit the efficient preparation and editing of written documents.
  B. Keyboard keys
     1. Alphanumeric: Keystrokes that represent letters, numbers, or symbols.
     2. Numeric keypad: Numbered keys that are arranged in a 10-key (adding) machine format.
     3. Escape (Esc): Allows you to exit a computer program.
     4. Cursor control (arrows): Allows you to move the cursor left, right, up, and down the screen.
     5. Delete (Del): Erases characters at the location of the cursor.
     6. Backspace: Allows the cursor to be moved in a leftward direction. Any characters backspaced over will be erased.
     7. Enter/Return: Pressed when inputting data.
     8. Shift: Places the alpha keys in uppercase and activates the symbols above the number keys.
     9. Caps lock: Holds the alpha keys in uppercase.
     10. Function keys (F1 to F12): Performs special computer functions such as retrieving, saving, or printing a document.
     11. Ctrl and Alt keys (control and alternate): Keys used in combination with the function keys to increase the number of available functions.
     12. Num Lock (number lock): Places the numeric keypad in a numbers-only mode.
     13. Tab: Moves the cursor to the right a predetermined number of spaces; used for indenting.
     14. Home: Moves the cursor to the left, right, upper, or lower margins.
     15. End: Moves the cursor to the end of a line.
     16. Insert: Toggle key that allows characters to be typed without erasing existing characters.
     17. Overstrike: Activated when the insert toggle key is pressed; allows characters to be typed over existing characters.
     18. Page up/Page down: Moves the cursor one page up or down.
     19. Pause/break: In some applications, it will immediately suspend computer operations.
     20. Print screen: Will print only what is displayed on the monitor screen.
     21. Space bar: Places spaces between letters, words, or numbers.
  C. Word processing functions
     1. Formatting: Determines the physical layout of a document.
        a. Margins: Sets the amount of space at the edges of the document.
        b. Tab set: Sets the number of spaces for each tab.
        c. Line spacing: Sets the number of blank lines between lines of text; usually single or double-spaced.
        d. Pitch: Sets the number of characters per inch of text.
           (1) Pica: Ten characters per horizontal inch.
           (2) Elite: Twelve characters per horizontal inch.
        e. Justification: Determines the alignment of text relative to the left or right margin.
        f. Header/Footer: Prints identical information at the top or bottom of each page.
        g. Pagination: Positions and prints page numbers.

h. Widow/orphans: Eliminates a widow or orphan.
   (1) A widow is the last paragraph line appearing alone at the top of a page.
   (2) An orphan is the first paragraph line appearing alone at the bottom of a page.
2. Editing: Allows for making changes in a document.
   a. Block: Using the cursor, text can be highlighted for manipulation.
   b. Delete: Blocked text will be erased.
   c. Copy and paste: A block of text is copied for placement elsewhere without erasing the original text.
   d. Cut and paste: A block of text is moved from one place within the document to another place.
3. Search: Instructs the computer to search for words or text for editing and replacing key words and phrases.
4. Printing: Recording the document on paper or hard copy.
5. Saving: Places data or information in storage on a floppy or hard disk.
6. Retrieval: Acquiring from storage, data, or information that has been saved on a disk.
D. Miscellaneous word processing terms and concepts
   1. Default: Predefined setting such as document format that is automatically loaded with each new document unless changed by the user.
   2. Directory: Index of files on a disk.
   3. Error message: A description of an error made by the user when entering data or commands.
   4. Menu: A screen display that provides a list of processing options that can be selected.
   5. Page break: The point where a new page begins; often designated by a broken line.
   6. Prompt/query: A message to the user that is displayed on the screen that provides helpful information or instructions regarding an entry to be made or action to be taken.
   7. Word wrap: As you approach the end of a line while typing text, the computer automatically moves to the beginning of the second and subsequent lines without having to press Enter or Return.
   8. Macro: A combination of time-saving key-strokes that when entered performs a specific function such as inserting a commonly used letter closing.
   9. Merge: Combining two or more files or documents together.
   10. Reveal codes: A set of coded instructions the word processing program invisibly records upon each keystroke. By pressing a designated function key, these codes can be revealed for fast editing.

11. Help screen: Upon pressing a designated function key, the computer will provide helpful explanations and instructions regarding the particular task you are currently performing.
12. Windows: An application that allows more than one application to be operational at one time.
13. Font: A typeface of a particular design and size.
14. Sort: Organize a list alphabetically or numerically in ascending or descending order.
15. Spell check: An added word processing application that checks for misspelled words.
16. Thesaurus: An added word processing application that identifies synonyms and antonyms of words.
17. Grammar check: An added word processing application that identifies grammar or punctuation errors.
18. Desktop publishing: Document presentation tool that permits the production of professional documents containing both text and graphics.

III. SPREADSHEETS

Numbers productivity tool.
A. Software programs that permit rapid calculations applied to a table of numerical data.
B. Changing one value in a spreadsheet will automatically change the other values associated with the changed value without having to recalculate the entire worksheet or report.
C. Worksheet: Working document that contains empty rows and columns for the input of data that can be numerically manipulated.
   1. Column headings are alphabetical.
   2. Row headings are numerical.
   3. Cell: Intersection of a row and column; e.g., cell A1 represents the space occupied at column A, row 1.
D. Data forms: The following types of data can be entered in a cell.
   1. Labels: Alphanumeric characters usually used as headings to identify the row or column.
   2. Values: Numerical data to which calculations can be applied.
   3. Formulas: Provide instructions for performing a mathematical calculation on data entered in other cells.
      a. For example, if at A4 the formula A1+A2+A3 was entered, it would direct the computer to add the values in cells A1, A2, and A3 and supply the total in A4.
      b. Formula symbols: $+$, addition; $-$, subtraction; $\times$, multiplication; $/$, division; $\char`\^$, exponents.
      c. Order of operations: When entering a formula, certain mathematical tasks will be carried out in a specified order. Calculations will be performed from left to right with parentheses first,

then exponents, multiplication and division, and finally addition and subtraction.

4. Special functions: Preprogrammed calculations or tasks.
   a. @SUM: Will add a group of values.
   b. @AVG: Will average a group of values.
   c. @SQR: Will determine the square root of a value.

E. Range: A designated group of cells being affected by a calculation or task; e.g., the notation (A1..C5) indicates that the task at hand should be applied to cells A1, A2, A3 through A15, B1, B2 through B15, C1, C2, C3, C4, and C5 only.

F. Operating modes
   1. Command mode: Pressing (/) key in some versions will display the menu for selection of command options. Windows versions will display the menu and icon shortcut buttons.
   2. Ready mode: Allows for the input of data and movement from cell to cell.
   3. Edit mode: Allows for changes in cells that already contain data.

G. Templates: A generic worksheet that is saved and repeatedly used for a similar application; e.g., a budget worksheet template that is used by each department to enter their individual department data to create a standardized budget document.

IV. DATABASE

Data management tool.

A. Software programs that facilitate the collection of data files that can be accessed, manipulated, rearranged, sorted, and categorized to meet user information needs.

B. Data hierarchy
   1. Fields: Basic piece of data such as a name, address, or course grade; usually arranged in columns.
      a. Alphanumeric: Data using any combination of letters, numbers, or symbols.
      b. Numeric: Numerical data used as codes or for calculations, or to express quantity.
      c. Logical: Data having one of two possible conditions; e.g., yes/no, male/female, true/false, etc.
      d. Memo: Provides further documentation or explanatory information for the user.
   2. Records: Collection of related fields, usually arranged in rows. Each record within a file will have the same collection of fields.
   3. Files: Collection of related records.

C. Entry operations
   1. Addition: Adding a field, record, or file to a database.
      a. Appending: Adding data at the end of a data set.
      b. Inserting: Adding data between data sets.

   2. Deletion: Removing a field, record, or file from a database.
   3. Modification: Changing an existing field, record, or file.

D. Database operations
   1. Sorting: Arranging data in a particular order or sequence; i.e., ascending or descending alphabetical or numerical order.
   2. Indexing: Creating a new file using existing fields and records without upsetting the original database file content and organization.

E. Database reports
   1. Summary reports: Reports that provide a count, subtotal, and total of various fields.
   2. Exception reports: Reports that identify fields or records that have a unique characteristic; commonly describes data that falls outside the norm or predetermined data set.
   3. Detail reports: Reports that list the records in each file.

F. Medical Practice Software
   1. Handles appointment scheduling, billing, and collection.
   2. The database contains demographic, financial, and insurance information.
   3. Each new patient's information is added to the database.
   4. Codes the service so the system can generate a claim for a third party payer or for the patient.
   5. The claim is sent electronically to either a payer or to a clearinghouse that then forwards it to a payer.
   6. When claims are paid, post them into the system.
   7. Can run financial reports.
   8. May include a code-checker to prevent improperly coded claims.
   9. Software includes the rules for submitting claims to most of the major managed care plans so you don't have to wait for denials to understand plan requirements.
   10. Able to sort tasks and triage them to the appropriate staff for action, e.g. new patient appointment—electronic message to send out new information packages relayed.
   11. Information may be input by using a hand-held device, voice recognition, or tablet.
   12. You can access information related to a particular patient and/or to groups of patients.
   13. E-prescribe: Provides reminders and alerts, and promotes compliance with guidelines and formularies.
       a. Integrates patient data from an electronic health record.
       b. Website can enable collection of patient information prior to visit.
       c. Allows patients to request appointments, prescription renewals, obtain test results, and pay bills online.

14. Planning and implementation of information technology (IT):
    a. Considered the future of medical decision-making.
    b. Information offers tools, not solutions.
    c. The success or failure of IT applications is related to change management.
    d. Treat IT decisions as cyclical.
    e. Ensure adequate financial commitment.
    f. Educate and train your staff on IT.
    g. IT applications are dependent on people.
    h. Don't try to do everything yourself.
15. Considerations:
    a. Needs and wants.
    b. Time frame for the IT applications.
    c. Who will be responsible?
    d. Learn about the future direction for IT in medical practices.
    e. What process will you use to evaluate your options and make a decision?
    f. How will you evaluate the results of your purchase?
16. Steps:
    a. HIPAA Security Rule compliance.
    b. Set goals and priorities.
    c. Create a task force.
    d. Develop a practice profile.
    e. Identify and solicit vendors.
    f. Develop a request for proposal.
    g. Compare and rank vendor responses.
    h. Make site visits and check references.
    i. Select the vendors and sign agreements.
    j. Develop an implementation plan.
    k. Evaluate the results.
    l. Start again.
17. Keys to success:
    a. Identify a champion who is able and willing to coach others through the transition process.
    b. Enlist the commitment of all physicians in the practice.
    c. Plan the timing to suit practice needs.
    d. Retain control of training and transition.
    e. Purchase an adequate level of support.

V. MISCELLANEOUS CONSIDERATIONS

A. Data communications: Connectivity tool
   1. Transfer of data from one point to another such as between computers in a room, or over long distances.
   2. Data transmission: Movement of data across communication lines.
      a. Serial transmission: Data is transmitted one bit at a time sequentially.
      b. Parallel transmission: All bits in a byte are transmitted simultaneously.
      c. Asynchronous: Bytes are transmitted one at a time.
      d. Synchronous transmission: Bytes are transmitted in groups.
      e. Simplex: Data is transmitted in one direction only.
      f. Half duplex: Data is transmitted to and from the point of origin, but only one direction at a time.
      g. Full duplex: Data can be transmitted in both directions simultaneously.
   3. Modem: Hardware component known as a modulator-demodulator that connects computers to communication lines.
   4. E-mail: Electronic mail. Messages and documents can be transmitted among users having the proper hardware and software.
   5. Voice mail: Voice messages that are electronically stored and transmitted over telephone equipment.
   6. Facsimile (fax): Machine that electronically transmits and receives documents across telephone lines.
   7. Telecommuting: Working outside the confines of organizational facilities via electronic communication technology.
   8. Networks: Collection of terminals, computers, and other equipment that uses communication channels to share data, information, hardware, and software.
      a. Local area network (LAN): Privately owned communication network that covers a limited geographic area such as an office, building, or group of buildings.
      b. Metropolitan area network (MAN): Privately owned communication network that covers a large citywide operation.
      c. Wide area network (WAN): Communication networks that are privately or publicly owned covering a wide geographic area through the use of telephone lines, microwaves, and satellites.

B. Integrated software: Combination productivity tool. Software package that combines applications such as word processing, spreadsheet, database, desktop publishing, and data communications programs to offer a powerful and flexible data processing tool.

C. Security and confidentiality
   1. Computer crime
      a. Software piracy: Illegally acquiring and using computer software (bootleg software) in violation of copyright laws. Site licensing generally must be purchased to copy software for multiple users in an organization.
      b. Computer embezzlement: Using computer technology to illegally divert funds.
      c. Salami shaving: A form of computer embezzlement that diverts small amounts of money from private accounts into one's own account.

d. Time bombs: Computer programs that are designed to erase files or compromise data integrity.

e. Data diddling: Changing data for one's own benefit; e.g., credit reports.

f. Trojan horse/trap door: A computer program designed to acquire access codes and passwords for illegal entry into a computer system.

g. Computer virus: A program created by another computer user that adversely affects the integrity of data or proper functioning of a computer.

h. Phishing: Using e-mail to illegally solicit private user information for the purpose of identify theft.

2. As most healthcare professionals are not computer programmers, medical data is highly vulnerable to computer crime and confidentiality breaches.

3. Electronic Communications Privacy Act of 1986: Protects against illegal interception of data communications.

4. Security measures
   a. Properly store and secure secondary storage devices.
   b. Passwords: Control access to sensitive patient data by requiring the assignment of secret individual access codes.
   c. Perform periodic inventory audits to prevent theft.
   d. Provide periodic employee training on computer crime and security methods.
   e. Fade-out screen: Information displayed on a monitor will disappear after a short period of nonuse. This prevents unauthorized persons from reading information displayed on a monitor.

VI. MEDICAL RECORDS

A. Review Medical Chart, Chapter 16.

B. Electronic Health Record
   1. Complex system of coordinated hardware, software, people, policies, and processes in support of patient care.
   2. The ideal EHR system will capture data from multiple sources and is used at the point-of-care (POC) to support clinical decision-making.
   3. A fully realized EHR system will provide:
      a. Seamless information interchange among providers at all levels of the health care continuum.
      b. Support for fully integrated evidence-based medicine.
      c. Embedded medical terminology to assist with documentation.

C. EHR Benefits
   1. EHR may be used at the point of care (POC), interacting directly with the system as they care for patients.
   2. Provide documentation of clinical findings and procedures.
   3. Active reminders for medication administration.
   4. Suggestions for less expensive drugs.
   5. Protocols for medical procedures.
   6. Alerts to duplicate services.
   7. Combined scheduling, registration, and billing system.
   8. Data and information can be exchanged with other providers and systems.
   9. CCR: Continuity of Care Record: Standard content physicians agree should be in a referral.

D. EHR Technology
   1. Databases: Organized collection of data in a standardized format.
   2. Data exchange: Protocols that ensure data transmitted from one system to another remains comparable. Standards that allow data from multiple sources to be integrated.
   3. Images: Electronically store and view documents and clinical images.
   4. Workflow systems: Any work process that must be handled by more than one person. Allowing access to the same information by multiple users.
   5. Data retrieval technology: Viewing data in a flexible format.
   6. Data capture technology: Human-computer interfaces; e.g. templates, macros, speech/handwriting recognition, handheld/wireless devices, patient devices, etc.
   7. System communications and networks: Hardware and architecture, LAN, WLAN, and WANs.
   8. Storage technology: Capable of archiving enormous amounts of data that can be retrieved in real-time.
   9. Workstations: Output devices that allow the retrieval, storage, and use of healthcare data.

E. Health Care Data Sets
   1. Data element: Single fact or measurement.
   2. Information: Data that has been collected, combined, analyzed, interpreted, and/or converted into a form that is meaningful.
   3. Aggregate data: Used to develop information about groups of patients.
   4. Data set: list of recommended data elements having uniform definitions.
   5. Purpose
      a. Identify the data elements that should be collected for each patient.
      b. Provide uniform definitions for common terms.

c. Allows for comparison of data collected at different facilities.
d. Uses of comparison data: accreditation, performance improvement, and research.

6. Common Data Sets
   a. Uniform Hospital Discharge Data Set (UHDDS): Inpatient hospital care.
   b. Uniform Ambulatory Care Data Set (UACDS): Care provided to patients who return home on day of service.
   c. Minimum Data Set for Long-Term Care (MDS): Nursing home residents.
   d. Outcome and Assessment Information Set (OASIS): Medicare beneficiaries receiving services from a home health agency.
   e. Data Elements for Emergency Department Systems (DEEDS)
   f. Essential Medical Data Set (EMDS): Complements DEEDS; concise medical history data set for each patient.
   g. Health Plan Employer Data and Information Set (HEDIS): Provides consumers with information needed to compare the performance of managed care plans.

VII. RECORDS MANAGEMENT

A. General
   1. Purpose: System of classifying, arranging, and storing documents in an orderly, efficient, and easily accessible manner.
   2. Common records
      a. Medical records.
      b. Financial records.
      c. Correspondence.
      d. Research records.
      e. Business records.
   3. Common storage media
      a. Hardcopy.
      b. Microfiche/microfilm.
      c. Computer.
   4. Equipment and supplies
      a. Storage cabinet
         (1) Vertical: File cabinet style.
         (2) Lateral: Chest of drawers style.
         (3) Shelf
            (a) Open or closed.
            (b) Stationary or pullout shelves.
      b. Guides
         (1) Cardboard or plastic dividers that permit grouping and subgrouping of related files.
         (2) Out guide: A guide used to replace a chart that has been temporarily removed from the cabinet, identifying the location or person in possession of the record.
         (3) Out folder: A folder that serves as an out guide but can hold patient documents

temporarily until the medical record is returned.
   c. Folders: Cardboard or plastic holders that contain a file's documents. Folders are often equipped with tabs to aid in the identification of their contents.
   d. Labels: Small stickers affixed to folders, drawers, and shelves to identify their contents.

B. Filing process
   1. Conditioning
      a. Documents are checked for damage and repaired as needed.
      b. Date and time stamped if required.
      c. Information potentially stored in more than one place is copied and cross-referenced.
   2. Inspecting and releasing
      a. Documents are not filed until responsible parties have seen and taken action on them.
      b. A release mark, initials or "TO FILE" stamp, is noted on the document's upper right corner.
   3. Indexing and coding
      a. Indexing: Determining where the document should be filed and deciding on a filing caption.
      b. Coding: Identifying on the document the caption to be used.
   4. Sorting: Arranging the documents according to the filing system used.
   5. Storing: Documents are placed in the appropriate file folder and placed in the file cabinet.

C. Alphabetical indexing rules
   1. Normally used with respect to names of persons, businesses, or organizations.
   2. Folder captions are restricted to only one subject with the documents arranged in reverse chronological order.
   3. Names are divided into units and filed alphabetically from left to right.
   4. A person's name is indexed with the surname as unit 1, the given name as unit 2, and the middle name as unit 3.
      a. Names are alphabetized according to the first unit letter by letter.
      b. The second unit is considered only after the first unit is the same. The third unit is considered only if unit one and two are the same.
      c. A fourth unit, usually date of birth is used for identical names—indexed chronologically.

Example:

Unit 1	Unit 2	Unit 3
Hicke	James	Earl
Hickey	Joanna	Jean
Hickey	William	Lee
Hicks	Paul	M.
Hicks	Peter	M.

5. Initials come before complete names starting with the same letter.

Unit 1	Unit 2	Unit 3
Koop	Beryl	Elizabeth
Koop	C.	Everett
Koop	Carl	Earl
Koop	Cary	Eastwood

6. Units having no name come before those that do.

Unit 1	Unit 2	Unit 3
Able	W.	A.
Able	Warren	Seth
Able	William	
Able	William	Charles

7. A hyphenated name is considered a single unit, e.g. Michael-Smith is indexed Michaelsmith. and The hyphen is disregarded unless it is a business name; in this case, they are placed in separate units at the hyphen.

Unit 1	Unit 2	Unit 3
Bagley	Jason	Peter
Linnis	Bagley	Logistics
Linnis	Jonathan	David
Linnis-Bagley	Joseph	Carson

8. Apostrophes in a name are disregarded, e.g. O'brian is indexed Obrian.

Unit 1	Unit 2	Unit 3
Oreck	Herbert	Hoover
O'reilly	Sean	Patrick
Oren	Candace	Michelle
Oster	Hans	Jan

9. Names with prefixes are filed as a single unit., e.g. De Narr is indexed Denarr.

Unit 1	Unit 2	Unit 3
De La Salle	Janice	Lesly
Du Pont	Abigail	S.
La Port	Joanna	Jean
La Salle	Candy	Rose

10. Abbreviations are indexed as if written in full., e.g. Wm is indexed William.

Unit 1	Unit 2	Unit 3
Saincere	Betty	Amie
St. Paul	Wm	Joseph
St. Paul	Winifred	Sarah
Sainze	Natasha	Natalie

11. Numbers as part of a name are indexed as if written out.

12. Titles, degrees, and terms for seniority usually are not considered in filing but may be indexed last , or may be placed in parenthesis at the end of the name for identification purposes, e.g., Dr., Pastor, Professor, Ph.D., M.S., B.S., A.S., Sr., Jr., I, II, III.

13. Married women who have adopted their husband's surname (family name or last name) are indexed according to their given name (first name) not the husband's., e.g., Mrs. John Jean would be indexed as Dianna Jean.

14. Identical names: When names are identical, the DOB is used as the distinguishing indexing unit. Identical names and birth dates are then indexed according to address.
Index in the following order:
Name, state, city, street, and house number from lowest to highest.

15. Names of organizations
  a. Indexed in the same order as written except when they include a person's name. In this case, the name is indexed according to surname, and then given name.
  b. Numbers are indexed as if written out.
  c. Disregard all punctuation.
  d. Directional terms (east, west, north, south) are indexed as separate units.
  e. Prepositions, conjunctions, and articles are disregarded unless *the* is the first word, then it is indexed as the last unit.

16. Numbers: Numbers as part of a name are indexed as if written out, e.g., 4th is indexed fourth.

Unit 1	Unit 2	Unit 3
Pharmacy	III	Drugs
Route	55	Pediatrics
2nd	Street	Clinic
21st	Avenue	Orthopedists

D. Numerical filing
  1. General
    a. Each patient is assigned a number that is identified on their medical chart.
    b. Each patient's number is cross-referenced with the patient's name and filed alphabetically.
    c. Commonly used in hospitals, group practices, and large clinics.
  2. Consecutive numerical system
    a. Each patient is assigned a number in the order of their first visit.
    b. Simplest numerical system often employed in practices of 10,000 patients or less.
  3. Terminal digit system
    a. Patients are assigned consecutive numbers as they visit the clinic , e.g., 1400.
    b. The numbers are separated into groups of two or three , e.g. 00 - 14 - 00.
    c. The numbers are read in groups from right to left and filed in this manner.

Individual #	Secondary #	Primary #
0	14	00

    d. Terminal Digit Filing: Index by primary number in ascending order. Then by secondary number in ascending order. Finally by individual number in ascending order.

Individual	Secondary	Primary
00	00	15
21	00	15
01	90	15
02	90	15
03	90	15

E. Subject filing
   1. Documents are indexed according to subject and then filed alphabetically, numerically, or both.
   2. Generally not applied to medical records, but often used on operational and research files.
F. Geographic filing
   1. Documents are indexed according to geographic location.
   2. May be integrated with a subject filing system; not common in health care organizations except perhaps for research activities.
G. Phonetic filing: Records are filed according to the sound of names rather than on spelling. Consonant sounds are assigned a code number and filed accordingly.
H. Electronic filing systems
   1. Bar codes: Medical records may be labeled with bar codes that can be read and tracked by computer software.
   2. Scanners: Scanning devices may be used to scan and index insurance documents and the like.
   3. Databases: Electronic files that can be accessed according to some search criteria.
I. Record protection, retention, and storage
   1. Use out guides whenever a chart is removed.
   2. Subpoenaed records, ideally, should be microfilmed or copied in case of loss.
   3. Maintain a log of all charts removed from the office indicating the date, time removed, and the location or holder. Follow through on all records not returned within 10 days.
   4. After hours all medical records should be properly stored and locked.
   5. Maintain a list and separately store inactive charts.
   6. Medical records should be maintained for a period of time consistent with federal, state, and accrediting agency guidelines, or for a period equal to the statute of limitations beyond a person's death.
J. Miscellaneous filing considerations
   1. Color coding
      a. Colored tabs may be employed to represent information about a chart or a patient at a glance.
      b. Most color coding systems are used on letters of the patient's surname to identify misfiled charts.
      c. For example, assume the first two letters of the patient's surname will be color coded as follows:

A through D = Red
E through H = Lavender
I through M = Yellow
N through Q = Blue
R through Z = Green

Persons with surnames that start with "CR" will have color tabs red, green. All persons with the surname starting with CR will have the same red, green pattern. If patient Clark is inadvertently filed between patient charts Craft and Crane, the color pattern red, green will be interrupted, indicating a misfiled chart.

   2. Tickler file: A general filing system that organizes items chronologically for follow-up such as appointments, accounts payable due dates, or insurance tracking.

VIII. MAIL PROCESSING

A. Equipment and supplies
   1. Postal scale: Used to weigh mail to determine correct postage.
      a. Available in spring, beam, pendulum, or electronic models.
      b. Quality control: Scale can be quality controlled by verifying that nine pennies equal one ounce.
   2. Postage meter: Machine used to print prepaid postage directly on envelopes or adhesive strips.
      a. May be used for any class of mail.
      b. Serves as postage payment, postmark, and cancellation mark.
      c. Setting meter: The appropriate buttons are pressed to indicate the date and amount of postage to be printed.
   3. Stationery
      a. It is recommended that paper and envelopes be light colored with dark print, and in standard dimensions to eliminate unnecessary charges.
      b. Open-window envelopes should be avoided because they often catch the corners of other mail and tear.
   4. Rubber stamps: To indicate date of receipt and to place restrictive endorsements on checks.
   5. Stapler, letter opener, labels, stickers, etc.
B. Common postal services
   1. Mail forwarding: First-class mail sent to the wrong address and returned can be forwarded to the correct address at no additional postage; simply cross out the incorrect address and write in the correct address. Other mail classes will require additional postage.
   2. Address change: Completing a change of address form at the post office will ensure that

all mail sent to the old address will be forwarded to the new address. Depending on the class of mail being delivered, this service may be provided from 3 months to a year.

3. Address correction: By writing *Address Correction Requested* beneath the return address, the sender can determine an addressee's new address. For a fee, the post office will forward first-class mail to the new address and return to the sender a card identifying the new address and a postage-due stamp indicating the fee.

4. Tracing mail: Mail that has not reached its destination can be traced by completing a postal form. Include a description of the mail and information identified on postal receipts (registered, certified mail, etc.) if applicable. First-class mail is not easily traced; however, the post office will attempt to do so.

5. Recalling mail: If mail has been sent in error, it may be returned if the mail has not been delivered to the recipient.
   a. A duplicate envelope identical to the one erroneously mailed will have to be prepared.
   b. Contact the local post office to determine where to take the envelope for mail recall.
   c. A *Sender's Application for Recall of Mail* form is completed and given to the postal clerk along with the duplicate envelope.
   d. If the mail is still at the post office, it will be returned; if, however, it has been delivered to another zip code, the postal clerk will attempt to intercept it before the mail reaches its destination.

C. Incoming mail
   1. A regular time each day should be scheduled to sort and distribute incoming mail.
   2. Letters marked *personal* or *confidential* are generally not opened by office staff; they are delivered directly to the addressee unless instructed to do otherwise.
   3. Mail inadvertently opened should be resealed with tape with a notation indicating it was opened in error.
   4. All checks received should be immediately stamped with a restrictive endorsement.
   5. Any enclosures mentioned in the correspondence not included in the letter should be notated next to the enclosure line and the sender contacted for the missing material.
   6. The contents of packages should be inspected to ensure that nothing is missing or damaged.
   7. Stamp the date received in the upper right corner.
   8. When a correspondent requests specific information or refers to past correspondence, that information is affixed to the letter for the appropriate party's review.
   9. The provider may request that certain correspondence be annotated; i.e., highlighting the who, what, why, and where.

D. Classifications
   1. First class: All letters and postcards less than 12 oz. Fastest air transport requiring no additional fee.
   2. Priority mail: First-class mail for items weighing greater than 13 oz to 70 lb. Envelopes with green diamond borders are often used.
   3. Second class: Periodicals. Includes delivery of newspapers, periodicals, and magazines.
   4. Third class: Media. Delivery of photographs, catalogs, printed circulars, booklets, or any printed material weighing less than 1 lb. Computer media, i.e., CDs, DVDs, and diskettes. Letters may not be included.
   5. Fourth class: Parcel post. Delivery of packages and printed material weighing 1 to 70 lb within specified physical dimensions (108 inches). Postage depends on weight and destination.
   6. Mixed class: Delivery of a letter sent with a parcel.
   7. Special fourth class: Delivery of books and manuscripts that have a minimum of 24 pages of which at least 22 must be text or illustrations without any form of advertising.
   8. Express mail: Overnight delivery of material to most metropolitan areas.
   9. Registered mail: First-class mail that is insured for a specific value.
   10. Certified mail: Delivery of mail requiring the receiver's signature as proof of delivery and receipt.
   11. Mailgram: A message transmitted electronically to a post office and then delivered by regular mail.
   12. Telegram: A message transmitted electronically to a telegram service for pickup by the recipient.
   13. Special delivery: Delivery beyond normal delivery hours, including Sundays and holidays. All classes of mail except express mail and bulk third-class mail are accepted.
   14. International mail: Letters, postcards, and parcels sent to foreign countries. Rates and restrictions apply.
   15. Delivery services: United Parcel Service (UPS), Federal Express (Fed Ex), and DHL Express (DHL) offer next-day, second-day, and regular shipping services. Delivery times and costs vary according to size, weight, and distance.

E. Mail security: Handling suspicious mail safely. During alerts, it is prudent to wear rubber gloves when handling incoming mail.

1. Examples of suspicious mail include the following:
   a. Postmark does not match the return address.
   b. Handwritten or poorly typed with no return address.
   c. Misspelled common words.
   d. Oddly sealed or excessively taped.
   e. Stamped with excessive postage.
   f. Excessive in weight.
   g. Exhibits signs of leakage.
   h. Lopsided or lumpy packaging.
   i. Protruding wires or aluminum foil.
   j. Exhibits odd sounds, e.g., ticking.
2. USPS recommendations
   a. Wash hands thoroughly after handling suspicious mail.
   b. Do not eat or drink around mail.
   c. Do not open, disturb, or sniff suspicious mail.
   d. Place the item in a plastic bag or container and isolate the area of the workplace.
   e. Do not allow anyone who might have touched the item to leave. Record a list of the people exposed and provide to public health authorities.
   f. Do not clean up any spilled material—cover with plastic or other material.
   g. Turn off fans and ventilation units that may aerosolize any contaminants.
   h. Immediately notify your supervisor and local law enforcement.

F. General considerations
1. Check outgoing letters for signatures and enclosures before sealing.
2. Avoid surcharges by keeping stationery within standard size limitations.
3. Indicate the proper mailing class to avoid being charged at the first-class rate.
4. Use window envelopes only if an address has four or fewer lines.
5. Mark the envelope to avoid damaging its contents (e.g., do not bend, hand stamp only, etc.).
6. With any computer disk, include a letter identifying its contents.
7. Place computer disks in protective cardboard or plastic before mailing.
8. Reduce expenses by using lightweight paper when sending international mail.
9. Include APO or FPO (Army/Air Force or Fleet Post Office) initials followed by the city and zip code when sending mail to selected military bases.
10. Mail log: An incoming and outgoing log may be established to record daily mail activity.

IX. WRITING MECHANICS

A. Parts of speech: Word categories that form sentences.
1. Noun: A word that names a person, place, thing, idea, living creature, quality, or action.
2. Verb: A word that describes an action, state of being, or relationship.
3. Adjective: A word that describes or limits a noun—tells you something about the noun.
4. Adverb: A word that describes, limits, or qualifies a verb, adjective, or other adverb—tells when, where, why, or how something was done.
5. Pronoun: Word that replaces a noun to avoid repeating the noun, e.g., I, you, he, she, it, we, they.
6. Conjunction: Joins two words, phrases, or clauses together, e.g., for, and, nor, but, or, yet, so.
7. Preposition: Joins a noun to some other part of the sentence—often describes the position, direction, location, time, or place of a noun.
8. Interjection: Words that provide transition (e.g., eh, okay, say, oh, no, ouch, yuck) or express emotion—usually followed by an exclamation point.
9. Article: A word that introduces a noun, e.g., a, an, the.

B. Sentence Structure
1. Phrase: A group of words that does not contain a subject (includes a noun) or a verb that complement each other, e.g., the medical assistant.
2. Clause: A group of words that contains both a subject and a verb that complement each other, e.g., the medical assistant collected.
3. Independent clause: The basic unit of a sentence. The subject and verb must form a complete thought, e.g., the medical assistant collected some blood.
4. Dependent clause: Contains a subject and verb, but the clause cannot stand independently.
   a. Often can be identified by the use of dependent clause markers, e.g., because, since, when, while, until, if, as, though, although, unless, after, before, once, whether.
   b. Clarifies and adds detail to an independent clause.
   c. May appear at the beginning, middle, or end of a sentence, e.g., Before lunch, the medical assistant collected some blood; the medical assistant, a competent professional, collected some blood; the medical assistant collected some blood, although she was exhausted.
5. Essential clause or phrase: Modifies a noun and is critical to the meaning of the sentence.
6. Nonessential clause or phrase: Adds extra information to a sentence. This information can be eliminated from the sentence without jeopardizing the meaning of the sentence.

7. Sentence: Has at least an independent clause—a subject and verb that expresses a complete thought.
8. Simple sentence: Includes one independent clause—a sentence that can stand alone, e.g., The medical assistant called in late.
9. Compound sentence: One that contains two independent clauses joined by a coordinating conjunction, e.g., *The medical assistant called in late* because *she was delayed by traffic.*
10. Complex sentence: Includes an independent clause and one or more dependent clauses—cannot stand alone as a sentence, but modifies or enhances the independent clause, e.g., The medical assistant, *who is not an early riser*, called in late.
11. Compound complex sentence: Includes two or more independent clauses and one or more dependent clauses, e.g., The medical assistant, who is not an early riser, called in late because she was delayed by traffic.

C. Capitalization
1. The first word of a sentence.
2. The pronoun "I."
3. Proper nouns, e.g., names of specific people, places, organizations.
4. Family relative names when used as a proper noun, e.g., Aunt, Mother, Sister.
5. Names of God (except the nonspecific use of the word "god"), specific deities, religious figures, and holy books, e.g., Jehovah, Apollo, Buddha, Koran.
6. Titles preceding names, e.g., Governor Daniels, Professor Johnson.
7. Directions when used as regions of the county, but not compass direction, e.g., Southern Maryland, south of Maryland.
8. Days of the week, months of the year, holidays, seasons when used as a title, but not seasons used generally, e.g., Monday, February, Easter, Fall semester, winter day.
9. Names of countries, nationalities, and specific languages, e.g., France, Dutch, English.
10. Major words in the titles of books, articles, songs, but not short prepositions or articles if not the first word, e.g., Harold and the Purple Crayon, Of Mice and Men.
11. Members of national, political, racial, social, civic, and athletic groups, e.g., Asian-American, Democrats, Minnesota Twins, Greenpeace.
12. Periods and events, but not century numbers, e.g., Great Depression, Constitutional Convention, seventeenth century.
13. Trademarks, e.g., Chevrolet, Nike, Coke.
14. Eponyms—things named after people unless generalized, e.g., Freudian, pasteurize, french fries, italics.

D. Numbers
1. Write out numbers in words when beginning a sentence.
2. Write out numbers less than 10 in words.
3. Identification numbers, Room 219, Interstate 70.
4. Page numbers and division of books and plays, e.g., page 5, chapter 20, act 3, scene 2.
5. Large round numbers can be written in numbers or words, e.g., five million, 5,000,000.
6. Use a combination of figures and words for clarity, e.g., five 13-year olds attended.

E. Punctuation: Marks used to separate groups of words for meaning, clarity, and emphasis.
1. Apostrophe (')
   a. Indicates the possessive of nouns, e.g., the girl's mother, Degas's art, birds' migration.
   b. Marks the omission of letters in contracted words, e.g., didn't, they're, he'd.
   c. Marks the omission of digits in numerals, e.g., class of '12, in the '80s.
   d. Forms plurals of letters, figures, abbreviations, symbols, and words referred to as words, e.g., dot your i's, three 4's, two Ph.D.'s, used &'s rather than and's.
2. Brackets ([ ])
   a. Encloses editorial comments within quoted material, e.g., He piqued [sic] outside the window.
   b. Enclose insertions that supply missing letters, e.g., She decide[d] otherwise.
   c. Serves as parentheses within parentheses, e.g., the Greek letter m (μ [mu])...
3. Colon (:)
   a. Introduces an amplifying word or phrase, e.g., There is only person who can do the job: Patrick.
   b. Introduces a list or series, e.g., there were three routes: north, south, or east.
   c. Introduces a phrase that explains, illustrates, simplifies, or restates the phrase before the colon, e.g., She did a fine job: effective, timely, and persuasive.
   d. Introduces lengthy quoted material set off from the rest of the text by indentation without quotation marks, or as running text with quotation marks.
      e.g., The procedure manual states the following:
      Cleanse the site with isopropyl alcohol...
      e.g., The procedure manual states the following: "Cleanse the site with isopropyl alcohol..."
   e. Separates elements in bibliographic data, in biblical citations, in time, and in ratios, e.g., New York: Cengage Learning, John 3:16, 5:00 p.m., ratio of 1:4.
   f. Separates titles and subtitles, e.g., Statistics: An Introduction.

g. Follows the salutation in formal letters, e.g., Dear Dr. Smith:

h. Follows headings in memoranda and business letters, e.g., To:, From:, Subject:

i. Placed outside quotation marks and parentheses when it punctuates the larger sentence, e.g., The advice is ineffective in "Test-taking Techniques": the tips don't apply.

4. Comma (,)
   a. Separates a series of three or more items, e.g., She passed the forceps, scalpel, and gauze in that order.
   b. Used in direct address, e.g., Dr. Smith, when shall we begin the operation?
   c. Sets off dates that include day and year, e.g., February 28, 1962.
   d. Separates state from city and the remaining sentence, e.g., She went to Vincennes, Indiana, to go to school.
   e. Used to surround appositives—phrases that explain a word, e.g., Dr Smith, the surgeon, canceled the operation.
   f. Sets off nonessential clauses or phrases, e.g., The medical assistants, Ashley and John, will arrive shortly.
   g. Separates independent clauses joined by a conjunction, e.g., Drs. Smith and Jones visited the hospital, but were unable to confer with the Chief of Staff.
   h. Used after an introductory clause or phrase, e.g., Although she was wrong, I should have respected her point of view.
   i. Sets off transition words, e.g., She had the facts right; however, she drew the wrong conclusion.
   j. Sets off parenthetical expressions, e.g., She had the facts right, the glucose was high and the WBC count was low; however, she drew the wrong conclusion.
   k. Sets off contrasting expressions, e.g., The surgery will take 2 hours, not 4.
   l. Sets off two or more adjectives that modify a noun, e.g., the medical assistant responded in a calm, reflective manner.
   m. Separates a direct quotation from its source, e.g., She said, "let us begin."
   n. Used to avoid ambiguity arising from adjacent words, e.g., Under Mr. George, Bush College prospered.
   o. Groups numerals into units of three, e.g., 1,235,000.
   p. Separates a surname from a following title, e.g., John Smith, M.D.
   q. Follows the salutation in an informal letter and follows the complimentary close, e.g., Dear Dr. Smith, Sincerely,

5. Dash (–)
   a. Marks an abrupt change in the sentence structure, e.g., Dr. Adams just arrived to the OR—what do you make of his choice of tie?
   b. Replaces commas or parentheses to emphasize a parenthetical phrase, e.g., She had the facts right—the glucose was high and the WBC count was low—however, she drew the wrong conclusion.
   c. Introduces defining phrases, e.g., A type I error—alpha.
   d. Precedes the attribution of a quotation, e.g., There are three kinds of lies: lies, damned lies and statistics.—Mark Twain
   e. Sets off an interrupting phrase, e.g., He was successful—to say the least—even in tough times.

6. Ellipsis (…)
   a. Indicates the omission of one or more words within a quotation, e.g., "Four score and seven…"
   b. Indicates faltering speech or an unfinished sentence, e.g., no, no, please don't…ugh.

7. Exclamation point (!)
   a. Rarely used—indicates strong emotion or after a command. Do not use a comma after an exclamation point.
   b. e.g., I said no!

8. Hyphen (-)
   a. Links elements in compound words, e.g., post-recovery, middle-of-the-road.
   b. Separates a prefix, suffix, or combining form from a base word if it is capitalized, or identical letters would be adjacent to each other, e.g., pre-Victorian, pus-like, anti-inflammatory.
   c. Used with the first of two prefixes having the same base word, e.g., pre- and postoperative care.
   d. Used with written out numbers between 21 and 99, e.g., twenty-two years old, twenty-first time.
   e. Used for a written out fraction, e.g., two-thirds.
   f. Used in numbers meaning "up to and including," e.g., pages 2-10, the years 1990-99.
   g. Used as the equivalent of *to, and,* or *versus* to indicate linkage or opposition, e.g., the New York-Paris flight, the Obama-Clinton debate, a score of 3-2.
   h. Marks an end-of-line division of a word. Although the patient presented with hypertension and angina pectoris, she refused to accept any medical treatment.

9. Parentheses (( )):
   a. Encloses phrases that provide illuminating information, e.g., Nurse Jones (an alumnus) gave the commencement address.

b. Encloses numerals to verify a spelled-out number, e.g., It will take four (4) weeks to complete.

c. Encloses numbers or letters representing a series, e.g., To be successful in this course, you should (1) read the text, (2) complete the practice exercises, (3) take the practice exam, and (4) review the exam study guide.

d. Encloses abbreviations or acronyms that follow the spelled-out form, e.g., The Department of Health and Human Services (DHHS).

e. Indicates alternative terms, e.g., Record what (s)he says during the deposition.

f. Encloses bibliographic or reference data, e.g., The 12 cranial nerves are illustrated (fig. 4)., exagiophobia (Cody, 1991) is the fear of tests.

g. Punctuate phrases in parentheses in accord with the general punctuation rules.

10. Period (.)

a. Marks the end of a sentence, e.g., Every day in every way, I am getting better and better.

b. Follows abbreviation, some contractions, separates letters in an acronym, e.g., ave., assn., Ph.D.

c. Follows outlining numerals and letters.
   1. Statistics
      a. Descriptive statistics
      b. Inferential statistics

d. Not used after headlines, heads or subheads, items in a column, index entries, or captions not in sentence form.

e. Not used before a question mark unless the period is used for an abbreviation.

f. Not used after an exclamation point or question mark.

g. Periods are placed inside quotation marks.

h. Periods are placed outside parentheses if the parenthetical sentence is part of a larger sentence. They are placed inside the parentheses if not part of another sentence.

i. Use it to end a rhetorical question.

11. Question mark (?)

a. Ends a direct question, e.g., When will the physician arrive?

b. Indicates uncertainty about a fact, e.g., The antique is circa 1880?–1900

c. Do not use a comma after a question mark.

12. Quotation marks, double (" "):

a. Encloses direct quotations but not indirect quotations, e.g., "The treatment is complete," he said. He said the treatment was complete.

b. Encloses words or phrases borrowed from others and informal words, e.g., She said she was "in charge." The patient appeared "shocky."

c. Encloses titles of poems, short stories, essays, articles, book chapters, as well as radio and television episodes, e.g., The title of this chapter is "Information Management."

d. Encloses lines of poetry included in the lines of the text, e.g., He began his serenade with "how do I love thee, let me count the ways."

e. A period or comma is used within the quotation marks.

f. A colon or semicolon is placed outside the quotation marks, e.g., The patient had a number of mental "issues": bipolar disorder and suicidal ideation.

g. A dash, question mark, or exclamation point is placed inside the quotation marks when it punctuates the quoted matter only, e.g., She asked, "What is his diagnosis?"

h. They are placed outside the quotation marks when it punctuates the whole sentence, e.g., What is the meaning of "distribution free statistics"?

13. Quotation marks, single (' ')

a. Encloses quoted material within quoted material, e.g., She said, "I distinctly heard the student ask, 'Will this be testable?'"

14. Semicolon (;)

a. Separates independent clauses joined without a conjunction, e.g., The principle diagnosis was heart murmur; no treatment was warranted.

b. Joins two clauses when the second includes a conjunctive adverb (however, thus, indeed, as a result, on the other hand, in that case), e.g., The patient was diagnosed with cholelithiasis; as a result, a cholecystectomy was ordered.

c. Used before introductory expressions (for example, that is, and namely), e.g. The researcher committed a Type I error; that is, he rejected a true null hypothesis.

d. Separates phrases or items in a series that contain commas, e.g., Unit 1 includes terms, measurement scales, and graphs; Unit 2 includes probability theories, distributions, and confidence intervals.

e. Placed outside quotation marks and parentheses, e.g., The researcher committed a Type I error (alpha error); that is, he rejected a true null hypothesis. The patient had a number of mental "issues"; that is, bipolar disorder, and suicidal ideation.

15. Slash (/)

a. Separates alternatives that represent "or," as well as "and/or," e.g., his/her.

b. Replaces the word "to" or "and" in some compound words and ranges, e.g., 2008/9, May/June.

c. Separates elements in numerical dates and fraction numerator and denominator, e.g., 9/11/01, 4/5.

d. Represents the words "per" or "to" when used between units of measure or a ratio, e.g., 400 mg/mL, 20/40 vision.

e. Included in some abbreviations, e.g., w/o, c/o, I/O.

f. Included in internet addresses, e.g., http://vinu.edu/directory.

F. Grammar in brief

1. The number of the subject should match that of the verb: If the noun is singular so should the verb; if the noun is plural, the verb is plural.
   a. <u>Mary</u> is a medical assistant
   b. <u>Mary and Jane</u> <u>are</u> medical assistants.

2. Use the proper case of pronoun.
   a. The physician was she (not her because "she was the physician" not "her was the physician").
   b. Who (not whom) did the procedure? (not whom because "he did the procedure" not "him did the procedure").
   c. Of whom (not who) do you speak? (not who because "I speak of him" not "I speak of he").
   d. I am taller than he ("than he is" not "than him is").

3. A participial phrase at the beginning of a sentence should refer to the grammatical subject.
   a. Experiencing much pain, the doctor treated the patient. The sentence literally means the doctor is experiencing the pain, not the patient. It should be recast to "The patient, experiencing much pain, was treated by the doctor."
   b. On arriving in New York, his friends met him at the airport. Who arrived in New York, he or his friends? On arriving in New York, he was met by his friends at the airport.

4. Rely more on the active voice than the passive.

5. Cast expressions in the positive form.

6. Use definite, specific, concrete language.

7. Omit needless words.

8. Keep related words together.

9. Select and stick to the general design of your writing: Plan the organization and format of your writing before you compose.

10. Make the paragraph the unit of composition.
    a. Subjects generally must be divided into topics.
    b. The paragraph is useful in addressing each topic and aids the reader by identifying the development of each topic as it supports the subject.

G. Commonly misused words

1. A vs. An: Use "a" before words starting with a consonant-type sound. Use "an" before words starting with a vowel-type sound, e.g., a hemostat, a scalpel, a union, an honorary degree, an appendectomy.

2. Aggravate v. irritate. The former means to worsen, the latter means to annoy.

3. All right. Written as two words meaning agreed, go ahead, or OK.

4. Allude v. elude. The former means an indirect mention. The latter means to avoid.

5. Allusion v. illusion. The former means an indirect reference. The latter, an unreal image.

6. Alternate v. alternative. The former means every other one in a series, or a substitute. The latter means the other one of a series of two.

7. Among v. between. When more than two things are involved use among.

8. Can v. may. The former means is able. The latter is asking permission.

9. Disinterested v. uninterested. The former means impartial. The latter means not interested in.

10. Effect v. affect. The former means result (noun) or bring about (verb). The latter means to influence.

11. Farther v. further. The former relates to distance. The latter relates to time or quantity.

12. Flammable v. inflammable. Both mean combustible.

13. Imply v. infer. The former is suggested but not expressed. The latter means to deduce.

14. Less v. fewer. The former refers to quantity (amount). The latter refers to number (countable).

15. Lend v. borrow. The one making the loan is lending. The one receiving is borrowing.

16. Nauseous v. nauseated. The former means sickening to contemplate. The latter means sick to the stomach.

17. That v. which. The former defines or restricts the pronoun. The latter does not.

18. Oral v. verbal. The former means transmitted by speech. The latter means transmitted by words, usually in writing.

H. General rules of style

1. Write in a way that comes naturally.

2. Design before you write.

3. Write with nouns and verbs.

4. Revise as necessary.

5. Do not overwrite.

6. Do not overstate.

7. Avoid the use of qualifiers.

8. Use orthodox spelling.

9. Do not explain too much.

10. Make sure the reader knows who is speaking.

11. Avoid fancy words.

12. Be clear.

13. Do not inject opinion unless appropriate.

14. Avoid figures of speech.

15. Avoid foreign expressions.

16. Use the standard rather than the unusual.

X. LETTERS

1. Letter structure (see Figure 10-5)

  a. Heading

    (1) Usually composed of preprinted letterhead within the upper 2 inches of the page.

    (2) Dateline: Date of correspondence should be placed at least three lines below the letterhead or somewhere between lines 12 and 15.

  b. Opening

    (1) Inside address

      (a) Placed four lines below the dateline.

      (b) Includes the name, title, and address of the receiver.

      (c) Street, avenue, boulevard, east, west, north, and south are spelled out.

      (d) Street names 1 through 10 are spelled out.

      (e) Street names 11 and above use figures.

      (f) City: Spelled out and followed by a comma.

      (g) State: Use two-letter abbreviation without period.

      (h) Zip code: Five or nine digits one space after the state.

    (2) Attention line: Optional; placed two lines below the inside address. Directs the letter to a particular person or department when the letter is addressed to an organization.

    (3) Salutation: The opening greeting; placed two lines below attention line or inside address as appropriate.

      (a) Recipient's title and name followed by a colon.

      (b) Informal (personal) correspondence permits a comma.

      (c) Mixed punctuation: Colon follows salutation.

      (d) Open punctuation: No terminal punctuation mark follows the salutation.

    (4) Subject line: Optional; placed two lines below the salutation. Indicates what the letter is about.

  c. Body: Placed two lines below the salutation.

    (1) Contains the message; each line is single-spaced.

    (2) Paragraphs are double-spaced.

  d. Closing

    (1) Complimentary close: Placed two lines below the last line of the body.

      (a) Only the first letter of the first word is capitalized.

      (b) Formal: Truly yours and Very truly yours.

      (c) Common: Sincerely and Sincerely yours.

      (d) Mixed punctuation: Comma follows the complimentary close.

      (e) Open punctuation: No terminal punctuation.

    (2) Signature line: Placed four to five lines below the complimentary close.

      (a) The typed name of person composing the letter.

      (b) The author's title, if short, should follow her name separated by a comma; otherwise, it should be placed directly below her name on the next line.

      (c) The author signs his name above the signature line.

    (3) Reference notation: Placed two lines below the signature line.

      (a) Identifies the letter's author and transcriber; for example: JC:eg or JC/eg

      (b) It is becoming conventional to omit the author's initials as the signature line is adequate.

      (c) It is becoming conventional that all terminal notations be separated by a single space.

    (4) Enclosure notation: Placed one or two lines below the reference notation.

      (a) Identifies any material accompanying the correspondence; for example:
Enc: Autopsy report
Enclosure: Autopsy report
Enclosure (3): Indicates the number of enclosures.

    (5) Copy notation: Placed one or two lines below enclosure notation.

      (a) Indicates a copy of the letter was provided to a third party.

      (b) Multiple parties are to be listed alphabetically or in order of authority; for example:
c: Jake Applebee.

      (c) bc: Blind copy. Indicates a copy has been sent to a third party without the recipient's knowledge.

    (6) Postscript: An afterthought. Placed two lines below the last typed line; for example:
P.S. Please don't forget to contact me regarding Ms. Jones.

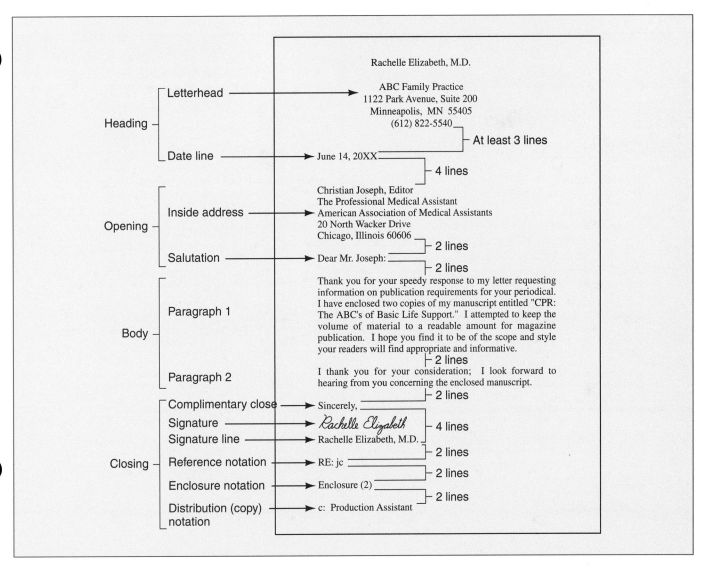

Figure 10-5

Parts of a letter—Full block style. Delmar/Cengage Learning.

2. Letter styles (see Figures 10-6A to D)
   a. Full block: All lines begin flush at the left margin.
   b. Modified block: All lines begin flush at the left margin except the dateline and complimentary close, which begin at the center of the page.
   c. Semiblock: Same as modified block except the beginning of each paragraph is indented five spaces.
   d. Hanging identification: Same as modified block except all lines of each paragraph are indented five spaces except the first line of each paragraph.
   e. Simplified: Same as full block except there is no salutation or complimentary close.
3. Margins: Free space along the four edges of the page.
   a. Short letter (less than 100 words): Use 2-inch margins.
   b. Medium letter (100 to 200 words): Use 1.5-inch margins.
   c. Long letter (more than 200 words): Use 1-inch margins.
4. Multiple pages
   a. Use plain bond paper of the same stock as the letterhead.
   b. Type the recipient's name seven lines from the top edge of the page.
   c. Type the page number one line below the recipient's name.
   d. Type the date one line below the page number; for example:

   Elaine Kramer
   Page 2
   May 10, 20XX

Letter (a) Modified Block Style

Rachelle Elizabeth, M.D.

ABC Family Practice
1122 Park Avenue, Suite 200
Minneapolis, MN 55405
(612) 822-5540

June 14, 20XX

Kevin James, Editor
The Professional Medical Assistant
American Association of Medical Assistants
20 North Wacker Drive
Chicago, Illinois 60606

Dear Mr. James:

Thank you for your speedy response to my letter requesting information on publication requirements for your periodical. I have enclosed two copies of my manuscript entitled "CPR: The ABC's of Basic Life Support." I attempted to keep the volume of material to a readable amount for magazine publication. I hope you find it to be of the scope and style your readers will find appropriate and informative.

I thank you for your consideration; I look forward to hearing from you concerning the enclosed manuscript.

Sincerely,

Rachelle Elizabeth

Rachelle Elizabeth, M.D

RE: jc

Enclosure (2)

c: Production Assistant

(a) Modified Block Style

Letter (b) Semiblock Style

Rachelle Elizabeth, M.D.

ABC Family Practice
1122 Park Avenue, Suite 200
Minneapolis, MN 55405
(612) 822-5540

June 14, 20XX

Brian David, Editor
The Professional Medical Assistant
American Association of Medical Assistants
20 North Wacker Drive
Chicago, Illinois 60606

Dear Mr. David:

Thank you for your speedy response to my letter requesting information on publication requirements for your periodical. I have enclosed two copies of my manuscript entitled "CPR: The ABC's of Basic Life Support." I attempted to keep the volume of material to a readable amount for magazine publication. I hope you find it to be of the scope and style your readers will find appropriate and informative.

I thank you for your consideration; I look forward to hearing from you concerning the enclosed manuscript.

Sincerely,

Rachelle Elizabeth

Rachelle Elizabeth, M.D

RE: jc

Enclosure (2)

c: Production Assistant

(b) Semiblock Style

Figure 10-6A

Letter styles—Modified block style. Delmar/Cengage Learning.

5. Spacing
   a. Six lines (seven returns) equal 1 inch.
   b. Pitch: Number of characters per inch of horizontal document space.
      (1) Pica: 10 characters per inch.
      (2) Elite: 12 characters per inch.
6. Folding for insertion into envelope (see Figure 10-7).
   a. #10 envelope
      (1) Fold the bottom one-third of the page up and crease.
      (2) Fold the top one-third over the bottom one-third and crease.
      (3) The last creased edge is inserted into the envelope first.
   b. #6 3/4 envelope
      (1) Fold the page in half, bottom up and crease.

Figure 10-6B

Letter styles—Semiblock style. Delmar/Cengage Learning.

      (2) Fold the right one-third to the left and crease.
      (3) Fold the left one-third over the right and crease.
      (4) The last creased edge is inserted into the envelope first.

XI. ENVELOPES

1. Common sizes (see Figure 10-8)
   a. #6 3/4: 6 1/2 inch × 3 5/8 inch.
   b. #10: 9 1/2 inch × 4 1/8 inch.
2. Return address: Sender's address.
   a. Placed three lines from top edge and five spaces from the left edge.
   b. Use all capital letters without punctuation; for example:

(c) Simplified Style

Thomas Arthur, M.D.

ABC Family Practice
1122 Park Avenue, Suite 200
Minneapolis, MN 55405
(612) 822-5540

June 14, 20XX

Paul Allen, Editor
The Professional Medical Assistant
American Association of Medical Assistants
20 North Wacker Drive
Chicago, Illinois 60606

Thank you for your speedy response to my letter requesting information on publication requirements for your periodical. I have enclosed two copies of my manuscript entitled "CPR: The ABC's of Basic Life Support." I attempted to keep the volume of material to a readable amount for magazine publication. I hope you find it to be of the scope and style your readers will find appropriate and informative.

I thank you for your consideration; I look forward to hearing from you concerning the enclosed manuscript.

Thomas Arthur
Thomas Arthur, M.D.

RE: jc

Enclosure (2)

c: Production Assistant

(d) Hanging Identification Style

Ian Francisco, M.D.

ABC Family Practice
1122 Park Avenue, Suite 200
Minneapolis, MN 55405
(612) 822-5540

June 14, 20XX

Matthew Earl, Editor
The Professional Medical Assistant
American Association of Medical Assistants
20 North Wacker Drive
Chicago, Illinois 60606

Dear Mr. Earl:

Thank you for your speedy response to my letter requesting information on publication requirements for your periodical. I have enclosed two copies of my manuscript entitled "CPR: The ABC's of Basic Life Support." I attempted to keep the volume of material to a readable amount for magazine publication. I hope you find it to be of the scope and style your readers will find appropriate and informative.

I thank you for your consideration; I look forward to hearing from you concerning the enclosed manuscript.

Sincerely,

Ian Francisco
Ian Francisco, M.D.

RE: jc

Enclosure (2)

c: Production Assistant

Figure 10-6C
Letter styles—Simplified style. Delmar/Cengage Learning.

Figure 10-6D
Letter styles—Hanging identification style. Delmar/Cengage Learning.

ELAINE KRAMER
1401 W 76 ST
RICHFIELD MN 55423

3. Recipient's address
   a. Placement
      (1) #6 3/4: Two inches from top edge, and 2.5 inches from left edge.
      (2) #10: Two inches from top edge, and 4 inches from left edge.
      (3) Leave a bottom margin of at least 5/8 inch.
   b. Use all capital letters without punctuation.
   c. An attention line (ATTN), if used, should be typed between the company name and address.
   d. Use the two-letter state abbreviation.
   e. If possible, the last line should include the city, state, and zip code.
   f. Nothing should be printed below or to the right of the recipient's address block; for example:

   ELAINE KRAMER
   AAMA
   20 N WACKER DR
   CHICAGO IL 60606

   g. Optical character reader (OCR) guidelines:
      (1) Use all upper case.
      (2) Maintain a uniform left margin for all lines.
      (3) Eliminate all punctuation except a hyphen in the zip + 4 code.
      (4) Leave a space between the city and state, as well as between the state and zip code.

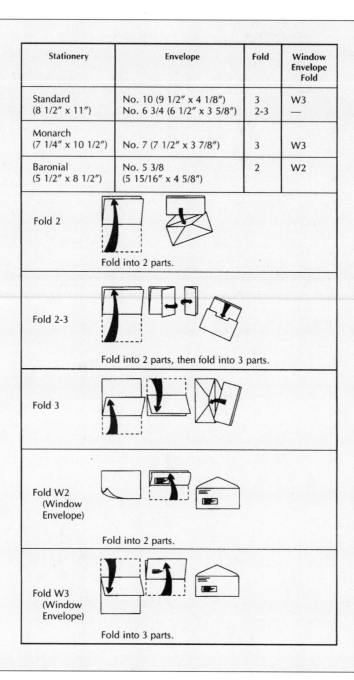

Stationery	Envelope	Fold	Window Envelope Fold
Standard (8 1/2" x 11")	No. 10 (9 1/2" x 4 1/8") No. 6 3/4 (6 1/2" x 3 5/8")	3 2-3	W3 —
Monarch (7 1/4" x 10 1/2")	No. 7 (7 1/2" x 3 7/8")	3	W3
Baronial (5 1/2" x 8 1/2")	No. 5 3/8 (5 15/16" x 4 5/8")	2	W2

Fold 2 — Fold into 2 parts.

Fold 2-3 — Fold into 2 parts, then fold into 3 parts.

Fold 3

Fold W2 (Window Envelope) — Fold into 2 parts.

Fold W3 (Window Envelope) — Fold into 3 parts.

Figure 10-7

Folding and inserting letters into an envelope. Delmar/Cengage Learning.

4. Notations

   a. Directed toward the recipient

     (1) Words such as personal or confidential should be typed two lines below the return address in all capital letters; for example:

     ELAINE KRAMER
     1401 W 76 ST
     RICHFIELD MN 55423

     CONFIDENTIAL

   b. Directed toward the post office: Words such as *special delivery* or *certified mail* should be typed in all capitals in the upper right corner immediately below the stamp placement.

XII. MEMORANDA

1. Written communication among workers within an office or organization (see Figure 10-9).

2. Employs guide words indicating the date, sender, receiver(s), and subject of the memo.

3. The information following the guide words should be aligned with each other and at least two to three spaces after the colon.

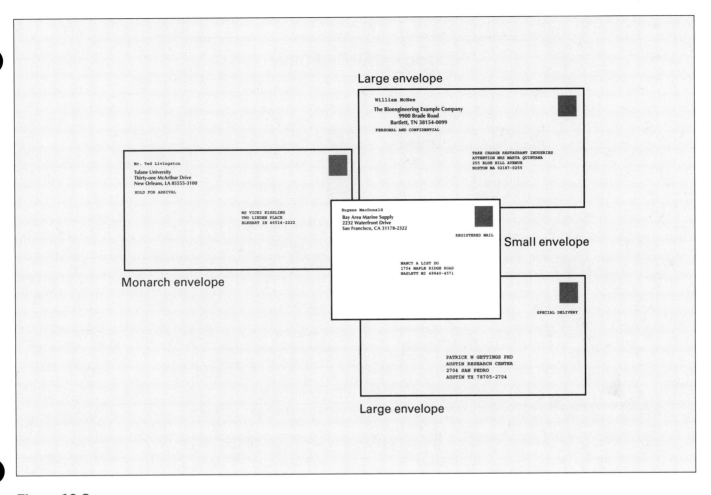

Figure 10-8

Preparing the envelope. Delmar/Cengage Learning.

4. The message should begin three lines below the last line of the guide words.
5. Reference notation
   a. Identifies the transcriber's initials.
   b. Placed two lines below the last line of the message.
6. Copy notation
   a. Indicates a copy of the memo that was provided to a third party.
   b. Placed two lines below last lines of message or reference notation.
   c. Multiple parties are to be listed alphabetically or in order of authority; for example:

TO: Elaine Kramer
FROM: J. P. Coutour
DATE: February 29, 20XX
SUBJ: OSHA Requirements

xxxxxxxxxxxxxxxxxxxxxxxxxxxxxxxxxxxxx
xxxxxxxxxxxxxxxxxxxxxxxxxxxxxxxxxxxxx
xxxxxxxxxxxxxxxxxxxxxxxxxxxxxxxxxxxxx
xxxxxxxxxxxxxxxxxxxxxxxxxxxxxxxxxxxxx
JC:eg
c: xxxxxxxxxxxxxx

7. Multiple pages
   a. Type the subject line seven lines from the top edge of the page.
   b. Type the page number one line below the subject line.
   c. Type the date one line below the page number; for example:

SUBJ: OSHA Requirements
Page 2
May 10, 20XX

XIII. MANUSCRIPTS

1. A written document that is submitted for publication.
2. Different professional organizations, e.g., American Medical Association (AMA) or American Psychological Association (APA), employ different standard formats for manuscript preparation and submission.
3. Title page

Gonzalez Medical Office

MEMORANDUM

TO: Dr. Jeff Brezner
            Obstetrics & Gynecology

FROM: Bettie Thompson   *B. Thompson*
            Human Resources

DATE: April 10, 20XX

SUBJECT: EMPLOYEE PICNIC

Note: Courtesy titles (Dr., Mr., Ms., Mrs., and Miss) are not used by the writer.

Thank you for agreeing to serve on our committee to organize the employee picnic next month. With the group of individuals who will be working on the arrangements, I am sure our picnic this year will be the best ever!

Enclosed with this letter are the following items from last year's efforts:

           Planning Committee Report
           Picnic Budget
           Picnic Employee Flyer
           Picnic Program
           Picnic Evaluation

The first meeting of our planning committee will be in the executive dining room on Tuesday, July 17, 19–, at 2:00 o'clock. My office assistant will be calling you to confirm your attendance at this meeting.

Bring all of your best ideas–let's make this picnic one that will be long remembered.

mos

Enclosures (5)

pc Dr. Maria Hernandez

Figure 10-9

Memorandum. Delmar/Cengage Learning.

   a. Identifies the title or main theme of the manuscript.
   b. The title, names of the authors, and their credentials are usually centered vertically and horizontally.

4. Acknowledgments
   a. Identifies those who have provided assistance in the research or preparation of the manuscript.
   b. Usually placed at the bottom of the title page or a separate page following the title page.

5. Abstract
   a. Summary of the manuscript in 100 to 200 words.
   b. Usually placed at the bottom half of the title page, by itself on the second page, or at the beginning of the text.

6. Text
   a. Title is typed in all capitals, 13 lines from the top edge.

   b. The body of the text begins three lines below the title.
   c. The text is usually double-spaced.

7. References: Identifying the published work of others in the text.
   a. References in text may be indicated with numerical superscripts or numbers in parentheses placed after the citation. The references would then be listed numerically at the end of the manuscript.
   b. References may also be cited using the author's last name, year of publication, and page numbers in parentheses; for example:
          (Cody, 2010, p. 45).
   The references would then be listed alphabetically by author at the end of the manuscript.

8. Footnotes: Cites references or other explanatory information near the bottom of the page on which the referenced material is printed rather than at the end of the manuscript.

9. Bibliography: A list of source material or references used in preparing a written work.
   a. Articles: Author, "title," *journal,* date, publication volume and number, pages. For example: Cody, J. P., "Measuring Your Study Skills," *The Professional Medical Assistant,* July/August, 1992, 35:4, pp. 13–17.
   b. Texts: Author, *title,* publisher, year, pages. For example: Cody, J. P., *The CMA Review Manual,* Delmar Cengage Learning, New York, 2005, p. 22.
10. Illustrations: Placed on separate sheets and assigned consecutive figure numbers.
11. Tables: Placed on separate sheets and assigned consecutive table numbers.
12. Reprints: Copies of a published article in pamphlet form to be given to interested colleagues.

XIV. PROOFREADERS' MARKS

A. After a rough draft has been reviewed, make all appropriate corrections before submitting it as final.
B. See Figure 10-10.

XV. CURRICULUM VITAE (CV)

A. Latin for "Study of Life."
B. Brief or detailed summary of a person's professional experience and activities.
C. CVs are a type of resume for selected professionals such as other healthcare providers and academicians, especially those having doctorate degrees.
D. Prepared on 8 1/2-by-11-inch bond paper having consistent formatting and balanced margins, i.e., 1 inch.
E. CVs are typically organized according to the following headings:
   1. Identifying information: Name, address, phone numbers.
   2. Family information: Although less common today, may identify name of spouse (including years of marriage) and names and ages of children.
   3. Education: Highest degree first. Degree, major, college, year of graduation.
   4. Internships/residencies: For physicians and other health professionals—specialty, sponsoring organization, and dates.
   5. Licenses and certifications: Name of license, number, and expiration date.
   6. Experience: Professional positions held in reverse chronological order.
   7. Memberships: Include professional membership level, e.g., member, fellow, diplomate, etc., and service posts, e.g., president, treasurer, secretary, etc.
   8. Community service: Work performed with community and nonprofit organizations, as well as service on boards and advisory committees.
   9. Research activity: Briefly describe past and current research work.
   10. Publications: Published articles and books, as well as unpublished manuscripts.
   11. Presentations: Speeches or papers given at seminars and conferences; other speaking engagements, panel discussions, and the like. Note title, place, and date.
   12. Awards and honors. Identify instances and tokens of special recognition.
   13. Personal interests and hobbies: Although less common today, this may be included as well.

XVI. INFORMATIONAL BROCHURES

A. Planning the brochure
   1. Identify available resources
      a. Determine who will write it.
      b. Determine who will have overall responsibility for its development.
      c. Determine who will produce it.
      d. Determine who will edit it.
      e. Determine who will design it.
      f. Determine the timeline for development.
      g. Determine the number of brochures needed.
   2. Define the target audience
      a. Consider age, gender, and culture.
      b. Identify their typical reading level.
      c. Identify their needs, interests, and behaviors.
      d. Solicit input from the target audience.
      e. Identify the distribution locations.
   3. Define goals
      a. Determine the brochure's purpose.
      b. Are new facts being taught—if so, what are they?
      c. Do attitudes need to be changed—if so, what are they?
      d. Do behaviors need to be changed—if so, what are they?
   4. Identify the key message and concepts:
      a. Identify the information the audience needs to know.
      b. Identify the concerns that need to be addressed.
      c. Identify any misconceptions that must be addressed.
      d. If there are too many messages and concepts, can some be deleted?
   5. Research the topic
      a. Determine whether everything that needs to be included is known.
      b. Collect the most current and accurate information available.

Change	Mark in Margin	Supplementary Mark in Text	After Change
Align	‖	‖words on a list	words on a list
Capitalize	cap	new york	New York
Close up space	⌒	win ter	winter
Delete	ℰ	leave out the	leave the
Delete and close up space	ℰ	peoople	people
Insert	out	leave ∧ the	leave out the
Insert apostrophe	⌄	Maries dress	Marie's dress
Insert asterisk	✱	the end, but	the end,* but
Insert brackets	[/]	run fast now ∧ ∧	run [fast] now
Insert colon	∧:	follow these steps∧	follow these steps:
Insert comma	∧	ham, eggs∧and toast	hams, eggs, and toast
Insert diagonal	Ⓘ	and∧or the former	and/or the former
Insert hyphen	⊝	do it yourself project ∧ ∧	do-it-yourself project
Insert parenthesis	(/)	run fast now ∧ ∧	run (fast) now
Insert period	⊙	the end∧	the end.
Insert quotation marks	⌄/⌄	the⌄end.⌄	the "end."
Insert semicolon	∧:	Row∧row∧row.	Row; row; row.
Insert space	#	the⌐space	the space
Let stand	Stet	best well-wisher	best well-wisher
Lowercase	lc	the Summer season	the summer season
Move down	⊔	n dow⊔	down
Move left	⊏	move ⊏left	move left
Move right	⊐	move right ⊐	move right
Move up	⊓	u⊓ p	up
Spell out	sp	wouldn't run	would not run
Begin a paragraph	¶	∧The first line and the seond	⠀⠀The first line and the second
Straighten the line	═	⎯⎯the straighten⠀⠀line	straighten the line
Transpose	tr	first to strike ↰	to strike first

Figure 10-10

Proofreaders' marks. Delmar/Cengage Learning.

c. Identify and solicit an available expert who can verify the facts.

6. Develop an outline
   a. Prepare a list of the topics and messages to be included.
   b. Organize the list logically to maximize comprehension.

7. Involve the target audience and experts
   a. Talk to members of the target audience to learn more about their knowledge, attitudes, practices, and opinions about the subject.
   b. Solicit the opinions of the target audience to assess what is most effective in communicating the key message and concepts.

8. Define the distribution plan
   a. Identify the locations members of the target audience visit.
   b. Identify where they get health-related information.
   c. Identify where the brochures can be displayed.
   d. Determine how many are needed at each location.
   e. Determine how each location will be stocked.

9. Determine the look and design
   a. Size:
   b. Font:
   c. Paper color:
   d. Paper type and weight:
   e. Graphics:
   f. Reproducibility:

B. Content considerations
   1. Timeliness: The information is up-to-date.
   2. Purpose and objectives: Limited and focused.
   3. Relevancy: Information is meaningful to the intended audience.
   4. Culture, gender, and age appropriate.
   5. Clarity: Clear and easy to understand; no chance for misunderstanding.
   6. Scope:
   a. Limit the content to "need to know" information.
   b. Limit the number of points, concepts, and messages.
   c. Focus on skills and how-to behaviors.
   d. Make the information action-oriented, not just factual.
   e. Repeat and summarize the main points.
   f. Use concrete examples rather abstract concepts.
      (1) Abstract: Safe sex reduces your chances of acquiring an STD.
      (2) Concrete: Use a condom when you have sex.
   7. Tone and appeal
   a. Present information in a truthful, sincere, positive manner.

b. Avoid biases, prejudices, or misleading concepts.

8. Recognition and contact information: Use the organization's logo with a phone number and address for more information.

C. Literacy considerations
   1. Health literacy: Many health and informational brochures use language that is too complex for most patients to understand.
   a. Typical: "A sodium restricted diet may be recommended to reduce hypertension."
   b. Needed: "If your blood pressure is high, eat less salt."
   c. Patient information must be developed at a reading level most people can understand.
   2. Use a readability test
   a. Aim for sixth-grade reading level or less.
   b. MS Word (1997-2003): Click on following: Tools, Spelling & Grammar, Options, Check "show readability statistics," OK. After completing spell-check, readability statistics will pop up on screen.
   c. MS Word (2007): Click on the following: Review, Spelling & Grammar, Options, Check "show readability statistics," OK. After completing spell-check, readability statistics will pop up on screen.
   3. Avoid the following
   a. Words with more than two syllables.
   b. Medical jargon.
   c. Technical terms.
   d. Unfamiliar acronyms or abbreviations.
   e. Statistics.
   f. Conceptual terms.
   g. Value laden terms.
   h. Negative words.
   i. Contractions.
   4. Use a conversational style and an active voice.
   5. Use short sentence: no more than 12 to 15 words.
   6. Use conventional, correct spelling.

D. Organization
   1. Context: Set the stage before giving new information
   a. State "if " before "then."
   b. E.g., Broccoli, carrots, sweet potatoes, peas, spinach, and squash have many nutrients.
   c. Improved: These foods have many nutrients: broccoli, carrots ... spinach, and squash.
   2. Sequencing
   a. Put important information first, last, or both.
   b. Present information or steps in a logical order
   c. E.g., How to use your metered-dose inhaler:
      (1) Make sure your inhaler has medicine in it.

(2) Take off the cap and hold the inhaler upright.

(3) Shake the can for 3 seconds.

(4) Tilt your head back and breathe out.

(5) ....

3. Grouping
   a. Put related ideas together.
   b. Use bullets instead of paragraphs.
4. Headings
   a. Organize the information under headings.
   b. Use short explanatory headings rather than single words.

E. Format
   1. Arrange the text according to how the eye reads a page, i.e., left to right, then next line from left to right.
   2. Do not hyphenate at the end of a line.
   3. Break sentences at natural pauses.
   4. Do not wrap text around pictures.
   5. Use plenty of white space.
   6. Justify on the left, leave the right ragged.
   7. Use at least a 12-point font.
   8. Use a serif font—do not use fancy fonts.
   9. Used mixed case—all caps and drop caps are hard to read.
   10. Add highlights and emphasis: Circles, color, boxes, bold, underlining, italics, arrows.

F. Graphics
   1. A picture is worth a thousand words—two-thousand if your audience cannot read.
   2. Should be relevant.
   3. Use basic line drawing with little detail.
   4. Familiar and easily recognizable.
   5. Avoid diagrams, graphs, and technical tables.
   6. Develop an attention-getting cover.
   7. Use action graphics that show the desired behavior—avoid showing the wrong behavior.
   8. Do not show body parts out of context.
   9. Use captions below graphics.
   10. Evenly placed throughout.

G. Audience Interaction
   1. Getting the audience involved encourages them to:
      a. Keep the brochure—not throw it away.
      b. Communicate with their providers.
      c. Share information with family and friends.
      d. Maintain mini-records of their health.
   2. Patients learn by doing: Insert items that encourage the patient to think, reflect, and act.
      a. Questions: e.g., Write down the name of your medicine: _____. What was your blood pressure today? ___/___ Date: _____.
      b. Problem solving: e.g., This is what I will do when I crave a cigarette: 1. _____, 2. _____, 3. _____, etc.

c. Word-picture association: e.g., Circle what you will do to get more aerobic exercise:

d. Personalization: e.g., This is your diet record. Write your name here: _____.

XVII. MEDICAL TRANSCRIPTION

A. General
   1. Organizations that engage in medical transcription adhere to published transcription formats and styles, or develop and document their own.
   2. Regardless of the format and style adopted, appearance, clarity, and legibility are the main considerations.

B. Equipment
   1. Transcriber.
   2. Foot pedal.
   3. Earphones.
   4. Audiocassettes.
   5. Computer hardware and software (word processing, etc.).
   6. Computerized digital voice processing machines: Dictator's voice is digitized by converting it into binary code that is displayed as type.

C. Format guidelines
   1. Document title: Centered in all capital letters on the first line. Underscoring optional.
   2. Identifying information
      a. The patient's name, record number, provider's name, date of admission, and other similar information is typed at the left margin as header titles in capital and boldface lowercase letters, followed by a colon.
      b. Each header title is double-spaced.
      c. The identifying information is typed two spaces after the colon.
   3. Headings
      a. Major headings: Typed in capital letters followed by a colon whether dictated or not. Underscoring, boldfacing, or typing on a separate line are optional.
         (1) HISTORY:
         (2) CHIEF COMPLAINT:
         (3) HISTORY OF PRESENT ILLNESS:
         (4) FAMILY HISTORY:
         (5) SOCIAL HISTORY:
         (6) PAST MEDICAL HISTORY:
         (7) REVIEW OF SYSTEMS:
         (8) GENERAL:
         (9) PHYSICAL EXAMINATION:
         (10) DIAGNOSIS:, IMPRESSION:, CONCLUSION:
         (11) SUBJECTIVE:, OBJECTIVE:, ASSESSMENT:, PLAN:
         (12) ADMITTING DIAGNOSIS:
         (13) SURGICAL PROCEDURES:
         (14) LABORATORY DATA:

b. Secondary subheadings: Typed in all capital letters followed by a colon and two spaces and inserted as dictated. Placement on a separate line is optional.

c. Tertiary subheadings: Typed in capital and lowercase letters followed by a colon and two spaces. They are typed only if dictated within the narrative following the secondary subheadings.

4. Format styles
   a. Full block
      (1) All headings except the report title, which is centered, are flush with the left margin.
      (2) Headings are double-spaced from the last line of the narrative from the previous heading.
      (3) Narrative text begins two spaces after the colon following the headings.
      (4) The second and subsequent lines of text are flush with the left margin.
   b. Indented
      (1) Subheadings are indented three to five spaces under the main headings.
      (2) Headings are double-spaced from the last line of the narrative from the previous heading.
      (3) Narrative data begins on the same line of the headings with the first two lines of text indented 23 to 27 spaces from the left margin.
      (4) The third and subsequent lines begin at the left margin.
      (5) If the third line completes the paragraph and is short, indent flush with the first two lines.
   c. Modified block
      (1) All headings begin at the left margin.
      (2) Headings are double-spaced from the last line of the narrative from the previous heading.
      (3) Narrative text begins on the same line as the headings indented 23 to 27 spaces.
      (4) Second and subsequent narrative lines are flush 23 to 27 spaces from the left margin.
   d. Run-on
      (1) All headings begin at the left margin.
      (2) There is no double-spacing between headings.
      (3) Narrative text begins on the same line as the headings.
      (4) The second and subsequent lines are flush with the left margin.

5. Signature line
   a. Type a solid line from the center of the page to the right margin four to six lines below the last line of completed narrative.
   b. Type the provider's name immediately below the line starting at the beginning of the line.

6. Reference notation and dates
   a. Typed two lines below the provider's name at the left margin.
   b. Identify the dictator and transcriber by typing the dictator's initials in all capital letters followed by a colon and the transcriber's initials in lowercase letters.
   c. Immediately below the reference notation, type the date the report was dictated using a D: followed by two spaces and the date, and below that the date the report was transcribed using a T: followed by two spaces and the date. For example:

       MFG: jpc
       D: 12/12/08
       T: 12/14/08

7. Multiple pages: A report that requires more than one page.
   a. Type the word "(Continued)" in parentheses two lines below the last line of narrative at the left margin.
   b. Do not begin a new page with just the signature line; include at least two lines from the ending narrative.
   c. Begin the next page with the patient's name, the reporting provider, date, and page number. For example:

       Jean Coutour
       Dr. Lance Boyle
       12/11/08
       Page 2

8. Syntax
   a. Most medical reports employ sentence fragments. Type fragmented sentences as dictated and punctuate accordingly.
   b. Follow the punctuation instructions given by the dictator.

D. Style guidelines
   1. Eponyms are capitalized: Hodgkin's disease, Foley catheter. Nouns following the eponym are usually not capitalized. Words derived from an eponym are not capitalized; e.g., parkinsonian, gram-positive.
   2. Drug/product trade names are capitalized, generic names are not: Tylenol, acetaminophen; Vicryl, catgut.
   3. Underscore or italicize the scientific names of organisms, except when used in the plural or as an adjective. The genus is capitalized, the species is not: *Staphylococcus aureus* or <u>Staphylococcus aureus</u>, staphylococci, staphylococcal.

4. Capitalize proper names of races, religions, languages, and sects: English, Hispanic, black, white, Jewish.

5. Patient allergies are underscored or in all capital letters: Allergies: PENICILLIN or penicillin.

6. Capitalize acronyms unless written out: MI, myocardial infarction.

7. Numbers from one to ten are spelled out when in narrative; use numerals for numbers 11 and higher.

8. Use numerals for numbers representing measurements: 150 mg, BP 120/80, PTT 25.

9. Use numerals when used with abbreviations or symbols: Pulses 2+, 100% oxygen.

10. Numbers less than one expressed as a decimal should be preceded by a zero: 0.9 retic.

11. Spell out ordinal numbers except when used with dates: First, second, third; February 2.

12. Vertebrae are abbreviated C1 to C7, T1 to T12, L1 to L5, and S1 to S5.

13. Cranial nerves are written in roman numerals I to XII.

14. Titers and ratios include a colon: 1:5 ratio, titer of 1:10.

15. Temperature reading: 98.6F, 37°C.

16. Suture material: 3-0 or 000 silk, No. 40 or #40.

17. Sub- and superscripts: H_2O or H2O, ^{198}Au or Au^{198}.

18. Use numbers for ECG leads, cancer grades, and military time: Leads V1-V6, grade 2 tumor, 1630 hours.

19. Virgule: Use the "/" to mean per or over. 100 mg/dL, 122/88

20. Lowercase "x" is used to indicate "by" in measuring dimensions, and to indicate "times" in magnification or frequency: 1 × 2 cm lesion, sponge count correct × 3, cells magnified × 100.

21. Abbreviate metric measurements without a terminal period: 5 cm, 125 mg, 1.5 mL.

22. Latin pharmacological abbreviations and acronyms are written in lowercase with periods: a.c., p.o., b.i.d.

CHAPTER 11

Front Office Management

I. RECEPTION

A. General
  1. The appearance of the reception area and receptionist, as well as the receptionist's disposition, sets the tone for the office visit.
  2. The receptionist should create a caring ambience.
  3. On the initial visit, all patients should complete a patient information/registration form.
  4. The patient should be presented with a clinic information brochure that describes the practice, office hours, medical staff, appointment scheduling, and procedures.

B. Reception room: Should be maintained, clean, and uncluttered.
  1. Counter: Should be high enough to maintain privacy for the receptionist and conceal records in close proximity.
  2. Reception desk: Should be at sitting level behind a counter. Reception materials should be neatly arranged, without clutter. Ideally, the receptionist should be able to observe the entire reception area.
  3. Periodicals: A variety of reading material should be available. Recommended subjects may include:
     a. Current events and news.
     b. Sporting events.
     c. Popular culture and entertainment.
     d. Travel.
     e. Special interest.
     f. Medical news.
     g. Children's literature if appropriate.
  4. Brochure rack: Pamphlets providing safety and health information.
  5. Television/VCR: Videos providing health news and information, or cartoons for children.
  6. Milieu: Lighting and temperature should be set at comfortable levels.
  7. Tables and chairs: Should be arranged for maximum patient comfort, movement, and decor.
  8. Coat rack: To store outerwear, hats, and umbrellas. Should reduce clutter.
  9. Play area: Toys and books may be appropriate especially in pediatric, obstetrical, and family practice clinics.

C. Receptionist: Is the first person seen in a clinic, thereby establishing the initial impression of the organization. This impression is based on:
  1. Attitude: MAs should demonstrate pride in themselves and their work. Their posture, demeanor, and communication skills should portray competence and a positive attitude.
  2. Appearance: The MA should be appropriately attired, with good personal hygiene.
  3. Etiquette: The MA should exhibit professionalism by portraying a friendly, cheerful, caring, courteous, and respectful demeanor.

D. Visitors
  1. The objective of a practice is to diagnose and treat patients; therefore, patients should take priority over most visitors.
  2. Other providers: The provider-visitor should be immediately announced, escorted to the healthcare provider's office, and asked to wait with an estimate of the waiting time.
  3. Pharmaceutical representatives (detail person)
     a. Secure the representative's business card, and check with the provider to see if there is time for a visit.
     b. If the provider is unable to meet with the representative, indicate this and request that an appointment be made.
     c. If the provider indicates that a visit can be made after a delay, indicate this with an estimate of the waiting time; allow the representative to decide whether to wait or to make an appointment for a later date.
  4. Vendors and sales representatives: Typically handled by the office manager or person responsible for purchases; can be handled in much the same manner as detail persons.
  5. Family and friends: Many providers discourage family and friends from visiting; however, if a visit is made, treat them similarly to visiting providers.

6. Former patients
  a. Ask the visitor to wait in the reception area and announce the visitor to the providers.
  b. If the provider is unable to meet with the visitor, explain the circumstances and encourage the visitor to leave a message.

II. TELECOMMUNICATION

A. General
  1. The vast majority of telephone contact occurs through incoming calls; the majority of which are made by patients.
  2. As an instrument, the telephone is a critical component of a successful practice. The manner in which the phone is used, and the demeanor of the in-house user, plays an important role in successful practice management.
  3. Effective communication and listening skills are an important requisite of telephone management.
B. Equipment and materials
  1. Six-button key set: Standard phone used in some offices.
    a. Up to four incoming lines.
      (1) Slow flashing light: Incoming call.
      (2) Fast flashing light: Call on hold.
      (3) Steady light: Call in progress.
    b. Intercom button: Allows for paging other offices or areas in a clinic.
    c. Hold button: When pushed places the call on hold.
  2. Speaker phone: Has the same features as the six-button key set including:
    a. Speaker mode: Allows you to talk without using the handset.
    b. Redial: Automatically dials the last number entered at the touch of a button.
    c. Speed dialing: Electronically stored numbers can be activated at the touch of a button or short code.
    d. Call forwarding: Incoming calls can be automatically directed to another number.
    e. Call waiting: Available for single-line phone systems only. When a call comes in while the phone is in use, a beep sounds. By pressing the phone, flash, or receiver key once quickly, you are switched to the second caller while placing the first caller on hold. The calls can be switched back by quickly depressing the same button again.
    f. Caller ID: Displays the name and phone number of an incoming call on a display panel.
    g. Call block: Disallows callers within the service area from reaching your telephone.
    h. Separate buttons for frequently dialed numbers.
      i. Volume control.
      j. Message display on a LCD screen.
      k. Built-in directories.
      l. Calendar display.
  3. Cellular phone: A transportable, mobile phone that permits telephone communication outside an office or in a car.
  4. Headset: An earphone-microphone device that is placed on the wearer's head over one or both ears, with the microphone adjusted in front of the mouth to permit hands-free telephone use.
  5. Telephone directories
    a. Local white pages: Alphabetical listing of names, addresses, and phone numbers of persons and businesses in a geographic area. Business phone numbers are usually marked near the back of the directory.
    b. Local yellow pages: Alphabetical listing of commercial enterprises advertising their products and services in a geographic area.
    c. Office directory: Compilation of frequently called numbers. Often in a Rolodex or 3- by 5-inch index card box.
  6. Telephone log
    a. A record of all incoming calls with name, number, reason for call, and action taken.
    b. Calls indicating that no action has been taken should be forwarded to the log sheet for the next day.
C. Incoming calls
  1. Responding to multiple lines:
    a. Never answer a call with "please hold."
    b. Indicate to the first caller that the other line is ringing and would she please hold; *wait for a response.*
    c. Thank the first caller and place her on hold.
    d. Answer the second caller and indicate that you are speaking to someone on another line and ask if the caller would please hold; *wait for a response* (ensure that it is not an emergency).
    e. Thank the second caller and place the caller on hold.
    f. Return to the first caller and thank the caller for holding.
    g. If the second call is an emergency, indicate that you need to place the caller on hold for just a moment, return to the first caller explaining the emergency and request that you call the person back in a few minutes. Return to the second caller and handle the emergency appropriately; do not forget to call the first caller at the first opportunity.
  2. Ending a call: Once a call is complete, avoid idle conversation by thanking the person for calling

and saying goodbye; wait for the caller to hang up first.

3. Telephone messages

  a. The message pad of choice is one that makes a carbon/carbonless copy of the message.

  b. Information recorded

    (1) Date and time of call.

    (2) Name of person called.

    (3) Caller's name and phone number(s).

    (4) Reason for call and message.

    (5) Notation of action taken.

    (6) Message taker's initials.

  c. Once the message has been recorded, forward it to the proper individual with attachments as necessary; calls regarding a patient may require pulling the medical record.

  d. Record a mark on the message pad that the message has been delivered.

4. Screening calls

  a. Judgment must be exercised in determining which calls to handle yourself and which to transfer to the provider or other staff members.

  b. If a patient requests to speak to the provider and:

    (1) the provider is not in, indicate so and offer to take a message or provide assistance.

    (2) the provider is with a patient, indicate so and offer assistance.

    (3) the provider is available to take calls, ask, "who may I say is calling, please?"

    (4) the provider is available but wants to minimize interruptions, indicate that you are unsure if he is free to take calls and ask, "who may I say is calling, please?"

  c. Calls that should be transferred to the provider include

    (1) Calls from other providers and professional colleagues. Obtain the patient's medical record if necessary.

    (2) Patients who refuse to discuss their condition with the MA.

    (3) Patients expressing problems associated with treatment or the result of treatment.

    (4) Patients requesting test results.

    (5) Patient problems the MA or other staff is unable to resolve.

    (6) Emergency situations.

    (7) Whenever there is doubt; especially regarding urgent patient conditions.

  d. Calls transferred to the provider regarding patient care should be accompanied by the patient's medical record.

  e. Unidentified callers: Those who refuse to describe the nature of the call should be handled by indicating that the provider is with a patient and cannot be disturbed and that you would be happy to take a message.

  f. Family and friends calling the provider: Handled according to the provider's wishes. Inform the provider of the call and carry out her instructions.

5. Angry callers

  a. Do not get caught up in the cycle of anger.

  b. Remain calm, diplomatic, and respectful.

  c. Determine and record the reason for the anger.

  d. If it is in your power, attempt to resolve the problem.

  e. If not, assure the caller that you will investigate and have the call returned by someone who can respond appropriately; follow through.

6. Telephone screening (triage): The manner in which calls are handled should, ideally, be identified in the practice's policy and procedures manual.

  a. Emergency calls

    (1) Remain calm and determine the nature of the emergency.

    (2) Life-threatening conditions such as shock, severe allergic reactions, cessation of breathing, myocardial infarction, cardiac arrest, and severe bleeding should be handled by the local EMS-911 provider network.

    (3) Typically, emergency calls should be transferred immediately to the provider. If the provider is unavailable, advise the patient to call 911.

  b. Urgent calls

    (1) The provider should be consulted immediately or as soon as possible depending on the circumstances.

    (2) Patients are typically seen by the provider or appropriately referred on the day they call or soon thereafter.

    (3) Includes such conditions as loss of consciousness, fever, vomiting, *severe* pain, allergic reactions to medications, *sudden* changes in condition, and *sudden* onset of unusual or critical signs and symptoms.

  c. Routine calls

    (1) Most routine calls can be handled by the MA or other office staff.

    (2) Includes simple medical inquiries (test results, advice), requests (refills),

appointments, business matters, and the like.

D. Local and long distance calls

1. When placing calls, know what you are going to say and how you are going to say it, while having all the necessary information at your fingertips.

2. Phone etiquette

   a. Because the caller cannot see you, your voice reflects your personality and demeanor. Your voice should convey the following characteristics:

      (1) Warmth, confidence, and friendliness.

      (2) Courteousness, diplomacy, and intelligence.

      (3) Caring, interest, and concern.

   b. Address the caller by name: Use formal address unless requested otherwise; this pleases the caller and helps you remember the conversation.

   c. Liberally use the terms "please" and "thank you."

   d. Attempt to smile while speaking on the phone; smiling affords a cheerful tone, as well as the characteristics identified above.

   e. Even though you may be quite busy, attempt not to appear rushed or impatient; do not rush the caller.

   f. Since confidentiality is paramount, use discretion when stating personal or medical information over the phone.

3. Returning calls

   a. To avoid interruptions, most providers will reserve one or two periods per day to return calls.

   b. When leaving return call messages for the provider, the patient's chart should be pulled and the message attached so the provider can refer to the chart upon returning the call.

4. Direct dial: 1 + area code + seven-digit number.

5. Operator assisted: 0 + area code + seven-digit number.

   a. Person-to-person: Request to speak to a specified person.

   b. Collect: The person called or person answering the call will be asked to accept the charge for the call; if accepted the call will go through.

   c. Third-number billing: A long-distance call is billed to a third number, usually the caller's home phone. Someone must be at the third number to accept charges.

6. Long-distance directory assistance within the United States: 411 or 1 + area code + 555-1212.

7. Be cognizant of differing time zones when calling long distance.

   a. Pacific time: 12:00—WA, OR, NV, and CA.

   b. Mountain time: 1:00—MT, UT, ID, WY, CO, NM, AZ; parts of ND, SD, NE, and KS.

   c. Central time: 2:00—MN, WI, IA, MO, AR, OK, TX, LA, MS, IL, AL; parts of TN, KY, ND, SD, NE, and KS.

   d. Eastern time: 3:00—all others.

8. WATS (800—Wide Area Telephone Service)

   a. Toll-free calls made anywhere within the United States 1-800-seven-digit number.

   b. 800 directory assistance: 1-800-555-1212.

9. International calls

   a. International access code (011) + country code + city code + local number + pound sign (#; if Touch-Tone).

   b. The call may take a minute or more to connect.

10. Wrong number

    a. Verify the number with the person answering the call.

    b. Apologize for the mistake.

    c. If long distance, call the local operator to credit your account.

11. Conference calls

    a. A telephone service that allows multiple people to have two-way phone communication with each other.

    b. Call the operator to request a conference call, providing the names and numbers of all persons participating.

12. Voice mail: Electronic communication system that digitizes and stores voice messages and informs the recipient of message availability, including guidelines for playback. Guidelines include

    a. Keep the recorded greeting and instruction menu short.

    b. Identify who to call in an emergency.

    c. Allow the caller to be able to select zero to speak to someone in person.

    d. Specify when calls will be received and returned.

    e. Provide clear after-hours instructions for medically related calls.

13. Prescription requests: Should be forwarded to the provider for approval.

E. Answering services

1. Providers must be able to be contacted at any time to respond to emergencies.

2. An answering service provides call coverage during times the clinic is closed.

3. A reliable means of being contacted should be chosen, because failure to respond to emergency

calls may cause the provider to be charged with abandonment (discussed in Chapter 6, Health Care Law).

4. Answering services may be with an agency that has trained staff to answer and screen emergency calls. The provider is informed of bona fide emergencies necessitating a return call to the patient.

5. An answering service may be as simple as an answering machine or voice mail recording that states, "In the event of emergency, contact the provider at (a particular number)."

6. Electronic pager: A device the provider carries that alerts the provider to call an answering service or call the number displayed on a small LCD screen.

F. Miscellaneous considerations

1. Answer the phone promptly; ideally on the first ring, but at least by the third ring.

2. Identify the office and yourself.

3. Determine who is calling; use the caller's name during the conversation; indicate how you may be of assistance.

4. Identify the caller to whom you are transferring the call.

5. Keep frequently called numbers within easy reach.

6. Minimize personal calls by confining them to important and urgent matters.

7. The handset should be held approximately two finger-breadths away from your mouth.

8. Enunciate clearly, using a moderate tone and rate; avoid slurring words and dropping your tone at the end of sentences.

9. Avoid the use of confusing medical jargon.

10. Spell out words or names that are phonetically ambiguous.

11. Do not eat, drink, or chew while managing the phones.

12. When calls cannot be transferred immediately, ask callers if they wish to wait, leave a message, or call back later.
    a. If the caller wishes to wait, provide an estimate of the expected waiting time.
    b. At intervals of one to two minutes, return to the caller to indicate that the person requested is still busy and ask if the caller wishes to continue holding.

13. Calls that require a wait of more than a few minutes should be handled by a return call.

14. Callers who refuse to identify themselves should generally not be transferred to the party requested.

15. Call back list: Patients who the provider wishes to call periodically to check on their progress such as the following patient situations:
    a. Prescribed new medication.

b. Unresponsive to prescribed drug.
c. Missed an appointment.
d. Depressed.
e. Experiencing a personal crisis that may affect one's illness or care.
f. Referred to a consulting provider.
g. Had outpatient surgery.

III. APPOINTMENTS

A. General

1. Process of determining which patient will see which provider, when, and for what period of time.

2. The scheduling system helps control time so that each clinic member can plan and carry out patient care.

3. Effective appointment scheduling requires familiarity with the practice philosophy, provider habits and preferences, and the needs of particular patients.

4. Effective appointment scheduling will provide greater efficiencies, may improve patient satisfaction, and possibly generate more revenue.

5. Waiting period: Twenty minutes is generally accepted as the maximum waiting period. Longer waits should be accompanied with an explanation and an estimate of the remaining delay.

6. Scheduling considerations
   a. Socioeconomic: Status of the patient population and the area being served, such as metropolitan, industrial, retirement, and rural communities.
   b. Patient need
      (1) Purpose of the visit.
      (2) Patient demographics (age, sex, education, etc.).
      (3) Procedures to be performed.
      (4) Patient schedule.
      (5) Insurance requirements.
   c. Provider preferences
      (1) Does the provider prefer to be busy all day, or have breaks periodically?
      (2) Does the provider wish to see fewer patients with more time spent with each, or the opposite?
      (3) Is the provider conscientious about starting on time?
      (4) Does the provider prefer to perform certain exams or procedures at specified times during the day or week?
   d. Facilities: Physical resources and facilities must be available at the time of the visit.
   e. Time: The time needed for different kinds of patients and procedures must be determined. Some providers spend differing amounts of time for similar procedures.

B. Materials
1. Appointment book
   a. Books are available for one or several providers and may show from one day to one week per page. Generally used for one calendar year at a time, they may be blank, lined, or have preprinted time slots; they may be spiral or loose-leaf bound.
   b. Daily log: Some practices may prefer a combination appointment book and journal page to record charges and payments.
   c. There should be enough space to record the patient's name and phone number, date, time, and purpose of visit.
   d. The appointment book should meet the needs of the practice, fit comfortably on the reception desk, be easily accessible, not moved constantly, and maintained in good condition as it serves as a backup legal document.
2. Writing instruments
   a. Most medical assistant literature will state that appointments should be written in blue or black indelible ink to preserve the appointment book's credibility as a legal document; however, many practices use pencil because it can be easily erased when appointments are changed or canceled and still be legible.
   b. Consistent with the information above, to verify information noted in the chart, erasing, scribbling, or whiting-out should not be done. Corrections should be done as described in Chapter 6, Health Care Law.
   c. Some clinics use another ink color such as red to denote new or special patients.
3. Appointment card
   a. Patients scheduling an appointment at the office after a visit should be provided with an appointment card.
   b. The standard appointment card is imprinted with the provider and clinic name, address, phone number, space for the patient's name, as well as the day, date, and time of the appointment.
4. Electronic appointment scheduling: Appointments are entered into a computer system, and daily appointment sheets can be printed.
C. Scheduling methods
1. Open office hours (tidal wave)
   a. The clinic is open for a specified time period and, barring emergencies, patients are seen in the order of arrival; the least efficient method.
   b. Not common in metropolitan areas, but may occasionally be used in rural clinics; more common among urgent care centers or emergicenters.
   c. This system may create long waits for some patients; there is the increased risk that most patients may not arrive until the afternoon.
2. Flexible office hours
   a. In addition to the typical office hours, 8 a.m. to 4:30 p.m., clinics may be open at odd hours one or more days per week to accommodate the varied work schedules of patients.
   b. Commonly employed in group practices, especially family practice and pediatrics.
3. Time specified (single-booking)
   a. Used when an appointment may take an extended period of time (an hour), e.g., psychiatry or physical therapy. Each patient is given an individual appointment time.
   b. This system, by itself, does not easily accommodate unplanned events; however, by using buffer times this problem can be minimized.
4. Stream (fixed interval): Each patient is given a specific appointment time, usually 15 minutes. Common among specialty and consulting practices.
5. Wave
   a. Considers unplanned deviations such as late patient arrivals, missed appointments, and underestimated time requirements.
   b. The objective is to begin and end each hour on time.
   c. The hour is divided by the average time typically spent with a patient. For example, if the average appointment is 15 minutes, four patients can, on average, be seen per hour.
   d. Four patients will be scheduled each hour and seen in the order of arrival.
   e. Tardiness and unplanned events will reduce the amount of provider idle time; however, variable waiting periods may result.
   f. Patients may come to realize that an appointment is not exclusively theirs, and complain.
6. Modified wave
   a. Instead of scheduling all of the patients that can be seen during an hour at the beginning of each hour, each patient appointment may be staggered throughout the hour.
   b. For example, two patients may be scheduled on the hour and two on the half-hour; two may be scheduled on the hour, one on the half-hour, and one 15 minutes later; two may be scheduled on the hour, one 15 minutes later, and one on the half-hour.
7. Double-booking
   a. Scheduling two patients simultaneously to see the same provider.
   b. Generally this is not a very efficient practice; however, a wavelike approach in which two

patients needing 5 minutes each may be scheduled for a 15-minute block with little to no disruption in the schedule.

c. Emergency patients may be scheduled during another patient's appointment time, thereby causing the routine patient to have to wait for the emergency to be handled. Advise the patient of the delay and provide an opportunity to reschedule the appointment.

8. Clustering (grouping): Scheduling similar appointments or procedures together during a day or week. For example, all well-baby checks are scheduled Wednesday morning; complete physicals are done each day between 9 a.m. and noon, etc.

D. Scheduling guidelines (see Figure 11-1 A and B)
1. Procedure
a. Develop the appointment matrix: Block out the time slots the provider(s) will be unavailable. Block out a buffer period for the morning and afternoon.
b. Chief complaint: Identify the reason for the visit to determine the level of urgency, amount of time, and available resources needed to schedule the appointment.
c. Determine whether the patient has been referred by another provider in case further information is needed.
d. Locate the first acceptable appointment time and perhaps an alternative. Offer the dates and times.
e. Enter the patient's name, phone number, and reason for the visit in the appointment book.
f. Explain any pertinent policies or instructions regarding the appointment.
g. Offer directions to the clinic.
h. Repeat the appointment date and time before bidding farewell.

2. New patients generally require more time to complete forms, go over policies, and undergo a complete physical examination.
3. When scheduling appointments 1 or 2 months in advance, always keep a few appointment slots open each day to accommodate patients with special needs or problems.
4. Buffer periods: One or two time slots should be scheduled each day to serve as catch-up periods.
5. When follow-up appointments are scheduled while patients are at the office, suggest an appointment time before soliciting their preference.
6. Complete an appointment card for the patient when scheduling return visits.

7. Appointment reminders: Although the appointment card serves this purpose, many practices call the patient a day prior to the appointment as a reminder.

E. Special problems
1. Habitually late: Patients who are habitually late for appointments may be scheduled at the end of the day so as not to disrupt work flow.
2. Return patients: Patients who have returned to the practice after an extended absence need to update their patient information forms.
3. Consecutive appointments: Attempt to schedule patients requiring appointments at periodic intervals (e.g., weekly or monthly) on the same day and at the same time to avoid confusion.
4. Cancellations: When a patient calls to cancel an appointment, attempt to offer an alternative appointment time while still on the phone.

F. Exception appointments: Certain events require adjustments in the schedule.
1. Emergency patients
a. Protocol must be developed regarding how emergencies will be handled in the office. Whenever there is any doubt, consult the provider.
b. The receptionist should always have a means of contacting the provider when absent from the office; however, if the provider is unavailable, err on the side of caution and treat as an emergency according to office protocol.
c. Emergency cases take precedence over all others; the patient should be seen immediately upon arrival.
d. Emergencies not falling within these protocols should be handled by local EMS-911 providers.

2. Acute-need patients
a. Patients experiencing acute illnesses should be seen on the day of their call unless determined otherwise by the provider.
b. Provide the first available appointment.
c. If all appointment and buffer times are taken, double-booking may be necessary.

3. Referrals
a. A referral describes the process of sending patients to other providers for diagnosis and treatment.
b. If the patient wishes to make the appointment, provide the provider's name, address, phone number, and appropriate documents needed by the consulting provider.
c. If speed is of the essence, the patient's provider should call the consulting provider to make the appointment.
d. Diagnostic studies

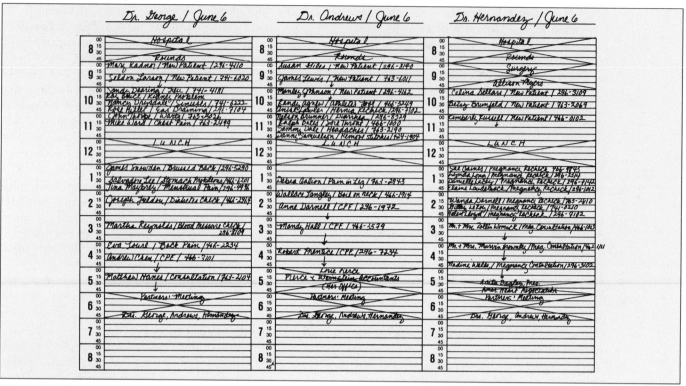

Figure 11-1 A

Appointment book page. Delmar/Cengage Learning.

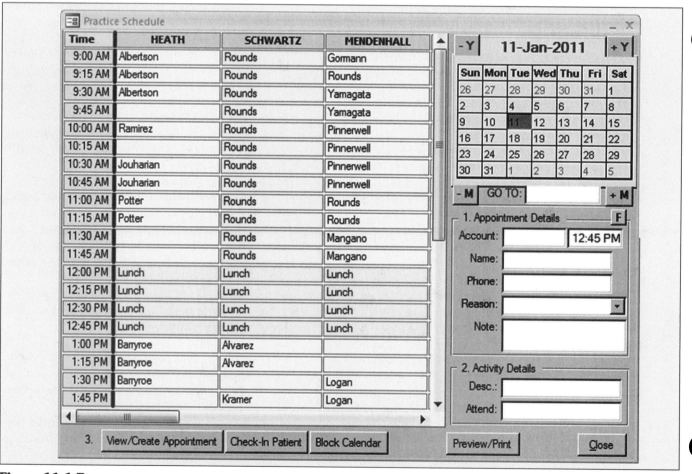

Figure 11-1 B

Electronic appointment schedule. Delmar/Cengage Learning.

(1) The diagnostic center should be provided with the patient's name, age/date of birth, insurance carrier, diagnosis, and studies to be done.

(2) Ensure that the patient is given the necessary instructions regarding such things as fasting and specimen collection.

4. Failed appointments (no-shows)

a. Patients who miss appointments because of forgetfulness may be reminded with a phone call the day before or with a postcard.

b. If the patient's condition requires continued treatment, a letter explaining this should be sent by certified mail.

c. If the patient's condition is serious enough, a call to the patient may be prudent; the provider should be notified of the failed appointment.

d. Although legally, a patient may be charged for a missed appointment that has not been cancelled, enforcing such policies may have a negative impact on patient-provider relations.

e. It may be advisable to discharge patients who habitually fail appointments.

f. All failed appointments should be noted in the chart and the appointment book.

5. Cancellations

a. Attempt to reschedule while the patient is on the phone.

b. Cancelled appointments may be filled by patients with advance appointments.

6. Delays

a. Occasionally, provider delays are inevitable; attempt to call patients who haven't arrived to come later or reschedule.

b. When the provider is called out on an emergency, a courteous explanation is in order. If the emergency is serious enough, all appointments for the day may be cancelled; attempt to call all patients to reschedule.

c. Waiting patients should be given an explanation, an estimate of the time of the delay, and the option to wait or reschedule.

7. Unscheduled patient visits

a. Patient visits without an appointment (walk-ins) should be avoided.

b. If the patient presents with an acute or emergency condition, the patient should be seen or EMS-911 provider contacted.

c. The provider may choose to see the patient briefly, with a more extensive follow-up visit scheduled for a later date.

G. Outside appointments

1. Occasionally, a provider may have appointments scheduled outside the clinic, such as at a hospital or home. When scheduling outside appointments, factor in travel time.

2. Hospital surgeries

a. Arrange the surgery with the hospital operating room secretary.

b. When doing so, have at hand the date and time, surgical procedure, OR time needed, patient's name, sex, age/DOB, phone number, and special needs of the provider.

c. Surgical flow sheet: Form that facilitates surgical scheduling by preventing scheduling problems, coordinating the details involving outside facilities, as well as adhering to insurance requirements.

(1) Patient identification and insurance information.

(2) Diagnostic scheduling.

(3) Clinical and preoperative results logged.

(4) Anticipated procedures identified and scheduled.

(5) Postoperative care plan.

3. House, hospital, and nursing home visits

a. House calls: House calls are rarely made; however, if scheduled, be sure to confirm the patient's name, address, major cross streets, directions, phone number, etc.

b. The provider may periodically visit long-term care patients in extended care facilities such as nursing homes. The scheduled appointment and travel time should be blocked in the appointment book.

CHAPTER 12

Financial Management

I. BANKING

A. General

1. A bank is a financial institution that receives deposits, lends money, makes collections, provides safety deposit boxes, and handles investment and trust funds for its customers.

2. Checks: The majority of transactions involve checks; commercial paper drawn on funds deposited and held in a bank account and payable on demand. A check is a written order to the bank to pay the amount specified.

   a. Drawer: The depositor; the person writing the check.

   b. Drawee: The bank in which the drawer has money on deposit.

   c. Payee: The party to receive the money as directed by the drawer.

3. Types of checks

   a. Cashier's check: A check the bank prepares, signed by a bank official, that is directly drawn from a person's account. No stop payments permitted.

   b. Certified check: The bank authenticates and guarantees a check by setting aside the funds until it is presented for payment; rarely used.

   c. Counter check: A check the bank prepares as a substitute for a regular check to permit the drawer to withdraw funds; often used when the drawer forgets his or her checkbook.

   d. Limited check: Check that is limited by amount and time of negotiability.

   e. Money order: Similar to a cashier's check, but can be purchased at the post office as well as convenience stores.

   f. Traveler's check: Special check prepared for those who are traveling or where personal checks may not be accepted or where carrying cash is not prudent.

B. Checking accounts

1. Checks are negotiable instruments: The right to receive money on deposit can be transferred to someone else if it meets the following criteria:

   a. In writing.

   b. Signed by the drawer.

   c. Payable to the order of another party.

      (1) The payee acknowledges the right to receive the money by endorsing (signing) the back of the check.

      (2) Blank endorsement: The check has only the payee's signature, thus making it payable to any bearer.

      (3) Restrictive endorsement: An endorsement that directs how the check is to be made payable; e.g., for deposit only, pay to the order of . . . , etc.

2. Opening a checking account

   a. Requires approval from a bank official and an initial minimum deposit.

   b. Signature card: All persons authorized to write checks for an organization must fill out and sign a form as an aid in verifying a depositor's signature.

3. Making deposits

   a. Paper money: Arranged in order of denomination with smallest denominations near the top. The bills should be stacked face up and top up. All checks must be endorsed.

   b. Coins: In considerable quantity should be placed in coin wrappers with the depositor's name and account number written on each.

   c. Checks: Checks should be examined for complete information and restrictively endorsed.

   d. Deposit ticket: A printed bank form that identifies the money items being deposited.

      (1) Preprinted forms containing MICR (magnetic ink character recognition) characters that can be read by a machine.

      (2) The MICR characters include an ABA (American Banking Association) number that indicates where the bank is located and information needed to sort and route deposit tickets and checks.

      (3) Preparation

(a) Enter the date in the designated space.

(b) Enter the total amount of bills and the total amount of coins separately.

(c) Enter each check individually along with their respective ABA numbers; for example:

   (i) 12-19/750

   (ii) Enter the numerator only.

(d) Record the total amount to be deposited in the designated space.

(e) Cash may be withdrawn by entering this amount in the designated space and subtracting this from the total amount listed.

(f) When making a withdrawal, a signature is required on the deposit slip accompanied by proper identification.

4. Dishonored checks: A check the bank refuses to pay generally because of insufficient funds deposited (NSF—not sufficient funds).

a. A depositor, upon writing a check, guarantees that funds are on deposit to cover the check amount.

b. If the drawer writes a check that is dishonored, the drawer's bank will send a notice (debit memo) to the drawer indicating that the check was dishonored, the reason, any fees assessed, and the current balance of the account.

c. If a check is deposited that is dishonored, the payee's bank will submit the dishonored check along with a debit memo explaining the reason the check was dishonored.

d. Overdraft: Issuing a check without sufficient funds. Illegal in most states.

e. Postdated checks: Checks dated after the date it was written.

(1) The check is not considered payable until the date written on the check.

(2) Banks may dishonor postdated checks.

5. Checkbook: Checks are bound individually or two to four to a page with perforations for ease of removal.

a. Check stub: Small form to the left of each check that contains space to record all relevant information about a check and checking account balance.

b. Check register: Information recorded on the check stub is, instead, recorded in a booklet maintained with the bound checks.

c. The drawer's name and address along with check number and account number in MICR characters are printed on each check.

d. Some checkbooks come with a blank page between each check made of specially treated NCR (no carbon required) paper for retaining a copy of the issued check.

6. Writing a check

a. Complete the check stub or register.

b. Write the name of the payee.

c. Write the amount in figures and words

(1) If the amount in figures and words do not agree, the bank may contact the drawer for the correct amount or return the check unpaid.

(2) If the difference is negligible, the bank should allow the check to clear based on the amount in words.

(3) Write the amount in figures with no space between the dollar sign and the first figure of the amount.

(4) The amount written in words should begin at the extreme left.

(5) Cents should be written in the form of a fraction or with no/100.

(6) A line should be stricken to cover any space remaining after the amount in words.

(7) Write the purpose of the check in the lower left corner where the word *Memo* is printed.

(8) Sign the check in the lower right corner.

7. Cancelled checks: After a bank has honored a check, the check is stamped (cancelled) so that it cannot be issued again.

C. Bank statements

1. Statement of account rendered to each depositor once a month by a bank. It identifies the following information:

a. Balance on deposit at the beginning of the period.

b. Amount of deposits credited during the period.

c. Amount of checks honored (debited) during the period.

d. Other items debited or credited during the period.

e. Balance on deposit at the end of the period.

2. Depending on the type of account and bank policies, cancelled (paid) checks and other documents representing debits and credits to the account may be enclosed with the bank statement.

3. Bank statement reconciliation

a. Because it takes two or more days from statement preparation by the bank to receipt by the depositor transactions may have occurred that make the current balance as stated on the bank statement disagree with the balance shown on the check register. Reasons for this include the following:

- (1) Outstanding checks: Checks that have been written between bank statement periods.
- (2) Outstanding deposits: Also known as deposits in transit; funds deposited in the account between bank statement periods.
- (3) Service fees: Fees assessed by the bank between bank statement periods.
- (4) Debits: Amounts that have been deducted from the account between bank statement periods.
- (5) Credits: Amounts that have been added to the account between bank statement periods.

b. Reconciliation is the process of adjusting both balances to reflect the transactions not represented by both the bank statement and check register in order to determine the true balance of the account. If done properly, the check register balance and the bank statement balance should agree after the adjustments have been made.

4. Reconciliation procedure

a. Compare the deposited amounts recorded on the check register with those shown on the bank statement.
- (1) Place a check mark in the register next to all deposits that are also shown on the bank statement.
- (2) Those that do not have a check mark are identified as outstanding deposits and should be added to the bank statement balance.

b. Compare the cancelled check amounts with those stated on the bank statement and check register.
- (1) Place a check mark in the register next to all checks that are also shown on the bank statement.
- (2) Those that do not have a check mark are identified as outstanding checks and should be deducted from the bank statement balance.

c. Identify all debits and credits to the account listed on the bank statement.
- (1) All amounts credited on the bank statement should be added to the check register.
- (2) All amounts debited on the bank statement should be deducted from the check register.

d. Identify any errors found on the bank statement or check register.

- (1) Errors found on the check register that mistakenly elevate or lower the account balance should be deducted or added to the check register, respectively.
- (2) Errors found on the bank statement should be reported to the bank promptly and adjusted accordingly.

e. Add and subtract all of the adjustments made to the bank statement and check register. Both adjusted balances should be equal.

f. For example, bank statement balance, $460.00; check register balance, 876.00; outstanding checks, 10.00, 20.00, 30.00; outstanding deposit, 500.00; service fee, 15.00; interest income, 12.00; check register error, check written for 25.00 was erroneously recorded as 52.00.

- (1) Bank statement balance

	$460.00
Outstanding deposit	+500.00
Outstanding checks (10+20+30)	− 60.00
Adjusted Bank Statement Balance	$900.00

- (2) Check register balance

	$876.00
Error (52−25)	+ 27.00
Interest income	+ 12.00
Service fee	− 15.00
Adjusted Check Register Balance	$900.00

II. ACCOUNTING AND BOOKKEEPING

A. Introduction

1. Described as the language of business, it is the process of recording, classifying, summarizing, reporting, analyzing, and interpreting financial and economic data.

2. Purpose: Provide financial information regarding the current business operation to interested parties, especially outsiders.
   a. Financial condition of a business: Profitability and solvency.
   b. Managerial performance.
   c. Effectiveness and efficiency of operations.
   d. Compliance with directives and regulations.

3. Users of accounting information
   a. Owners/managers.
   b. Creditors.
   c. Government agencies.
   d. Accrediting agencies.
   e. Third-party payers.

4. Accounting elements
   a. Assets: Property of value owned or controlled by a business.

(1) Money.
(2) Land/building/fixtures/furnishings.
(3) Machinery/equipment.
(4) Merchandise: Products to be sold.
(5) Accounts receivable: Fees owed to the clinic.
(6) Securities: Stocks and bonds.
    b. Liabilities: Debt obligations; creditor interest.
       (1) Accounts payable: Supplier/vendor debts.
       (2) Notes payable: Bank debts.
    c. Owners' equity: The amount by which assets exceed liabilities; net worth; ownership interest; capital.
       (1) Revenue: Inflow of assets through sale of products or services. Has the effect of increasing owner's equity.
       (2) Expense: Outflow of assets to generate revenue. Has the effect of reducing owner's equity.
       (3) Drawing: Withdrawal of assets for personal use. Has the effect of reducing owner's equity.
5. Accounting equation
   a. Assets = Liabilities + Owners' Equity
   b. Liabilities = Assets − Owners' Equity
   c. Owners' Equity = Assets − Liabilities
B. Bookkeeping systems
   1. Single-entry system: All transactions are recorded once using a pegboard system (see Figure 12-1).
      a. Materials and documents
         (1) Pegboard: Lightweight metal or plastic board that contains pegs along the left edge to hold the corresponding perforated accounting documents.
         (2) Journal: A page that approximates the size of the pegboard also known as the daysheet, daybook, or daily log. Maintains a record of all daily charges (fees) and receipts.
         (3) Ledger cards: Record of all fees and payments for each patient.
         (4) Charge slip/receipt
             (a) A form used to record a charge to serve as a bill, or as a receipt given to the patient for a fee payment.
             (b) Superbill: Multicopy charge slip that may be retained by the clinic, patient, and insurance carrier.
      b. Mechanics
         (1) The journal is affixed to the pegboard with the perforations along the left edge of the sheet placed on the pegs.
         (2) Each patient ledger card is placed on the journal page, over the pegs with the columns and rows of the ledger card aligned with the journal page.

(3) The charge slip/receipt is placed over the ledger card in the same fashion.
(4) The entries are made with information recorded simultaneously on the three forms described above.
2. Double entry system
   a. Each transaction is recorded in a way that maintains a balancing of the accounting elements.
   b. Account: A record used to keep track of the increases and decreases to each element of the accounting equation. Consists of the following:
      (1) Title and account number.
      (2) Debit and credit columns.
      (3) Date column.
      (4) Posting reference.
   c. Each business transaction requiring an entry affects at least two accounts: One account will be debited, the other will be credited.
      (1) Accounts that are debited are recorded in the left-hand column, such as the following:
          (a) Increases in assets.
          (b) Decreases in liabilities.
          (c) Incurred in expenses.
      (2) Accounts that are credited are recorded in the right-hand column, such as the following:
          (a) Decreases in assets.
          (b) Increases in liabilities.
          (c) Generation of revenue.
   d. Trial balance: A list of all accounts by title and their respective debit or credit balances.
   e. Financial statements
      (1) Income statement (profit-loss statement): Summarizes revenue and expenses to determine the level of profit or loss.
      (2) Balance sheet: Summarizes the assets, liabilities, and owners' equity at a specified date.
   f. Accounting documents
      (1) Source documents: Any document that indicates a transaction has occurred, such as a receipt.
      (2) Chart of accounts: A list and numbering of all accounts.
      (3) Journal: A book of original entry that serves as a chronological record of daily business transactions.
      (4) Ledger: A collection of individual records of each account.
          (a) General ledger: Asset, liability, and capital accounts grouped together.
          (b) Accounts receivable ledger: A ledger of all persons and businesses that owe money to the company.

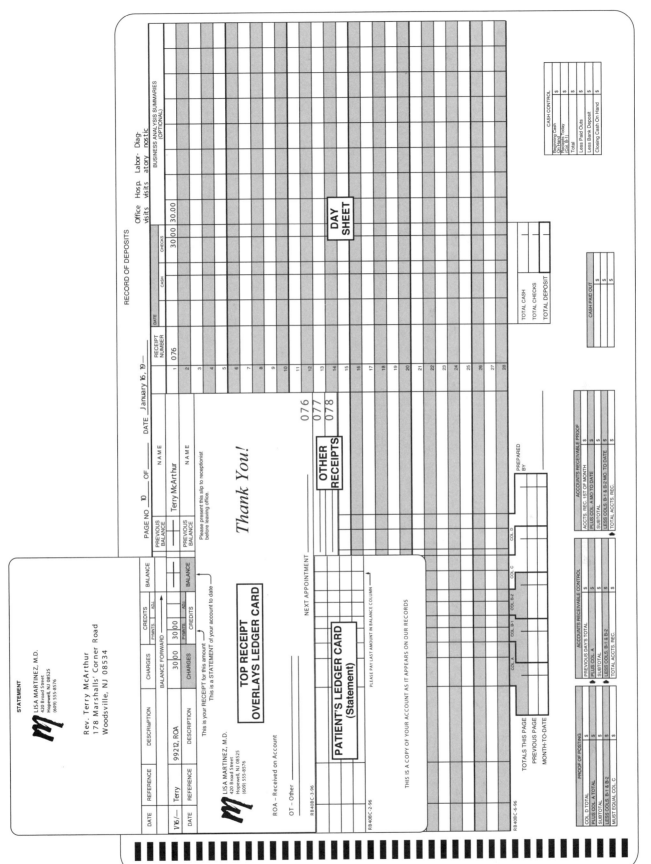

Figure 12-1

Pegboard and forms. Delmar/Cengage Learning.

(c) Accounts payable ledger: A ledger of all businesses the company owes money to.

g. Accounting process
(1) The source document is reviewed to determine whether it should be recorded as a transaction.
(2) Journalize: Daily transactions are recorded in the journal as debits and credits.
(3) Posting: Periodically, the information recorded in the journal is transferred to each ledger record reserved for the account debited or credited in the journal.
(4) Adjustments: Accounts are adjusted for any changes in the amounts not already recorded.
(5) Closing: Expense and revenue accounts are closed (zeroed out) at the end of the accounting period.
(6) Trial balance: At the end of an accounting period (month or year), a trial balance is prepared.
(7) Accounting statements: From the trial balance an income statement and balance sheet is prepared.

C. Accounts receivable: Fees owed by patients for services rendered.
1. Because most receipts are through third-party payments, it is not uncommon for payment to be received 30 to 90 days after the service has been rendered.
2. Often clinics receive less than the total charge for patient services due to:
a. Uncollectible accounts allowance: Bad debts, unpaid fees.
b. Charity allowance: Discounts given to indigent patients.
c. Contractual allowance (discounts): Lower fees paid by third-party payers.
d. Courtesy allowance: Discounts given to employees, physicians, and clergy.
3. Aging accounts receivable
a. Process of classifying each account receivable according to the amount of time the balance is unpaid.
b. Typical aging categories include current, 31 to 60, 61 to 90, 91 to 120, and greater than 120 days past due.
c. Serves as a measure of collection effectiveness.
d. The day that statements are sent for current charges begins day 1 of the aging process.
e. A patient's account may cover more than one aging period. If a partial payment is made, the payment is applied to the oldest category balance.

f. Category percentage = Age category total / total accounts receivable $\times$ 100.

D. Accounts payable: Money owed to outside businesses for sales and services rendered.
1. When purchases are received, a packing slip is usually enclosed itemizing the contents of the package.
2. An invoice may also be included that lists the items ordered, and the quantity and price of each. Verify that invoice, packing slip, and package contents agree.
3. Place the unpaid invoice in an accounts payable tickler file to ensure timely payments.
4. When an account is paid, an entry needs to be made in the appropriate accounts payable ledger or expense disbursement record.

E. Petty cash fund: A cash amount maintained in the office to pay minor expenses, eliminating the need to write a check.
1. To establish a petty cash fund, a check is written for the amount that is to be set aside for the fund. The check is usually made payable to the person responsible for controlling the fund.
2. When the check is cashed by the bank, the money is placed in a cash drawer or office safe. A designated person is authorized to make payments from the fund.
3. Petty cash voucher: A special form of receipt showing the name of the payee, the amount, the purpose of the payment, and the account to be charged is generally required to aid in controlling the fund.
4. Petty cash register: A record having multiple columns used to record petty cash disbursements.
5. Replenishment: When the fund has reached a low enough level, a check is written to cover all of the disbursements since the last replenishment period to bring the fund back up to the designated amount.

III. BILLING AND COLLECTIONS

A. General
1. Purpose: Maintain consistent generation of revenue and even, steady cash flow.
2. Financial policies must be clearly defined and made known to the patient.
B. Professional fee structure
1. Professional fees should reflect the revenue needed to maintain the financial stability of a practice.
a. Fees are influenced by the time and degree of difficulty in providing the service.
b. Fees should cover operating expenses such as labor, materials, and overhead.
2. Fee schedule

a. A list of common services with accompanying code numbers, descriptions, and prices.

b. Under federal regulations, the fee schedule must be available to all patients. A sign explaining this patient right should be posted in the office.

3. Fee profile: Record of customary fees collected and compiled by third-party payers. The fee profile influences what insurance companies will allow and pay for services.

4. Usual, customary, and reasonable charges (UCR)

a. Usual fee: Fee that a provider most frequently charges for a service.

b. Customary fee: Range of usual fees charged for the same service by practitioners of similar training and experience within a geographic area.

c. Reasonable: A fee assigned to a service that has some unusual or complex features. It typically meets the criteria of both usual and customary.

5. Fee discounts and allowances

a. It is better to adjust a fee before rather than after treatment.

(1) Reducing the fee after treatment may imply that a lower quality of care was rendered.

(2) Avoid reducing a fee on the basis of a poor treatment outcome.

(3) Reducing the fee in response to a dispute should be done "without prejudice" and indicated in writing; i.e., the right to sue for the original amount is not waived if the patient fails to pay the reduced fee.

b. Discounts may be commonly given to fee-for-service patients or for cash payments.

c. Uncollectible accounts allowance: Bad debts, unpaid fees.

d. Charity allowance: Discounts given to indigent patients.

e. Contractual allowance (discounts): Lower fees paid by third-party payers.

f. Courtesy allowance: Discounts given to employees, physicians, and clergy.

C. Forms

1. Patient information

a. Used to collect general information about the patient to facilitate efficient billing and collection activities.

b. Common information includes:

(1) Patient's name, home address, phone number.

(2) Occupation, business address, phone number.

(3) Date of birth, Social Security number, driver's license number.

(4) Insured's name, insurance carrier, policy numbers.

(5) Spouse's name, occupation, business phone number.

(6) Person to contact in emergencies.

2. Release of information

a. Used to request information from other providers and to authorize third parties such as an insurance company to be given information about a patient.

b. The release is usually good for approximately 1 year after it is signed, although some states have specific guidelines.

3. Assignment of benefits: Requests insurance payments to be sent directly to the provider rather than the patient.

D. Billing systems

1. Methods

a. Time-of-service: Fees are collected when the service is rendered. Improves cash flow and reduces collection costs.

b. Monthly billing: Sending the patient a bill on a monthly basis.

c. Cycle billing: Billing segments of the patient population at different times consistently each month; e.g., patient names starting A through F are billed the first week of each month, G through L, the second week, and so on.

d. Credit/debit card billing: Payment is made using a major credit card or debit card.

e. Billing service: The clinic contracts with an outside agency to prepare and mail patient bills.

2. Billing statements

a. Statements must be neat and accurate.

b. Typed statements: Each bill is individually typed. Out-of-date and time-consuming process.

c. Ledger cards: Photocopied and mailed to the patient.

d. Superbill: Given to the patient at the visit for payment or remitted at a later time usually within 30 days.

e. Computerized: Financial data is keyed into a computer and statements are automatically prepared.

E. Fidelity bond: Insurance against embezzlement.

1. Employees handling money should be bonded. The insurance or bonding agency replaces an amount that is stolen or lost.

2. Personal bond: Covers an individual; requires a thorough background investigation and is usually done for persons handling large sums.

3. Position-schedule bond: Covers a specific job title, such as bookkeeper, rather than a named individual.

4. Blanket-position bond: Covers all employees.

F. Credit arrangements

1. A service rendered before payment is an extension of credit.

2. Equal Credit Opportunity Act
   a. Federal law requiring equal extension of credit to all persons demonstrating ability to pay. Prohibits discrimination in extending credit based on the following:
      (1) Race, color, religion, national origin, gender, marital status, or age.
      (2) Receipt of money through public assistance.
      (3) Exercising rights under consumer credit laws.
   b. The patient must be informed of credit denial.
   c. The patient has 60 days to request, in writing, the reason credit was denied.

3. Federal Truth in Lending Act
   a. Enforced by the Federal Trade Commission (FTC).
   b. Governs interest charges or installment agreements of more than four payments.
   c. Regulation Z: Requires completing a form disclosing information regarding finance charges.

4. Fair Debt Collection Practices Act: Federal law prohibiting abusive, deceptive, and unfair debt collection activities.

G. Collections

1. General
   a. The difficulty in collecting an account increases proportionately to its age.
   b. Do not attempt to collect a debt through a third party.
   c. It is illegal to harass the debtor.
   d. It is illegal to threaten action that cannot legally be taken or is not intended to be taken.

2. Rationale
   a. Revenue must be collected to cover expenses.
   b. Potential loss of patient: Patients may not keep appointments out of embarrassment or may change providers.
   c. Noncollection may imply guilt: The patient may perceive that inadequate care was provided.
   d. Noncollection encourages nonpayment: The added costs of nonpayment may be unfairly shifted to paying patients.

3. Telephone collection
   a. May be more effective than a collection letter.
   b. Making the call will bring in more money than not calling.
   c. It is illegal to make threatening, frightening, or verbally abusive collection calls.
   d. It is illegal to call at odd times in the day, usually between 8 p.m. and 8 a.m. It may also be illegal to call people at work.
   e. Determine the identity of the person with whom you are speaking by using the person's full name. It is illegal to discuss debts with third parties.
   f. Assume a positive and respectful attitude.
   g. Ask if it is a convenient time to speak; if not, ask to call at a specified time or get a commitment for a return call.
   h. State the purpose of the call by being brief and concise.
   i. Attempt to get a commitment for settling the past-due account (time and amount).
   j. Follow up on promises.

4. Collection mailings
   a. Never use postcards.
   b. Prepare collection correspondence to suit the situation.
   c. Dun message: Derived from Old English word *dunnen* meaning "to make a loud noise." A dun message is a reminder to the patient regarding payment of a debt.
   d. Attempt to imply the good intentions of the patient to settle the account.
   e. After a few friendly reminders, employ an increasingly firmer tone in subsequent correspondence.
   f. Collection letters should be signed by the business manager or person responsible for collections, not the provider.
   g. Inform patient regarding legal action or use of collection agency, using certified mail with return receipt.

5. Progressive collection process: A color or written code should be developed to keep track of collection efforts. At a minimum, create a coding system to symbolize the following actions:
   a. First bill sent pending receipt of payment.
   b. A friendly reminder or two sent after 1 month past due.
   c. Telephone calls requesting payment.
   d. Collection letters sent.
   e. Final notice sent.
   f. Forwarding account to collection agency.
   g. Updates on collection agency attempts.
   h. Legal action such as small claims, lawsuit, etc.

6. Disputed charges: The patient does not agree with the amount billed.
   a. If the patient was billed in error, locate the error and correct it; follow up with a letter of apology.

b. If the amount is disputed, attempt to explain that the fee is usual for the service and locale.

c. Avoid reducing the fee.

d. If a serious dispute exists, arbitration may be necessary.

7. Tracing skips

a. Skip: Person who has moved purposely to avoid collection efforts.

b. Call the phone numbers and references identified on the patient information form to locate the patient.

c. Check the local phone book for the phone numbers of neighbors to inquire regarding the patient's whereabouts.

d. Check with the patient's employer and leave a message.

e. It is illegal to communicate with a third party more than once.

f. Check with the Department of Motor Vehicles for an address change.

g. When the above efforts prove futile, immediately forward the account to a collection agency.

8. Claims against estates

a. A bill owed by a deceased patient requires the filing of a claim against the patient's estate.

b. A creditor's claim form should be filed with the patient's attorney or estate executor, or the county probate clerk.

c. The claim should show an itemization of the bill, the total amount due, and the provider's signature.

d. The claim should be sent certified mail, return receipt requested.

e. The estate executor will mail a letter accepting or rejecting the claim; if accepted, the account will be settled eventually.

f. If the claim is rejected, it must be filed within a specified period of time with the county probate court.

g. Once the claim is filed, all collection efforts must be suspended; follow up if after 60 days there has been no notification.

9. Bankruptcy: Filed under federal law when a business or individual has debts that exceed assets.

a. Once notified of a bankruptcy proceeding, suspend all collection efforts.

b. The notification will advise you of the amount the patient claims to owe the provider. If it is the correct amount, you simply await the court's decision.

c. If you disagree with the amount, you must appear at the hearing or submit a notarized document itemizing the charges and the balance due.

d. Chapter VII: Because the debtor has few to no assets, the debtor is relieved of all debts. As medical bills represent unsecured debts, you can expect to receive no payment.

e. Chapter XIII: Typically, reorganized debts set up with a debt payment plan. Although the court may reduce or eliminate some debt, it is advisable to file a claim with the court for even a small amount.

10. Collection through small claims court

a. There is a limit, defined by each state, on the amount that can be collected through small claims. As of this writing, most states pose a limit of less than $5000.

b. Does not require attorney representation; the provider or clinic representative and patient present their own case before a judge, who makes a decision and informs both parties in a short period of time, usually 2 to 4 weeks.

c. Only a judgment is made, you must still collect the money.

d. The patient-defendant can appeal, but the provider-plaintiff cannot.

e. Has the advantage of cost and time savings.

11. Collection through attorney-directed suits is rare unless the amount owed is large because of the time and cost expended. It is common for an attorney to prepare a collection letter on behalf of a provider or clinic.

12. Collection agencies

a. Once an account has been determined uncollectible, forward it immediately to a collection agency.

b. Once an account has been given to a collection agency, the clinic must suspend all collection efforts. Patients should be directed to the agency for payments on the account.

c. Typically, collection agencies will retain 40% to 60% of the amount collected as their collection fee. This is a minor expense considering the efforts of the clinic have resulted in no payment at all.

d. If the agency determines that a collection case warrants special consideration, it will consult the provider before proceeding further.

e. Care must be exercised in selecting a reliable, ethical collection agency, because a clinic can be held liable for the illegal acts of a collection agency.

13. Billing minors: Determine the person financially responsible for the minor's care at the first visit. Unless the minor is emancipated in some fashion or can receive care without parental consent (e.g., birth control, substance abuse, etc.), a legal guardian should be billed.

14. Billing third parties: In some instances, a person or organization will request examination or treatment of a patient.
    a. Commonly requested by insurance companies to include health, life, and workers' compensation; social service agencies such as for federal disability benefits; and attorneys for criminal, malpractice, or insurance claim actions.
    b. The person or organization requesting the service is financially responsible for payment of the fee.
15. Garnishment: Attaching personal assets, especially wages, to pay debts.
    a. The Consumer Credit Protection Act limits the amount of employee earnings withheld for garnishment.
    b. It protects the employee from termination for garnishment to settle one's debt.
    c. Only disposable income (net pay) is subject to garnishment.
    d. Generally garnishment cannot exceed 25% of disposable income.

IV. PAYROLL

A. General
  1. Payroll accounting has become one of the most important components of an organization's accounting system.
  2. Payroll may be a considerable operating expense as the total federal and state tax may exceed 10% of the wages paid to employees.
  3. Nearly all aspects of payroll are affected by government laws and regulations. Lack of compliance may result in both fines and back-pay awards.
  4. Income tax amounts withheld from employees must be paid at regular intervals to the IRS or to authorized banks. Although the tax money is temporarily held by the organization, it is a federal fund and must be accounted for.
  5. Payroll responsibilities
    a. Explain payroll procedures to new employees.
    b. Collect payroll data and process payroll records, reports, and payments.
    c. Understand and comply with all laws and regulations.
B. Payroll laws and regulations
  1. Employers must keep detailed records for each employee with the following information:
    a. Name, address, date of birth, and Social Security number.
    b. Amount and date of each wage payment and the period covered by the payment.
    c. The amount of wages subject to the various taxes.
    d. The amount of taxes withheld.
    e. When and why an employee leaves the organization.
  2. Fair Labor Standards Act (FLSA): Also known as the federal wage and hour law.
    a. Affects any organization involved in interstate commerce (doing business in more than one state).
    b. Sets the minimum wage employers are required to pay employees.
    c. Requires employers to pay one and one-half times the regular wage for work in excess of 40 hours per week.
  3. Title VII—Civil Rights Act of 1964: Prohibits discrimination in hiring, firing, or promoting employees because of race, color, religion, national origin, or gender.
  4. Age Discrimination in Employment Act (ADEA): Prohibits the use of unfair employment practices regarding people over 40 years of age.
  5. Americans with Disabilities Act of 1990 (ADA): Prohibits unfair employment practices regarding occupationally qualified persons with disabilities. The law requires that employers make reasonable accommodations for such disabilities.
  6. Employee Retirement Income Security Act (ERISA): Protects pension funds and regulates pension fund operations.
  7. Immigration Reform Act of 1985: Employers must certify that newly hired employees are either United States citizens or authorized to work in the United States.
  8. State minimum wage law: Some states set their own minimum wage rate; state rates must be higher than the federal rate.
  9. Workers' compensation laws: Most states have laws requiring employers to provide employees with workers' compensation insurance, which protects employees from losses associated with job-related illnesses, injuries, or death. Employers must purchase such insurance or contribute to a state fund.
  10. State disability benefit laws: California, Hawaii, New Jersey, New York, Rhode Island, and Puerto Rico have laws intended to provide disability insurance to employees who are absent from work because of illnesses or injuries that are not job-related.
  11. Immigration and Nationality Act: Employers are required to verify that all employees, U.S. citizens or not, are authorized to work.
    a. Employment Eligibility Verification Form I-9 is completed for each new hire and filed with the Immigration and Naturalization Service (INS) within three business days.

b. Using Form I-9, the employer must verify the documents presented by the employee authorizing employment in the United States. Although the form identifies the mix of documents necessary to confirm eligibility, typically this includes a government issued identification card and a Social Security card.

C. Gross earnings

1. General

    a. Absences: Although some states may have specific requirements, FLSA does not require employers to pay employees for hours not worked because of illness.

    b. Tardiness: Unless required by state law, FLSA does not require employers to pay employees for periods of tardiness.

    c. Rest periods/coffee breaks: Unless required by state law, FLSA does not require that employees be given rest periods; however, if the time spent on a rest period is 20 minutes or less, the time must be counted as hours worked.

    d. Meal periods: Unless determined otherwise by state law, only meal periods during which the employee is relieved from duty may be considered nonworking time and does not require compensation.

2. Employment designations

    a. Employer: A person or organization who hires one or more persons to perform specified job duties in the United States.

    b. Employee: A person who performs specified job duties in the United States.

        (1) The employee is under the control and direction of an employer with regard to the performance of a job. An employee can be told what to do and how to do it.

        (2) If the employee meets the criteria above, the employer must assess payroll deductions.

        (3) Salary: Compensation for administrative, managerial, or professional work.

            (a) Exempt: A salaried employee is exempt from the FLSA rule requiring overtime at time and a half. The employer is not required to pay time and a half for overtime.

            (b) Nonexempt: The employer is required to pay time and a half for overtime.

        (4) Wage: Compensation for skilled or unskilled labor. Generally, wage employees must be paid a minimum of time and a half for overtime.

    c. Independent contractor: One who provides a service for a fee.

        (1) Independent contractors are generally hired to solve a problem. They may be told what needs to be done; i.e., the desired end result, but not how it should be done.

        (2) By definition, independent contractors are not employees; they receive a fee, not a wage or salary. Therefore, no payroll deductions will be assessed.

        (3) Independent contractors are responsible for paying their own payroll taxes.

3. Earnings calculations

    a. Wage

        (1) Data

            (a) Regular wage rate = $8/hour

            (b) Regular hours worked = 40 hours/week

            (c) Saturday overtime = 8 hours ($\times 1.5$)

            (d) Sunday overtime = 8 hours ($\times 2$)

        (2) Calculation

            (a) $8 $\times$ 40 hours = $320 regular earnings

            (b) $8 $\times$ 1.5 = $12/hour Saturday

            (c) $8 $\times$ 2 = $16/hour Sunday

            (d) $12 $\times$ 8 hours = $96 Saturday overtime

            (e) $16 $\times$ 8 hours = $128 Sunday overtime

            (f) $320 + $96 + $128 = $544 total earnings for the week

    b. Salary (nonexempt)

        (1) Data

            (a) Monthly salary = $1,600

            (b) Regular hours worked = 40 hours/week

            (c) Saturday overtime = 8 hours ($\times 1.5$)

            (d) Sunday overtime = 8 hours ($\times 2$)

        (2) Calculation

            (a) $1,600 $\times$ 12 = $19,200/year

            (b) $19,200 / 52 = $369.23/week regular earnings

            (c) $369.23 / 40 = $9.23/hour

            (d) $9.23 $\times$ 1.5 = $13.85/hour Saturday

            (e) $9.23 $\times$ 2 = $18.46/hour Sunday

            (f) $13.85 $\times$ 8 hours = $110.80 Saturday overtime

            (g) $18.46 $\times$ 8 hours = $147.68 Sunday overtime

            (h) $369.23 + $110.80 + $147.68 = $627.71 total earnings for the week.

D. Payroll taxes
   1. Income tax
      a. The Current Tax Payment Act of 1943: Requires employers to withhold income tax on a pay-as-you-go basis.
      b. The amount of tax withheld is not the exact annual tax liability. Because the tax is based on graduated withholding rates, the annual tax return will adjust for overages or shortages of taxes withheld.
      c. Advances such as traveling or business expenses and educational assistance such as tuition are generally not taxable.
   2. Federal Insurance Contributions Act (FICA): Social Security and Medicare tax.
      a. FICA consists of two main parts that are reported separately.
         (1) Old-age survivors, and disability insurance (OASDI).
         (2) Hospital insurance (Medicare).
      b. Taxable wage base: Maximum amount of wages subject to FICA tax during a calendar year. As of this writing, the taxable wage base is $106,800 for OASDI and all earnings are subject to Medicare.
      c. Tax rates: OASDI = 6.2%, Medicare = 1.45%; FICA total is 7.65%.
      d. Employers are required to collect FICA tax from employees and make payment to the IRS when the employer taxes are paid.
      e. Once the employer deducts the tax from the employee's earnings every pay period, the employees are no longer liable for payment of the tax.
      f. Every dollar contributed by the employee must be matched by the employer; therefore, a combined rate of 15.3% (7.65% × 2) of total taxable employee earnings will be paid.
   3. Unemployment compensation tax
      a. Federal and state programs established by the Social Security Act of 1935 to provide economic security during periods of temporary unemployment.
      b. Federal Unemployment Tax Act (FUTA): Requires most employers to pay a tax to support the federal unemployment insurance program.
      c. Only employers are subject to FUTA; however, FUTA is computed based on employee earnings even though employees do not pay FUTA tax.
      d. Taxable wage base: As of this writing, it is $7000.
      e. FUTA rate: As of this writing, it is 6.2%.
      f. State unemployment tax (SUTA): Nearly all states have an unemployment tax; few require an employee contribution.
         (1) All states have an experience-rating (or merit-rating) system. Employers who provide steady work for their employees pay lower rates.
         (2) Employers experiencing episodes of unemployment will pay a higher rate.

E. Payroll tax returns, reports, and forms
   1. Form SS-4: Application for Employer Identification Number. Federal tax identification number application. Required for employers withholding taxes from employees. States may require a separate number for state withholdings.
   2. Form SS-5: Social Security number application. All employees are required to have a Social Security number.
   3. Form W-2: Wages and Tax Statement. Given to employees to identify earnings and taxes withheld, as well as to prepare personal tax returns.
      a. Must be prepared for all employees who earned more than a specified amount or had federal income tax or FICA tax withheld during the year.
      b. Must be provided to employees no later than January 31 of the following year.
      c. Consists of a packet of six sheets bound together
         (1) Copy A: Sent to the Social Security Administration.
         (2) Copy 1: Sent to state tax department.
         (3) Copy B: Filed with employee's federal tax return.
         (4) Copy C: Kept by employee for personal record.
         (5) Copy 2: Filed with employee's state tax return.
         (6) Copy D: Kept by the employer.
   4. Form W-3: Transmittal of Income and Tax Statements.
      a. Employers must file Copy A of all W-2s with the Social Security Administration by February 28 along with Form W-3.
      b. Used to report the total amount of federal income tax and FICA tax withheld during the year and the number of W-2s being sent to the government.
      c. The amounts shown on the W-2s and the quarterly tax returns, Form 941, must all agree with the amounts shown on Form W-3.
   5. Form W-4: Employee's Withholding Allowance Certificate.
      a. Identifies the number of withholding allowances the employee claims regarding federal income tax.
      b. Withholding allowances consist of personal allowances and special tax credits.
      c. Each taxpayer can claim a personal allowance and one for each dependent. Tax credits

cover allowable expenses such as child care and disability expenses.

d. If the employee fails to file Form W-4, the employer must withhold taxes as if the employee were single and claimed no allowances.

e. Must be maintained for at least 4 years after the employee's employment is terminated.

f. Must be filed with the IRS if the employee claims 14 or more allowances or earns $200 or more and claims the exempt status.

6. Form 940: Employer's Annual Federal Unemployment Tax Return. Must be filed by January 31.

7. Form 941: Employer's Quarterly Federal Tax Return.

a. Reports all federal income tax and FUTA tax withheld on each quarter ending March 31, June 30, September 30, and December 31.

b. Form 941 should be filed by April 30, July 31, October 31, and January 31, annually.

8. Form 8109: Federal Tax Deposit Coupon Book. Used to make quarterly federal income tax and FUTA tax deposits.

F. Payroll deductions

1. Income tax: The most common is the wage-bracket (tax table) method.

a. Federal income tax: Requires the use of the Employer's Tax Guide, Publication 15, Circular E.

b. State income tax: Requires a tax table provided by the state.

c. Use of the tax table depends on four factors:

(1) Length of payroll period: Daily, weekly, biweekly, semimonthly, monthly, and miscellaneous.

(2) Gross earnings during the period.

(3) Marital status.

(4) Number of withholding allowances claimed.

d. Locate the table covering the payroll period and marital status of the employee. On the table, identify where the amount of earnings noted on the left column intersect with the number of withholding allowances across the top. This is the amount of tax to be withheld.

e. Computerized payroll systems typically use the percentage method; i.e., the amount of tax is calculated using a percentage formula.

2. FICA, FUTA, and SUTA: Typically, the percentage rate is multiplied by the taxable gross earnings.

3. Garnishments: Deductions authorized by a court of law for overdue debts.

4. Tax levies: Garnishments imposed by the IRS for overdue taxes. Usually requires the employee to complete a form to help the employer determine the amount of garnishment.

5. Union contracts: Such as union initiation fees, dues, and assessments.

6. Insurance: Such as life, medical, or dental insurance.

7. Pension: Deductions that contribute to a retirement fund.

8. Miscellaneous: Includes such deductions as savings plans, charitable contributions, or stock or bond purchase plans.

9. Net earnings (pay) is computed by subtracting all deductions from gross earnings.

G. Payroll system

1. System methods

a. Manual: Most common method for small organizations.

(1) Payroll is computed and processed by hand, using a calculator, typewriter, and forms.

(2) Pegboard payroll system: Similar to pegboard system described earlier.

(a) A payroll register is placed on a board containing alignment pegs.

(b) The employee earnings record is placed over the payroll register and aligned on the pegs.

(c) The check and stub are placed over the employee earnings record where the information is recorded on each form simultaneously.

b. Computerized: Payroll data is entered into the computer, where the necessary calculation, records, and reports are prepared automatically.

c. Payroll processing service bureau: Payroll data is sent to the service bureau. The service bureau processes the data by computer and delivers the completed payroll records and checks.

2. Payroll register

a. Provides a summary of hours worked, earnings, deductions, and net pay for all employees each payroll period.

b. Once all payroll data has been recorded, each column and row is totaled and proved.

3. Employee earnings record

a. Provides detailed annual payroll data on each employee.

b. It contains the same data as the payroll register, but is specific to each employee.

4. Payroll accounting: Payroll records are sent to the accountant or bookkeeper to be entered in the journal and posted to the ledgers, so that timely and accurate financial statements and tax returns can be prepared.

CHAPTER 13

Insurance Claims Management

I. INTRODUCTION

A. Purpose: A medical coding system enables the translation of verbal descriptions of diseases, injuries, illnesses, and procedures into numerical codes.
   1. Tracking: Systematic method of monitoring progress of disease processes.
   2. Classification: Allows for grouping related diagnoses and procedures.
   3. Research: Provides comparable data for compiling research information.
   4. Evaluation: Permits analysis of medical utilization.
   5. Standardization: Simplifies reimbursement functions.

B. Types of coding systems
   1. ICD-9-CM: International Classification of Diseases, 9th Revision, Clinical Modification. Used to code diagnosis or disease conditions.
   2. CPT: Current Procedural Terminology. Used to code medical services and procedures provided by physicians.
   3. Health Care Common Procedural Coding System. A national coding system for reporting medical services to the Medicare program.
   4. RBRVS: Resource-Based Relative Value System. Medicare fee schedule (MFS) for services based on the level of resources needed to provide a service.
   5. DRG: Diagnosis Related Groups. A prospective fixed Medicare fee structure for hospital billing of inpatient services based on principal diagnosis.
   6. MS-DRG: Medical Severity DRG. Weighted by the severity of diagnosis, paying more for sicker patients.
   7. RVS: Relative Value Study. A point value is assigned to the service performed based on the time, knowledge, and skill required of the provider. This point value is multiplied by a standard dollar factor to arrive at a final fee amount.

C. The International Statistical Classification of Diseases and Related Health Problems (ICD-10-CM)
   1. Will employ a new alphanumeric coding system.
   2. Will include more codes and apply to more users than ICD-9-CM because it is designed to collect data on every type of healthcare encounter.
   3. E codes and V codes will use other alphanumeric designations and will not be listed separately but will be incorporated throughout.
   4. The change from ICD-9-CM to ICD-10-CM and ICD-10-PCS (Procedure Coding System) may be mandated for 2012 or later.

II. ICD-9-CM (INTERNATIONAL CLASSIFICATION OF DISEASES, 9TH REVISION, CLINICAL MODIFICATION)

A. Assigns numeric codes to diseases, illnesses, injuries, and health-related conditions.

B. Description of the ICD-9-CM coding system
   1. ICD-9-CM is organized in three volumes.
      a. Volume I (Tabular List of Diseases): Numerical arrangement of conditions.
      b. Volume II (Alphabetical Index of Diseases): Diseases and conditions arranged alphabetically.
      c. Volume III (Tabular List and Alphabetical Index of Procedures): Medical procedures arranged both numerically and alphabetically. Commonly used by hospitals to code inpatient procedures.
   2. Volume I: Numerical arrangement.
      a. 001 to 799: Codes referring to specific health conditions by body system.
      b. 800 to 959, 990 to 999: Codes referring to injuries.
      c. 960 to 989: Codes referring to poisonings.
      d. V Codes (V01 to V89): Codes referring to factors that influence health status. A definitive diagnosis cannot be stated; however, there is a valid reason for seeking medical care.
         (1) Preoperative evaluations.
         (2) Annual physical exams.
         (3) Well-baby checks.
      e. E Codes: External causes of injury and poisoning (associated with 800 + level codes.)
      f. M Codes: On Appendix A. Morphology of Neoplasms.

g. Glossary of Mental Disorders: Appendix B. Alphabetical list of terms and definitions associated with mental disorders (codes 290 to 319).

h. Classification of Drugs by AHFS (American Hospital Formulary Services): Appendix C. Organized in AHFS numerical order along with its ICD-9-CM equivalent.

i. Classification of Industrial Accidents According to Agency: Appendix D.

j. List of Three-Digit Categories: Appendix E. Identifies the three-digit category codes organized by section headings.

3. Volume II: Three-part index to Volume I.

a. Section 1

(1) Alphabetical index of diseases and injuries.

(2) Hypertension chart.

(3) Neoplasm chart.

b. Section 2: Table of Adverse Effects to Drugs and Chemicals. Identifies the types of external causes of adverse effects (see Figure 13-1).

(1) Accidental poisoning.

(2) Assault.

(3) Misadventure in therapeutic use.

(4) Suicide attempt.

(5) Undetermined.

c. Section 3: The Index to External Causes (E codes). Codes the circumstances surrounding an accident or act of violence that resulted in an injury.

C. Organization of Volume I (see Figure 13-2A)

1. Codes 001 to 999 use a three-digit main number with further clinical specificity identified by adding a fourth- and fifth-digit modifier.

2. Chapter headings are printed in bold uppercase letters after a chapter number.

Substance	Poisoning	External Cause (E Code)				
		Accident	Therapeutic Use	Suicide Attempt	Assault	Undetermined
1-propanol	980.3	E860.4	—	E950.9	E962.1	E980.9
2-propanol	980.2	E860.3	—	E950.9	E962.1	E980.9
2, 4-D (dichlorophenoxyacetic acid)	989.4	E863.5	—	E950.6	E962.1	E980.7
2, 4-toluene diisocyanate	983.0	E864.0	—	E950.7	E962.1	E980.6
2, 4, 5-T (trichlorophenoxyacetic acid)	989.2	E863.5	—	E950.6	E962.1	E980.7
14-hydroxydihydromorphinone	965.09	E850.2	E935.2	E950.0	E962.0	E980.0
A						
ABOB	961.7	E857	E931.7	E950.4	E962.0	E980.4
Abrus (seed)	988.2	E865.3	—	E950.9	E962.1	E980.9
Absinthe	980.0	E860.0	—	E950.9	E962.1	E980.9
beverage	980.0	E860.0	E934.2	E950.4	E962.0	E980.4
Acenocoumarin, acenocoumarol	964.2	E858.2	E934.2	E950.4	E962.0	E980.3
Acepromazine	969.1	E853.0	E939.1	E950.3	E962.0	E980.3
Acetal	982.8	E862.4	—	E950.9	E962.1	E980.9
Acetaldehyde (vapor)	987.8	E869.8	—	E952.8	E962.2	E982.8
liquid	989.89	E866.8	—	E950.9	E962.1	E980.9
Acetaminophen	965.4	E850.4	E935.4	E950.0	E962.0	E980.0
Acetaminosalol	965.1	E850.3	E935.3	E950.0	E962.0	E980.0
Acetanilid(e)	965.4	E850.4	E935.4	E950.0	E962.0	E980.0
Acetarsol, acetarsone	961.1	E857	E931.1	E950.4	E962.0	E980.4
Acetazolamide	974.2	E858.5	E944.2	E950.4	E962.0	E980.4
Acetic						
acid	983.1	E864.1	—	E950.7	E962.1	E980.6
with sodium acetate (ointment)	976.3	E858.7	E946.3	E950.4	E962.0	E980.4
irrigating solution	974.5	E858.5	E944.5	E950.4	E962.0	E980.4
lotion	976.2	E858.7	E946.2	E950.4	E962.0	E980.4
anhydride	983.1	E864.1	—	E950.7	E962.1	E980.6
ether						

Figure 13-1

ICD-9-CM Table of Drugs and Chemicals (partial). From ICD-9-CM for Hospitals—Volumes 1, 2 & 3, 2005 Professional. Reprinted with permission of Ingenix.

3. Notes that follow the chapter heading provide guidelines for coding within the chapter. When a note includes an exclusion statement, the exclusion applies to the entire chapter.

4. Major topic headings are indicated by upper-case letters followed by the inclusive codes in parentheses. Exclusions below the topic heading apply only to those codes identified in parentheses.

5. Category headings further divide the major topic headings. Subcategory headings are indented and include a fourth-digit modifier.

6. Fifth-digit modifiers further divide subcategory headings and are generally preceded by a section mark (§), or other fifth-digit marker or flag.

D. Organization of Volume II (see Figure 13-2B)
   1. Volume II is an alphabetical listing of conditions that may be expressed as nouns, adjectives, or eponyms.
   2. Main terms are printed in boldface followed by a code number. Modifiers in parentheses may be present between the main term and code number.
   3. Subterms are indented providing further subclassifications.
   4. Special main terms may be consulted when the main condition is not obvious.

E. ICD-9-CM coding conventions
   1. Volume I
      a. Colon (:): Each modifier after the colon completes the main statement before the colon.
      b. Brace (}): The term after the brace is a required modifier of the statement to the left of the brace.
      c. Section mark (§): Identifies a code that requires a fifth-digit modifier.
      d. Excludes (enclosed in a rectangle): Conditions listed do not qualify for the code assignment.
      e. Includes: Clarifies a code description, but does not have to be constrained by it.
   2. Volume II
      a. Diagnoses, are organized by main terms printed in boldface type: Chronic bronchitis would be found under **Bronchitis, chronic.**
         (1) Obstetric conditions: Indexed under **Delivery, Pregnancy, or Puerperal.**
         (2) Medical/surgical complications: Indexed under **Complications.**
         (3) Secondary disorders caused by the original condition: Indexed under **Late Effects.**
      b. Modifiers: Specific factors that influence a diagnosis code.
         (1) Nonessential modifier: Main terms followed by terms in parentheses.
            (a) The terms in parentheses may be included with the main term; e.g., **Bronchitis** (diffuse) (hypostatic) . . . 490.
            (b) The code 490 can be used for bronchitis; diffuse bronchitis, or hypostatic bronchitis, etc.
         (2) Subterm modifier: Specific manifestations of a condition that have a specified code.
            (a) These terms are indented below the main term and represent different diagnoses;
            (b) e.g., **Hernia**
                Hernia (acquired). . .553.9
                appendix 553.8
                brain 348.4
                colostomy (stoma) 569.69
         (3) Adjectives: Such as acute, chronic; or anatomical names will appear as main terms with no code and a reference to "see condition."
      c. See also: Direction to consider another code.
      d. See category: Directions to look into a synonym for the condition.
      e. See condition: Indicates that you are looking up the wrong word such as an adjective. You would not look up the diagnosis *acute pericarditis* under the term "acute," but under pericarditis and then the subterm "acute."
   3. Conventions common to both Volumes I and II
      a. Bracket ([]): Enclosed terms are synonyms, alternative words, explanatory phrases, or secondary codes.
      b. Parentheses (()): Enclosed terms may or may not affect a main term, but in Volume II are essential modifiers when following a subterm.
      c. NEC (Not Elsewhere Classified): Used for ill-defined terms where more precise information is not available.
      d. NOS (Not Otherwise Specified): A generalized diagnosis term that may require greater specificity.
      e. Note: Defines terms or provides instructions (fifth-digit modifier use).
      f. See: Directions to investigate another code.

F. Basic ICD-9-CM coding steps
   1. Locate the main term in the Alphabetical Index of Volume II.
   2. If you cannot find the main term, look up major terms such as syndrome, disease, disorder, derangement of, abnormal, etc.
   3. Read through and act on notes printed after the boldface main term.

| Chapter heading | **3. ENDOCRINE, NUTRITIONAL AND METABOLIC DISEASES, AND IMMUNITY DISORDERS (240-279)** |

Chapter heading

3. ENDOCRINE, NUTRITIONAL AND METABOLIC DISEASES, AND IMMUNITY DISORDERS (240-279)

Excludes statement

EXCLUDES *endocrine and metabolic disturbances specific to the fetus and newborn (775.0-775.9)*

Instructional note

Note: All neoplasms, whether functionally active or not, are classified in Chapter 2. Codes in Chapter 3 (i.e., 242.8, 246.0, 251-253, 2555-259) may be used to identify such functional activity associated with any neoplasm, or by ectopic endocrine tissue.

Major topic heading

DISORDERS OF THYROID GLAND (240-246)

Category code

√4th 240 Simple and unspecified goiter
DEF: An enlarged thyroid gland often caused by an inadequate dietary intake of iodine.

Subcategory code

240.0 Goiter, specified as simple
Any condition classifiable to 240.9, specified as simple

240.9 Goiter, unspecified

Description statements

Enlargement of thyroid
Goiter or struma:
   NOS
   diffuse colloid
   endemic

Goiter or struma:
   hyperplastic
   nontoxic (diffuse)
   parenchymatous
   sporadic

EXCLUDES *congenital (dyshormonogenic) goiter (246.1)*

DISEASES OF OTHER ENDOCRINE GLANDS (250-259)

√4th 250 Diabetes mellitus

EXCLUDES *gestational diabetes (648.8)*
hyperglycemia NOS (790.6)
neonatal diabetes mellitus (775.1)
nonclinical diabetes (790.29)

Subclassification codes for 5th digit assignment

The following fifth-digit subclassification is for use with category 250:
▲ **0 type II or unspecified type, not stated as uncontrolled**
   Fifth-digit 0 is for use for type II patients, even if the patient requires insulin
   ▶ Use additional code, if applicable, for associated long-term (current) insulin use V58.67 ◀
▲ **1 type I (juvenile type), not stated as uncontrolled**
▲ **2 type II or unspecified type, uncontrolled**
   Fifth-digit 2 is for use for type II patients, even if the patient requires insulin
   ▶ Use additional code, if applicable, for associated long-term (current) insulin use V58.67 ◀
▲ **3 type I (juvenile type), uncontrolled**

AHA: 2Q, '02, 13; 2Q, '01, 16; 2Q, '98, 15; 4Q, '97, 32; 2Q, '97, 14; 3Q, '96, 5; 4Q, '93, 19; 2Q, '92, 5; 3Q, '91, 3; 2Q, '90, 22; N-D, '85, 11

DEF: Diabetes mellitus: Inability to metabolize carbohydrates, proteins, and fats with insufficient secretion of insulin. Symptoms may be unremarkable, with long-term complications, involving kidneys, nerves, blood vessels, and eyes.
DEF: Uncontrolled diabetes: A nonspecific term indicating that the current treatment regimen does not keep the blood sugar level of a patient within acceptable levels.

√5th 250.0 Diabetes mellitus without mention of complication
   Diabetes mellitus without mention of complication or manifestation classifiable to 250.1-250.9
   Diabetes (mellitus) NOS
CC Excl: For code 250.01-250.03: 250.00-250.93, 251.0-251.3, 259.8-259.9

AHA: 4Q, '97, 32; 3Q, '91, 3, 12; N-D, '85, 11;
   For Code 250.00;
   4Q, '03, 105, 108; 2Q, '03, 16 1Q, '02, 7, 11;
   For Code 250.01:
   4Q, '03, 110; 2Q, '03, 6 **For Code 250.02:** 1Q, '03, 5

Figure 13-2A

ICD-9-CM Diseases Tabular List. From ICD-9-CM for Hospitals—Volumes 1, 2 & 3, 2005 Professional. Reprinted with permission of Ingenix.

Dextrocardia (corrected) (false) (isolated)
(secondary) (true) 746.87
with
complete transposition of viscera 759.3
situs inversus 759.3
Dextroversion, kidney (left) 753.3
Dhobie itch 110.3
Diabetes, diabetic (brittle) (congenital) (familial)
(mellitus) (poorly controlled) (severe) (slight)
(without complication) 250.0 ☑

---

*Note - Use the following fifth-digit
subclassification with category 250:*

▸ *0   type II or unspecified type, not stated
as uncontrolled
Fifth-digit 0 is for use for type II patients,
even if the patient requires insulin*

*1   type 1 (juvenile type), not stated as
uncontrolled*

*2   type II or unspecified type,
uncontrolled
Fifth-digit 2 is for use for type II patients,
even if the patient requires insulin*

3   type I (juvenile type), uncontrolled ◂

---

with
coma (with ketoacidosis) 250.3 ☑
hyperosmolar (nonketotic) 250.2 ☑
complication NEC 250.9 ☑
specified NEC 250.8 ☑
gangrene 250.7 ☑ (785.4)
hyperosmolarity 250.2 ☑
ketosis, ketoacidosis 250.1 ☑
osteomyelitis 250.8 ☑ (731.8)
specified manisfestations NEC 250.8 ☑
acetonemia 250.1 ☑

Figure 13-2B

*ICD-9-CM Diseases Tabular List. From ICD-9-CM for Hospitals—
Volumes 1, 2 & 3, 2005 Professional.* Reprinted with permission
of Ingenix.

4. Consider and apply conventions for any modifiers of the main term.
5. Follow any cross-references; i.e., "see," "see also," "see category."
6. Verify the code number in Volume I and make modifications as instructed.
7. Record the final code assignment.
G. ICD-9-CM coding guidelines
   1. Never code qualified diagnoses such as *suspected, suspicion of, questionable,* or *rule out.* You may, however, code symptoms of the patient's chief complaint.
   2. Never assign a code without verifying it in Volume I.
   3. Never guess: When in doubt, check it out.
   4. A few diagnoses cannot be verified in Volume I.
   5. Use of the fourth- and fifth-digit modifiers is not optional.
   6. Avoid, whenever possible, the use of fourth-digit modifiers that represent a nonspecific diagnosis.

7. Differentiate between acute and chronic.
8. The phrase "with mention of" should not be interpreted to mean "due to" or "as a result of."
9. The word "and" written between two separate conditions should be read as "and/or."
10. Etiology determinations may be required. Is the condition acquired or congenital, traumatic or nontraumatic, or is it a gynecological or obstetrical case?
H. Coding table guidelines
   1. There are two coding tables in Volume II
      a. Hypertension.
      b. Neoplasms.
   2. Hypertension table: The table has three main column headings. Found under the main term **Hypertension** (see Figure 13-3).
      a. Malignant: Severe form with vascular damage and a diastole of >130 mmHg.
      b. Benign: Mild and in control.
      c. Unspecified: No notation of benign or malignant.
   3. Neoplasm table: Arranged by anatomical site and six tumor classifications. Found under the main term **Neoplasm** (see Figure 13-4).
      a. Primary malignancy: The original tumor site where it began.
      b. Secondary malignancy: The tumor has metastasized.
      c. Carcinoma in situ: A malignant tumor that is localized, circumscribed, and noninvasive.
      d. Benign: A noninvasive, nonspreading, nonmalignant tumor.
      e. Uncertain behavior: Impossible to predict morphology or behavior.
      f. Unspecified nature: A neoplasm with no indication of histology or nature.

III. CPT (CURRENT PROCEDURAL TERMINOLOGY)

A. Systematic listing and coding of procedures and services performed by healthcare providers.
   1. Each procedure or service is identified by a five-digit code.
   2. CPT codes simplifies the reporting of services to insurance carriers.
   3. The CPT book is divided into six sections. Within each section are subsections with anatomical, procedural, condition, and descriptor subheadings.
      a. Evaluation and Management (E & M): 99201 to 99600.
      b. Anesthesia: 00100 to 01999.
      c. Surgery: 10040 to 69990.
      d. Radiology: 70010 to 79999.
      e. Pathology and Laboratory: 80048 to 89399.
      f. Medicine: 90281 to 99199.

	Malignant	Benign	Unspecified
Hypertension, hypertensive (arterial) (arteriolar) (crisis) (degeneration) (disease) (essential) (fluctuating) (idiopathic) (intermittent) (labile) (low renin) (orthostatic) (paroxysmal) (primary) (systemic) (uncontrolled) (vascular)	401.0	401.1	401.9
with			
heart involvement ▶(conditions classifiable to 429.0-429.3, 429.8, 429.9 due to hypertension) ◀ (see also Hypertension, heart..	402.00	402.10	402.90
with kidney involvement — see Hypertension, cardiorenal			
renal involvement (only conditions classifiable to 585, 586, 587) (excludes conditions classifiable to 584) (see also Hypertension, kidney..	403.00	403.10	403.90
renal sclerosis or failure..	403.00	403.10	403.90
with heart involvement — see Hypertension, cardiorenal			
failure (and sclerosis) (see also Hypertension, kidney)...........	403.01	403.11	403.91
sclerosis without failure (see also Hypertension, kidney).......	403.00	403.10	403.90
accelerated — (see also Hypertension, by type, malignant)..............	401.0	——	——
antepartum — see Hypertension, complicating pregnancy, childbirth, or the puerperium			
cardiorenal (disease)..	404.00	404.10	404.90
with			
heart failure..	404.01	404.11	404.91
and renal failure..	404.03	404.13	404.93
renal failure..	404.02	404.12	404.92
and heart failure..	404.03	404.13	404.93
cardiovascular disease (arteriosclerotic) (sclerotic).........................	402.00	402.10	402.90
with			
heart failure..	402.01	402.11	402.91
renal involvement (conditions classifiable to 403) (see also Hypertension, cardiorenal)...	404.00	404.10	404.90

Figure 13-3

ICD-9-CM Hypertension table (partial). From ICD-9-CM for Hospitals—Volumes 1, 2 & 3, 2005 Professional. Reprinted with permission of Ingenix.

B. CPT format and conventions
1. A main statement followed by a semicolon and, in most cases, a subordinate statement describing the site's special procedure or statement of the extent of the services. E.g: 55700
   Biopsy, prostate; needle or punch, single or multiple . . .
2. Terms indented below the main statement represent additional subordinate statements. E.g.: 55700 Biopsy, prostate; needle or punch. . . 55705 incisional, any approach
3. Guidelines: Specific directions located at the beginning of each of the six sections necessary to code accurately.
4. CPT symbols
   a. Bullet (●): Located on the left side of a code number indicates a new procedure.
   b. Triangle (▲): Indicates a code description has been revised.
   c. Horizontal triangles (▶ . . . ◀): Surrounds revised guidelines and notes.
   d. Asterisk (*): Located after a code number indicates variable preoperative and postoperative services.
   e. Plus (+): Identifies add-on codes for procedures that are commonly performed at the same time.
   f. Circle with slash (∅): Identifies codes that are not to be used with modifier-51.
5. Modifiers: Terminal, two-digit code that represents an alteration in the circumstances or employment of the procedure.
   a. −21: Prolonged E & M Services.
   b. −22: Unusual Procedural Services.
   c. −23: Unusual Anesthesia.
   d. −24: Unrelated E & M Service.
   e. −25: Significant, Separately Identifiable E & M Service by the Same Physician on the Day of a Procedure.

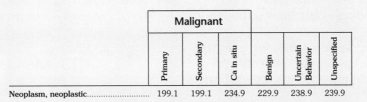

	Malignant					
	Primary	Secondary	Ca in situ	Benign	Uncertain Behavior	Unspecified
Neoplasm, neoplastic........................	199.1	199.1	234.9	229.9	238.9	239.9

> *Notes — 1. The list below gives the code numbers for neoplasms by anatomical site. For each site there are six possible code numbers according to whether the neoplasm in question is malignant, benign, in situ, of uncertain behavior, or of unspecified nature. The description of the neoplasm will often indicate which of the six columns is appropriate; e.g., malignant melanoma of skin, benign fibroadenoma of breast, carcinaoma in situ of cervix uteri.*
>
> *Where such descriptors are not present, the remainder of the Index should be consulted where guidance is given to the appropriate column for each morphological (histologic) variety listed; e.g., Mesonephroma — see Neoplasm, malignant; Embryoma — see also Neoplasm, uncertain behavior; Disease, Bowen's — see Neoplasm, skin, in situ. However, the guidance in the Index can be overridden if one of the descriptors mentioned above is present; e.g., malignant adenoma of colon is coded to 153.9 and not to 211.3 as the adjective "malignant" overrides the Index entry "Adenoma — see also Neoplasm, benign."*
>
> *2. Sites marked with the sign * (e.g., face NEC*) should be classified to malignant neoplasm of skin of these sites if the variety of neoplasm is a squamous cell carcinoma or an epidermoid carcinoma, and to benign neoplasm of skin of these sites if the variety of neoplasm is a papilloma (any type).*

	Primary	Secondary	Ca in situ	Benign	Uncertain Behavior	Unspecified
abdomen, abdominal.............................	195.2	198.89	234.8	229.8	238.8	239.8
cavity..	195.2	198.89	234.8	229.8	238.8	239.8
organ..	195.2	198.89	234.8	229.8	238.8	239.8
viscera..	195.2	198.89	234.8	229.8	238.8	239.8
wall...	173.5	198.2	232.5	216.5	238.2	239.2
connective tissue................	171.5	198.89	—	215.5	238.1	239.2
abdominopelvic..................................	195.8	198.89	234.8	229.8	238.8	239.8
accessory sinus — see Neoplasm, sinus....						
acoustic nerve..................................	192.0	198.4	—	225.1	237.9	239.7
acromion (process).............................	170.4	198.5	—	213.4	238.0	239.2

Figure 13-4

ICD-9-CM Neoplasm table (partial). From ICD-9-CM for Hospitals—Volumes 1, 2 & 3, 2005 Professional. Reprinted with permission of Ingenix.

f. −26: Professional Component.

g. −27: Multiple Outpatient Hospital E/M Encounters on the Date.

h. −32: Third-Party Mandated Service.

i. −47: Anesthesia by Surgeon.

j. −50: Bilateral Procedure.

k. −51: Multiple Procedures.

l. −52: Reduced Services.

m. −53: Discontinued Procedure.

n. −54: Surgical Care Only.

o. −55: Postoperative Management Only.

p. −56: Preoperative Management Only.

q. −57: Decision for Surgery.

r. −58: Stages or Related Procedure or Service by the Same Physician During the Postoperative Period.

s. −59: Distinct Procedural Service.

t. −62: Two Surgeons.

u. −63: Procedure on Infant Less Than 4 kg.

v. −66: Surgical Team.

w. −73: Discontinued Outpatient Procedure Prior to Anesthesia Administration.

x. −74: Discontinued Outpatient Procedure After Anesthesia Administered.

y. −76: Repeat Procedure by Same Physician.

z. −77: Repeat Procedure by Another Physician.

aa. −78: Return to the Operating Room for a Related Procedure During the Postoperative Period.

bb. −79: Unrelated Procedure or Service by the Same Physician During the Postoperative Period.

cc. −80: Assistant Surgeon.

dd. −81: Minimum Assistant Surgeon.

ee. −82: Assistant Surgeon (when qualified resident surgeon not available).

ff. −90: Reference (Outside) Laboratory.

gg. −91: Repeat Clinical Diagnostic Laboratory Test.

hh. −99: Multiple Modifiers.

6. Major headings are in boldface type.
7. Notes: Provide coding instructions throughout the book.
   a. Blocked paragraphs: Appearing at the beginning of a heading or subheading provides general information regarding those headings.
   b. Indented paragraphs: Within parentheses provide directions to review other codes.
   c. E.g. statements: Within parentheses provide examples of conditions a code applies to.
8. Descriptive qualifiers: Narrative descriptions surrounding, sometimes in parentheses, a code description that provides more detailed information about the code.

C. Basic CPT coding steps
1. Review the guidelines beginning each section.
2. Upon reading the medical documentation, familiarize yourself with the type and circumstances of the procedures being coded.
3. Turn to the index. Locate the main term. If the main term is not listed, locate synonyms for the main term or anatomical sites, etc. E & M services are listed under *Evaluation and Management.*
4. Locate any subterm and follow cross-references.
5. Read the code descriptions of all code numbers listed in the Index.
6. Record the proper code. If the proper code cannot be located, follow CPT guidelines for handling *unlisted services.*

D. Evaluation and management
1. Includes basic diagnostic and treatment service such as clinic visits, examinations, and the like.
2. The E & M section is divided into broad categories thats have two or more subdivisions.
3. Common E & M terminology
   a. New patient is defined as "a patient who is new to the practice or has not received any professional services by the provider or another provider of the same specialty who belongs to the same group practice, for 3 or more years."
   b. Established patient is "a patient who has received professional services from the provider or another provider of the same specialty who belongs to the same group practice, within the past 3 years."
   c. Concurrent care: The rendering of similar services to the same patient by more than one provider on the same day.
   d. Counseling: Discussion with a patient and/or family regarding diagnosis, treatment, and patient education.

4. Within each category, the following must be determined to properly select an E & M code. The first three are the key components:
   a. History
      (1) Problem focused: Includes chief complaint and brief history of presenting problem.
      (2) Expanded problem focused: Chief complaint, brief history of presenting problem, and review of system affected by the presenting problem.
      (3) Detailed: Chief complaint, extended history of presenting problem, extended review of system affected by the presenting problem, and pertinent past, family, and/or social history.
      (4) Comprehensive: Chief complaint, extended history of presenting problem, complete review of systems, and complete past, family, and social history.
   b. Examination
      (1) Problem focused: Examination is limited to the affected body area or organ system.
      (2) Expanded problem focused: Examination is limited to the affected body area or organ system and other symptomatic or related organ systems.
      (3) Detailed: Extended examination of the affected body area or organ system and other symptomatic or related organ systems.
      (4) Comprehensive: Complete single system specialty examination or a complete multisystem examination.
   c. Complexity of medical decision making: Complexity of determining a diagnosis and/or selecting a management strategy.
      (1) Within each of four complexity levels, there are three criteria to consider:
         (a) The number of diagnoses or management options possible.
         (b) The amount and/or complexity of data to be reviewed.
         (c) The risk of complication, morbidity, and/or mortality.
      (2) Complexity levels
         (a) Straightforward: All three criteria are minimal.
         (b) Low complexity: Low degree in each.
         (c) Moderate complexity: Moderate degree.
         (d) High complexity: High degree.
   d. Contributing components: Counseling, coordination of care, nature of presenting

problem, and time. Four additional contributing factors to consider in choosing the proper E & M code.

E. HCPCS (Healthcare Common Procedural Coding System)
  1. Tri-level coding system that expands the existing CPT system to provide a temporary listing of newly developed codes before inclusion in the CPT system.
  2. Level I: Existing CPT codes.
  3. Level II: Additional codes that permit greater precision of coding within the more broadly defined CPT categories, as well as reporting nonprovider services.
     a. Originally developed for use by the Medicare system, it has been nationally accepted and used.
     b. Includes codes not found within the existing CPT system such as injection of specific therapeutic drugs, chiropractic services, and surgical supplies.
     c. Uses a five-character alphanumeric coding system. The codes are grouped into related procedures ranging from A0000 to V5999.
     d. HCPCS uses a two-letter modifier that can also be used with regular CPT codes.
  4. Level III: Codes used by private insurance companies contracted to process government insurance claims such as Medicare. No longer required.

IV. HEALTH INSURANCE

A. Insurance is economic protection against financial loss caused by possible, but unplanned events affecting an individual or business.
B. Medicare and Medicaid Anti-Fraud and Abuse Act of 1977: Prohibits intentional misrepresentation or concealment of facts and acts that lead to improper reimbursement, as well as inappropriate or poor quality of care.
C. Coordination of benefits: Insurance policy clauses that restrict the overpayment of benefits because more than one medical insurance policy is in force.
D. Commercial insurance: Insurance policies created and sold by general insurance companies.
E. Self-insured plans: Organizations that establish insurance accounts in a financial institution for their employees or members.
F. Managed care: Programs that oversee the delivery of services to ensure that care is appropriate, necessary, and cost-effective.
  1. Capitation: Managed care is financed according to a fixed, prepaid payment for each enrolled patient during a fixed period, usually annually.
  2. Primary care provider (PCP): Enrollees receive care from a primary care physician identified on an approved list of providers. The PCP provides primary care services as well as supervises and coordinates the care of enrollees.
  3. Quality assurance: Federally qualified programs must have a quality assurance program to assess the quality of care rendered.
  4. Utilization management/review (UM/UR): Method of controlling healthcare costs and quality by reviewing the appropriateness and necessity of care before (prospectively) and after (retrospectively) the care is provided.
     a. Preadmission certification: Determining medical necessity before a hospital admission is approved.
     b. Preauthorization: Determining whether a service will be reimbursed before its delivery.
     c. Concurrent review: Determines medical necessity for services during a hospital admission.
     d. Discharge planning: Arranging appropriate services following patient discharge.
  5. Case management: Cost-effective plan development and coordination of care for complicated cases.
  6. Second surgical opinions: Opinion from a second surgeon to determine the appropriateness, necessity, and cost-effectiveness of surgical care.
  7. Physician incentives: Financial reward to physicians who are able to provide appropriate services at reduced costs.
G. Managed care models
  1. Exclusive provider organization (EPO): Plan that provides benefits to patient subscribers if they receive care from a network provider (physician or facility under contract with the EPO).
  2. Integrated delivery system (IDS): Organization of affiliated providers, such as hospitals, clinics, physician groups, and surgical centers, offering joint services to subscribers.
  3. Health maintenance organization (HMO): Capitated managed care organization that emphasizes preventive medicine.
     a. Group model: Physicians form an independent group and contract with an HMO to provide services to its members.
     b. Individual (independent) practice association (IPA): Several providers who agree to provide services to HMO members.
     c. Network model: HMO contracts with two or more group practices to provide services to its members.
     d. Staff model: HMO hires physicians and pays them a salary to provide services to its members.
  4. Preferred provider organization (PPO): Network of physicians and hospitals who contract with insurance companies or employers to provide services to subscribers at a discounted fee.

5. Point of service plan (POS): HMOs and PPOs that allow patients to either use the HMO/PPO panel of providers or seek care outside the network if so authorized, or for an additional charge if not authorized.
6. Triple option plan (cafeteria plan): Insurance plans that offer a choice among HMO, PPO, or traditional health insurance plans.

H. General plan options: There are many possible components of a health insurance policy. Specific options can be chosen to meet the needs of the insured.
1. Basic benefits: Basic benefits of the average policy will include the following:
   a. Diagnostic studies.
   b. Hospitalization.
   c. Surgical treatment.
   d. Obstetrical and neonatal care.
   e. Intensive care and chemotherapy.
2. Major medical: Includes services not covered by a basic plan such as the following:
   a. Outpatient visits including minor surgical care.
   b. Physical and occupational therapy.
   c. Cost of durable medical equipment (DME).
   d. Mental health care.
   e. Prescription drugs and dental care.
3. Companion plan: Policy provision designed to pay the fees not covered by conventional insurance plans.

I. Payment methods
1. Payment terminology
   a. Fee charged: The total amount the provider charges for the service.
   b. Allowable fee: The maximum amount the carrier will consider for reimbursement.
   c. Reimbursed fee: The amount the carrier will actually pay for the service; usually a percentage of the allowable fee, e.g., provider charges $100 for a service; the carrier considers the allowable charge to be $80 for the service; the reimbursed fee is 80% of the allowable fee resulting in a $64 payment to the provider.
2. Provider fee profile and UCR: See Chapter 12.
3. Assignment of benefits (AOB): An instruction to the carrier to send payment directly to the provider.
   a. Most commercial carriers will reimburse the patient unless instructed to do otherwise.
   b. Depending on the carrier, the patient may indicate AOB by completing a form or signing the appropriate box on the insurance claim form.
   c. The assignment does not necessarily absolve the patient from paying the difference between what is billed and what is reimbursed.

d. If the provider accepts assignment, the carrier will remit payment to the provider. With government claims, the provider must indicate on the claim form whether or not assignment is accepted or rejected.
e. Generally, if assignment is accepted, the provider can bill only the difference between the allowed charge and the allowed fee.
f. Providers who reject assignment are free to bill the patient the difference between the fee charged and the fee reimbursed unless a limit is imposed. (Except for Tricare or Medicare.)
g. Providers who elect to treat Medicaid and workers' compensation patients must accept the reimbursement as payment in full without further billing the patient.
h. BC/BS participating providers (PAR) must also accept the carriers' determined fees when treating certain BC/BS subscribers. Patients are responsible for deductibles and copayments.

J. Patient responsibilities
1. Patients should be aware of the services covered by their policies and the payment methods.
2. Never make the statement, "I'm sure your insurance will cover this."
3. Avoid reviewing the patient's insurance literature to determine coverage. Ask the patient to call the carrier for this information, or verify the coverage by calling the carrier.
4. The contract for care is between the provider and patient, not the provider and carrier.
5. Most commercial policies pay a fixed percentage of allowed charges. This must be carefully explained to the patient because what is billed and what is allowed are rarely the same.

K. Common terminology
1. Carrier (insurer): Insurance company that sells or administers an insurance contract.
2. Insured (subscriber): Policyholder or person contracting with a carrier for insurance coverage.
3. Provider: Health professionals who provide medical services; usually a physician.
4. Beneficiary: Persons designated by the insured to receive the benefits of an insurance policy.
5. Premiums: Fixed, periodic fees paid to keep an insurance policy in force.
6. Deductible: A specified annual amount initially paid for covered services before insurance benefits are paid.
7. Copayment: A percentage of the cost of service paid by the insured.
8. Exclusion: Conditions or treatment not covered by the policy.
9. Group policy: Policy purchased by an organization for the benefit of its members.

10. Individual policy: A policy or added coverage over and above a group policy purchased by an individual.
11. Preexisting condition: Medical conditions present or being treated at the time a policy application is made. Some policies will not cover preexisting conditions.
12. Subrogation: Assuming an obligation or duty a third party is liable for.
13. Explanation of benefits (EOB): A document prepared by the carrier that accompanies payment identifying the services rendered, the amount billed, allowed, and paid, and any explanatory information as appropriate.
14. Rider: Contractual clauses designating coverage items in addition to the standard contract.
15. Balance billing: Billing the patient for the difference between the provider's fee and the carrier's allowed fee.
16. Capitation: A fixed, prepaid fee per person enrolled per time period for services regardless of type or volume.
17. Fee-for-service: Provider bills for each service rendered rather than a capitation arrangement.
18. Indemnity plan: Commercial fee-for-service insurance policy.

V. INSURANCE SOURCES

A. Medicare
1. Federal program administered by CMS (Centers for Medicare and Medicaid Services). Established in 1965 as Title 18 of the Social Security Act.
2. Eligibility: Generally available to the aged and disabled.
   a. Persons age 65 or older, retired on Social Security benefits, or on railroad retirement including spouses age 65 or older.
   b. Spouses, age 65 or older, of persons currently contributing FICA tax.
   c. Persons receiving Social Security disability income (SSDI) for at least 2 years.
   d. Workers afflicted with end-stage renal disease (ESRD) who contribute FICA tax, and their ESRD-afflicted spouses or dependents.
   e. Disabled dependents of workers contributing FICA tax, and their ESRD-afflicted spouses or dependents.
   f. The Cost to Donors of kidneys transplanted into eligible ESRD patients.
   g. Retired federal employees enrolled in the Civil Service Retirement System (CSRS) and their spouses age 65 or older.
3. Benefits
   a. Part A: Automatic benefit covering the provision of certain institutional (inpatient) care.

All fees are generally paid once the deductible has been satisfied.
   b. Part B: Voluntary program requiring a monthly premium covering the provision of certain outpatient services. Eighty percent of allowable charges are generally paid, with the remaining 20% of allowable charges due from the patient once the annual deductible has been satisfied.
   c. Part C: Medicare Advantage. Allows Medicare beneficiaries to join managed care plans rather than participating in Parts A or B.
   d. Part D: Medicare Prescription Drug Benefit. Voluntary program requiring a monthly premium and deductible covering prescription medications.
4. Medigap: Commercial individual policy that covers deductible and coinsurance and, in some cases, items not covered by Medicare.

B. Medicaid
1. Federal program administered by each state. Established in 1965 as Title 19 of the Social Security Act.
2. Federal government funds a major portion of the Medicaid program with remaining funding provided by the state.
   a. Each state administers, determines eligibility requirements, available benefits, and payment levels according to minimum federal requirements.
   b. Eligible patients receive an official identification card for the periods they remain eligible or, in some states, for life.
3. Eligibility: Generally available to persons with income below the federal poverty level.
   a. Persons receiving Supplementary Security Income (SSI) for the aged and disabled.
   b. Persons receiving TANF (temporary assistance to needy families) benefits.
   c. Certain low-income individuals and families who meet federal and state eligibility guidelines.
4. Medi/Medi: Some patients may be covered by both Medicare and Medicaid. In such case, Medicare is the primary carrier and billed first. Medicaid is the payer of last resort.
5. MediCal: Medicaid program of California.

C. Tricare/CHAMPVA: Civilian Health and Medical Program of the Veterans Administration.
1. Federal medical care programs benefitting military dependents and veterans of the Air Force, Navy, Marine Corps, Army, Coast Guard, and uniformed branches of the Public Health Service, National Oceanic and Atmospheric Administration (NOAA), and North Atlantic Treaty Organization (NATO).

2. Tricare is designed for military dependents and retirees and their dependents who are eligible to be treated in military healthcare facilities.
3. Tricare eligibility
   a. Dependents of personnel employed by the organizations identified above.
   b. Retired persons and their dependents.
   c. Disabled dependents of affiliated personnel.
   d. Dependents of deceased personnel or retirees.
   e. Dependents of reservists called to active duty for more than 30 days are eligible during the active duty status.
4. CHAMPVA eligibility
   a. Dependents of a permanently disabled veteran with a service-related disability.
   b. Dependents of a deceased veteran who died as a result of a service-related condition.
   c. Dependents of a person who died in the line of military duty.
5. Tricare/CHAMPVA are secondary payers to all commercial and government insurance programs except Medicaid.
D. Workers' Compensation
   1. State-administered program established to defray the cost of medical care and lost wages associated with work-related illnesses and injuries.
   2. Philosophically, Workers' Compensation laws were designed to expedite the employee's return to work to avoid the provision of welfare benefits.
   3. Typically, Workers' Compensation patients are compensated in full for medical expenses and perhaps a portion of lost wages.
   4. Coverage types
      a. State compensation fund: State government body serves as the carrier where employers pay premiums to cover claims.
      b. Self-insured program: An employer may establish its own insurance fund upon meeting specific state requirements.
      c. Private, commercial program: Employers purchase commercial insurance meeting state requirements.
      d. Combination program: Any combination of the three arrangements described above.
   5. Eligibility: A person must incur an illness or injury while carrying out the duties of a job as required by an employer.
   6. Case classifications
      a. Medical treatment: Filed for minor illnesses or injuries where the employee is able to return to work in a few days.
      b. Temporary disability: Filed for illnesses or injuries that require more than a few days of

rehabilitation or recuperation before returning to work.
      c. Permanent disability: Filed for illnesses or injuries resulting in diminished capacity to return to work. Typically ranges from 10% to 100% disability.
      d. Vocational rehabilitation: Filed for temporary and permanently disabled persons who require education and training to return to work.
      e. Survivor benefits: Claims provide death benefits to eligible dependents according to the decedent-employee's earning capacity.
E. Blue Cross/Blue Shield
   1. Independent membership associations that provide prepaid healthcare services.
   2. Blue Cross was originally designed to cover hospital services, whereas Blue Shield covered provider services. More recently this coverage distinction has become blurred.
   3. Fiscal intermediary: BC/BS may contract with the federal government to administer Medicare, Medicaid, and Tricare.
      a. Blue Cross will handle Medicare Part A claims.
      b. Blue Shield will handle Medicare Part B claims.
      c. In some states BC and BS handle both.
F. Independent commercial insurance carriers: Have their own individual requirements, but the principles are essentially the same as those described thus far.

VI. INSURANCE CLAIMS

A. CMS-1500 Claim Form: Universal claim form developed by CMS that standardizes the data required by most carriers to process insurance claims (see Figure 13-5).
   1. Block 1—Insurance program designator: Check all of the appropriate boxes. Use CHAMPUS for Tricare. Use *Other* for commercial carriers and BC/BS. Use *FECA* (Federal Employee Compensation Act) for Workers' Compensation.
   2. Block 1a—Insured's I.D. number: Enter insurance identification number as it appears on the insurance card. Enter Medicare number for Medi/Medi claims. Enter sponsor's SSN for Tricare/CHAMPVA.
   3. Block 2—Patient's name: Enter the patient's last, first, and middle initial.
   4. Block 3—Patient's birth date/sex: Enter two digits each for month, day, and year (after year 2000, four digits will be used); check appropriate box for sex (gender).
   5. Block 4—Insured's name: Enter *Same* if patient and policyholder are the same; otherwise, enter

the insured's last, first, and middle initial. Enter sponsor's name for Tricare/CHAMPVA.

6. Block 5—Patient's address/telephone: Self-explanatory.
7. Block 6—Patient relationship to insured: Check the appropriate box.
8. Block 7—Insured's address/telephone: If the same as the patient enter *Same;* otherwise, enter the insured's address. Enter the active duty sponsor's military base address.
9. Block 8—Patient status: Check the appropriate box.
10. Blocks 9a to 9d—Other insured's information: Enter other policy information supplementing the primary policy.
11. Block 10a—Patient's condition related to employment: If *Yes,* complete a Workers' Compensation claim.
12. Block 10b—Auto accident: If an auto accident, include the two-letter state abbreviation.
13. Block 10c—Other accident: Self-explanatory.
14. Block 10d—Reserved for local use: Enter the word *Attachment* if any supporting documents will be included with the claim.
15. Blocks 11 to 11d—Insured's information: Reserved for a second primary policy.
16. Block 12—Patient's or authorized person's signature authorizing release of medical information, or enter SIGNATURE ON FILE.
17. Block 13—Patient's or authorized person's signature authorizing assignment of benefits, or enter SIGNATURE ON FILE.
18. Block 14—Date of first illness/injury/pregnancy: Enter the date according to the patient's medical chart.
19. Block 15—If patient has had same or similar illness, give first date: Self-explanatory.
20. Block 16—Dates patient unable to work in current occupation: Enter dates for Workers' Compensation; otherwise, leave blank.
21. Block 17—Name of referring physician or other source: Enter the name of the referring provider or primary surgeon on claims for assistant surgeon services.
22. Block 17a—I.D. number of referring physician: Medicare requires the provider's UPIN (Unique Provider's Identification Number); commercial carriers may require the provider's tax I.D. number, or PAR's PIN; otherwise, leave blank.
23. Block 18—Hospitalization dates related to current services: Enter admission and discharge dates for any inpatient services included on the CMS-1500.
24. Block 19—Reserved for local use: Some carriers may have specific instruction regarding the use of this block.

25. Block 20—Outside laboratory: Check *No* if all laboratory work was done in the provider's office; check *Yes* if an outside laboratory performed the tests and billed the provider.
26. Block 21—Diagnosis or nature of illness or injury: Enter up to four ICD-9-CM codes without decimal points.
27. Block 22—Medicaid resubmission code: Generally left blank.
28. Block 23—Prior authorization number: Enter the number assigned for preauthorizations given for any procedures listed.
29. Block 24A—Dates of service: For single procedures, enter the date it was performed in the *From* column. If a procedure was performed on consecutive days, also enter the last day it was performed in the *To* column. Use eight-digit date, e.g., 08012004.
30. Block 24B—Place of service: Enter the code number from the standard list provided by the particular carrier.
31. Block 24C—Type of service: Enter the code number from the standard list if necessary.
32. Block 24D—Procedures, services, or supplies: Enter the appropriate CPT or HCPCS code before the solid line; enter the first of up to three modifiers between the solid and broken line and no more than two other modifiers two spaces apart after the broken line.
33. Block 24E—Diagnosis code: Enter the reference number identifying the diagnosis in block 21 that is most closely associated with the procedure listed.
34. Block 24F—Charges: Enter the fee charged for the listed procedure.
35. Block 24G—Days or units: Enter the number of times or the number of days over which the procedure was performed.
36. Block 24H—EPSDT Family Plan: For Medicaid claims, enter an E if the service is part of the Early and Periodic Screening, Diagnosis and Treatment program; enter an F for family planning services or B for both.
37. Block 24I—EMG: Check this box if the services were provided in a hospital emergency department.
38. Block 24J—COB: Coordination of benefits. Check this box if the patient is covered by one or more primary policies. (Enter the data required for all of block 11.)
39. Block 24K—Reserved for local use: For Medicare, enter the provider's PIN (Provider Information Number) if it is different from the group practice PIN entered in block 33.
40. Block 25—Federal Tax I.D. number: Enter the provider's EIN (Employer's Tax Identification Number).

1500

HEALTH INSURANCE CLAIM FORM

APPROVED BY NATIONAL UNIFORM CLAIM COMMITTEE 08/05

| | PICA | | | | | | | | PICA | |

1. MEDICARE ☐ (Medicare #) MEDICAID ☐ (Medicaid #) TRICARE CHAMPUS ☐ (Sponsor's SSN) CHAMPVA ☐ (Member ID#) GROUP HEALTH PLAN ☐ (SSN or ID) FECA BLK LUNG ☐ (SSN) OTHER ☒ (ID)

1a. INSURED'S I.D. NUMBER (For Program in Item 1)
555-55-555

2. PATIENT'S NAME (Last Name, First Name, Middle Initial)
MCKAY, LEO M

3. PATIENT'S BIRTH DATE MM 04 DD 01 YY 1963 SEX M ☒ F ☐

4. INSURED'S NAME (Last Name, First Name, Middle Initial)
MCKAY, LEO M.

5. PATIENT'S ADDRESS (No., Street)
123 W FIRST STREET

6. PATIENT RELATIONSHIP TO INSURED
Self ☒ Spouse ☐ Child ☐ Other ☐

7. INSURED'S ADDRESS (No., Street)
123 W FIRST STREET

CITY ANYWHERE STATE PA

8. PATIENT STATUS
Single ☒ Married ☐ Other ☐
Employed ☐ Full-Time Student ☐ Part-Time Student ☐

CITY ANYWHERE STATE PA

ZIP CODE 11666 TELEPHONE (Include Area Code) (824) 556-6189

ZIP CODE 11666 TELEPHONE (Include Area Code) (824) 556-6789

9. OTHER INSURED'S NAME (Last Name, First Name, Middle Initial)

10. IS PATIENT'S CONDITION RELATED TO:

11. INSURED'S POLICY GROUP OR FECA NUMBER
1122334

a. OTHER INSURED'S POLICY OR GROUP NUMBER

a. EMPLOYMENT? (Current or Previous) YES ☐ NO ☒

a. INSURED'S DATE OF BIRTH MM 04 DD 01 YY 1963 SEX M ☒ F ☐

b. OTHER INSURED'S DATE OF BIRTH MM DD YY SEX M ☐ F ☐

b. AUTO ACCIDENT? YES ☐ NO ☒ PLACE (State)

b. EMPLOYER'S NAME OR SCHOOL NAME
ABC MANUFACTURING COMPANY

c. EMPLOYER'S NAME OR SCHOOL NAME

c. OTHER ACCIDENT? YES ☐ NO ☒

c. INSURANCE PLAN NAME OR PROGRAM NAME
HOW MUCH INSURANCE COMPANY

d. INSURANCE PLAN NAME OR PROGRAM NAME

10d. RESERVED FOR LOCAL USE

d. IS THERE ANOTHER HEALTH BENEFIT PLAN? YES ☐ NO ☒ *If yes*, return to and complete item 9 a-d.

READ BACK OF FORM BEFORE COMPLETING & SIGNING THIS FORM.

12. PATIENT'S OR AUTHORIZED PERSON'S SIGNATURE I authorize the release of any medical or other information necessary to process this claim. I also request payment of government benefits either to myself or to the party who accepts assignment below.

SIGNED Signature on File DATE 01/14/XXXX

13. INSURED'S OR AUTHORIZED PERSON'S SIGNATURE I authorize payment of medical benefits to the undersigned physician or supplier for services described below.

SIGNED Signature on File

14. DATE OF CURRENT: MM 01 DD 10 YY XXXX ILLNESS (First symptom) OR INJURY (Accident) OR PREGNANCY(LMP)

15. IF PATIENT HAS HAD SAME OR SIMILAR ILLNESS. GIVE FIRST DATE MM DD YY

16. DATES PATIENT UNABLE TO WORK IN CURRENT OCCUPATION FROM MM DD YY TO MM DD YY

17. NAME OF REFERRING PROVIDER OR OTHER SOURCE
17a.
17b. NPI

18. HOSPITALIZATION DATES RELATED TO CURRENT SERVICES FROM MM DD YY TO MM DD YY

19. RESERVED FOR LOCAL USE

20. OUTSIDE LAB? YES ☐ NO ☐ $ CHARGES

21. DIAGNOSIS OR NATURE OF ILLNESS OR INJURY (Relate Items 1, 2, 3 or 4 to Item 24E by Line)
1. 789 . 0
2. 558 . 9
3. 783 . 0
4.

22. MEDICAID RESUBMISSION CODE ORIGINAL REF. NO.

23. PRIOR AUTHORIZATION NUMBER

24. A. DATE(S) OF SERVICE From MM DD YY	To MM DD YY	B. PLACE OF SERVICE	C. EMG	D. PROCEDURES, SERVICES, OR SUPPLIES (Explain Unusual Circumstances) CPT/HCPCS	MODIFIER	E. DIAGNOSIS POINTER	F. $ CHARGES	G. DAYS OR UNITS	H. EPSDT Family Plan	I. ID. QUAL.	J. RENDERING PROVIDER ID. #
1	01 10 XXXX		3		99214		1,2,3	85 00	1		NPI	1543298760
2	01 10 XXXX		3		82270		1,2	13 00	1		NPI	1543298760
3											NPI	
4											NPI	
5											NPI	
6											NPI	

25. FEDERAL TAX I.D. NUMBER SSN ☐ EIN ☒
91-1234432

26. PATIENT'S ACCOUNT NO.
MCK111

27. ACCEPT ASSIGNMENT? (For govt. claims, see back) YES ☐ NO ☒

28. TOTAL CHARGE $ 98 00

29. AMOUNT PAID $

30. BALANCE DUE $ 98 00

31. SIGNATURE OF PHYSICIAN OR SUPPLIER INCLUDING DEGREES OR CREDENTIALS (I certify that the statements on the reverse apply to this bill and are made a part thereof.)
Mark Wos MD
SIGNED DATE 01/14/XXX

32. SERVICE FACILITY LOCATION INFORMATION
a. NPI b.

33. BILLING PROVIDER INFO & PH # (814) 555-1155
INNER CITY HEALTH CARE
222 S FIRST AVE
CANTON PA 11666
a. R09876543 b.

NUCC Instruction Manual available at: www.nucc.org

APPROVED OMB-0938-0999 FORM CMS-1500 (08/05)

Figure 13-5

Completed CMS-1500 claim. Courtesy of the Centers for Medicare and Medicaid Services.

41. Block 26—Patient's account number: Optional; enter the patient's account number as desired.
42. Block 27—Accept assignment: Check *Yes* or *No* as appropriate. For Medicaid and Workers' Compensation, you must check *Yes.*
43. Block 28—Total charge: Enter the sum of all the charges on this claim.
44. Block 29—Amount paid: If appropriate, enter the amount collected as applied toward the deductible, or copayments for services listed on the claim.
45. Block 30—Balance due: Enter the difference of blocks 28 and 29.
46. Block 31—Signature of physician or supplier including degrees or credentials: Have the provider sign.
47. Block 32—Name and address of facility where services were rendered: Enter this information when the services were provided at a site other than the provider's office or patient's home. A *Yes* in block 20 requires the same information regarding the outside laboratory.
48. Block 33—Physician's supplier's billing name, address, zip code, phone number, and PIN#/GRP#: Enter the appropriate information. Enter the phone number after the phrase *and PHONE #.*

B. Insurance claim development
   1. Preregister the patient who calls for an appointment—obtain the following information:
      a. Patient's full name.
      b. Address and phone number.
      c. Employer, address, and phone number.
      d. Date of birth.
      e. Guarantor: Person responsible for covering charges.
      f. Social Security number.
      g. Spouse name, occupation, and employer.
      h. Referring provider's name.
      i. Emergency contact.
      j. Health insurance information.
   2. Upon arrival, have the patient complete a patient registration form.
   3. Photocopy the patient's insurance card and file in the financial record.
   4. Confirm the patient's insurance information and coverage.
   5. Enter all information into the computer management system.
   6. Have the patient sign a consent to payment form.
   7. Create a new patient's medical record.
   8. Generate the patient's encounter form (superbill).
   9. After care, assign diagnosis and procedure codes.
   10. Enter and total charges on the encounter form.
   11. Post the charges to the patient's ledger account.
   12. Collect payment from the patient as warranted.
   13. Post payment to the patient's account.
   14. Complete the insurance claim form.
   15. Log and file a copy of the claim form and any attachments.
   16. Submit claim to the carrier.

C. Carrier claim processing
   1. Patient and policy identification is confirmed.
   2. Procedure codes are matched with the policy's benefit list.
   3. Procedure codes are matched against the diagnosis code.
   4. The claim is checked against data from the patient's past claims.
   5. Determination is made concerning "allowed charges."
   6. Determination of patient's annual deductible.
   7. Determination of copayment or coinsurance requirements.
   8. Explanation of benefits and transmittal notice forms are generated.
   9. EOB, transmittal notice, and benefit check (if payment approved) are sent.

D. General guidelines
   1. Ensure that appropriate information release forms are current before submitting a claim.
   2. Inpatient medical services are itemized and charged separately.
   3. Global surgical charges will include preoperative and postoperative care; however, additional surgical services resulting from postoperative complications may be charged separately.
   4. CPT surgical codes followed by an * are charged on a fee-for-service basis.
   5. Claims that require additional documentation describing unusual circumstances or justifying the care rendered should include the patient and policy identification information on an attachment submitted with the claim.
   6. CMS-1500 is designed for optical character readers (OCR) for electronic processing. Submit claims that have attachments by mail, not electronically.
      a. Type out the information using only capital letters and pica pitch (10 characters per inch).
      b. Do not use periods, hyphens, commas, dollar signs, or slashes.
      c. Use two zeros (00) in the cents column to represent whole dollar amounts.
      d. Dates should be typed in eight digits; e.g., April 4, 1996 is typed 04/04/1996.
      e. Checked boxes should have an "x" within the box.

BWC
Better Workers' Compensation
Built with *you* in mind.

First Report of an Injury, Occupational Disease or Death

WARNING:
Any person who obtains compensation from BWC or self-insuring employers by: knowingly misrepresenting or concealing facts, making false statements, or accepting compensation to which he/she is not entitled, is subject to felony criminal prosecution for fraud.

(R.C. 2913.48)

Injured Worker and Injury/Disease/Death Info.

Last name, first name, middle initial		Social Security number	Marital status ☐ Single ☐ Married ☐ Divorced ☐ Separated ☐ Widowed	Date of birth
Home mailing address		Sex ☐ Male ☐ Female		Number of dependents
City	State	9-digit ZIP code	Country if different from USA	Department name

Wage rate $ _____ Per: ☐ Hour ☐ Month ☐ Week ☐ Year ☐ Other

What days of the week do you usually work? ☐ Sun ☐ Mon ☐ Tues ☐ Wed ☐ Thur ☐ Fri ☐ Sat

Regular work hours From _____ To _____

Have you been offered or do you expect to receive payment or wages for this claim from anyone other than the Ohio Bureau of Workers' Compensation? ☐ YES ☐ NO If yes, please explain.

Occupation or job title

Employer name

Mailing address (number and street, city or town, state, ZIP code and county)

Location, if different from mailing address

Was place of accident or exposure on employer's premises? ☐ YES ☐ NO
If no, give accident location, street address, city, state and ZIP code)

Date of injury/disease	Time of injury _____ ☐ AM ☐ PM	If fatal, give date of death	Time employee began work _____ ☐ AM ☐ PM	Date last worked	Date returned to work
Date hired		State where hired		Date employer notified	

Description of accident (Describe the sequence of events that directly injured the employee, or caused the disease or death

Type of injury/disease and part(s) of body affected (For example: sprain of lower left back, etc.)

Benefit Application/Medical Release – I am applying for recognition of my claim under the Ohio Workers' Compensation Act for work-related injuries that I did not purposely inflict. I request payment for compensation and/or medical expenses as allowable. Direct payment(s) to the providers of any medical services are authorized. I understand that I am allowing any provider who attends to, treats or examines me to release all medical, psychological, and/or psychiatric information that is related causally or historically to physical or mental injuries relevant to issues necessary to the administration of my workers' compensation claim to the Ohio Bureau of Workers' Compensation, the Industrial Commission of Ohio, the employer listed in this claim, that employer's managed care organization, and any authorized representatives. I further authorize the Ohio Rehabilitation Services Commission to release information about my physical, mental, vocational and social conditions that is related causally and historically to physical or mental injuries relevant to issues necessary for the administration of my workers' compensation claim to the aforementioned parties.

Injured worker signature	Date	Telephone number ( )	Work number ( )

Treatment Info.

Health care provider name	Telephone number ( )	Fax number ( )	Initial treatment date
Street address	City	State	9-digit ZIP code

Diagnosis(es): Include ICD code(s)

Will the incident cause the injured worker to miss eight or more days of work? ☐ YES ☐ NO

Is the injury causally related to the industrial incident? ☐ YES ☐ NO

Health care provider signature	11-digit BWC provider number	Date

Employer Info.

Employer policy number

CHECK IF ☐ Employer is self-insuring
☐ Injured worker is Owner/Partner/Member of Firm

Telephone number ( )	Fax number ( )	E-mail address	Federal ID number	Manual number

Was employee treated in an emergency room? ☐ YES ☐ NO

Was employee hospitalized overnight as an in-patient? ☐ YES ☐ NO

If treatment was given away from worksite, provide the facility name, street address, city, state, ZIP code

☐ **CERTIFICATION** - The employer **certifies** that the facts in this application are correct and valid.	☐ **REJECTION** - The employer **rejects** the validity of this claim for the following reason(s) below:	**FOR SELF-INSURING EMPLOYERS ONLY** ☐ **CLARIFICATION** - The employer **clarifies and allows** the claim for the condition(s) below:

Employer signature and title	Date	OSHA case number

BWC-1101 (Rev. 7/23/2002)
FROI-1 (Combines C-1, C-2, C-3, C-6, C-50, OD-1, OD-1-22)

This form meets **OSHA 301** requirements

Figure 13-6

First report form for Workers' Compensation for payment of medical fee only. Courtesy of Ohio Bureau of Workers' Compensation.

f. Corrections should be made with permanent correction methods, not removable methods.

g. List only one procedure per line.

h. Photocopies cannot be optically read.

7. The federal Consolidated Omnibus Budget Reconciliation Act of 1987 (COBRA) requires that providers maintain government claim forms and attachments for at least 5 years.

8. Insurance log: Maintain a log for recording the status of each claim form completed and submitted identifying the patient's name, diagnosis, insurance carrier, and date of submission.

E. Carrier guidelines

1. Medicare
   a. CMS requires all providers to report the primary carrier (blocks 4, 7, 11 to 11C) when Medicare secondary payers (MSP) claims are filed and Medicare/Medicaid crossover coverage (MCD) on the claim form.
      (1) Medicaid should always be treated as the payer of last resort.
      (2) Medicare will usually be treated as the next to the last payer.
   b. The filing deadline is December 31 of the year following the date of service.

2. Medicaid
   a. As filing deadlines vary across the nation, it is important to file the claim as soon as possible.
   b. Providers treating Medicaid patients must accept assignment and accept reimbursement as payment in full.
   c. Patients cannot be billed for qualified services regardless of the reimbursed amount, even for those patients who fail to reveal their Medicaid eligibility at time of service.
   d. Services not covered by Medicaid can be billed directly to the patient.
   e. Maintain a current photocopy of the patient's identification card.

3. Tricare/CHAMPVA
   a. DD Form 1251-Nonavailability Statement must be obtained as authorization for medical services in civilian community.
   b. Filing deadline is September 30 of the year following the date of service.
   c. Inpatient mental health care requires a Treatment Report every 30 days.
   d. Mental health care requires a Treatment Report for more than 23 outpatient visits per calendar year.
   e. DD Form 2517 Statement of Personal Injury-Possible Third-Party Liability must be attached to claims for covered treatments of injury having ICD-9-CM codes 800 to 959.
   f. The deductible period runs from October 1 to September 30.

g. Request a DEERS (Defense Enrollment Eligibility Reporting System) check to verify Tricare eligibility.

h. Maintain a current photocopy of the patient's identification card.

4. Workers' compensation
   a. First report of injury: Form should be completed in quadruplicate at the first visit and distributed to the following parties (see Figure 13-6):
      (1) State Workers' Compensation Commission/Board.
      (2) Employer-designated compensation carrier.
      (3) Employer.
      (4) Patient's chart.
   b. Filing deadlines vary by state, ranging from 24 hours to 10 days.
   c. Progress reports: A narrative progress report should be filed indicating any significant change in the patient's status and upon discharge.
   d. If an established patient seeks treatment for a work-related condition, a separate chart and ledger card must be established.
   e. Providers treating workers' compensation patients must accept assignment and accept reimbursement as payment in full.

5. Blue Cross/Blue Shield
   a. PAR: Participating provider. A provider who contracts with BC/BS to accept approved reimbursements as payment in full and not bill the subscriber for the difference between the service charge and the allowed fee.
   b. Claims must be filed within 12 to 15 months from date of service depending on the particular plan and state.
   c. Rebill claims not paid within 40 days.
   d. Maintain a current photocopy of the patient's identification card.

F. Causes for delayed and rejected claims

1. Typographical errors.
2. Coding errors.
3. Diagnosis does not support medical necessity of the treatment rendered.
4. Incorrect identification and policy numbers.
5. Names not matching with those shown on policy.
6. Incorrectly calculated fee total.
7. Missing data.
8. Dates of treatment not corresponding with dates shown on support documents or attachments.
9. Missing or inadequate attachments.
10. Staples or defacement of bar code area of the form.
11. Submission of claims to the wrong carrier.
12. The patient is not eligible for benefits.

CHAPTER 14

Facilities Management

I. OFFICE ARRANGEMENT

A. Locate desks so that people who use them will have enough light but no glare.

B. There should be as much air as possible at a desk without locating anyone in a draft.

C. Place equipment where it can be easily used and where work will flow in one direction—not criss-crossing the room.

D. Arrange tables or counters to handle supplies or to assemble papers.

E. Place files where they can be easily accessed but out of the flow of general office traffic.

F. Use bookcases and special shelves for books, magazines, and pamphlets to keep these items from using up workspace on desks and tables.

G. While striving for orderliness and good appearance, the best arrangement is the one that gets the work done.

H. The appearance of an office is improved by simple practices, such as the following:

1. Putting things away from day to day.
2. Clearing correspondence baskets daily to avoid the accumulation or misplacement of documents.
3. Properly storing supplies that may stain documents or deteriorate rapidly.
4. Not storing cleaning or hazardous materials in desks.
5. Removing equipment from desks that might be damaged when the office is cleaned.
6. Avoiding accumulations of loose paper or trash in the office. They may create a fire hazard.
7. When securing equipment or supplies that others have been using, exercising good judgment to avoid loss or misplacement of material. What may look like complete confusion to one person may have complete order and meaning to another.

II. CAPITAL RESOURCE MANAGEMENT

A. Facilities management
1. A clean, comfortable, and tastefully decorated office reflects an effective and efficient clinic.

2. Climate control: Temperature range of 68° to 74°F is most comfortable with proper ventilation.
3. Lighting: Fluorescent lights are ideal because they provide uniform light and little to no heat.
4. Floor covering: Wall-to-wall carpeting is well-suited for all areas except where spills are likely to occur such as in the laboratory and treatment rooms, where vinyl or tile is best. For safety reasons there should be no loose rugs or mats.
5. Wall covering: Soft-color or pastel paints or wallpaper minimizes eyestrain.
6. Traffic control: Patients and staff should be able to move easily about without crowding or causing bottlenecks.
7. Storage: Adequate space with locks must be available to maintain supplies and equipment in a neat and orderly fashion.
8. Sound control: Rooms should be constructed and arranged to minimize echoing and sounds emanating from them.
9. Patient rooms: Should be arranged so that the patient cannot be seen when the door is opened.
10. Reception space: Discussed in Chapter 11, Reception.
11. Administrative space: Should be separate from areas frequented by patients. Locks should be installed as appropriate.
12. Clinical space: Should be checked between each patient and kept clean, neatly organized, and well-stocked.
13. Laboratory space: Should be well-ventilated to prevent the accumulation of fumes, and contaminated items should be well-controlled.
14. Lavatories: Ideally separate facilities should be available for staff and patients.
15. Maintenance and janitorial services
    a. Each person should keep their respective work areas neat, clean, and in good repair.
    b. Agree on a list of services and schedule that will be provided by the housekeeping service.
    c. Identify any and all areas that are not to be accessed.

d. Be mindful of the service's performance and immediately notify the service of any problems noted.

16. Safety
   a. The clinic environment should be continuously monitored for potential safety hazards.
   b. Fire extinguishers/smoke alarms: Should be strategically placed for optimum effectiveness as well as quick and easy access; they should be periodically checked to ensure proper functioning.
   c. Fire exits: Should be clearly marked; staff should be aware of evacuation procedures.

17. Security
   a. The phone number of security personnel or services should be readily available.
   b. Burglar proof the clinic by installing locks and properly securing rooms and areas from unauthorized access.
   c. Secure all valuable and personal belongings to prevent pilferage.
   d. Install alarms as appropriate; display a security system sign as a deterrent to would-be thieves.

18. Waste disposal: Regular waste, biohazard waste, and sharps waste should be disposed of separately.

B. Office equipment
   1. Warranty: Most equipment will come with a limited warranty; keep this information filed away for future need.
   2. Service agreements: May be included with a purchase or paid for separately; maintain a file for reference as needed.
   3. Inventory
      a. An inventory of all capital items, such as equipment, should be prepared every year or two.
      b. An inventory will be needed to prepare the fixed assets portion of the balance sheet.
      c. For each item, include its name, serial number, date of purchase or lease, and price. This information should be kept on file.
      d. Include all clinical, laboratory, and office equipment, furniture, instruments, artwork, and anything of value not normally consumed.
   4. Capital purchases versus leases
      a. Purchased equipment usually includes a limited warranty covering the costs associated with defects in materials or craftsmanship for a limited period of time after purchase.
      b. An extended warranty may be purchased with the equipment that covers specified repairs for a longer period of time after purchase.
      c. Maintain a file for each piece of equipment which includes:
         (1) Sales receipt.
         (2) Operating manual.
         (3) Warranty information.
         (4) Service contracts.
         (5) Repair and maintenance invoices.
      d. For a fixed fee, a service contract may be purchased to cover both maintenance and repair costs over a period of time, usually 1 to 5 years.
      e. Rather than purchasing equipment, it can be leased (rented) for a period of time. Usually during this time a service contract is in force to effect maintenance and repairs. Leasing may be more financially feasible than outright purchase.
      f. At the end of the lease period, the equipment may be discounted for purchase at its fair market or scrap value, or a current model may be leased.

   5. Ten key machine: An office calculator that can print data on a paper tape.
      a. The keys are arranged in a three-by-three keypad with the top row consisting of 7, 8, 9; the middle row or home-row keys consisting of 4, 5, 6; and the bottom row consisting of 1, 2, and 3.
      b. The middle three fingers are lightly placed on the home-row keys.
         (1) The index finger is placed over the 4 key, middle finger over the 5 key, and the ring finger over the 6 key.
         (2) The 5 key typically has a small bump to help locate the home-row.
      c. Each finger operates the key directly above and below the home-row key it rests on.
         (1) Index finger controls 7, 4, and 1.
         (2) Middle finger controls 8, 5, and 2.
         (3) Ring finger controls 9, 6, and 3.
         (4) Thumb controls 0.

   6. Photocopier: A machine that photographically reproduces multiple copies of original documents.
      a. Most photocopiers have a variety of adjustments to include:
         (1) Number of copies selector.
         (2) Paper size selector: Commonly 8½- by 11-inch and 11- by 14-inch.
         (3) Feeder control that can copy a stack of documents automatically.
         (4) Collating by copying a stack of documents in the proper sequence.
         (5) Sorting by making multiple copies of a stack of documents.
         (6) Making the copy darker or lighter than the original.

(7) Stapling.

(8) Reduction/enlargement of the original.

b. Operating guidelines

   (1) Review the operating manual before usage.

   (2) Allow the machine to warm up when first turned on.

   (3) Keep the machine in a well-ventilated area to avoid overheating.

   (4) Close the lid before making copies to avoid wasting toner.

   (5) Do not place documents containing paper clips or staples on the glass platen as they may scratch the glass.

7. Facsimile (fax): An electronic machine that permits the transmission of documents via telephone line.

a. Review the operating manual before usage.

b. Prepare a transmittal sheet with each fax, which includes:

   (1) Name, address, phone/fax number of sender.

   (2) Name and title of recipient.

   (3) Date, total number of pages.

   (4) Room for messages.

c. Be cautious of confidentiality when transmitting medical information.

C. Supplies

1. Includes all consumable items (anything that is consumed or used up) needed by the practice to operate such as office, housekeeping, and medical supplies.

2. Supplies are generally ordered on an ongoing basis to replace the quantity that is consumed.

3. It is probably best to designate one person to inventory, maintain, and order supplies.

4. Doing business with a particular vendor on price alone is usually not prudent, as service may not be adequate. Developing a sound business relationship with a vendor that meets your needs will usually save time and money.

5. Factors to consider for supply inventory and requisition:

a. Lead-time usage: Considering the amount of time needed for delivery, the amount of stock used during the delivery period. For example, if it takes about 5 days from requisition to receive an order, and approximately five items are used a day, the lead-time usage will be 25 items (5 days $\times$ 5 items/day).

b. Stock-outs: Running out of supplies.

c. Safety stock: The amount of buffer stock that for the vast majority of times will prevent stock-outs resulting from delivery delays, back orders, etc. This is usually determined through trial and error; e.g., 18 items.

d. Order point: Usually lead-time usage quantity plus safety stock quantity. For example, when 43 items (25 + 18) remain in inventory a supply order should be made. The 25 items will cover the delivery period and the other 18 will cover unplanned delays.

6. Receipt and storage

a. Supplies should be delivered to the same holding location that is out of the way of patient care activities.

b. The contents of the package should be checked against the purchase order and invoice. Note discrepancies and back orders.

c. Store the materials in a neat and orderly fashion out of reach of unauthorized persons.

III. ACCESSIBILITY

A. General

1. Americans with Disabilities Act (ADA): Federal civil rights law that prohibits the exclusion of people with disabilities from engaging in everyday activities in the community as well as conducting commerce.

2. The Department of Justice operates a toll-free ADA Information Line (800-514-0301 voice and 800-514-0383 TDD).

3. In addition, tax credits and deductions were established that can be used annually to offset many costs of providing access to people with disabilities.

4. Public accommodations: Private businesses that provide goods or services to the public.

5. If one owns, operates, leases, or leases to a business that serves the public, then the person is subject to ADA regulations, including existing facilities as well as for compliance when a facility is altered or a new facility is constructed.

6. The ADA requires that accessibility be improved without taking on excessive expenses that could harm a business.

7. A business that serves the public must remove physical "barriers" that are "readily achievable," which means *easily accomplishable without undue difficulty or expense.*

a. The requirement is based on the size and resources of the business.

b. Larger businesses with more resources are expected to take a more active role in removing barriers than are small businesses.

c. Because economic conditions vary, when a business has resources to remove barriers, it is expected to do so; but when profits are down, barrier removal may be reduced or delayed.

B. Architectural Barriers
  1. Physical features that limit or prevent people with disabilities from obtaining the goods or services offered, such as:
     a. Parking spaces that are too narrow to accommodate people who use wheelchairs.
     b. A step or steps at the entrance.
     c. Round doorknobs or door hardware that is difficult to grasp.
     d. Aisles that are too narrow for a person using a wheelchair.
  2. When a business removes barriers, it should follow the design requirements for new construction in the ADA Standards for Accessible Design.
  3. Priorities for barrier removal include the following:
     a. First, provide access to the business from public sidewalks, parking, and public transportation.
     b. Then provide access to the areas where goods and services are made available to the public.
     c. Once these barriers are removed, provide access to public toilet rooms.
     d. When these barriers have been removed, it may be necessary to remove any remaining barriers including those that limit use of public telephones and drinking fountains.
C. Accessible parking
  1. When parking is provided for the public, designated accessible parking spaces must be provided, if doing so is readily achievable.
  2. Space must be provided for the vehicle and an additional space located either to the right or to the left of the space that serves as an access aisle.
  3. A sign with the international symbol of accessibility must be located in front of the parking space and mounted high enough so it is not hidden by a vehicle parked in the space.
  4. The designated spaces should be the spaces closest to the accessible entrance and be located on level ground.
  5. An accessible route must be provided between the access aisle and the accessible building entrance. This route must have no steps or steeply sloped surfaces, and must have a firm, stable, slip-resistant surface.
  6. Van-accessible spaces must have an access aisle that is at least 8 feet wide. There should be a vertical clearance of at least 98 inches on the vehicular route to the space, at the parking space, and along the vehicular route to an exit.
  7. Accessible parking spaces for cars must have an access aisle that is at least 5 feet wide.

  8. The number of accessible parking spaces that should be provided is based on the total number of parking spaces provided or according to the type of business.
  9. In general the following conditions must be met:
     a. In a parking lot with 25 or fewer spaces, 1 space should be an accessible parking space.
     b. If it has 50 or fewer spaces, it should have 2 accessible parking spaces.
     c. If only 1 accessible parking space is provided, it also must be a van accessible space.
     d. When more than 1 accessible parking space is required, 1 of 8 accessible parking spaces must be van accessible.
     e. Where parking is provided in several locations near building entrances, the accessible parking should also be dispersed, if doing so is readily achievable.
  10. Outpatient facilities: 10% of the parking spaces must be accessible.
  11. Facilities that specialize in servicing persons with mobility impairments: 20% must be accessible.
D. Accessible Entrance
  1. Providing physical access to a facility from public sidewalks, public transportation, or parking is basic to making goods and services available to people with disabilities.
  2. Where one or two steps exist at an entrance, access can be achieved by:
     a. Using an alternative accessible entrance.
     b. Adding a short ramp.
     c. Modifying the area in front or to the side of the entrance to eliminate a step or installing a lift.
  3. When a business has two public entrances, in most cases, only one must be accessible.
  4. In such cases, a sign must provide direction to the accessible entrance.
  5. The alternative entrance must be open during hours of operation.
  6. When a ramp is added to provide an accessible entrance, the slope of the ramp should be as shallow as possible but not more than 1:12. It is also important to provide handrails whenever the slope is more than 1:20 and the vertical rise is greater than 6 inches (a slope of 1:20 means that for every 20 units of horizontal length there is 1 unit of vertical rise or fall).
E. Doors
  1. Doors must be wide enough to be accessible, usually at least 36 inches.
  2. Disabilities that limit grasping make some door hardware inaccessible. In such cases, they must be made accessible.

a. Panel-type handles can be replaced with loop-type handles.

b. A round door knob can be replaced with a lever handle or clamp-on lever.

c. A thumb latch can be disabled so the door can be pulled open without depressing the latch.

F. Service counters

1. Counters must be accessible, if making them so is readily achievable.

2. A counter that is at least 36 inches long and that is not more than 36 inches above the floor will be accessible.

3. It is also possible to provide an auxiliary counter nearby or to use a folding shelf or area next to the counter, if doing so is readily achievable.

4. A clear floor space must be present in front of the accessible surface that permits a customer using a wheelchair to pull alongside.

   a. This space is at least 30 inches by 48 inches and may be parallel or perpendicular to the counter.

   b. It is also connected to the accessible route that connects to the accessible entrance.

   c. A clipboard or lapboard may be provided for use until a more permanent solution can be implemented.

G. Policies and procedures: Businesses must review their policies and procedures for serving customers and change those that exclude or limit participation by people with disabilities.

H. Communicating with customers

1. When communication by speech is not possible, simple questions may be handled with pen and paper, by exchanging written notes or a mixture of speech and written notes.

2. When more complex or lengthy communications are needed, it may be necessary to provide a sign language interpreter.

3. Many people with hearing or speech disabilities use a telecommunications device for the deaf (TDD) instead of a standard telephone.

4. The ADA established a free state-by-state relay network nationwide that handles voice-to-TDD and TDD-to-voice calls.

IV. OFFICE SAFETY

A. OSHA standards

1. Hazard communication standard (employee right-to-know standard [ERTK])

   a. Employers must evaluate their workplace for the existence of any hazardous agents and provide training and information to employees who are routinely exposed to such agents.

      (1) Hazardous substances: Chemicals and gases.

      (2) Harmful physical agents: Noise, heat, and radiation.

      (3) Infectious agents: Bacterial, viral, fungal, parasitic, and rickettsial agents.

   b. Written ERTK program: Must include the following provisions.

      (1) Training outline provided to all affected employees.

      (2) A list of known hazardous agents and corresponding MSDS forms accessible to the employee.

      (3) A labeling and warning system used in the workplace.

      (4) Method of informing employees of the above.

   c. Material safety data sheet (MSDS) (see Figure 14-1)

      (1) Form prepared by the manufacturer that describes a substance's physical and chemical properties, health hazards, precautions, and first aid measures.

      (2) An MSDS must be kept for each hazardous substance and easily accessible to employees.

   d. Labeling: All hazardous agents must be properly labeled with the following information:

      (1) Name of the hazardous substance.

      (2) Specific hazard warnings.

      (3) Name and address of manufacturer.

2. Bloodborne pathogen standard

   a. OSHA Section 1910.1030 requires employers to take steps to ensure employee safety and to provide annual training regarding occupational exposure to bloodborne pathogens.

   b. Bloodborne pathogens: Disease-causing microorganisms that may be present in blood or body fluids; principally, hepatitis B virus (HBV) and human immunodeficiency virus (HIV).

   c. Transmission

      (1) Bloodborne pathogens are transmitted when blood or other potentially infectious material (OPIM) come in contact with mucous membranes, nonintact skin, or by touching or handling contaminated items or surfaces.

      (2) Most HIV transmissions have occurred through puncture injuries.

      (3) HBV is more persistent than HIV and is able to survive for at least a week in dried blood.

   d. Prevention: There are four strategies for prevention.

      (1) Engineering controls: Structural or mechanical devices that are designed to minimize exposure to bloodborne

MATERIAL SAFETY DATA SHEET

I – PRODUCT IDENTIFICATION

COMPANY NAME: We Wash Inc.

ADDRESS: 5035 Manchester Avenue
         Freedom, Texas 79430

Tel No:	(314) 621-1818
Nights:	(314) 621-1399
CHEMTREC:	(800) 424-9343

PRODUCT NAME: Spotfree

Product No.: 2190

Synonyms: Warewashing Detergent

II – HAZARDOUS INGREDIENTS OF MIXTURES

MATERIAL:	(CAS#)	% By Wt.	TLV	PEL
According to the OSHA Hazard Communication Standard, 29CFR 1910.1200, this product contains no hazardous ingredients.		N/A	N/A	NA

III – PHYSICAL DATA

Vapor Pressure, mm Hg: N/A
Evaporation Rate (ether=1): N/A
Solubility in H2O: Complete
Freezing Point F: N/A
Boiling Point F: N/A
Specific Gravity H2O=1 @25C: N/A

Vapor Density (Air=1) 60–90F: N/A
% Volatile by wt N/A
pH @ 1%   Solution 9.3–9.8
pH as Distributed: N/A
Appearance: Off-White granular powder
Odor: Mild Chemical Odor

IV – FIRE AND EXPLOSION

Flash Point F: N/AV

Flammable Limits: N/A

Extinguishing Media: The product is not flammable or combustible. Use media appropriate for the primary source of fire.

Special Fire Fighting Procedures: Use caution when fighting any fire involving chemicals. A self-contained breathing apparatus is essential.

Unusual Fire and Explosion Hazards: None Known

V – REACTIVITY DATA

Stability - Conditions to avoid: None Known

Incompatibility: Contact of carbonates or bicarbonates with acids can release large quantities of carbon dioxide and heat.

Hazardous Decomposition Products: In fire situations heat decomposition may result in the release of sulfur oxides.

Conditions Contributing to Hazardous Polymerization: N / A

Figure 14-1

Material safety data sheet. Delmar/Cengage Learning.

Spotfree
VI – HEALTH HAZARD DATA

EFFECTS OF OVEREXPOSURE (Medical Conditions Aggravated/Target Organ Effects,
A. ACUTE (Primary Route of Exposure)   EYES: Product granules may cause mechanical irritation to eyes.
   SKIN (Primary Route of Exposure): Prolonged repeated contact with skin may result in drying of skin.
   INGESTION: Not expected to be toxic if swallowed, however, gastrointestinal discomfort may occur.
B. SUBCHRONIC, CHRONIC, OTHER: None known.

VII – EMERGENCY AND FIRST AID PROCEDURES

EYES: In case of contact, flush thoroughly with water for 15 minutes. Get medical attention if irritation persists.
SKIN: Flush any dry Spotfree from skin with flowing water. A lways wash hands after use.
INGESTION: If swallowed, drink large quantities of water and call a physician.

VIII – SPILL OR LEAK PROCEDURES

Spill Management: S weep up material and repackage if possible.
   Spill residue may be flushed to the sewer with water.

Waste Disposal Methods: Dispose of in accordance with federal, state and local regulations.

IX – PROTECTION INFORMATION/CONTROL MEASURES

Respiratory: None needed   Eye: Safety   Glove: Not
                                                                      glasses   required

Other Clothing and Equipment: None required

Ventilation: Normal

X – SPECIAL PRECAUTIONS

Precautions to be taken in Handling and Storing: Avoid contact with eyes. Avoid prolonged or repeated contact with skin.
   Wash thoroughly after handling. Keep container closed when not in use.
Additional Information: Store away from acids.

Prepared by: D. Martinez   Revision Date: 04/11/_ _

Seller makes no warranty, expressed or implied, concerning the use of this product other than indicated on the label. Buyer assumes all risk of use and/or handling of this material when such use and/or handling is contrary to label instructions.

While Seller believes that the information contained herein is accurate, such information is offered solely for its customers consideration and verification under their specific use conditions. This information is not to be deemed a warranty or representation of any kind for which Seller assumes legal responsibility.

Figure 14-1
Material safety data sheet (continued). Delmar/Cengage Learning.

pathogens. Common engineering controls include:

(a) Handwashing facilities.
(b) Eyewash stations.
(c) Sharps containers.
(d) Biohazard labels.

(2) Work practice controls: Protocols that promote the behaviors necessary to properly use engineering controls and personal protective equipment.

(3) Personal protective equipment (PPE): Equipment that minimizes exposure beyond the limits of engineering and work practice controls.

(a) Laboratory coats.
(b) Face shields.
(c) Gloves.

(4) Standard Precautions: Application of the concept that all blood, body fluids, secretions, excretions, and moist body substances are to be treated as if contaminated by medically important pathogens regardless of their actual pathogenicity. Examples of materials requiring the use of standard precautions include:

(a) Intravascular fluids
  (i) Blood.
  (ii) Body fluids containing blood.

(b) Extravascular fluids
  (i) Semen.
  (ii) Cerebrospinal fluid.
  (iii) Synovial fluid.
  (iv) Pleural fluid.
  (v) Unidentifiable body fluid.

(c) Secretions
  (i) Saliva.
  (ii) Nasal secretions.
  (iii) Sputum.
  (iv) Tears.
  (v) Vaginal secretions.

(d) Excretions
  (i) Feces.
  (ii) Sweat.
  (iii) Urine.

(e) Vomitus.

e. Immunization: All people who have routine occupational exposure to blood or OPIM have the right to receive the immunization series against hepatitis B during normal working hours and at no personal expense.

f. Exposure control: Enforcement of exposure control policies is required.

(1) Engineering and work practice controls: Policies must be enforced regarding the use of engineering controls, work practice controls, and PPE.

(2) PPE, when warranted, is required to be furnished, cleaned, laundered, disposed, and replaced, free of charge, and used by the employee.

(3) Contaminated sharps (any contaminated object that can cause a cut or puncture wound) must be placed in clearly labeled, puncture-resistant, leak-proof containers immediately after use. Bending, shearing, or recapping needles is prohibited.

(4) Biohazard labels must be placed on all devices used to contain blood or OPIM.

(5) Work surfaces and equipment must be cleaned and decontaminated using an acceptable disinfectant.

(6) Contaminated waste, other than sharps, must be placed in biohazard waste containers located in each laboratory.

(7) Contaminated laundry must be placed in a biohazard container marked "Laundry bag for decontamination."

(8) The above controls must be periodically evaluated.

g. Postexposure evaluation and follow-up: When an employee incurs an exposure incident, it must be reported to that person's supervisor and properly followed up.

3. Maintain records of any hazardous waste and chemical disposal.

B. Falls

1. Most common office accident. Common causes include the following:

a. Tripping over an open desk or file drawer.
b. Tripping over electrical cords or wires.
c. Using a chair or stack of boxes in place of a ladder.
d. Slipping on wet floors.
e. Loose carpeting.
f. Objects stored in halls or walkways.
g. Inadequate lighting.

2. Preventing falls

a. Be sure the pathway is clear before you walk.
b. Close drawers completely after every use.
c. Avoid excessive bending, twisting, and leaning backward while seated.
d. Secure electrical cords and wires away from walkways.
e. Always use a stepladder for overhead reaching. Chairs should never be used as ladders.
f. Clean up spills immediately.
g. Pick up objects co-workers may have left on the floor.
h. Report loose carpeting or damaged flooring.

      i. Never carry anything that obscures your vision.

      j. Wear stable shoes with non-slip soles.

3. To avoid or minimize injury when falling, roll, do not reach.

C. Body mechanics and lifting

1. Most back injuries result from improper lifting.

2. Assume a balanced stance, feet placed shoulder-width apart. When lifting something from the floor, squat close to the load.

3. Keep your back in its neutral or straight position. Tuck in your chin so your head and neck continue the straight back line.

4. Grip the object with your whole hand, rather than only with your fingers. Draw the object close to you, holding your elbows close to your body to keep the load and your body weight centered.

5. Lift by straightening your legs. Let your leg muscles, not your back muscles, do the work. Tighten your stomach muscles to help support your back. Maintain your neutral back position as you lift.

6. Never twist when lifting. When you must turn with a load, turn your whole body, feet first.

7. Never carry a load that blocks your vision.

8. To set something down, use the same body mechanics designed for lifting.

9. If you are doing a lot of twisting while lifting, try to rearrange the space to avoid this. People who have to twist under a load are more likely to suffer back injury.

10. Rotate through tasks so that periods of standing alternate with moving or sitting. Ask for stools or footrests for stationary jobs.

11. Store materials at knee level whenever possible instead of on the floor. Make shelves shallower (12 to 18 inches) so you do not have to reach forward to lift the object. Break up loads so each weighs less.

12. If you must carry a heavy object some distance, consider storing it closer, request a table to rest it on, or try to use a hand truck or cart to transport it.

D. Supply storage

1. Office materials that are improperly stored can lead to objects falling on workers, make for poor visibility, and create a fire hazard.

2. A good housekeeping program will reduce or eliminate hazards associated with improper storage of materials.

3. Boxes, papers, and other materials should not be stored on top of lockers or file cabinets because they can cause landslide problems.

4. Boxes and cartons should all be of uniform size in any pile or stack.

5. Always stack material in such a way that it will not fall over.

6. Store heavy objects on lower shelves.

7. Try to store materials inside cabinets, files, and lockers.

8. Office equipment such as typewriters, index files, lights, or calculators should not be placed on the edges of a desk, filing cabinet, or table.

9. Aisles, corners, and passageways must remain unobstructed. There should be no stacking of materials in these areas.

10. Storage areas should be designated and used only for that purpose.

11. Store heavy materials so you do not have to reach across something to retrieve them.

12. Fire equipment, extinguishers, fire door exits, and sprinkler heads should remain unobstructed. Materials should be, at a minimum, at least 18 inches from sprinkler heads.

E. Ergonomics

1. Fitting the workplace to the workers by modifying or redesigning the job, workstation, tools, or environment.

2. Workstation design can have a big impact on office workers' health and well-being.

3. There are a multitude of discomforts that can result from ergonomically incorrect computer workstation setups.

4. The key to comfort is in maintaining the body in a relaxed, neutral position.

5. The ideal work position is to have the arms hanging relaxed from the shoulders.

6. If a keyboard is used, arms should be bent at right angles at the elbow, with the hands held in a straight line with forearms and elbows close to the body.

7. The head should be in line with the body and slightly forward.

8. Adjust the height of the chair's seat so that the thighs are horizontal while the feet are flat on the floor.

9. Adjust the seat pan depth so that your back is supported by the chair back rest while the back of the knee is comfortable relative to the front of the seat.

10. Adjust the back rest vertically so that it supports/fits the curvature of your lower back.

11. With your arms at your sides and the elbow joint approximately 90 degrees, adjust the height/position of the chair armrests to support the forearms.

12. Adjust the height of the keyboard so that the fingers rest on the keyboard home row when the arm is to the side, the elbow at 90 degrees, and the wrist straight.

13. Place the mouse, trackball, or special keypads next to the keyboard tray. Keep the wrist in a neutral position with the arm and hand close to the body.

14. Adjust the height of the monitor so that the top of the screen is at eye level. If bifocals or trifocals are used, place the monitor at a height that allows easy viewing without tipping the head back.
15. Place reference documents on a document holder close to the screen and at the same distance from the eye.
16. A footrest may be necessary if the operator cannot rest his or her feet comfortably on the floor.

F. Safe work practices
1. Adjust the drapes or blinds.
2. Move the monitor away from sources of glare or direct light.
3. Tip the monitor slightly downward.
4. Use diffusers on overhead lighting.
5. Place an anti-glare filter on the screen.
6. Clean the monitor screen on a regular basis.
7. Avoid cradling the telephone between the head and shoulder. Hold the phone with your hand, use the speaker phone, or use a headset.
8. Keep frequently used items such as the telephone, reference materials, and pens and pencils within easy reach.
9. Position the monitor directly in front of the user.
10. Move between different postures regularly.
11. Apply task lighting as to your needs.
12. Use the minimum force necessary to strike the keyboard/10-key keys.
13. Use the minimum force necessary to activate the hole punch and stapler.
14. Vary your tasks to avoid a long period of one activity.
15. Take mini-breaks to rest the eyes and muscles.
16. Neutralize distracting noise by using ear plugs, playing soft music, or turning on a fan.
17. Maintain a comfortable workplace temperature by using layers of clothing or a fan.

G. Indoor air quality
1. Most likely problem sources: Poor ventilation, poor thermal conditions, too much or not enough humidity, emissions from office machines and copiers and other building contaminants, and poor ergonomic layout of workstations.
2. Generally there should be 20 cubic feet of outside air per minute per person for an office environment.
3. This is a sufficient amount of air to dilute building contaminants and maintain a healthy environment.
4. Indoor air quality complaints increase significantly in offices that are not supplied sufficient outside air.
5. Recommended humidity range: 30% to 60%; humidity above 50% can promote mold growth.

6. Recommended temperature range: 68.5° to 80° F.
7. All ventilation systems should receive periodic cleaning, and filters should be changed on a regular basis.
8. The ventilation system should introduce an adequate supply of fresh outside air into the office and capture and vent point air pollutant sources to the outside.
9. Office machinery should be operated in well-ventilated areas.
10. Photocopiers should be placed away from workers' desks.
11. Workers should vary work tasks to avoid using machines excessively.
12. Office equipment should be cleaned and maintained according to the manufacturers' recommendations.
13. Special attention should be given to special operations that may generate air contaminants (such as painting, pesticide spraying, and heavy cleaning).
14. Provisions for adequate ventilation must be made during these operations or other procedures, such as performing work during off-hours or removing employees from the immediate area.

H. Lighting
1. Poor office lighting can cause eye strain and irritation, fatigue, double vision, watering and reddening of the eyelids, and a decrease in the power of focus and visual acuity.
2. Headaches as well as neck and back pains may occur as a result of workers straining to see small or detailed items.
3. Poor lighting in the workplace is also associated with an increase in accidents.
4. Regular maintenance of the lighting system should be carried out to clean or replace old bulbs and faulty lamp circuits.
5. A light-colored matte finish on walls, ceilings, and floors to reduce glare is recommended.
6. Whenever possible, office workers should not face windows, unshielded lamps, or other sources of glare.
7. Adjustable shades should be used if workers face a window.
8. Diffuse light will help reduce shadows. Indirect lighting and task lighting are recommended, especially when work spaces are separated by dividers.
9. Task lamps are very effective in supplementing general office lighting for those who require or prefer additional lighting. Some task lamps permit several light levels.

I. Noise
1. In an office setting, OSHA noise standards are rarely approached or exceeded.

2. When employees are subjected to sound levels exceeding OSHA standards, feasible administrative or engineering controls must be utilized.

3. If such controls fail to reduce sound levels, personal protective equipment must be provided and used to reduce sound levels.

4. Select the quietest equipment if possible. When there is a choice between two or more products, sound levels should be included as a consideration for purchase and use.

5. Provide for proper maintenance of equipment, such as lubrication and tightening of loose parts that can cause noise.

6. Locate loud equipment in areas where its effects are less detrimental. For example, place impact printers away from areas where people must use the phone.

7. Use barrier walls or dividers to isolate noise sources. Use of buffers or acoustically treated materials can absorb noise that might otherwise travel further. Rubber pads to insulate vibrating equipment can also help reduce noise.

8. Enclose equipment, such as printers, with acoustical covers or housings.

9. Schedule noisy tasks at times when it will have less of an effect on the other tasks in the office.

J. Electrical safety
   1. Electrical systems should be grounded as warranted.
   2. By grounding an electrical system, a low-resistance path to earth through a ground connection is intentionally created.
   3. When properly done, this path offers sufficiently low resistance and has sufficient current-carrying capacity to prevent the build-up of hazardous voltages.
   4. Most fixed equipment such as large, stationary machines must be grounded. Cord and plug connected equipment must be grounded if it is located in hazardous or wet locations.
   5. Never remove the third (grounding) prong from any three-prong piece of equipment.
   6. Overloading electrical circuits and extension cords can result in a fire.
   7. Floor-mounted outlets should be carefully placed to prevent tripping hazards.
   8. Equipment and cords should be inspected regularly, and a qualified individual should make repairs.
   9. Electrical cords should be examined on a routine basis for fraying and exposed wiring.
   10. A cord should not be pulled or dragged over nails, hooks, or other sharp objects that may cause cuts in the insulation.
   11. Cords should never be placed on radiators, steam pipes, walls, and windows.
   12. Particular attention should be placed on connections behind furniture, because files and bookcases may be pushed tightly against electric outlets, severely bending the cord at the plug.
   13. An adequate number of outlet sockets should be provided. Extension cords should only be used in only situations where fixed wiring is not feasible.
   14. If it is necessary to use an extension cord, never run it across walkways or aisles because of the potential tripping hazard. If you must run a cord across a walkway, either tape it down or purchase a cord runner.
   15. Wall receptacles should be designed and installed so that no current-carrying parts are exposed, and outlet plates should be kept tight to eliminate the possibility of shock.
   16. Switches to turn equipment on and off should be provided, either in the equipment or in the cords, so that it is not necessary to pull the plugs to shut off the power.
   17. To remove a plug from an outlet, take a firm grip on and pull the plug itself. Never pull a plug out by the cord.
   18. Disconnect electrical machines before cleaning, adjusting, or applying flammable solutions.
   19. If a guard is removed to clean or repair parts, replace it before testing the equipment and returning the machine to service.
   20. Electrical panel doors should always be kept closed, to prevent "electrical flashover" in the event of an electrical malfunction.

K. Fire safety
   1. Learn the location of fire escape routes and how to activate the fire alarm.
   2. Participate in practice fire drills on a regular basis.
   3. Become familiar with stairway exits because elevators may not function during a fire or may expose passengers to heat, gas, and smoke.
   4. Heat-producing equipment such as copiers, work processors, coffeemakers, and hot plates are often overlooked as a potential fire hazard. Keep them away from anything that might burn.
   5. Be sure to turn off all appliances at the end of the day. Use only grounded appliances plugged into grounded outlets (three-prong plug).
   6. If electrical equipment malfunctions or gives off a strange odor, disconnect it and call the appropriate maintenance personnel.
   7. Promptly disconnect and replace cracked, frayed, or broken electrical cords.
   8. Keep extension cords clear of doorways and other areas where they can be stepped on or chafed.
   9. Never plug one extension cord into another.

10. Do not allow combustible material (boxes, paper, etc.) to build up in inappropriate storage locations (near sources of ignition).
11. Develop a program of scheduled inspections.

L. Emergency preparedness

1. Office workers should be able to recognize the signal to evacuate their work area and know how to exit in an expedient manner.
2. For emergency evacuation, the use of floor plans or workplace maps that clearly show the emergency escape routes and safe or refuge areas should be included in the plan.
3. All employees must understand the actions they are to take in the work area and assemble in a safe zone.
4. All new employees should discuss how they should respond to emergencies with their supervisors shortly after starting work and whenever their responsibilities under the plan change. This orientation should include the following:
   a. Identifying the individuals responsible for various aspects of the plan (chain of command) so that in an emergency, confusion will be minimized and employees will have no doubt about who has authority for making decisions.
   b. Identifying the method of communication that will be used to alert employees that an evacuation or some other action is required as well as how employees can report emergencies (such as manual pull stations, public address systems, or telephones).
   c. Identifying the evacuation routes from the building and locations where employees will gather.
5. If you discover a fire or see or smell smoke, immediately follow these procedures:
   a. Notify the local fire department.
   b. Activate the building alarm (fire pull station). If not available or operational, verbally notify people in the building.
   c. Isolate the area by closing windows and doors and evacuate the building, if you can do so safely.
   d. Shut down equipment in the immediate area, if possible.
   e. If possible and if you have received appropriate training, use a portable fire extinguisher to assist evacuation, assist another to evacuate, or control a small fire.
   f. Do not collect personal or official items; leave the area of the fire immediately and walk, do not run to the exit and designated gathering area.
   g. You should provide the fire and police teams with the details of the problem upon their arrival. Special hazard information you might know is essential for the safety of the emergency responders.
   h. You should not re-enter the building until directed to do so. Follow any special procedures established for your unit.
   i. If the fire alarms are ringing in your building, you must evacuate the building and stay out until notified to return.
   j. Move to your designated meeting location or upwind from the building, staying clear of streets, driveways, sidewalks, and other access ways to the building.
   k. If you are a supervisor, try to account for your employees, keep them together, and report any missing persons to the emergency personnel at the scene.
6. If an individual is overexposed to smoke or chemical vapors, remove the person to an uncontaminated area and treat for shock.
7. Do not enter the area if you suspect that a life-threatening condition still exists (such as heavy smoke or toxic gases).
8. Follow standard CPR protocols. Get medical attention promptly.
9. If your or another person's clothing catches fire, extinguish the burning clothing by using the drop-and-roll technique, wrap the victim in a fire blanket, or douse the victim with cold water (use an emergency shower if it is immediately available).
10. Carefully remove contaminated clothing; however, avoid further damage to the burned area.
11. Cover injured person to prevent shock. Get medical attention promptly.

CHAPTER 15

Operations Management

I. OPENING A MEDICAL PRACTICE

A. First month
1. Determine the start-up date
   a. Allow 6 to 9 months to put everything in place.
   b. Make the decision on attorney, accountant, banker, realtor, and practice management consultant (if desired).
2. Select business structure: Obtain legal advice.
3. Decide what services will be provided: Make it early in your process because this will drive many other decisions.
4. Draft the fee schedule
   a. Identify the CPT codes that will be used to bill for services.
   b. Decide what fees will be charged as soon as possible.
   c. When applying for credentialing and network status, ask each payer for its reimbursement by specific code.
   d. Begin work on your practice logo and other identity pieces (stationary, business card).
5. Decide on information technology: Practice management systems, website, electronic health records system, e-prescribing, and the integration among these applications.
6. Determine space and location requirements and select a site: Work with a real estate consultant.
7. Obtain telephone and fax numbers, an email address, and a practice website: Most managed care plans will not process your application for credentialing until they have all these details.
8. Develop a compliance plan: Get assistance from an attorney re: Stark, anti-fraud and abuse, HIPAA Privacy and Security, and other government programs.
9. Familiarize yourself with the requirements of the HIPAA Privacy and Security Rules to help make informed decisions about building and interior design.
10. Design the office layout and décor: Consult with an interior design firm.

B. Second month
1. Obtain/amend the physicians state medical license: Required for medical staff privileges, malpractice insurance, and participation in the various managed care provider networks.
2. Obtain/amend the physician's medical malpractice coverage.
   a. Ask your state Medical Society or Department of Insurance for carrier names and then comparison shop for coverage and price.
   b. Make sure you purchase the level of coverage that the payers require, and be careful about tail coverage.
3. Obtain a federal tax ID number.
   a. www.irs.gov/business/small/index.html
   b. Required by managed care companies and other payers.
4. Register the practice with the Secretary of State and other appropriate state and local agencies.
5. Submit/amend application(s) for hospital privileges.
   a. The medical staff office at each hospital will provide guidance.
   b. Requires recommendations, copies of licenses and board certification, drug enforcement administration (DEA) numbers, verification of professional liability insurance, and documentation and proof of expertise in certain procedures.
   c. May take several months, so start as soon as possible.
   d. Managed care companies may not review your applications for credentialing until the physician has hospital privileges.
   e. Ensure the physician is credentialed at one or more hospitals before opening the practice.
6. Obtain a national provider identification (NPI) number.
   a. Will enable you to conduct electronic claims and other HIPAA-regulated transactions.
   b. Contact the NPI Enumerator by phone (800-465-3203 or 800-692-2326), by email (customerservice@npienumerator.com) or

by writing to NPE Enumerator, PO Box 6059, Fargo, ND 58108-6059.

7. Apply to become part of the networks for one or more managed care plans.
   a. Without this, patients will not come to your practice and/or medical colleagues will not refer to you.
   b. Seek advice from the state Medical Society or colleagues in the community.

8. Apply for participation in Medicare and Medicaid.
   a. Contact your Medicare intermediary and your state Medicaid agency to get information about credentialing and claims submission.
   b. Make sure you know the rules for both programs.

9. Obtain/amend the physician's federal and state narcotic licenses.
   a. Both are required to prescribe narcotics.
   b. The Department of Justice Drug Enforcement Administration Form 224 is available at www.usdoj.gov/dea.

10. Select a banker and arrange for a bank loan if necessary: One experienced in dealing with medical practices.

C. Third month
1. Review the office lease or other documents with an attorney: Decide whether to build, purchase, or lease.
2. Prepare a list of the fixed assets that you should purchase and get price quotations.
3. Prepare a strategic business plan for the practice:
   a. Develop the supporting financial information (i.e., budget, operating statement, cash flow projections and balance sheet) and implementation plan.
   b. It should contain your mission, vision, goals and objectives, strategies, actions steps, timing and delegation of responsibilities.
   c. Collaborate with an external consultant, your accountant, and your banker to prepare this document.
4. Open a business checking account: Specify who in your practice will have signatory authority.
5. Obtain a state(s) unemployment tax identification number.
   a. Register with your state's Department of Employment Security.
   b. Check the IRS website for state-specific information (www.irs.gov/business/small/index/html)
6. Develop an employee compensation package.
   a. An insurance broker can provide information on health and dental insurance.
   b. Decide on wages, salaries, and benefits before hiring employees so you can make this information part of the offer.
7. Develop job descriptions and advertise and interview multiple candidates for each position.
8. Schedule implementation and training for the practice management system, web-based communications, and electronic health records.
9. Clarify the requirements for Medicare and Medicaid billing.
   a. Understand the coding and billing requirements for each of these programs.
   b. Pay a personal visit to representatives of each program to make sure you are clear.
   c. Each year, the Office of Inspector General publishes a work plan that lays out priorities.
   d. Remain current on new developments.
10. Test the claims submission processes for every government and private payer.
    a. Take advantage of opportunities for direct claims submission that bypass clearinghouse intervention; will result in faster reimbursement.
    b. If claims go through a clearinghouse, understand the relationship between the clearinghouse and the practice management system.

D. Fourth month
1. Determine payment and collection policies: Get input from the accountant regarding billing cycles, collection letters, timing for sending overdue accounts to a collection agency, and write-offs.
2. Schedule training on billing and collections.
3. Order patient account statements.
   a. Make sure the language is clear.
   b. Your patients might confuse statements with bills.
4. Purchase equipment and supplies: Investigate purchasing discounts that are available through professional associations and/or directly from vendors.
5. Purchase office furniture and supplies.
6. Activate and test the website.
7. Test e-prescribing capability.
8. Develop a practice brochure, introductory letter, and other materials to announce the opening or new location of the practice.
   a. It communicates your mission, your qualifications, the way in which your office works, and information about the physicians and staff.
   b. Keep a hard copy of the brochure in the waiting room and mail it out to announce the opening of your practice.
   c. Post the information in the brochure on the practice website.

9. Order business cards, stationary, practice brochure, and other print material:
   a. Take advantage of quantity discounts.
   b. Order materials for report preparation and filing: If paper records rather than paperless office is preferred, order the specific materials required.
10. Select and engage answering and paging services.
    a. Should be compatible with any other methods of communication that have already been selected.
    b. Test them ahead of time to make sure they meet expectations.

E. Fifth month
1. Draft and finalize an Employee Handbook.
   a. Reduce exposure to potential legal issues: Develop written policies and procedures for hiring, compensation package (wage, and salary, benefits), performance evaluation, termination, and conditions of employment.
   b. Put this information in an Employee Handbook that is given to all new employees during orientation.
2. Develop a patient information package.
   a. Ensures patients understand how the practice works.
   b. Include services provided, how to make appointments, how to get medical advice and test results, and how to renew prescriptions.
   c. Include policies regarding confidentiality and financial policies, including payment plans, charging for missed appointments, and collections.
   d. Give patients a hard copy of the package and make it available on the website.
3. Determine appointment scheduling methods: Ensure online features work.
4. Decide on the opening date.
5. Draft and order cards announcing the opening of the practice.
6. Draft an announcement and place ads in local newspapers.
   a. Include name, address, phone, email address, and welcome message to new patients (if accepting them).
   b. Mention the physician's training and experience and/or participation in managed care plans and government programs.
   c. Ensure ad runs 2 weeks before the opening date.
7. Develop a list of names to whom the announcement will be sent.
   a. New and potential patients, referring physicians, health-care organizations, and the community.

b. Chambers of Commerce and other local organizations may also have information.
8. Meet with referring physicians.
9. Obtain/order periodicals and educational materials for your waiting room.
   a. Keep the age and gender of patient population in mind when you order materials.
   b. Start this task at least 9 weeks before you open or move.
10. Obtain/amend membership in state and county medical societies and in professional associations.

F. Sixth to ninth month
1. Train employees on the practice management system, web-based communication, EHR, and e-prescribing systems.
   a. Cross train people so they can cover for each other when someone is out sick or on vacation.
   b. Ask the vendors to do the training at the practice site.
   c. You will have employee turnover and your vendors will upgrade their systems, so repeat this training regularly.
2. Train employees on the billing system.
3. Train employees on HIPAA compliance.
   a. Designate HIPAA Privacy and HIPAA Security Officials.
   b. Incorporate HIPAA training into orientation for new employees and do a refresher at least annually.
4. Obtain any manuals needed for the office: Maintain written documentation for Medicare, Medicaid, coding, and on each managed care plan with which you contract.
5. Set up accounting systems for accounts payable, petty cash, and bank reconciliations.
6. Train employees on the accounting systems.
7. Prepare employee personnel files
   a. Keep them in a secure place.
   b. Restrict access to employee files other than the practice manager and one of the physician owners.
8. Train employees on operating policies and procedures.
   a. Ensure operating policies and procedures are clear to all your employees.
   b. Clarify entire work flow process before the practice is opened.
   c. Begin developing a Quality Improvement plan: Expect to benchmark the practice against others and against evidence-based standards.
9. Plan the details of the opening: Plan a nice celebration for the opening.
10. Opening day!

II. MANAGEMENT AND SUPERVISION

A. General
   1. Management: The process of developing, implementing, and achieving organizational objectives.
      a. Administration: Process of managing non-human resources to achieve organizational objectives.
      b. Leadership: The process of managing human resources to achieve organizational objectives.
   2. Chain of authority: There should be a clear line of authority within the clinic by which reporting to more than one supervisor is avoided.
   3. Effectiveness versus efficiency.
      a. Effectiveness describes achieving goals and objectives in a timely fashion; i.e., doing the right things.
      b. Efficiency describes achieving goals and objectives using the least amount of resources possible; i.e., doing things right.

B. Management process
   1. Planning: Developing a department's or organization's goals or objectives.
   2. Organizing: Assembling and coordinating the necessary human, physical, and capital resources necessary to carry out the objectives of an organization.
   3. Directing: Supervising the use of resources to achieve organizational objectives.
   4. Controlling: Comparing actual results with planned results, and making the necessary adjustments to achieve organizational objectives.

C. Supervision
   1. Leadership: The process of working with and through people to achieve organizational objectives willingly.
   2. Leadership comprises two types of behavior.
      a. Task behavior: The extent to which the leader tells the employee what, how, when, where, and who is to perform a specific task.
      b. Relationship behavior: The extent to which the leader engages in listening, communicating, facilitating, and supportive behaviors.
   3. Assess the employee's levels of ability and willingness.
      a. Ability is a function of:
         (1) Knowledge: The employee understands the task to be performed.
         (2) Experience: The employee has experience carrying out the task or related tasks.
         (3) Performance: The employee has demonstrated skill in successfully completing the same or similar tasks.
      b. Willingness is a function of:
         (1) Confidence: Employees feel they can perform tasks.
         (2) Commitment: Employees feel they will perform tasks.
         (3) Motivation: Employees feel they want to perform tasks.
   4. Readiness levels: R1 to R4.
      a. R1: Unable and unwilling.
      b. R2: Unable but willing.
      c. R3: Able but unwilling.
      d. R4: Able and willing.
   5. Select the appropriate leadership style
      a. Telling: Supervisor makes decisions providing specific instructions and closely supervises performance. High task and low relationship behavior. Most appropriate for employees having low ability and willingness (R1).
      b. Selling: Supervisor makes and explains decisions and provides opportunity for clarification. High task and relationship behavior. Most appropriate for employees with some ability and willingness (R2).
      c. Participating: Supervisor shares ideas and facilitates decision making. Low task and high relationship behavior. Most appropriate for employees with a fair amount of ability and low willingness (R3).
      d. Delegating: Supervisor turns over responsibility for making and implementing decisions. Low task and relationship behavior. Most appropriate for employees with high ability and willingness (R4).
   6. Work plans
      a. Consistent with organizational and department objectives, employees develop their own goals to be achieved within a certain period of time.
      b. It is the supervisor's responsibility to meet with employees periodically to review and offer support in the achievement of work-plan goals.

D. Self management
   1. To Do lists: Don't trust your memory, write it down.
      a. At the end of the day, make a laundry list of things to do the next day.
      b. Prioritize the list according to urgency or importance.
         (1) A items: Items of sufficiently high importance or requiring immediate attention.
            (a) Comprises approximately 20% of all that must be done.
            (b) Typically takes up to 80% of your time to complete.
         (2) B items: Items of moderate importance.

(3) C items: Routine items of least importance.
  (a) B and C items make up approximately 80% of all that must be accomplished.
  (b) Typically consumes approximately 20% of your time.
  c. Check off each item as it is completed. Add items as appropriate.

2. Objectives and goals
  a. At the beginning of each year or planning period, review the organization's philosophy, vision, mission, and organizational plans.
  b. Based on this review, prepare a list of three to five major objectives that can be realistically achieved within the period.
  c. For each objective, prepare a list of short-term goals that, if completed in a timely fashion, will allow you to achieve each major objective.
  d. Make every effort to meet your goals, making modifications as the need arises.

3. Day planners: Keep a day planner or small calendar book to record appointments, to-do lists, and important phone numbers, and as a means of organizing your work activities.

E. Teamwork
  1. Consists of two or more people working together to achieve a goal.
  2. Teams are generally formed to develop and execute a project, analyze a situation, formulate a recommendation, solve a problem, manage resources, or the like.
  3. Team development (Bruce Tuckman, 1977):
    a. Forming: The team meets and learns about the opportunity and challenges, then agrees on goals and begins to tackle the tasks. Supervisors of the team will probably need to be directive during this phase.
    b. Storming: Different ideas compete for consideration. The team addresses issues such as what problems they are really supposed to solve, how they will function independently and together, and what leadership model they will accept.
    c. Norming: Team members adjust their behavior to each other as they develop work habits that make teamwork seem more natural and fluid. Team members begin to trust each other. Motivation increases as the team gets more acquainted with the project. Supervisors of the team during this phase tend to be more participative than in earlier stages.
    d. Performing: Teams are able to function as a unit as they find ways to get the job done smoothly and effectively without inappropriate conflict or the need for external supervision. Supervisors of the team during this phase are almost always participative.
    e. Adjourning: Completing the task and breaking up the team.
    f. Transforming: A team that lasts may transcend to a higher phase of achievement.

4. Team player: One who subordinates personal aspirations and works in a coordinated effort with other members of a group, or team, in striving for a common goal.

5. Leadership: A team leader should be appointed. Depending on the experience and functionality of the team, a formal leader may be unnecessary; however, agreement on how the team will be held accountable should be determined.

6. The team's work objectives must be determined, as well as the timetable in which to achieve them, and the criteria by which success will be measured.

7. The last 15 minutes of team meetings should be reserved to summarize what was decided or concluded, to agree on work assignments, and to discuss the purpose of the next meeting.

8. To maintain momentum and a sense of urgency, teams should adopt interim deadlines for completion of tasks.

9. Brainstorming:
  a. A nonjudgmental form of idea generation, sifting, and selection.
  b. Everyone agrees to suspend judgment about any idea initially forwarded.
  c. Everyone agrees to keep in mind that there is probably more than one "answer" for the task at hand.
  d. Everyone attempts to listen naively, as though they possess no prior knowledge.
  e. Prior agreement on objective criteria is reached before value judgments are engaged by the team.

10. Values that support trust within a team:
  a. Avoid looking good at another's expense.
  b. Accept that people will be wrong in the beginning.
  c. Demonstrate respect for facts, data, and objective analysis.
  d. Tolerance of the mess and chaos inherent in the innovation process.
  e. Managers should welcome and embrace criticism.
  f. Members should evaluate the team's efforts.
  g. Rewards should be based on team results and product.

III. HUMAN RESOURCES MANAGEMENT

1. Hiring process
   a. Recruiting: When a position becomes available, potential internal and external candidates are notified through company postings and advertisements.
   b. Interviewing: Meeting with selected candidates to exchange employment information.
   c. Checking references: Calling references to verify employment and other job information as appropriate.
   d. Candidate selection: Choosing the best candidate based on education, training, experience, references, and "fit" within the organization.
   e. Employment offer: Offering the job to the selected candidate to include compensation and benefits.
   f. Post-offer negotiation: Negotiating terms of employment not acceptable at the initial offer.
   g. Acceptance/rejection: If the offer is not accepted, another candidate is offered the position or the process begins again.
2. Recruitment: When selecting potential employees consider the following:
   a. Job duties versus the applicant's training and experience.
   b. Employee characteristics being sought.
   c. Compensation and benefit requirements.
   d. Availability.
3. Interviewing
   a. Purpose: Gather pertinent information about the applicant by facilitating the candidate's willingness to talk.
   b. Conduct the interview in a comfortable, private setting without interruption; ideally, the interviewer should sit with the applicant at a table rather than behind a desk.
   c. Set the applicant at ease by explaining the agenda of the interview.
   d. Ask open-ended questions rather than yes/no questions, leading questions that suggest the proper answer, or questions already answered on the resume.
   e. Attempt to identify experience and training that will impact success or failure on the job.
   f. Avoid personal questions, especially those that have little to do with bonafide occupational qualifications.
   g. Illegal questions to avoid
      (1) Questions regarding sexual preference, national origin, race, and religion.
      (2) Age: Verifying whether the applicant is 18 years or older is permitted.
      (3) Marital status and number of dependents or children.

4. Job description: Should include the following:
   a. Job title.
   b. Job summary: A brief narrative description of the position.
   c. The supervisor's job title.
   d. Job duties and responsibilities.
   e. Job specifications: The level of education and training, as well as required skills and abilities.
5. Orientation and training
   a. Purpose: To make a smooth transition from candidate to employee status to include:
      (1) Imparting the philosophy, vision, and mission of the organization.
      (2) Identifying performance expectations.
      (3) Facilitating identification of the new employee as a member of the team.
      (4) Providing a protected period of time to learn a new job.
      (5) Assessing the employee's skills and learning needs.
   b. Assignment of a preceptor: To help the new employee navigate through the system.
   c. Staff introductions.
   d. Tour of the facility.
   e. Review of policies and procedures.
   f. Specific job training.
6. Probation: New employees should be placed on 60- to 90-day probation to determine whether an adequate employment match has been made. At the end of this period, a performance appraisal should be prepared and reviewed with the employee.
7. Performance appraisal
   a. Should be an objective assessment regarding an employee's quality and quantity of work, dependability, efficiency, teamwork, attitude, and appearance.
   b. The appraisal should occur regularly once or twice a year.
   c. The results of the appraisal should be discussed with the employee.
   d. Together, the supervisor and employee should agree on strengths and weaknesses with a plan of action to overcome weaknesses.
   e. Often used as a basis for reviewing salary changes.
8. Compensation and benefits: Should be determined based on the following criteria:
   a. Job tasks and responsibilities.
   b. Typical compensation for the same or comparable jobs in the local market.
   c. Employee experience, accomplishments, and performance.
9. Employee discipline: All disciplinary actions should be recorded in the employee's personnel file.

a. Progressive discipline: Increasing degrees of discipline should be imposed for repeated performance problems or violations.
   (1) First offense: Oral warning.
   (2) Second offense: Written warning.
   (3) Third offense: Suspension—written warning with loss of pay.
   (4) Fourth and subsequent offense: Termination.
   (5) Disciplinary probation: A step that may be included anywhere in the process.
b. Employee due process: Employees have the following rights:
   (1) To know what is expected of them and the consequences for not meeting expectations.
   (2) To consistent and predictable employer responses to violation of rules.
   (3) To fair discipline based on the facts.
   (4) To question the facts and present a defense.
   (5) To appeal disciplinary actions.
   (6) To progressive discipline.
   (7) To be considered as individuals.
10. Professional development
   a. As an employer you should encourage and help subsidize activities that promote professional development among your employees.
   b. Membership in professional organizations.
   c. Attendance at seminars, workshops, conventions, as well as college courses.
   d. Completion of continuing education units (CEUs).
F. Policies and procedures
   1. Purpose: Identifies what is expected and how to handle specific circumstances.
   2. Content
      a. Statement of an organization's mission, vision, and philosophy.
      b. Orientation.
      c. Dress code.
      d. Department/job responsibilities and expectations.
      e. Holidays, leave, paid time off, and vacation.
      f. Payroll, professional development, and benefits.
      g. Disciplinary actions.

IV. RISK MANAGEMENT

A. Risk management defined: The process of planning, organizing, directing, and controlling organizational activities to economically minimize the adverse effects of accidental losses.
B. Goals
   1. Prevent and manage liability exposure.
   2. Improve the quality of patient care.
   3. Protect financial assets—prevent, eliminate, or reduce financial loss.
   4. Train all employees and volunteers.
   5. Reduce the incidence of injury.
   6. Identify and neutralize hazards.
   7. Monitor and evaluate adverse events.
   8. Manage potential claims.
   9. Integrate with quality assurance and utilization management review.
C. Quality assurance
   1. In 1989, the Joint Commission, formerly JCAHO, required operational linkages between risk management (RM) and quality assurance (QA).
   2. QA measures ensure that patients receive safe, appropriate care leading to the most successful outcomes possible.
   3. Prevention of patient injuries is the greatest interaction between RM and QA.
D. Risk concepts
   1. Risk: The probability of an adverse outcome that leads to a loss.
   2. Risk management: The process of identifying, analyzing, and neutralizing factors potentially resulting in financial loss to the practice, thereby improving quality of care.
   3. Types of risk
      a. Speculative risk: Probability of gain or loss that is intended to provide patient benefits (e.g., diagnostic and treatment services, research and experimentation).
      b. Pure risk: Probability of loss only—primary focus of RM (e.g., hazardous practices).
   4. Potential compensable event (PCE): Any event that may result in compensation to another party. Often described as a complaint, incident, or occurrence.
E. Risk management process
   1. Risk identification: Discover potential areas of risk.
      a. Review clinical and medical staff committee minutes (e.g., morbidity/mortality, infection control, safety, transfusion, QA reports, etc.).
      b. Chart reviews: Evaluating a department's standard for documentation. Observing for key indicators.
      c. Inspection of patient care areas: Observe for safety hazards, noncompliance, and monitoring of patients.
      d. Provider interviews: Heightens awareness of RM and assessing standards of care.
   2. Risk assessment
      a. Frequency: How often has the event occurred? Are there any patterns or relationships that appear to be common?

b. Severity: What is the potential level of financial loss?

c. Highly frequent or severe events should take priority.

d. Almost impossible to insure against high-frequency, high-severity events.

3. Risk control

a. Four strategies

(1) Risk elimination: Discontinue services creating the risk (e.g., high-frequency/high-severity losses).

(2) Risk avoidance: Change factors creating the risk (e.g., behavior, facilities, policies, etc.).

(3) Risk retention: Endure low frequency/low severity losses (e.g., lost patient property).

(4) Risk transfer: Insure against low-frequency/high-severity losses (e.g., fire, malpractice).

b. Common control methods

(1) Staff education.

(2) Patient education (i.e., detailed written instructions).

(3) Patient representative: Valuable resource to address patient complaints, concerns, and suggestions.

4. Risk transfer

a. Risks that are not eliminated or avoided are retained and financed if possible. Financing involves transferring the risk for financial loss to an insurance carrier.

b. Entails commercial and/or self-insurance.

c. Choose deductible-premium mix.

d. Consider pros and cons of carrier claims management versus in-house claims management.

5. Claims management

a. Purpose: Early identification, investigation, and resolution of PCEs.

b. Classify the incident

(1) Incident: Adverse outcome with no loss potential.

(2) Investigative incident: Some loss potential.

(3) Potential claim: Definite loss potential—investigation warranted.

(4) Claim: Written demand for compensation—potential lawsuit.

(5) Suit: Legal remediation.

c. Establish claims file: Prepared when there is a possibility of loss, liability, or exposure.

d. Prepare investigative brief

(1) Claimant information: Demographics.

(2) Insured information.

(3) Allegations and injuries.

(4) Result of medical records review.

(5) Interviews.

(6) Copies of relevant policies and procedures.

(7) Results of peer/expert review.

(8) Evaluation of damages.

(9) Evaluation of liability.

(10) Settlement value and strategy.

e. Conduct investigation.

f. Evaluate potential bill abatement (reduction).

g. Communicate with administration.

h. Settlement negotiations.

i. Litigation management.

F. Insurance concepts

1. Insurance: Device for the transfer of risk through the accumulation of funds.

2. Insurer: Insurance company.

3. Insured: Beneficiary of insurance policy.

4. Peril: Cause of loss that can be insured against.

5. Hazard: Operating condition that increases the chance of loss of a covered peril.

6. Risk (exposure): Likelihood that a covered peril will cause a loss.

7. Accident: Sudden, unforeseen, unintended event.

8. Insurable interest: Financial interest the insured must possess at time of loss.

9. Indemnity: One party (insurer) legally standing in the place of another (insured).

10. Deductible: Initial amount of loss the insured suffers before the insurer indemnifies.

11. Limits of liability: Maximum amount the insurer will pay to cover a loss. Limits apply to each occurrence and aggregate occurrences during the policy period.

12. Liability coverage: Policy that pays sums for which an insured is liable to third parties for personal or property damage.

13. Warranties: Specific claims made by the insured that allow coverage or reduce the cost of coverage.

14. Coinsurance: Policy that covers only a portion of the loss.

15. Parts of a policy

a. Declarations: Information about the insured and the insured's interests to be covered.

b. Insurance agreement: The insurer's promise to indemnify covered perils.

c. Exclusions: Limitations, restrictions, or items not covered.

d. Conditions: Requirements for keeping the policy in force and recovering for claims.

e. Endorsements (riders): Additions or limitations that change the standard policy.

16. Insurance types

a. Property: Protects insured's plant and equipment and/or loss of revenue resulting from business interruptions.

    b. Liability: Covers employee negligence.
    c. Health professional liability (HPL): Covers malpractice.
    d. Comprehensive general liability (CGL): Covers risks resulting from public use of property.
      (1) HPL is restricted to personal injury; CGL covers property damage as well.
      (2) HPL covers damage resulting from health services.
      (3) HPL requires the insured's consent for settlement; not so for CGL.
    e. Director's and officer's (D&O) liability: Covers D&O risks or negligence.
    f. Blanket crime (bonding): Covers embezzlement and employee dishonesty.
    g. Automobile: Covers damage and/or personal injury.
    h. Excess liability: Increases limits of malpractice insurance.
    i. Error and omissions (E&O): Covers nonmedical professional liability such as accounting and legal services.
    j. Umbrella insurance
      (1) Increases limits and broadens coverage of named policies to cover catastrophic losses.
      (2) When underlying policy limits are met, the umbrella is activated for injuries, defense, and related costs.
      (3) Covers risks not normally included in typical liability policies such as intentional torts.
17. Claims made policy: A claim to be covered must be submitted within the policy period even though the incident did not occur within the policy period—common for HPL.
18. Occurrence policy: Coverage requires the incident to have occurred during the policy period even though the claim was filed outside the policy period—CGL and HPL.

V. MEETINGS MANAGEMENT

A. General
    1. Maintain a calendar of all meetings scheduled identifying the topic, date, time, and place.
    2. The MA may be called upon to assist in organizing, scheduling, and recording the minutes of professional society meetings for which the physician is responsible.
    3. Rules of Order: The manner in which meetings are conducted depends on the type of meeting and preferences of administrators; a typical order of business follows:
      a. Reading minutes from last meeting.
      b. Officer/committee/department reports.
      c. Special business.

      d. Unfinished business.
      e. New business.
B. Chairing/facilitating
    1. The person chairing the meeting is responsible for ensuring that all facets of the process from planning to execution are effectively and efficiently carried out.
    2. The major function of the chairperson is to ensure that the objectives of the meeting are achieved.
    3. Start and end the meeting on time: It is advisable to end on time even if the purpose of the meeting is not complete. If not, schedule another meeting.
    4. Keep the meeting participants focused on the meeting's objectives.
    5. Encourage full participation without fear of criticism.
    6. Enforce meeting rules, protocol, and etiquette.
C. Scheduling
    1. Factors to consider:
      a. Objectives of the meeting.
      b. Time, place, duration.
      c. Expected attendance.
      d. Refreshments.
    2. Informing attendees: Send a letter or memo identifying the meeting logistics.
D. Agenda: Typed list identifying the items or topics to be discussed under each section of the rules of order (see Figure 15-1A).
E. Minutes: Record of the contents of a meeting (see Figure 15-1B).
    1. Introductory matter includes:
      a. The name of the organization.
      b. The kind of meeting.
      c. Place, date, and time of meeting.
      d. Those in attendance and absent. Identification of the chairperson or acceptable delegate.
      e. Whether the minutes of the last meeting was read and approved.
    2. Each issue should have its own paragraph, to include as appropriate:
      a. Statement of each motion.
      b. Name of the person making the motion.
      c. The results of the motion.
    3. Statement regarding the time of adjournment.
    4. Signature of recorder.
F. Brainstorming: Method of generating ideas without judgment or criticism.
    1. An issue or problem is identified and defined.
    2. Members of the group contribute as many ideas as possible.
    3. All ideas, regardless of worth, are written down by a recorder.
    4. No one is allowed to judge, criticize, or evaluate any idea until the brainstorming session is complete.

```
                        AGENDA

                  Chicago Medical Society
                    Monthly Meeting
                    October 14, 20XX



  1.   Reading of the minutes of the previous meeting (approved or changed).

  2.   Reading of correspondence.

  3.   Presentation of the Treasurer's report.

  4.   Old business:

       a.    Filling the vacancy of the office of Vice President.

       b.    Reviewing applications of new members.

  5.   New business:

       a.    Reviewing officer nominations for next year.

       b.    Voting on increase of membership dues for next year.

  6.   Program: Dr. Tia Wong of University Hospital Cardiology Department,
       "A Program of Diet and Exercise After Cardiac Surgery."

  7.   Announcements.

  8.   Adjournment.
```

Figure 15-1A

Meeting agenda. © Delmar/Cengage Learning.

5. As a group, organize the ideas into logical categories.
6. Ask each member to select the top three to five ideas and rate them on a scale of one to three or five.
7. Based on the individual rankings, select the top three or five ideas.

VI. TRAVEL

A. General
   1. Although the use of travel agents is common, the provider may prefer the MA alone, or the MA working with an agent, to arrange travel and accommodations.
   2. Travel agents: Arranging travel with an agent is probably more effective and efficient than handling it yourself, unless you are experienced in such matters.
      a. Agents are able to arrange and coordinate air and ground transportation for smooth travel.
      b. They are better able to secure competitive rates.
      c. They are good resources for suggesting local entertainment, and sight-seeing packages, as well as providing valuable travel advice.
   3. Itinerary: Once all arrangements have been made, prepare a typed schedule of events and activities, departure and arrival times, phone numbers, etc. Maintain a copy in the office in case the provider needs to be contacted.
   4. Travel is not for the timid. Anything can go wrong and it often does. Always leave ample time for contingencies such as delays, lost confirmations, etc.
B. Speaking engagements
   1. Confirm in writing the place and time of the engagement, as well as the topic to be discussed.

MINUTES OF THE MEETING
CHICAGO MEDICAL SOCIETY

October 14, 20XX
University Hospital, Room 254C

THE CALL TO
ORDER

The monthly meeting of the Chicago Medical Society was held on October 14, 20XX in Room 254C at University Hospital. The meeting was called to order at 7:30 p.m. by President Dr. Lee Wentworth.

ATTENDANCE

The following members were present:

Dr. Ernest Dodd	Dr. Mark Newman
Dr. Brian Frieze	Dr. Peter Schmidt
Dr. Rose Garcia	Dr. Yen Tuo
Dr. Marvin Kaser	Dr. Lisa Twan
Dr. Carol Mason	Dr. Lee Wentworth
Dr. Jane Meyer	

MINUTES READING

Upon motion made, seconded, and unanimously passed, the reading of the minutes from the last meeting were waived.

TREASURER'S
REPORT

The Treasurer reported that the society's bank balance as of October 12, 20XX was $1,254.72. There is one outstanding bill of $62.50 to the University Hospital Catering Service. A motion was made, seconded, and unanimously made to pay the bill.

VICE PRESIDENCY
VACANCY

The next matter of business was obtaining nominations for the office of Vice President. After discussion concerning the elections to be held in December for officers for next year, it was decided that the Treasurer would assume the duties of the Vice President until the elections are held.

MEMBERSHIP
APPLICANTS

Dr. Ernest Dodd of the Membership Committee reported on the three physicians who made application for membership. These included Dr. Galen Becker, Dr. Monica Hover and Dr. Mia Song. Their credentials were presented. A motion was made, seconded, and unanimously carried to admit the three applicants to the society. Dr. Dodd will notify the applicants in writing.

OFFICER
ELECTIONS

A Nomination Committee was formed to meet in two weeks to review the officer nominations. Doctors Kaser, Tuo, and Wentworth volunteered for the committee.

MEMBERSHIP
DUES

A motion was made to increase membership dues by $25.00 for the next year. This was seconded, and unanimously carried to apply the increase for next year.

ADJOURNMENT

Upon motion, the meeting was adjourned at 8:45 p.m.

_____   _____
Recording Secretary   President

Figure 15-1B

Meeting minutes. Delmar/Cengage Learning.

2. Ensure arrangements are made for audiovisual supports, copy services, handouts, display tables, and the like.

3. Honorarium: A gratuitous payment for professional service for which custom or propriety forbids a price to be set. Confirm any honoraria.

C. Flight arrangements

  1. The travel or ticket agent will require the following:

    a. Passenger's name, address, and phone number.

    b. Point of origin and destination.

    c. Departure and return dates.

    d. Preferences: Class, seating, direct or connecting flights, etc.

    e. Method of payment.

  2. Check with the airlines before leaving for the airport in case there are any delays or cancellations.

  3. E-tickets: Electronically generated airline ticket. Perhaps the most convenient ticketing arrangements because, for many airlines, check-in can be done over the Internet or at each airline's electronic check-in machines rather than at the ticket counter. The electronic check-in machine will issue a boarding pass upon completion.

  4. Security: Given the heightened security at airports, a boarding pass is usually required to proceed through security checkpoints. Allow an extra 45 to 60 minutes for security processing.

  5. Exit seating: Such assignments cannot be made at the time of ticket purchase. You must check in at the flight counter and request an exit seat. Your seat assignment will be changed if available, provided you understand, are physically capable, and are willing to carry out emergency evacuation instructions as identified by the airline.

  6. Luggage: Should be checked in at least one hour before scheduled departure. Always keep luggage within sight, because any contraband discovered will be considered your property and may have serious legal consequences.

  7. Always confirm connecting flight information with the agent meeting passengers departing the plane.

D. Ground transportation

  1. Courtesy car: Many major hotel chains will provide transportation services to and from the airport; although there is no fee, gratuities are expected.

  2. If a courtesy car is not available, some major airports may have round-trip taxi service for a fixed, prepaid fee. Generally, you must provide 24-hour advance notice for the place and time of pick up for transportation back to the airport.

  3. Car rental

    a. Car rental agencies require the following:

      (1) Customer's name, address, and phone number.

      (2) Rental dates.

      (3) Valid driver's license.

      (4) Major credit card: Often a specified amount will be held on the card as a security deposit.

    b. Gas consumption: The tank may be filled up before drop-off, or the rental agency will fill the car for a fee that is usually about twice the going price per gallon.

    c. Insurance: Unless your personal or business auto insurance will cover damage and liability expenses, it may be advisable to purchase insurance with the rental for a nominal fee.

    d. Drop-off: Returning the car at an agency site other than the pickup point will result in an extra charge.

    e. If your flight is delayed and arrival is scheduled after closing time, contact the agency for arrangements.

E. Hotel accommodations

  1. Confirm with the provider any preferences regarding hotel amenities such as smoking/nonsmoking, pool, spa, sauna, weight room, restaurant, cable television, etc.

  2. When booking hotel accommodations, the following information will be provided to the hotel clerk:

    a. Provider-customer's name, address, and phone number.

    b. Dates of the stay.

    c. Major credit card number and expiration date to confirm (hold) the room(s). The hotel may hold up to 125% of the expected charges.

    d. Special requests, such as courtesy car pickup, and similar services.

  3. Be sure to obtain the confirmation number as proof of confirmation.

F. Foreign travel

  1. Passport: For travel abroad, a passport is required.

    a. A passport can be acquired at selected travel agencies, major post offices, or from a county clerk.

    b. If the passport is lost, notify Passport Services at the State Department immediately. If abroad, notify the nearest U.S. consulate or embassy.

    c. If the provider travels abroad extensively, request a 48-page passport rather than the 24-page version.

  2. Visa: Written permission to enter a country.

    a. A visa is an endorsement on the passport indicating the traveler has been examined by the proper authorities—usually the local consulate —and is permitted to enter the country.

   b. Because visa applications are at the personal discretion of embassy personnel, it may be advisable to secure the services of a visa agency.

VII. COMMUNITY RESOURCES

A. Counseling services

   1. The MA may have agency names and numbers available as a referral source for patients.

   2. Many counseling agencies will provide services on a weighted scale based on income and ability to pay.

   3. Referral information for the following services is recommended:

      a. Family/marriage.

      b. Behavioral.

      c. Addiction.

      d. Career.

      e. Abuse.

      f. Financial.

      g. Genetic.

      h. Legal.

B. Child Protective Services: The address and numbers of local child protective services should be readily available for making the necessary reports.

C. Emergency Medical Services

   1. In case of emergencies not handled by the clinic, local EMS information should be available as needed.

   2. Keep in mind that not all communities have a 911 responder network, so keep the appropriate numbers handy.

D. Professional organizations: Information such as the name, address, and phone number of organizations important to the practice should be readily available.

   1. American Medical Association.

   2. Local medical society.

   3. Pertinent medical specialty organizations.

   4. American Association of Medical Assistants and local chapters.

   5. American Academy of Physicians Assistants.

   6. American College of Health Care Executives.

   7. State board of medicine and nursing.

   8. American Nurses Association.

   9. Pertinent allied health organizations.

E. Education and training services: A handy reference for local providers of continuing education activities is useful; such agencies may include hospitals, medical suppliers and vendors, pharmaceutical companies, and such organizations as the American Heart Association, and American Red Cross.

F. Employment agencies: Reference information on local employment, professional placement, and temporary agencies may be helpful to fill vacancies.

G. Public health service: Local public health department information should be available for making necessary reports.

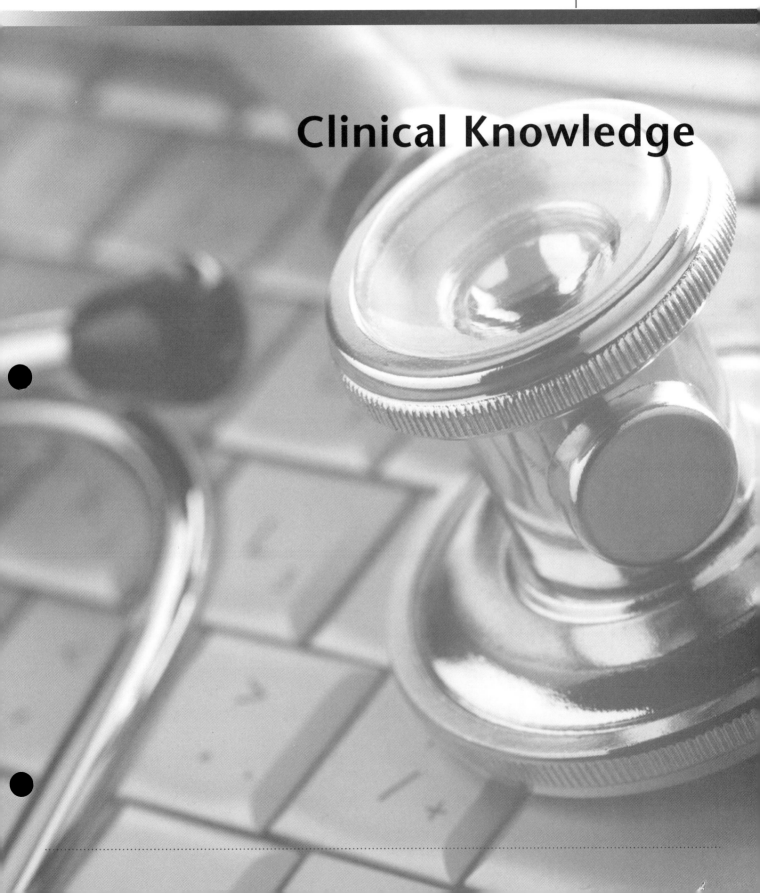

SECTION V

Clinical Knowledge

CHAPTER 16

Diagnostic and Treatment Services

I. THE MEDICAL CHART

A. Introduction
   1. The medical chart is a chronological system for recording each patient's medical care.
   2. Establishing a chart and maintaining its continuity ensures that the patient receives competent, comprehensive medical care.
   3. All patient contact related to medical care, office visits, conversations, and correspondence must be documented in the medical chart.

B. Purpose: To establish a database on each patient consisting of information concerning the patient's life, history, illness, and treatment.
   1. Serves to provide a communication link between the healthcare provider and office staff.
   2. Serves as a document for planning patient care.
   3. Provides evidence of the type and quality of care received by the patient so as to legally protect both the provider and patient.
   4. Provides clinical data for research and education.

C. Content: Depends on the type of practice and the provider's preferences; however, the following is generally included in the chart.
   1. Chief complaint (CC): Primary reason for seeking medical care.
   2. Past medical history (PH/PMH): This document may be prepared by the MA, provider, or patient. Questions relate to usual childhood diseases (UCD), past illnesses, past surgeries, and current health status.
   3. Family history (FH): Includes details regarding the patient's parents and siblings such as health status, age and causes of death, hereditary diseases, etc.
   4. Present illness (PI): Details associated with the chief complaint.

5. Social history (SH): Information regarding personal habits such as exercise, sleep, diet, alcohol/tobacco/drug use, sexual activity, hobbies, etc.
6. Occupational history (OH): Information regarding the patient's employment.
7. Physical examination (PE): A complete physical exam may be performed to assess the status of each body system. This documentation will serve as a base reference for future diagnosis and treatment.
8. Diagnostic and laboratory tests: Test results are usually arranged in reverse chronological order.
9. Consultation reports: Evaluations made by other practitioners at the request of the provider.
10. Past medical records.
11. Correspondence: As related to the patient's care.
12. Provider's notes: Notes written in the chart by the health care provider regarding a patient's diagnoses and treatment.
13. Termination summary: Documents that serve to identify discontinuation of care either by a consulting or primary provider.

D. Organization: The chart's organization will depend on the needs of the practice and the provider's preferences. Two organizational methods are commonly employed:
   1. Source: Medical data are categorized according to its source.
      a. Medical history: Whereby personal and family history may be included or recorded separately.
      b. Progress notes: The first forms presented, directly related to the patient's care, prepared by the health care provider, and arranged in reverse chronological order.
      c. Diagnostic reports: Usually follow the progress notes and may be shingled.
      d. Correspondence: Follows the diagnostic reports.

2. Problem oriented medical record (POMR): Medical data are organized and identified according to disease, situation, or condition.

    a. Database: Includes the patient's history, chief complaint, physical exam findings, and laboratory results. An additional page is prepared for each condition requiring diagnosis and treatment.

    b. Problem list: Consists of physical, psychological, and social problems related to the condition. The chart may distinguish between short- and long-term problem lists.

    c. Plans: Detailed description of diagnostic and treatment measures to include instruction, teaching, and perhaps further evaluations.

    d. Progress notes: Uses the SOAP approach.

       (1) S: *Subjective* data related to the patient's signs, symptoms and feelings as described by the patient.

       (2) O: *Objective* data as determined by the provider's examination and diagnostic tests.

       (3) A: *Assessment* (S+O) describing the provider's impression of the problem and ultimately the diagnosis after considering the subjective and objective data.

       (4) P: *Plan* (S+O+A) of action to solve the problem; may include treatment, medication, consultation, surgery, evaluations, etc.

E. Documentation guidelines

    1. All notations made by the MA should be in ink, dated, and initialed.

    2. All visits and phone calls require a chart notation.

    3. No-show appointments or uncooperativeness should be recorded.

    4. The patient's name and date, at a minimum, should be recorded on each page of the chart.

    5. Errors are never obliterated. Corrections are made by drawing a line through the error and recording the correct data next to it with the date and corrector's initials or signature.

    6. Any correspondence sent to the patient requires a chart notation to include the date of mailing.

    7. Medical activities outside the office as prescribed by the provider require a chart notation.

F. General considerations

    1. The provider should initial or sign documents flagged for review after reading it.

    2. The MA is an agent of the provider and must safeguard both the provider's and patient's rights. In so doing, the integrity of the medical chart must be maintained.

    3. All entries must conform to professional standards such that humorous, sarcastic, or casual remarks be excluded.

4. If progress notes are typed, they should be signed by the provider before filing.

5. The patient may exhibit anxiety when entries are made in the chart. The MA can relieve this anxiety by explaining the purpose of such entries.

6. The contents of the medical record are confidential and privileged information.

7. The patient owns the information contained in the chart, but the provider owns the record. Any information concerning its contents requires consent from both the provider and the patient before its release.

8. Omissions of information can be legally as damaging as improper or false inclusions. If it is not recorded, it was not done.

II. PATIENT HISTORY

A. Introduction

    1. The history is a systematic process of recording relevant past medical data that affects the patient's medical care.

    2. The interview includes written and oral questions to ascertain the patient's health status.

    3. Approaches to obtaining the patient history

       a. The patient history can be obtained by the provider, whereby the patient communicates the information once.

       b. The history can be obtained by the MA, thus economizing the provider's time; however, the patient may have to repeat information when the provider performs the physical exam.

       c. The patient may be asked to complete a self-directed health history questionnaire while awaiting the physical exam.

B. Content of the patient history

    1. Demographics: Name, date of birth (DOB), marital status, children, occupation, education, and social information.

    2. Personal habits: To determine any correlation between the patient's health and lifestyle.

       a. Diet/nutrition.

       b. Weight patterns.

       c. Exercise.

       d. Tobacco, alcohol, and drug use (legal and illegal).

       e. Sleeping patterns.

    3. Family history: The patient is asked to identify the health habits, illnesses, and diseases of parents, siblings, and sometimes grandparents. Time and cause of death of family members may also be required.

    4. Past illnesses: The patient will identify all past illnesses, diseases, surgeries, injuries, childhood conditions, hospitalizations, drug sensitivities, and allergies.

5. Female patients will be asked questions concerning menses, pregnancies, and birth outcomes.
6. Patient statement describing general health.
7. Review of systems (ROS): Questions regarding each of the major body systems and parts.
   a. Head: Aches, pains, and tension.
      (1) Eyes: Pain, vision, strain, drainage, and tearing.
      (2) Ears, nose, and throat: Hearing, pain, vertigo, tinnitus, congestion, hoarseness, swallowing, epistaxis, etc.
      (3) Mouth: Pain, teeth, gums, sores, bleeding, etc.
   b. Cardiovascular system: Palpitations, pain, blood pressure, edema, arrhythmia, etc.
   c. Respiratory system: Shortness of breath (SOB), pain, irregularities, asthma, cough, allergies, etc.
   d. Urinary system: Voiding habits, discharges, pain, frequency, odor, color, etc.
   e. Gastrointestinal system: Diet, weight, pain, indigestion, nausea, vomiting, bowel movements, hemorrhoids, etc.
   f. Menses: Interval, regularity, discharge, cramps, flow volume, etc.
   g. Neurological system: Vertigo, weakness, coordination, tremors, memory, concentration, etc.
   h. Musculoskeletal system: Pain, deformity, mobility, swelling, etc.

C. Obtaining the health history
   1. The attitude of the MA must be professional while exhibiting interest.
   2. The purpose of the interview should be explained.
   3. The MA should be personable and make eye contact, and provide positive feedback.
   4. Remain nonjudgmental.
   5. Use short, direct questions.
   6. Respond appropriately.
   7. Speak in terms the patient can understand.
   8. Mirror the patient's important statements.
   9. Pinpoint vague responses and descriptions: Ask who, why, what, where, and how.
   10. Ask what treatment has been attempted in the past and by whom. What impact does the condition have on the patient's physical, psychological, and social well-being?
   11. Condense the patient's responses into a brief summary.
   12. Where there is poor recall, attempt to place the event in time or sequence.

D. Recording patient information
   1. Most of the information discussed thus far will be recorded in the progress notes.
   2. The patient's descriptions should be converted into proper medical terminology.

3. The MA should quantify as much of the data as possible when appropriate.
4. The MA should use qualitatively appropriate language.
5. The notations should be brief and relevant, avoiding word-for-word descriptions.
6. Patient's feelings, where relevant, should be quoted as much as possible.
7. The MA should not record conjecture or judgmental statements and avoid the use of the word "appears."
8. All notations should be dated and initialed.
9. Collect the following information regarding severe pain:
   a. P: *Provoke* the patient to reveal what seems to cause the pain.
   b. Q: *Quality* of the pain should be elicited; stabbing, dull, throbbing, etc.
   c. R: *Region* where the pain is located.
   d. S: *Signs and symptoms* that accompany the pain such as nausea, redness, swelling, etc.
   e. T: *Time* of onset, frequency, and duration.

E. Common charting terminology: Review also the pathophysiology for each body system in Chapter 5, Anatomy and Physiology, as well as the pharmacological terms in Chapter 18, Pharmacology and Drug Therapy.
   1. Ab: Abortio; abortion.
   2. Abnl: Abnormal.
   3. Abx: Antibiotics.
   4. AD: Auris dextra; right ear.
   5. AS: Auris sinistra; left ear.
   6. AU: Auris unitas; both ears.
   7. AJ: Ankle joint.
   8. AMA: Against medical advice.
   9. A&O: Awake and oriented.
   10. A&P: Auscultation and palpation/percussion.
   11. A/R: Apical/radial.
   12. ASAP: As soon as possible.
   13. AMAP: As much as possible.
   14. ASE: Axilla, shoulder, elbow.
   15. ATR: Achilles tendon reflex.
   16. (B): Both.
   17. Bx: Biopsy.
   18. Cath: Catheterize.
   19. CCE: Clubbing, cyanosis, edema (of extremities).
   20. CHD: Childhood diseases.
   21. CIG: Cigarettes.
   22. C/O: Complains of.
   23. COD: Cause of death.
   24. CPE: Clubbing and pitting edema (of extremities).
   25. CXR: Chest X-ray.
   26. D/C: Discontinue.
   27. Ddx: Differential diagnosis.
   28. DOA: Dead on arrival.

29. DOB: Date of birth.
30. DOC: Date of conception.
31. DRE: Digital rectal exam.
32. DTR: Deep tendon reflexes.
33. EENT: Eye, ear, nose, throat.
34. EOMI: Extraocular movements intact.
35. F/U: Follow up.
36. Fx: Fracture.
37. G&D: Growth and development.
38. GRAV: Gravida; pregnancy.
39. GSW: Gunshot wound.
40. HCM: Health care maintenance.
41. H/O: History of.
42. H&P: History and physical.
43. I&D: Incision and drainage.
44. I/O: Input and output (urine).
45. IOP: Intraocular pressure.
46. JVD: Jugular venous distension.
47. (L): Left.
48. LBP: Low back pain; low blood pressure.
49. LBW: Low birth weight.
50. LMP: Last menstrual period.
51. (M): Murmur.
52. NKA: No known allergies.
53. OD: Oculus dextra; right eye.
54. OS: Oculus sinistra; left eye.
55. OU: Oculus unitas; both eyes.
56. PARA: Live, viable births.
57. PERRLA: Pupils equal, round, and reactive to light and accommodation.
58. PP&A: Palpation, percussion, and auscultation.
59. PPD: Packs per day (cigarettes).
60. (R): Right.
61. ROM: Range of motion.
62. SOB: Shortness of breath.
63. SUD: Sudden unexplained/unexpected death.
64. Sz: Seizure.
65. T&A: Tonsillectomy and adenoidectomy.
66. T&T: Tone and turgor.
67. UCD: Usual childhood diseases.
68. V&V: Vulva and vagina.
69. Y/O: Year(s) old.

III. ASEPSIS AND INFECTION CONTROL

A. Handwashing
   1. Appropriate handwashing is the most important defense against disease transmission.
   2. Use a surgical scrub containing chlorhexidine.
   3. Proper handwashing requires both friction and running water.
   4. Hands should be washed between patients, after handling laboratory specimens, before and after using the bathroom, after touching contaminated materials, and before leaving the lab or clinic.
   5. Procedure
      a. Remove all jewelry except wedding bands.
      b. Adjust the water temperature to lukewarm and allow your hands to get completely wet; apply soap from a dispenser and lather while keeping the fingers pointed downward toward the drain. Do not allow your hands to come into contact with the sink while washing.
      c. Rub, using friction, between fingers and over hands for 30 seconds.
      d. Rinse so that the water flows from the wrist downward to the fingertips.
      e. Apply soap and scrub for an additional 15 seconds; rinse as before. Inspect for cleanliness.
      f. If the faucet is not foot-operated, turn the faucet off with a paper towel and discard the towel. Dry hands with a new paper towel and discard.
B. Sanitization: Process of cleaning or freeing materials, especially instruments, from dirt. Requires scrubbing materials with brushes and detergents.
   1. Detergents: Wetting agents that mechanically remove bacteria, emulsify fats and oils, as well as dissolve high protein substances such as blood.
   2. Ultrasound: Instruments may be placed in an ultrasonic bath containing a detergent solution. The ultrasonic bath is a device that passes sound waves through the liquid causing vibration which loosen contaminants, blood, and dirt.
   3. Antiseptics: Agents of sanitization used on the skin.
C. Disinfection: Process of removing infectious material from selected objects.
   1. Chemical: Surface germicides used on inanimate materials that are sensitive to heat.
      a. Soap: Mechanically removes some infectious material such as bacteria, but does not generally destroy them unless it contains a germicide.
      b. Alcohol: Isopropyl alcohol is commonly used on skin as it has some germicidal properties; iodine sometimes added for strength.
      c. Acids: Phenol is an excellent germicidal.
      d. Alkalies: 10% sodium hypochlorite (bleach) is commonly used on laboratory surfaces and selected equipment.
      e. Formaldehyde: 5% formalin is effective but requires thorough rinsing with water.
   2. Ultraviolet radiation: Ultraviolet light has a germicidal effect on surfaces and airborne microbes, but has no penetrating power.
   3. Desiccation: Drying inhibits bacterial growth and is commonly used as a preservative; spores are highly resistant.

4. Boiling: Kills most bacteria, except some spore-forming bacteria and viruses.

D. Sterilization: Complete destruction of all microorganisms or infectious agents.

   1. Chemical: Agents such as glutaraldehyde may be used for heat-sensitive material, but material must be submerged for extended periods.

   2. Steam under pressure (autoclave): Most common and effective means of sterilization.

   3. Gas: Special sterilization chamber that uses a sterilizing gas and sometimes pressure.

   4. Oven: Dry heat at a temperature and time interval necessary to destroy all microorganisms.

E. OSHA standards

   1. Bloodborne pathogens: Disease-causing microorganisms that may be present in blood or body fluids; principally, hepatitis B virus (HBV) and human immunodeficiency virus (HIV).

   2. Transmission

     a. Bloodborne pathogens are transmitted when blood or an other potentially infectious material (OPIM) comes in contact with mucous membranes, non-intact skin, or by touching or handling contaminated items or surfaces.

     b. Most HIV transmissions have occurred through puncture injuries.

     c. HBV is more persistent than HIV and is able to survive for at least a week in dried blood.

   3. Prevention: There are four strategies for prevention.

     a. Engineering controls: Structural or mechanical devices that are designed to minimize exposure to bloodborne pathogens. Common engineering controls include:

       (1) Handwashing facilities.

       (2) Eyewash stations.

       (3) Sharps containers.

       (4) Biohazard labels.

     b. Work practice controls: Protocols that promote the behaviors necessary to properly use engineering controls.

     c. Personal protective equipment: Equipment that minimizes exposure beyond the limits of engineering and work practice controls.

       (1) Lab coats.

       (2) Face shields.

       (3) Gloves.

     d. Standard precautions: Application of the concept that all blood, body fluids, secretions, excretions, and moist body substances are to be treated as if contaminated by medically important pathogens regardless of their actual pathogenicity. Examples of materials requiring the use of standard precautions include:

       (1) Blood.

       (2) Semen.

       (3) Vaginal secretions.

       (4) Cerebrospinal fluid.

       (5) Synovial fluid.

       (6) Pleural fluid.

       (7) Body fluid containing blood.

       (8) Unidentifiable body fluid.

       (9) Saliva.

      (10) Feces.

      (11) Nasal secretions.

      (12) Sputum.

      (13) Sweat.

      (14) Tears.

      (15) Urine.

      (16) Vomitus.

   4. Immunization: All people who have routine occupational exposure to blood or OPIM have the right to receive the immunization series against hepatitis B during normal working hours and at no personal expense.

   5. Exposure control

     a. Engineering and work practice controls: Engineering and work practice controls must be used to eliminate or minimize exposure. Where occupational exposure remains after institution of these controls, personal protective equipment (PPE) must be used.

     b. PPE to be used by the employee, when warranted, is required to be furnished, cleaned, laundered, disposed, and replaced, free of charge.

     c. Contaminated sharps (any contaminated object that can cause a cut or puncture wound) shall be placed in clearly labeled, puncture-resistant, leak-proof containers immediately after use. Bending, shearing, or recapping needles is prohibited.

     d. Biohazard labels will be placed on all devices used to contain blood or OPIM.

     e. Work surfaces and equipment must be cleaned and decontaminated using an acceptable disinfectant.

     f. Contaminated waste, other than sharps, shall be placed in biohazard waste containers located in each laboratory.

     g. Contaminated laundry will be placed in a biohazard marked *Laundry bag for decontamination.*

     h. The above controls will be periodically evaluated.

   6. Postexposure evaluation and follow-up: When an employee incurs an exposure incident, it must be reported to that person's supervisor and properly followed up.

IV. VITAL SIGNS AND ANTHROPOMETRY

A. Introduction
1. Vital signs, also known as cardinal signs, are measurements that indicate the state of health of the human body (fr. L. *vita* meaning life).
2. Together with the results of the patient history, physical exam, laboratory, and other diagnostic tests, vital signs enable the provider to determine a diagnosis.
3. Vital signs include temperature, pulse, respiration, and blood pressure (TPR, BP).

B. Temperature (T)
1. General
   a. Temperature reflects the balance between heat loss and heat production. Heat gain is generated through a process known as metabolism.
   b. Illness upsets the metabolic process disturbing the amount of heat that is produced. Most diseases increase metabolism.
   c. Some disorders, however, decrease body temperature such as syncope, dehydration, and CNS injury.
   d. Periods of growth also increase metabolism and therefore body temperature.
      (1) Children generally have a slightly higher body temperature because of growth and because their bodies have less surface area to release heat.
      (2) There is an inverse relationship between body size and metabolic rate.
   e. Heat is regulated via skin receptors and the hypothalamus. As the body overheats, the nervous system sends signals to release perspiration in the skin and to dilate superficial blood vessels to release heat.
   f. Temperature conversion formula
      (1) C to F: (C × 9 ÷ 5) + 32 = F
          For example: (37°C × 9 ÷ 5) + 32 = 66.6 + 32 = 98.6°F
      (2) F to C: (F − 32) × 5 ÷ 9 = C
          For example: (102°F − 32) × 5 ÷ 9 = 70 × 5 ÷ 9 = 38.9°C
2. Factors affecting body temperature
   a. Age
      (1) Infants = 97.7 to 99.5°F, 36.5 to 37.5°C.
      (2) Old age = below 97°F.
   b. Environment: Length of exposure, humidity, temperature, and windchill.
   c. Activity: Physical activity increases temperature.
   d. Diurnal variation: Normal variations throughout the day; lowest in the morning.
   e. Emotional state: Depression decreases temperature; agitation increases temperature.
   f. Physiological processes: e.g., digestion, pregnancy, ovulation, and hormonal activities.
3. Normal temperature
   a. Oral: 97 to 99°F, 36 to 37.8°C.
   b. Rectal: One degree F higher than oral.
   c. Axillary: One degree F lower than oral.
4. Fever characteristics
   a. Fever (pyrexia or hyperthermia) is a temperature over 100°F. It can be caused by infection, brain tumors, and hyperthyroidism. Untreated high fevers (≥ 105°F, 40.5°C) can cause brain damage or death.
   b. Febrile: Having a fever.
   c. Afebrile: Without a fever.
   d. Onset (invasion): Period when fever began.
   e. Continuous: Relatively constant elevated temperature.
   f. Defervescence: Fever subsides.
   g. Intermittent: Fluctuation between normal/subnormal and fever.
   h. Remittent: Elevated fluctuations not returning to normal.
   i. Subsiding: Phase during which temperature is returning to normal.
   j. Lysis: Gradual return of elevated temperature to normal.
   k. Crisis: Sudden return of elevated temperature to normal.
5. Thermometer: Instrument used to measure temperature; calibrated in either Fahrenheit or Celsius (centigrade) (see Figures 16-1A to D). *[Federal legislation has been proposed to ban the sale of mercury thermometers, except by prescription, and to provide federal monies for the exchange of the thermometers at the state and local levels. In many states, the sale of such thermometers has already been prohibited and arrangements provided for proper disposal of these instruments. However, there remains the possibility that an examination question could be presented in reference to these thermometers.]*
   a. Oral thermometers: Have a long slender bulb and are either placed under the tongue (sublingual) or in the axilla. Color coded blue.
   b. Rectal thermometers: Have a shorter, blunter bulb to prevent rectal injury or perforation. Color coded red.
   c. Security bulb thermometer: Has a shatterproof encasement to prevent breakage and is used for disoriented patients.
   d. Electronic thermometers: Consist of a stylus that is covered with a disposable plastic sheath. The temperature is displayed digitally.
   e. Aural (tympanic) thermometer: Placed in the ear to measure the temperature

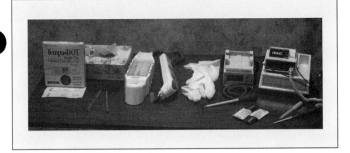

Figure 16-1A

Different types of thermometers. Delmar/Cengage Learning.

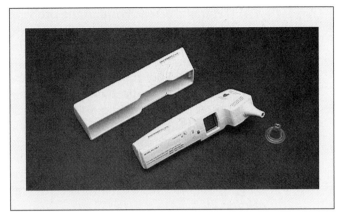

Figure 16-1C

Aural (tympanic) thermometer. Delmar/Cengage Learning.

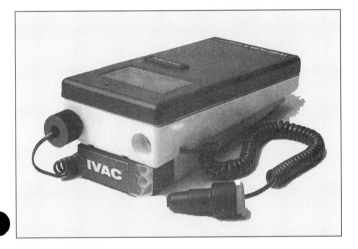

Figure 16-1B

Electronic thermometer. Delmar/Cengage Learning.

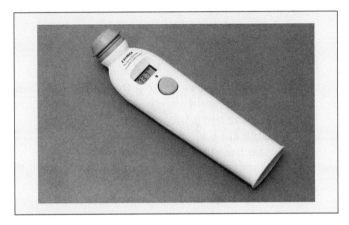

Figure 16-1D

Temporal artery thermometer. Delmar/Cengage Learning.

immediately by picking up infrared energy from the tympanic membrane; is especially handy for children.

   f. Temporal artery (TA) thermometer: Measures the temperature of the skin surface over the temporal artery. A probe is slid across the midline of the patient's forehead, whereafter the temperature is digitally displayed.

6. Care of the glass thermometer

   a. Breakage should be handled with thorough and careful cleanup as mercury is toxic.

   b. Cleaning and disinfecting

     (1) Wipe with dry gauze, cotton, or paper towel.

     (2) Wash in cool sudsy water and rinse in cool water. Dry thoroughly.

     (3) Immerse in 70% methanol, isopropyl alcohol, or benzalkonium chloride (Zephiran) for at least 20 minutes. Rinse under cool water.

     (4) Store in container with gauze fitted at the bottom. Oral and rectal thermometers are kept separate and labeled.

     (5) If stored in solution, rinse with cool water and shake mercury down around 94°F.

7. When recording the patient's temperature, indicate whether it was oral (O), rectal (R), or axillary (A).

8. Procedure

   a. Observe standard precautions; wash hands; identify the patient.

   b. Shake the thermometer down to around 95°F; place a sheath over the thermometer.

   c. Appropriately place the thermometer.

     (1) Oral: Place under the patient's tongue; instruct patient to close lips around thermometer and breathe through the nose. Keep in place for 5 minutes.

     (2) Axillary: Wipe the axilla dry; place the thermometer under the armpit for 10 minutes.

     (3) Rectal: Apply lubricating gel to the thermometer; insert into the rectum 0.5 inch for infant, 1 inch for children, and 1.5 inches for adults and keep in place 2 to 3 minutes.

(4) Temporal artery: Position the probe at the midline of the forehead. Keeping the probe in contact with the skin, press and hold the scan button while slowly sliding the probe across the forehead until reaching the hairline. When the scan is complete, release the scan button and lift the probe off the skin. Note the reading and record.

d. Remove the thermometer and wipe dry; make the reading and record (see Figure 16-2).

e. Rinse the thermometer, sterilize, and store according to clinic protocol; clean up.

C. Pulse (P)

1. General
   a. The rate and characteristics of the pulse provide clues as to the condition of the cardiovascular system.
   b. The pulse is defined as the wave of alternating expansion and relaxation of the arterial walls with each contraction of the left ventricle.
   c. Normally the pulse in any of the arteries will be the same as the heartbeat.

2. Factors affecting pulse
   a. Disease
      (1) Pain, atherosclerosis, hyperthyroidism, infection, and fever will increase the pulse rate.
      (2) Hypothyroidism, mental depression, chronic pain, and CNS disorders may decrease the pulse rate.
   b. Age: Increasing age makes the heart less efficient, thus reducing cardiac output.
   c. Physical activity
      (1) Exercise will increase the pulse rate.
      (2) Certain postures may decrease the pulse rate.
   d. Emotional status: Agitation increases pulse; depression may decrease it.
   e. Medications: May have either effect.

3. Pulse characteristics
   a. Rate: Number of beats per unit time, usually a minute.
      (1) Infants = 100 to 160/min
      (2) 1 to 7 years = 80 to 120/min
      (3) 7 to 12 years = 80 to 90/min
      (4) 12 years and older = 60 to 100/min
      (5) Elderly = 60 to 90/min
      (6) Athletes = 50 to 70/min
   b. Rhythm: Interval of time between beats (tempo).
   c. Volume: Force or strength of the pulse.
   d. Texture: Texture of the arterial wall should be smooth and soft.

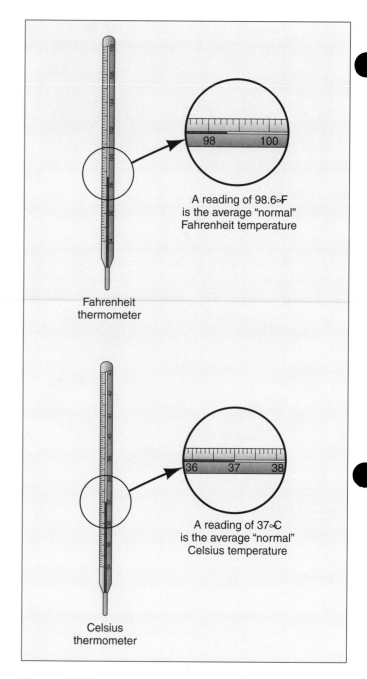

Figure 16-2

Fahrenheit and Celsius thermometers. Delmar/Cengage Learning.

4. Arrhythmias/dysrrhythmias: The absence of rhythm; irregular.
   a. Tachycardia: Rapid pulse > 100/min.
   b. Bradycardia: Slow pulse < 60/min.
   c. Extrasystole: Extra contraction commonly described as a skipped beat.
   d. Atrial fibrillation: Atrial rate 400 beats/min or more; usually associated with myocardial infarction.
   e. Ventricular fibrillation: Ventricular rate 350 beats/min or more; usually indicates that an arrest is imminent.

5. Pulse sites: The pulse may be taken anywhere on the body where there is a superficial artery that lies over a bone (see Figure 16-3).

   a. Radial: Pulse located at the wrist on the thumb side.

   b. Carotid: Pulse located in the groove of the neck between the trachea and sternocleido-mastoid.

   c. Brachial: Pulse located on the medial arm at the fold of the elbow.

   d. Femoral: Pulse located in the groin region.

   e. Temporal: Pulse located over the temporal bone.

   f. Popliteal: Pulse located at the back of the knee.

   g. Dorsalis pedis: Pulse located on the superior surface of the foot.

   h. Apical: Pulse taken with the stethoscope just below the left nipple. Often performed on infants and cardiac patients.

6. Procedure

   a. Radial pulse

     (1) Wash hands; identify the patient.

     (2) Have patient assume a sitting or lying position.

     (3) Gently compress the radial artery until the pulse is felt.

     (4) If there are no known heart problems and the beat is regular, count the number of beats for 30 seconds and multiply by two; if not, count for 1 minute.

     (5) Make note of rhythm, strength, and arterial elasticity; record findings.

   b. Apical pulse

     (1) Wash hands; identify the patient.

     (2) Have patient assume a sitting or lying position.

     (3) Place a warmed stethoscope under the left nipple at the fifth intercostal space.

     (4) If the beat is regular, count for 1 minute; if irregular, count for 3 minutes and divide by three.

     (5) Make note of rhythm; record findings.

D. Respiration (R)

  1. General

   a. Respiration involves the exchange of the respiratory gases, oxygen, and carbon dioxide. One cycle of respiration consists of one inspiration and expiration.

   b. Respiration is both internal and external. External respiration involves the exchange of gases between the alveoli of the lungs and the capillaries. Internal respiration involves the exchange of gases between the capillaries and body cells.

   c. Respiratory control: The center of the brain that controls respiration is the medulla oblongata. The brain controls breathing as determined by the chemical content of the blood, most notably CO_2.

  2. Factors affecting respiration

   a. Disease: Pain, hyperthyroidism, respiratory infections, and fever will increase the respiratory rate.

   b. Age: Increasing age also affects the muscular tone of the diaphragm, thus decreasing the respiratory rate.

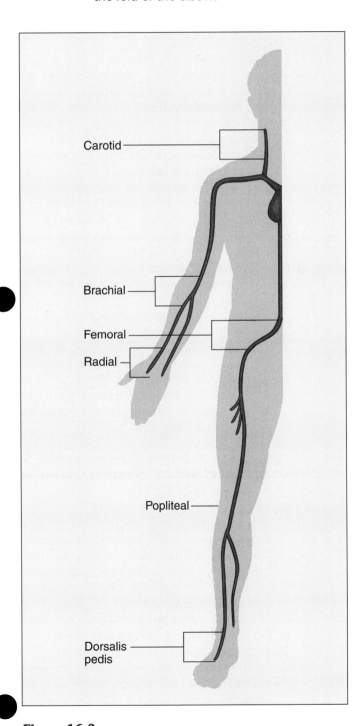

Figure 16-3

Pulse sites. Delmar/Cengage Learning.

c. Physical activity: Increases the respiratory rate.

d. Emotional status: Agitation and/or excitement increases respirations whereas depression decreases the rate.

e. Medications/drugs: May have either effect.

f. Body position: May have either effect depending on the respiratory status of the individual patient.

3. Characteristics of respiration

a. Normal rate
   (1) Newborn   = 30 to 80
   (2) 1 to 6 years = 20 to 40
   (3) 7 to 14 years = 15 to 25
   (4) Adults   = 12 to 20

b. Rhythm: Regular and even is normal. Respiratory rhythm is normally irregular in children.

c. Depth: Air volume inhaled and exhaled.

d. Audibility: Not easily audible except snoring.

4. Breathing patterns

a. Eupnea: Normal breathing.

b. Dyspnea: Difficult, labored breathing.

c. Apnea: Temporary cessation of breathing.

d. Orthopnea: Difficulty breathing in positions other than upright.

e. Hyperpnea: Increased depth of breathing.

f. Tachypnea: Increased rate of breathing.

g. Cheyne-Stokes: Alternating periods of apnea and tachypnea.

h. Rales: Crackling, gurgling breathing sound caused by excretions in the bronchi.

i. Rhonchi: Rattling in the throat as in snoring.

j. Stertor: Laborious breathing as in snoring.

5. Because respiration can be consciously controlled, the respiratory rate should be measured without the patient's knowledge.

6. Procedure

a. So that the patient is unaware of the respiratory rate measurement, the MA, after determining the pulse rate, should continue to act as if taking the pulse.

b. Watch the rise and fall of the chest; count each inhalation and exhalation as one respiration.

c. If respirations are regular, count for 30 seconds and multiply by two; if irregular, count for 1 minute.

d. Note depth, rhythm, and any irregularities; record findings.

E. Blood pressure (BP)

1. General

a. Measuring the BP is common with most visits as hypertension is often asymptomatic.

b. Blood pressure indirectly measures the force of pressure that the blood exerts on the walls of the arteries.

c. Systole: The force of pressure exerted when the heart is contracting is called the systolic phase.

d. Diastole: Pressure exerted when the heart relaxes is called the diastolic phase.

e. Expressed as a fraction: Systolic/diastolic.

2. Normal values (averages)

a. Newborn = 50/30

b. 6 years = 95/62

c. 10 years = 100/65

d. 16 years = 118/75

e. Adult = < 120/80

f. Elderly = 138/86

3. Factors affecting blood pressure

a. Age: As patients age, the elasticity of the blood vessels decreases, resulting in overall higher blood pressures.

b. Activity: During resting states the blood pressure is lower than during exercise.

c. Gender: Males generally have higher blood pressures than females.

d. Diurnal variation: Normal variations throughout the day, usually lower in the mornings.

e. Stress: Usually results in higher readings.

f. Disease and medication: May have either effect.

4. Descriptive terminology

a. Hypertension: High blood pressure; BP $\geqq$ 140/90.
   (1) Essential hypertension: High BP of unknown etiology.
   (2) Secondary hypertension: High BP associated with other disease processes.

b. Hypotension: Low BP; BP < 90/60.

c. Orthostatic hypotension: Temporary hypotension when one moves from a horizontal to vertical position.

d. Pulse pressure: Difference between the systolic and diastolic pressure. Average is 40 mmHg with a systolic:diastolic:pulse pressure ratio of 3:2:1.

5. Physiology of sphygmomanometry

a. The instrument used to measure BP is a sphygmomanometer; either of the mercury column or aneroid type, coming in small, medium, or large cuff sizes. [*Federal legislation has been proposed to ban the sale of mercury sphygmomanometers because of the health risk associated with mercury spillage. Many states have imposed a ban and provided for proper disposal of these instruments.*]

b. External pressure is applied by means of an inflated cuff placed approximately at heart level. Blood circulation in the distal artery ceases. The heart, however, continues to pump blood causing the proximal artery to increase in size.

c. At this point, no sound will be auscultated because the cuff's pressure is greater than that of the artery.

d. When the cuff is gradually deflated, blood will begin to circulate past the cuff. Sound (Korotkoff sounds) can now be auscultated.

e. As the cuff is further deflated, the sound will become fainter until it is no longer heard.

f. The systolic pressure is taken at the point at which the first discernable beat is heard upon auscultation.

g. The diastolic pressure is taken at the point at which the last beat is heard before disappearing.

6. Korotkoff sounds: Five phases of BP sound.
   a. Phase 1: Faint tappings that increase in intensity.
   b. Phase 2: Sounds develop into a squeaking quality.
   c. Phase 3: Crisp sounds that increase in volume (systolic reading).
   d. Phase 4: Sounds become muffled. If phase 4 is to be recorded as well: 120/110/80.
   e. Phase 5: Sounds disappear (diastolic reading).

7. Repeated BP reading in the same arm will increase the BP.

8. Indicate which arm is used for BP: Left or right.

9. Procedure
   a. Observe standard precautions; wash hands; identify the patient.
   b. Palpate the brachial artery at the medial aspect of the antecubital space.
   c. Place the BP cuff snugly around the upper arm with the arrow pointing at the brachial artery, and the lower edge about 1 inch above the elbow.
   d. Close the thumb valve and inflate the cuff smoothly to about 180 mmHg for patients with a history of normal BP; hypertensive patients will probably require a higher inflation pressure.
   e. Firmly place the stethoscope bell over the brachial artery.
   f. Deflate the cuff by slightly releasing the thumb valve until the gauge needle drops 2 mm per second.
   g. Note the gauge reading upon the first beat heard, the systolic reading (see Figure 16-4).
   h. Continue deflating until the last beat is heard, the diastolic.
   i. Fully release the thumb screw to deflate the cuff completely; remove the cuff.
   j. Record the BP; put instruments away.

F. Anthropometric measures
   1. Height
      a. May be measured in inches or centimeters.

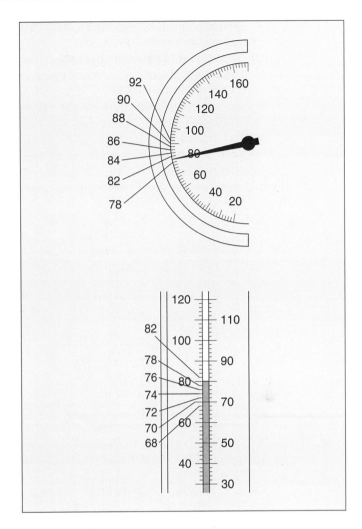

Figure 16-4

Blood pressure reading. Delmar/Cengage Learning.

   b. Procedure
      (1) Identify the patient; explain procedure.
      (2) Place a paper towel on the base of the scale; lift the height bar above the patient's head.
      (3) Instruct patient to remove shoes; assist the patient to step up to face you so that the patient's back is toward the height bar. Have the patient stand erect in the middle of the scale base.
      (4) Lower the height bar until it rests horizontally on the crown of the patient's head.
      (5) Note the height on the scale and record to the nearest one-quarter inch; return the bar to its original position (see Figure 16-5A).

2. Weight
   a. May be measured in pounds or kilograms.
   b. Procedure
      (1) After determining the patient's height, move the large weight to the 50 lb

notch nearest to, but still under the patient's weight.

(2) Move the smaller weight bar to the right until the pointed balance bar floats in the middle of the frame.

(3) Add the large and small weight values together.

(4) Record to the nearest one-quarter pound; return the weights to 0 position (see Figure 16-5B).

3. Skinfold thickness/arm circumference: Measures degree of body fat.

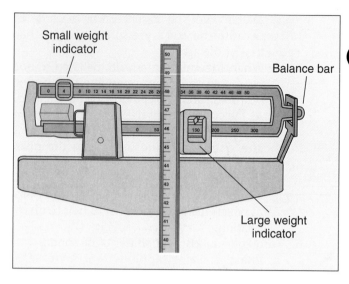

Figure 16-5B

Weight scale markings. Delmar/Cengage Learning.

4. Head, neck, and chest circumference: Often performed on children to monitor growth and development.

V. PHYSICAL EXAM PREPARATION

A. Introduction

   1. The medical assistant prepares patients for examination by gowning, positioning, and draping.

   2. The patient must disrobe and put on a gown that will facilitate performing the procedure by exposing only the body part to be examined.

B. Gowning

   1. Factors to be considered in determining the extent of undress and gowning required are as follows:

   a. The patient's comfort and need for privacy.

   b. The type of examination or procedure to be performed.

   c. The patient's age and gender.

   d. The accessibility of the body part to be examined.

   2. Types of gowns: Gowns can be made of cloth, which must be laundered, or of paper, which is disposable.

   a. Partial gowns: Cover only the shoulders, chest, and back, with street clothing worn from the waist down.

   b. Full gowns: Are at least knee length, with an opening extending the full length of the gown. They are closed by either ties or Velcro strips.

   3. Usually, all clothing is removed (underwear is sometimes an exception). The opening may be worn either in the back or in front, depending

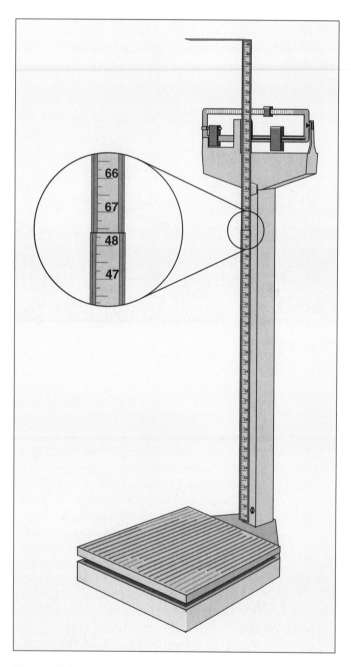

Figure 16-5A

Height scale markings. Delmar/Cengage Learning.

on the provider's preference and the ease of accessibility.

C. Positioning and draping

1. The examination table
   a. Well-padded vinyl table of sufficient width and length to support almost any size patient.
   b. Covered by a sheet of paper that extends the entire length of the table. After each patient, the paper is torn away and replaced from the roll.

2. Positioning (see Figures 16-6A to J):
   a. Explain the reason and procedure for assuming a particular position.
   b. Erect standing (anatomic): The patient stands upright with arms at sides and palms facing forward.
      (1) Used to examine the patient's musculoskeletal and nervous system. The patient may be instructed to bend over, walk, or move specific body parts in a particular manner.

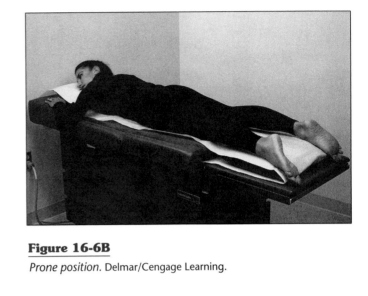

Figure 16-6B

Prone position. Delmar/Cengage Learning.

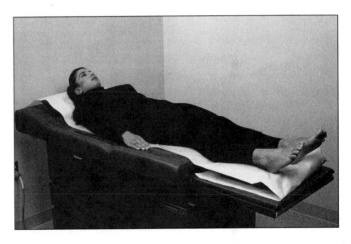

Figure 16-6C

Horizontal recumbent (supine) position. Delmar/Cengage Learning.

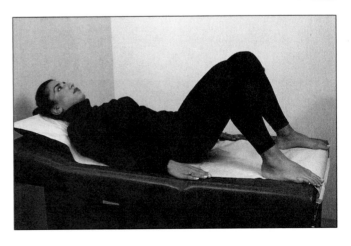

Figure 16-6D

Dorsal recumbent position. Delmar/Cengage Learning.

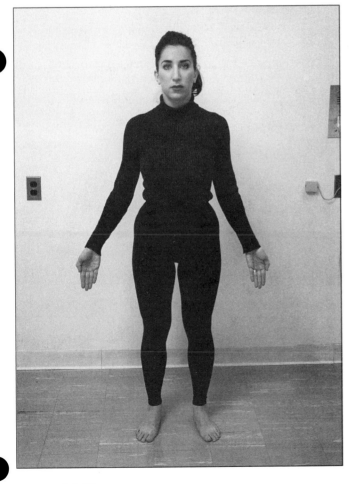

Figure 16-6A

Anatomical position. Delmar/Cengage Learning.

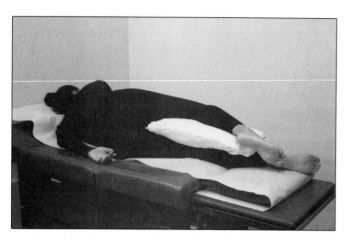

Figure 16-6E

Sims' position. Delmar/Cengage Learning.

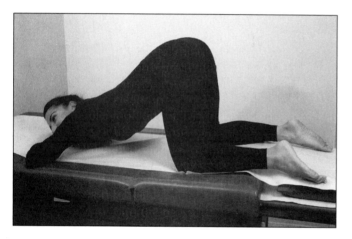

Figure 16-6F

Knee-chest (genupectoral) position. Delmar/Cengage Learning.

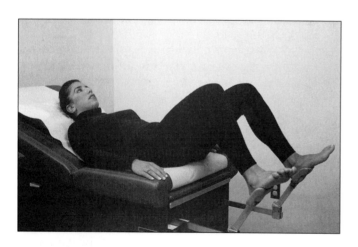

Figure 16-6G

Lithotomy position. Delmar/Cengage Learning.

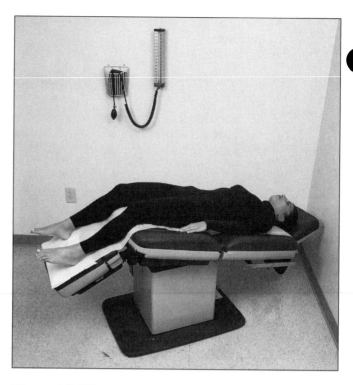

Figure 16-6H

Trendelenburg position. Delmar/Cengage Learning.

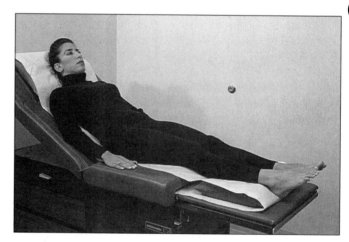

Figure 16-6I

Semi-Fowler's position. Delmar/Cengage Learning.

    (2) Assesses the patient's level of coordination, strength, flexibility, balance, and range of motion.

  c. Sitting: The patient sits upright on the examination table, with legs dangling over the side.

    (1) The patient is covered by a drape sheet across the lap.

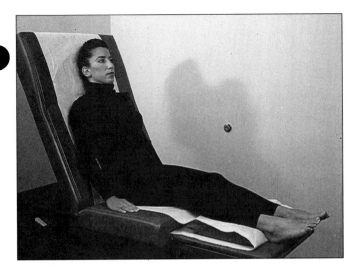

Figure 16-6J

High Fowler's position. Delmar/Cengage Learning.

    (2) The head, chest, back (heart, lungs), front (breasts, axilla), and upper extremities are examined.

d. Supine (horizontal recumbent): The patient is lying flat on the back with arms at the sides and is covered by a drape sheet extending from under the axilla. The chest, heart, abdomen, and extremities are examined.

e. Trendelenburg: Patient lies supine with foot of the table elevated. Draping is same as for supine; used to treat shock, or perform abdominal surgery.

f. Dorsal recumbent: The patient is supine with legs flexed at the knees and the feet flat on the table.

    (1) The drape sheet is placed over the patient in a diamond-shaped fashion with the lateral corners wrapped around each leg. The upper and lower corners cover the chest, abdomen, and the public area.

    (2) The genitals and rectum can be examined.

g. Lithotomy: The female patient assumes the dorsal recumbent posture with the feet placed in stirrups. The patient's knees are flexed, the buttocks are moved to the edge of the table, and the legs are spread apart.

    (1) Position of choice for the vaginal examination, pelvic exam, and the Pap smear procedure.

    (2) Draping is the same as the dorsal recumbent position.

h. Sims' (lateral): The patient lies on the left side with the left arm behind the body and the right arm forward, flexed at the elbow. Both legs are flexed at the knee, but the right leg is sharply flexed and positioned next to the left leg, which is slightly flexed. A drape sheet covers the patient from the breasts to the toes and is adjusted when necessary to expose the anal area.

i. Prone: The patient lies flat on the abdomen with the head turned slightly to the side. The arms can be positioned above the head and extended, or alongside the body.

    (1) The back, spine, and lower extremities can be examined in this position.

    (2) A drape sheet extends from the waist to the knees and is adjusted for adequate exposure when necessary.

j. Knee-chest (genupectoral): The patient assumes a kneeling position with buttocks elevated and head and chest on the table with arms extended above the head and flexed at the elbow. Used for proctologic exams.

k. Proctologic: The knee-chest position is assumed more sharply with the use of a special table. Draping is the same as in the knee-chest position. Proctologic examinations are performed in this position.

l. Jackknife (reclining): The patient lies on the back with shoulders elevated, knees flexed, and thighs flexed at right angles to the trunk. Used when passing a urethral sound.

m. Fowler's: The patient sits on the examination table with the back supported at approximately 90% and the legs slightly flexed on the table. A drape sheet covers the patient's legs; used for patients with dyspneic conditions.

n. Semi-Fowler's: Same as Fowler's except the back is supported at approximately 45 degrees.

3. General considerations

a. The patient should remain gowned and draped with breasts, abdomen, and pelvic area unexposed until the provider actually begins the examination. Only the body part being examined will be exposed.

b. The patient should not remain in an uncomfortable position any longer than is required to complete the examination or treatment procedure.

c. The medical assistant should be alert for ways of increasing the patient's comfort during positioning. Any position can be modified to alleviate the patient's discomfort or to accommodate a weakened or painful body part.

d. Providing the patient with a blanket will increase comfort and prevent chilling.

e. Offering a magazine to read is often appreciated.

f. Measures should be taken to prevent the patient from falling off the exam table.

g. When the medical assistant's absence is unavoidable, a family member should be present.

h. When female patients are examined by male providers, it is prudent for a female medical assistant to remain in the room during the examination to provide legal protection for the provider in the event he is accused of inappropriate behavior.

VI. THE PHYSICAL EXAMINATION

A. General

1. A general examination is normally performed on new patients in order to assess their state of health and establish some comparative base for future visits.

2. Objective: Early detection of disease or the signs indicating the potential for disease.

3. A general physical examination may be performed when the symptoms are not readily associated with a particular system or body part.

4. As a diagnostic tool, the MA must be familiar with the examination process, principles, and methods to prepare the patient and assist the health care provider.

5. Effective diagnosis requires integration of the data from the patient history, physical examination, vital signs, laboratory and diagnostic tests, patient's communications, and the provider's general perceptions.

6. Symptoms: Unobservable conditions and feelings experienced by the patient such as pain or nausea that cause medical treatment to be sought.

7. Signs: Observable characteristics or events, while sometimes noticed by the patient, are noticed by the provider.

B. Diagnostic levels

1. Differential diagnosis: Ruling out certain diseases by comparing them with others having similar signs and symptoms to determine the actual diagnosis; e.g., Rule out (R/O) cholecystitis.

2. Tentative diagnosis (impression): Temporary, working diagnosis that is subject to change as the provider collects additional data from other diagnostic tools; e.g., possible appendicitis.

3. Final diagnosis: The final conclusion the provider reaches after the results of all diagnostic tools have been integrated and evaluated; e.g., Final diagnosis—Amebic dysentery.

C. Examination methods

1. Inspection: Visually observing for abnormalities in size, shape, color, continuity, position, and symmetry.

2. Palpation: Process of touching and feeling to detect abnormalities of movement, size, shape, texture, temperature, and tenderness.

3. Percussion: The percussion hammer, fingers, or knuckles are used to tap body parts, especially the chest and abdomen to evaluate the internal structures based on vibration and sound.

4. Manipulation: Physically moving or probing body parts such as joints to check for abnormalities.

5. Auscultation: Listening to body parts through a stethoscope, especially the heart, lungs, and abdomen.

6. Mensuration: Measurements of body parts, movements, and body fluid constituents.

D. Common equipment (see Figure 16-7)

1. Ophthalmoscope: Instrument used to visually examine the internal eye.

2. Otoscope: Instrument used to visually examine the external and middle ear.

3. Pocket flashlight or headlight: Used to illuminate the mouth, throat, nares, and other body surfaces and orifices.

4. Ruler or flexible tape measure: To measure body structures and anomalies.

5. Tongue depressors: To control tongue movement while examining the mouth and throat.

6. Stethoscope: Instrument used to listen to the sounds emanating from various body parts and cavities.

7. Gloves and lubricant: Used for rectal and pelvic exams.

8. Vaginal speculum: Instrument that when inserted into the vagina allows visualization of the cervix.

9. Reflex hammer: Rubber hammer used to test reflex activity.

10. Tuning fork: Instrument that when struck vibrates to produce sound to test hearing.

11. Miscellaneous supplies: Cotton-tipped applicators, slides, slide fixative, and tissues.

E. Medical assistant role

1. Preparing the patient and the examination room.

2. Handing instruments to the provider and obtaining other instruments and materials as directed.

3. Assisting the patient to assume positions and exposing body areas for examination.

4. Offering the patient reassurance and providing comfort.

5. Preparing and cleaning room for next patient.

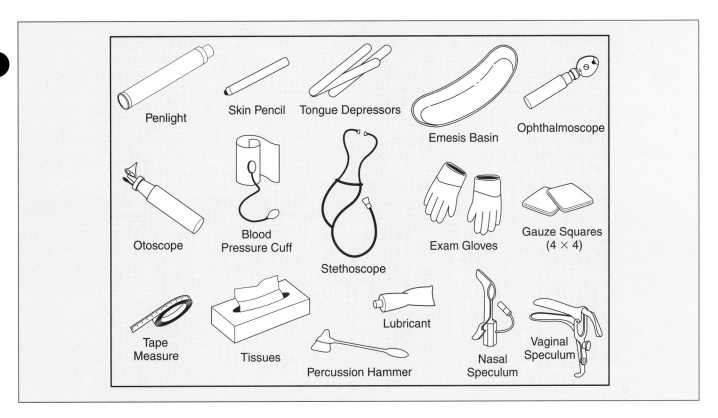

Figure 16-7

Common medical instruments. Delmar/Cengage Learning.

VII. PHYSICAL EXAMINATION PROCESS

A. Examination format: With some variation, this is the typical exam sequence.
1. Health history.
2. Specimen collection: Collection of urine, blood, and other body fluids may occur before the health history or after the physical examination.
3. Vital signs and anthropometric measurements: These usually occur before the health history.
4. Physical examination.
5. Other diagnostic procedures: Spirometry, audiometry, X-ray, ECG, etc. These procedures sometimes occur after the physical examination.
6. Postexam discussion: The provider discusses with the patient the outcome of the examination.

B. General assessment: Using one or all of the examination methods, the provider assesses the general state of health of the body parts and systems.
1. Signs of distress, skin color, stature, posture, motor activity, and gait.
2. Grooming, the presence of odors, facial expression, mood, body language, state of awareness, and speech are noted as the patient is interviewed.

C. Sitting position
1. Head: Examination of the hair, scalp, skull, and face.
2. Eyes: Ophthalmoscope used to examine the fundus and vessels. Visual acuity may also be measured.
3. Nose and sinuses: Otoscope or nasal speculum may be used to examine the nasal passages and sinus cavities.
4. Mouth and pharynx: The lips, interior mucosa, roof of the mouth, gums, teeth, tongue, and pharynx are inspected.
   a. The provider will use a light source and a tongue blade to visualize the pharynx. A laryngeal mirror is sometimes required.
   b. If the medical assistant hands the provider a tongue blade, it is held in the center to allow the provider to grasp either end.
5. Neck: The trachea, thyroid, and cervical lymph nodes are inspected and palpated. The carotid artery is auscultated bilaterally.
6. Back: The spine and muscles of the back are inspected and palpated.
7. Thorax and lungs: The chest wall and the lungs are examined.
   a. The chest is inspected for symmetry, the presence of masses or nipple discharge, and general appearance.

b. The axillary nodes are palpated. A stethoscope is used to auscultate breath sounds.

D. Supine position

1. Breasts: Examined when applicable for masses, nipple discharge, tenderness, etc.

2. Heart: Inspection of the anterior chest to observe pumping action. Auscultation to determine the apical pulse.

3. Abdomen: All exam methods are used to examine the abdomen.

   a. A stethoscope is used to auscultate bowel sounds and abdominal blood vessels.

   b. Inspection is used to determine the symmetry and contour of the abdomen.

   c. Percussion and manipulation is used to outline the borders of abdominal organs, and to detect the presence of air or fluid in the stomach or bowel.

4. Inguinal: Palpated for inguinal nodes and hernia.

5. Male genital and rectal examination: The penis, scrotal contents, prostate, anus, and rectum are inspected and palpated. A rectal examination for both men and women may also be performed while the patient is in the Sims' position.

6. Female genitalia and rectal examination: Examination of the external genitalia, vagina, cervix, and rectum can be accomplished while the patient is in the lithotomy or dorsal recumbent position.

   a. Pelvic examination: One gloved hand, inserted into the vagina, palpates the internal structures while the other hand palpates the external abdomen to examine the uterus, fallopian tubes, and ovaries.

   b. Papanicolaou smear: Use of the vaginal speculum is required to visualize the vaginal wall and cervix. A cervical scraper or brush is used to collect cells and mucus for detection of neoplasms.

   c. A wet mount (prep) is often requested by healthcare providers when vaginal discharge is present to detect the presence of candidiasis (yeast) and/or trichomoniasis (*Trichomonas vaginalis*).

7. Legs: Inspected and palpated; pulse sites are felt to check regularity and volume.

E. Standing position

1. Musculoskeletal system: Range of motion, muscle strength, gait, alignment of the legs, feet, arms, and hands are inspected.

2. Peripheral vascular system: The legs are inspected for varicosities. The femoral, popliteal, and dorsalis pedis pulses are also assessed.

3. Hernia. In men, the inguinal area is again inspected and palpated because a hernia may become pronounced when upright.

4. Neurologic examination: The patient's gait, ability to do knee bends, to hop, to walk on toes and heels, etc., help evaluate the neurological and musculoskeletal systems.

VIII. SPECIALTY EXAMINATIONS

Commonly performed when the patient has received a complete or general physical examination within an appropriate time period (usually 1 to 3 years) or when the patient has been referred to a specialist for a specific problem.

A. Dermatological: Diagnosis and treatment of disorders of the integumentary system.

1. Examination: Skin, hair, and nails are inspected and palpated for color, consistency, texture, erythema, eruptions, irregularities, and tenderness.

2. Diagnostics

   a. Tuberculin skin test: Tuberculosis antibody testing using either intradermal injection (Mantoux) or multipuncture (Tine) methods.

   b. Allergy hypersensitivity testing: Antigenic substances or commonly known allergens are injected intradermally to detect allergies.

      (1) Scratch test: Small scratches are made on the surface of the skin, and known allergens are applied to the scratch marks. If allergic, a wheal will usually form within 30 minutes.

      (2) Radioallergosorbent Test (RAST): Uses radioisotopes to measure the presence of antibodies in a blood sample.

      (3) Multiple radioallergosorbent Test (MAST): Uses an enzymatic detection system in place of a radioisotopes that have been treated with different allergens.

   c. Culture: Scrapings of superficial skin or cultures of wounds and lesions for microscopic examination and identification of organisms.

   d. Potassium hydroxide (KOH) preparation: Scrapings of superficial skin are combined with KOH for microscopic examination and identification of fungi or other microorganisms.

   e. Biopsy: Surgical removal of skin or lesions for microscopic analysis.

3. Treatment applications

a. Wart removal: Performed with cryosurgery using liquid-nitrogen–soaked sterile swabs.

b. Topical applications: Ointments, creams, and jellies.

B. Ophthalmological

1. Examination: Inspection and measurement of external eye, eyelids, accessory structures, eye movements, pupillary distance.

2. Diagnostics

a. Ophthalmoscopy: Using an ophthalmoscope to examine the fundus, vessels, macula, optic nerve, and other structures of the inner eye.

b. Visual acuity: Measures the degree of clarity or sharpness of vision.

(1) Snellen eye test (see Figures 16-8A and B)

(a) A chart composed of 11 rows of letters or objects.

(b) Each row's fraction contains the top number 20 because the test is being conducted at a distance of 20 feet from the chart.

(c) The bottom number signifies the distance at which people with normal acuity can read the row.

(d) If an individual standing 20 feet from the chart can read the row that is normally read at 100 feet, the patient has 20/100 vision in the eye examined.

(e) Each eye is measured as the degree of visual acuity in each may vary.

(f) For children compare the E to a "table with three legs." Children are then instructed to point in the direction the legs are pointing.

(2) Jaeger card: Usually used for testing in optometrists' and ophthalmologists' offices, tests near vision acuity. The patient holds the card approximately 18 inches from the body and is instructed to read the smallest line that can be seen clearly.

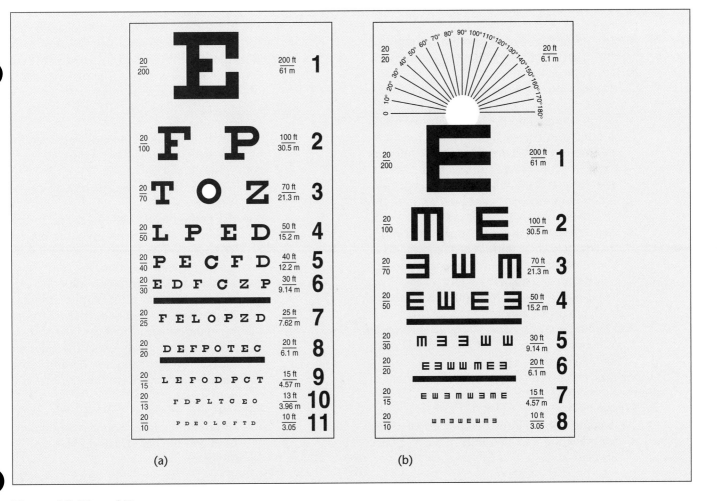

(a)   (b)

Figure 16-8A and B

Eye chart using letters for testing visual acuity. Delmar/Cengage Learning.

c. Retinoscopy: Using a retinoscope to measure the refractive error of children under 6 years old.

d. Ishihara color vision test: Tests the patient's ability to determine and differentiate among colors.

e. Tonometry: Using a tonometer to measure intraocular pressure to diagnose glaucoma.

3. Treatment applications

a. Eye irrigation

(1) Wash hands and don gloves; identify the patient; explain procedure.

(2) Have patient assume a sitting or lying position; drape towel to protect clothing.

(3) Ask patient to tilt head back and to the side with emesis basin placed against the head to catch irrigation solution.

(4) Gently wipe eye from bridge of nose outward with gauze; fill bulb syringe with irrigation solution.

(5) Gently spread the eye open and slowly expel the solution over the eye from its inner to outer canthus, catching the solution in the emesis basin; blot dry with gauze.

(6) Record procedure, noting the solution used and the eye irrigated; clean up.

b. Eye instillation

(1) Allow ophthalmic medications to warm to room temperature as needed; verify by comparing the order with the medication label.

(2) Wash hands and don gloves; identify the patient; explain procedure.

(3) Have the patient tilt back head; gently pull down lower eyelid and ask the patient to look up.

(4) Release the indicated number of drops on the inner portion of the lower lid at the center without touching the dropper to any tissue.

(5) Ask the patient to lightly close the eye for several minutes.

(6) Record procedure, noting the medication, dosage, and eye medicated; clean up.

C. Otorhinolaryngological: Diagnosis and treatment of disorders of the ear, nose, and throat.

1. Examination

a. Ear tenderness may be determined by gently grasping the ear lobe and moving it back and forth.

b. Inserting the otoscope

(1) Adult: Tilt the patient's head back, grasp the auricle gently, and pull it upward and back, to permit complete visualization of the eardrum.

(2) Child: The external canal is shorter and slants at an upward angle so the auricle will be pulled slightly down and back. It is best to insert the otoscope slightly before moving the external ear as outer ear movement affects the shape.

c. The nasal structures, sinuses, and throat will be examined.

2. Diagnostics

a. Otoscopy: Using an otoscope to examine the external ear and the tympanic membrane.

b. Audiometry: Tests hearing acuity using an electronic instrument that produces tones at selected frequencies in hertz (Hz) and intensities in decibels (dB).

(1) Weber test: Evaluates that hearing is the same in both ears.

(2) Rinne test: Compares bone and air conduction by placing a tuning fork on the mastoid bone until the patient no longer feels the vibrations and is then immediately placed near the ear canal to see if any further sounds can be heard.

c. Vestibular tests: Methods of evaluating disturbances in equilibrium. For the Romberg test, the patient is asked to stand with feet together and eyes closed. The patient is then observed for imbalance or swaying.

3. Treatment applications

a. Ear irrigation

(1) Wash hands and don gloves; identify the patient; explain procedure.

(2) Have patient assume a sitting or lying position; drape towel to protect clothing.

(3) Ask patient to tilt head back and to the side with ear or emesis basin placed against the head and under the ear to catch irrigation solution.

(4) Fill syringe with irrigation solution.

(5) Position the ear to straighten the ear canal (described above); place syringe tip in the ear and direct the flow of solution upward; slowly expel the solution into the ear, catching the solution in the basin as it drains from the ear; blot dry with gauze.

(6) Visualize the ear for desired result; record procedure, noting the solution used and the ear irrigated; clean up.

b. Ear instillation

(1) Wash hands and don gloves; identify the patient; explain procedure; verify by comparing order with medication label.

(2) Have patient assume a sitting or lying position; ask patient to tilt head back and to the side.

(3) Position the ear to straighten the ear canal (described above); expel the number of drops indicated without touching the dropper to tissue.

(4) Ask the patient to remain in this position for a few minutes; place a wick (cotton plug) in the ear canal as warranted; record procedure, noting the medication used, dosage, and the ear medicated.

D. Orthopedic: Diagnosis and treatment of musculoskeletal disorders.

1. Examination: Observes for decreased range of motion, swelling, tenderness, decreased or unequal strength, deformities, or growths.

2. Diagnostics

a. Diagnostic imaging: X-ray is commonly used for the diagnosis of fractures. Myelography is used to diagnose intervertebral disk conditions, arthrography for joint conditions, and bone scans for analysis of bone age, density, and growth.

b. Goniometry: Measures joint mobility. The goniometer is an orthopedic protractor calibrated to measure the range of motion of a joint.

c. Electromyography: Records the electrical activity of muscular tissue.

d. Muscle biopsy: Invasive procedure in which a small piece of muscle tissue is obtained for microscopic examination. This procedure is often done to differentiate between myopathic (muscle disease) and neurogenic (nerve origin) disorders.

e. Arthroscopy: Using a lighted instrument to examine the internal structures of a joint.

f. Bone mineral density (BMD): A test to measure how much calcium is in a specific region of the bones; useful because ordinary X-rays cannot detect mild bone loss. A bone must lose a minimum of a fourth of its weight before a regular X-ray will detect the abnormality.

3. Treatment applications

a. Wraps and splints: Cloth, gauze, ace material, and/or rigid materials used to support or immobilize injured limbs and joints.

b. Casting: Application of moldable material (plaster, plastic resin, or fiberglass) that hardens to hold a limb or joint in a fixed position.

(1) Clean and dry affected part.

(2) Cut stockinette material several inches longer than the affected part; gently slip stockinette over the affected limb.

(3) Apply several layers of padding over the stockinette.

(4) Submerge the casting material in water until saturated; squeeze excess water without loss of casting material.

(5) Wrap casting material over the padding; before completing the last few wraps, fold the stockinette and padding material back over the ends of the cast material and complete the wrapping to form soft-padded edges.

c. Physical therapy: The application of physical agents to reduce pain and edema; to increase range of motion and circulation; and to promote healing of injured body parts.

E. Cardiopulmonary: Diagnosis and treatment of heart, lungs, and blood vessels.

1. Examination

a. Listening to the heart with a stethoscope, noting heart sounds, rate, and rhythm.

b. Inspection of the face, nose, and throat and examination of the mucous membranes and visible respiratory system structures.

c. The provider then inspects and palpates the sinuses, neck, lymph nodes, and glands. The lungs are examined with a stethoscope, and the skin, rib cage, and lungs are inspected and percussed.

2. Diagnostics

a. Electrocardiography (ECG): Use of an ECG to measure the electrical activity of the heart.

b. Holtor monitor: Portable ECG recording device that can be worn to record a patient's heart activity over a 24-hour period.

c. Cardiac stress testing: Testing performed by a qualified provider to measure the amount of stress a patient's heart can tolerate before developing dysrhythmia or ischemia.

d. Diagnostic imaging: Chest and sinus X-ray, bronchography, fluoroscopy, angiocardiography, and echocardiography.

e. Throat/sputum culture: Identify pathogenic agents of the throat and secretions.

f. Bronchoscopy: Using a lighted instrument to examine the trachea and bronchi.

g. Pulmonary function tests (PFTs)

(1) Computerized diagnostic tool for measuring lung capacity and assessing pulmonary abnormalities figure (16–9).

(2) Patient should be instructed to withhold bronchodilators and/or nebulizers per the provider's instructions (usually 8 to 24 hours) before testing.

(3) The test should be repeated until three consistent results are obtained for comparison and subsequent interpretation.

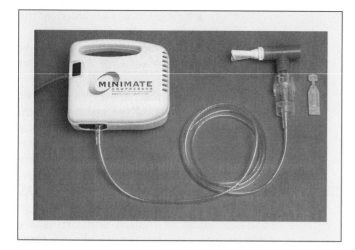

Figure 16-9

Spirometer. Delmar/Cengage Learning.

   h. Peak flow assessment (peak expiratory flow/ PEF)
     (1) Useful, inexpensive tool for asthmatics to assess lung condition at home.
     (2) Meter measures how quickly and easily air is moved out of the lungs.
     (3) Slow and difficult air movement indicates less than optimal lung function and may indicate a need for medication to prevent or lessen an asthmatic attack.
     (4) Measurement often used in providers' offices for screening asthmatic conditions.

F. Gastroenterological
  1. Examination: Direct examination of the mouth, abdomen, and rectum using inspection, palpation, and manipulation.
  2. Diagnostics
    a. Gastric content analysis.
    b. Occult blood (Guaiac): Test for blood in the rectum.
    c. Ova and parasites (O&P): Stool specimens for the detection and identification of intestinal parasites.
    d. Gastroscopy: Using a lighted instrument to examine the esophagus and stomach.
    e. Anoscopy: A cylindrical instrument used to visualize the terminal rectum and anus.
    f. Proctoscopy: Using a lighted instrument to examine the rectum.
    g. Sigmoidoscopy: Using a lighted instrument to examine the sigmoid colon.

G. Urological: Diagnosis and treatment of urinary disorders.
  1. Examination: Palpation of the kidneys and bladder. Inspection and palpation of the external genitalia.

Palpation of the prostate gland through the rectum.
  2. Diagnostics
    a. Diagnostic imaging: Intravenous pyelogram (IVP); Kidneys, ureters, and bladder (KUB) X-ray; CT scan and MRI.
    b. Cystoscopy: Using a lighted instrument to examine the internal bladder.
    c. Cystometry: Measures bladder capacity and intracystic pressure.
    d. Urinalysis: Physical, chemical, and microscopic examination of urine.
    e. Urine culture: Detection and identification of agents causing urinary tract infection (UTI).
    f. Semen analysis: Semen samples may be collected to determine quantity and mobility of sperm.

H. Obstetrics and Gynecological: Diagnosis and treatment of disorders associated with the female reproductive organs and pregnancy.
  1. Examination
    a. Breast: Inspection for asymmetry, misalignment, nipple discharge, erythema, and edema. Palpation for consistency, masses, tenderness, and axillary lymph nodes.
    b. Pelvic: Inspection of the external genitalia, vagina, and cervix; palpation of the Bartholin's glands, bimanual palpation and manipulation of the vagina, cervix, uterus, ovaries, and fallopian tubes.
    c. Rectovaginal: With the middle and index finger inserted into the rectum and vagina, respectively, the posterior pelvic region is palpated.
    d. Prenatal: Initial general, breast, and pelvic exam with periodic visits to monitor fetal growth and development.
  2. Diagnostics
    a. Diagnostic imaging: Hysterosalpingography X-ray.
    b. Papanicolaou smear: Microscopic analysis of the cells and mucus of the cervix is made to diagnose neoplasms.
    c. Colposcopy: A lighted instrument used to provide magnified visualization of the cervix.
    d. Laparoscopy: A lighted instrument inserted into the abdomen through an incision in the umbilicus to examine the abdominal and pelvic organs.
    e. Human chorionic gonadotropin (HCG) tests: Blood or urine pregnancy tests.
    f. Pelvimetry: Caliper device used to measure pelvic size.
    g. Ultrasonography: The use of sound waves to detect abnormal structure and function.

I. Neurological: Diagnosis and treatment of nervous system disorders.
  1. Examination
    a. Mental status survey: Cognitive abilities. Inspection of body posture and general appearance, intelligence, memory, orientation to person, time, and place.
    b. Evaluation of cranial nerves
      (1) Olfaction: Patient is asked to identify common odors.
      (2) Vision: Visual acuity and ophthalmoscopy.
      (3) Pupil motor reaction: A flashlight inspection is made to check pupillary dilation and constriction.
      (4) Palpation of the facial muscles as the patient clenches teeth.
      (5) Sensory: Objects are placed on the face to evaluate the sense of touch.
      (6) Facial motor ability: Observe facial symmetry and movement as the patient is given directions to frown, smile, puff out cheeks, clench teeth, etc.
      (7) Voice: Evaluate for hoarseness, speech, and movements.
      (8) Hearing: Various tones are created to test hearing capabilities.
    c. Motor nervous system: Coordination, muscle strength, and gait are evaluated as the patient is asked to walk, do knee bends, walk on toes, raise hands above head, flex extremities, do finger-to-nose movements. Romberg test.
    d. Sensory nervous system: Arms, trunk, legs. Inspection with pin and tuning fork, cotton balls.
    e. Reflexes: Reflex hammer used to test reflexes of the knees, elbows, ankles, etc.
  2. Diagnostics
    a. Diagnostic imaging: X-ray, CT, and MRI may be used to detect structural abnormalities.
    b. Electroencephalography (EEG): Through electrode placement on the head, the EEG records electrical brain waves helpful in diagnosing epilepsy.
    c. Lumbar puncture: Collection and analysis of cerebral spinal fluid (CSF).

IX. PEDIATRIC CONSIDERATIONS

A. Infant growth and development: Review Chapter 6, Human Development.
B. Growth chart (see Figure 16-10)
    a. A chart to plot the growth patterns of children's weight, height, and head circumference.
    b. The chart identifies statistically what percentile a child's growth falls in.
    c. Percentile increments are usually 10, 25, 50, 75, and 90 percentiles. The average is the 50th percentile.
    d. A 24-month child's weight falling in the 75th percentile means the child weighs more than does 75% of the population at 24 months.
C. The physical exam: Generally similar to a general exam; however, there are two general categories:
  1. Well-child visit: The provider progressively evaluates the growth and development of the child. A physical examination of the child is performed during each well-child visit and is directed toward discovering any abnormal conditions commonly associated with the stage of development reached by the child. The child will also receive any necessary immunizations during these visits.
  2. Sick-child visit: The child is exhibiting the signs and symptoms of disease, and the provider evaluates the patient's condition to arrive at a diagnosis and prescribe treatment.
D. Neonatal health assessment
  1. Apgar scale: Used to assess newborn health. One minute and 5 minutes after birth, the obstetrician or nurse gives the newborn a reading of 0, 1, or 2 on each of five signs.
  2. A high total score of 7 to 10 indicates that the newborn's condition is good; a score of 5 indicates that there may be developmental difficulties; and a score of 3 or below signals an emergency and indicates that survival may be in doubt.
  3. Apgar rating system
    a. Heart rate
      (1) Absent   = 0
      (2) Slow (<100)   = 1
      (3) Fast (100 to 140)   = 2
    b. Respiration
      (1) Absent (>1 min)   = 0
      (2) Irregular/slow   = 1
      (3) Good/normal cry   = 2
    c. Muscle tone
      (1) Limp/flaccid   = 0
      (2) Weak/some flexion   = 1
      (3) Strong/active   = 2
    d. Body color
      (1) Blue/pale   = 0
      (2) Pink body/blue extremities   = 1
      (3) Entire body pink   = 2
    e. Reflex irritability
      (1) No response   = 0
      (2) Grimace   = 1
      (3) Coughing/sneezing and crying   = 2

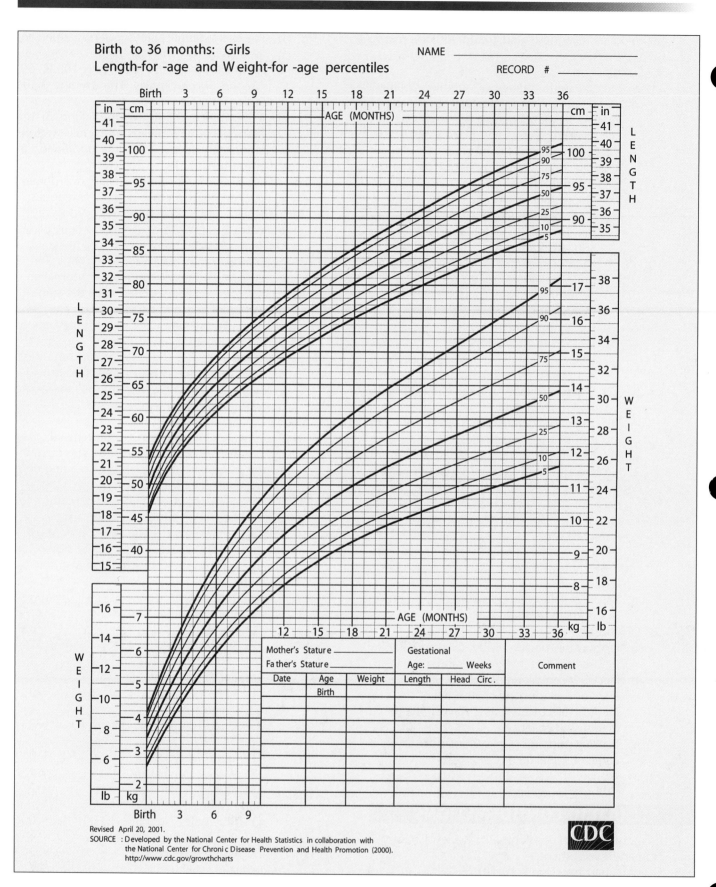

Figure 16-10

Growth chart for boys' height and weight, ages birth to 36 months. Courtesy of the Centers for Disease Control and Prevention.

E. Carrying the infant: The infant should be lifted and carried in a manner that is both safe and comfortable for the infant (see Figures 16-11A to C).
  1. Cradle position: Head rests on crook of one arm, while other arm supports the back.
  2. Football position: Infant is held at waist level with one arm around the infant's body while supporting the back and head.

  3. Upright position: One hand supports the infant's bottom, while the other hand and arm support the infant's head and upper back.
F. Immunizations: See Chapter 18, Pharmacology and Drug Therapy.

X. ELECTROCARDIOGRAPHY

A. Introduction
  1. Heart anatomy and physiology: Review chapter 5 on circulatory system.
  2. Cardiac electrophysiology
    a. The conduction system: Review circulatory system.
      (1) Sinoatrial (SA) node.
      (2) Atrioventricular (AV) node.
      (3) Bundle of His.
      (4) Right and left bundle branches.
      (5) Purkinje fibers.
    b. Two major electrical aspects of the heart
      (1) Automaticity: The heart's ability to generate its own electrical stimulus.
      (2) Conductivity: The ability of cardiac cells to receive a stimulus from a neighboring cell and pass it to the next cell, causing a wavelike motion to create a contraction.
  3. Electrical states
    a. Polarization: Cardiac cells are in a resting, negatively charged state.
    b. Depolarization: Cells are discharging a positively charged electrical impulse to create a contraction.

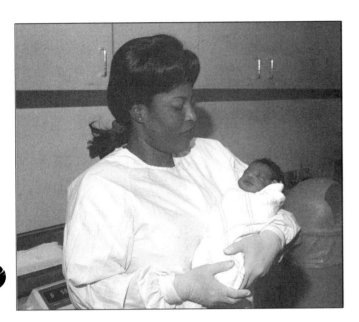

Figure 16-11A

Cradle hold. Delmar/Cengage Learning.

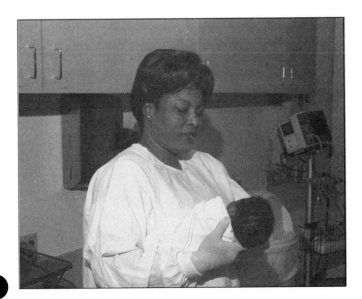

Figure 16-11B

Football hold. Delmar/Cengage Learning.

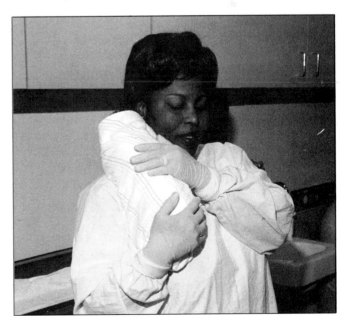

Figure 16-11C

Upright hold. Delmar/Cengage Learning.

c. Repolarization: Transformation of cells from a depolarized (active) to polarized (resting) state for recharging.

4. Cardiac electrical activity generates, via automaticity, and spreads, via conduction, through the heart, creating an electrical wave that can be measured with an ECG.

B. Normal ECG and heart anatomy

1. All beats appear as a similar pattern, equally spaced, comprising three major units: P wave, QRS complex, and T wave (see Figure 16-12).

   a. ECG waves: Each beat comprises five major waves: P, Q, R, S, and T.

   b. P wave: Reflects the impulse emanating from the atria.

   c. QRS complex: The Q, R, and S wave, as a unit, reflects the impulse passing through the ventricles.

   d. T wave: Reflects repolarization of the ventricles.

2. ECG wave increments

   a. Isoelectric line (baseline or zero-voltage line): The point on the ECG wave where no (upward or downward) deflection is present indicating no electrical activity (voltage).

   b. Wave: Any upward or downward deflection from the isoelectric line.

   c. Segment: Lines between waves; distance between selected wave marks, but not including them; e.g., the ST segment is the distance between the S and T waves, but not including the S or T wave.

   d. Interval: Lines that contain waves; distance covering the beginning of one wave mark to the end of a second wave mark; e.g., the PR interval is the distance between the beginning of the P wave to the end of the R wave.

   e. Complex: Any arrangement of the QRS waves or PQRST waves in their entirety.

3. P wave: The first upward deflection representing atrial depolarization (atrial contraction).

   a. Normal P wave: Three small blocks high and wide or fewer.

   b. Enlarged P wave: Found in mitral stenosis or chronic obstructive pulmonary disease, which would cause atrial hypertrophy.

4. PR interval: Extends from the beginning of the P wave to the onset of the QRS. It represents conduction of the impulse through the atria from the SA to the AV node.

   a. Normal: Three to five small blocks wide (0.12 to 0.20 second).

   b. Lengthened PR interval: Seen when the impulse is forced to travel at a slower rate, which can occur in arteriosclerosis, inflammation, insufficient oxygen supply, or

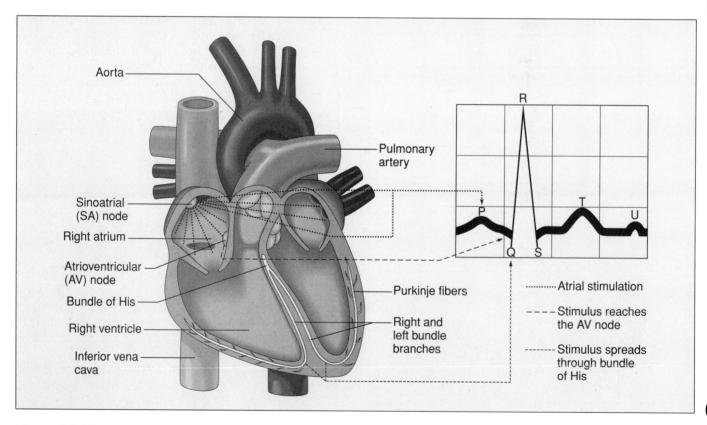

Figure 16-12

Normal ECG wave pattern. Delmar/Cengage Learning.

scarring from rheumatic heart disease. It can also occur as an effect of depressant drugs or digitalis.

5. QRS complex
   a. Consists of three deflections
      (1) Q wave: The downstroke before the R wave.
      (2) R wave: The first upward deflection.
      (3) S wave: The downstroke following the R wave.
   b. Not every QRS complex shows a discrete Q, R, and S wave, but the configuration is still referred to as the QRS complex to denote a ventricular impulse. It represents transmission of the impulse from the AV node to the Purkinje fibers.
   c. Normal: Duration is 2.5 small squares or fewer (0.10 second).
   d. Enlarged Q wave: Over a small square wide or greater in depth than one-third the height of the QRS complex may indicate a myocardial infarction.
   e. Tall R wave: Usually indicates enlarged ventricles.

6. ST segment
   a. The ST segment begins at the end of the S wave (the point where the line turns right) and ends at the beginning of the T wave. It represents the transition from ventricular depolarization to repolarization.
   b. ST elevation: Seen in an acute myocardial infarction or muscle injury.
   c. ST depression: Seen when the heart muscle is not getting a sufficient supply of oxygen, or as an effect of digitalis; usually transient.

7. T wave
   a. Represents electrical recovery (repolarization) to allow cells to recharge in preparation for ventricular depolarization (contraction).
   b. Normal: No more than 10 small blocks (10 mm) high in the precordial (chest) leads and five small blocks (5 mm) high in the remaining leads.
   c. Flat/inverted T wave: Seen in response to ischemia, position change, food intake, or certain drugs.
   d. Elevated T wave: Seen when the serum potassium is elevated.

8. QT interval
   a. Represents the time from the beginning of the Q wave (downward deflection following the P wave) through the QRS and the T wave. It includes the time until the T wave is completed (goes back to the baseline). It demonstrates the impulse from the beginning of ventricular contraction to complete recovery.
   b. Normal: Should be less than one-half of the R-R interval (from the peak of one R wave to the peak of the next R wave).
   c. Prolonged QT interval: Drugs such as quinidine, procainamide hydrochloride (Pronestyl) and disopyramide phosphate (Norpace) can prolong the QT interval predisposing one to ventricular tachycardia.
   d. A prolonged QT time presents an extended opportunity for stray impulses to excite the heart tissue and trigger dangerous ventricular rhythms.

9. U wave: Small upward deflection following the T wave. It is seldom present, but may occur when the serum potassium level is low.

10. Rest period: Following the U wave the stylus returns to the baseline representing no electrical activity (polarized state) or rest period between beats.

C. ECG leads
   1. Electrical flow in the heart is measured by externally applied electrodes relative to a direct line, called an axis, between two poles.
   2. A lead comprises one negative pole, one positive pole, and one ground.
   3. Leads create an electrical picture of the heart taken at different angles.
   4. Sensors (electrodes): Uses 10 sensors—4 limb sensors and 6 chest to create 12 leads.
   5. Limb leads: Six of the 12 leads are called limb leads.
      a. Bipolar (standard) limb leads: Measures cardiac electrical activity between two extremities; between a negative and positive electrode (pole) (see Figure 16-13A).
         (1) Lead I: Measures electrical activity from the right arm to the left arm (RA to LA).
         (2) Lead II: From right arm to left leg (RA to LL).
         (3) Lead II: From left arm to left leg (LA to LL). The right-leg position is not displayed as part of the flow of current through the heart, as it is used for grounding the system.
      b. Unipolar (augmented) limb leads: Measures electrical activity between the heart and one extremity. Each lead measures activity from the posterior heart to the positive pole (the positive electrode) on the anterior chest (see Figure 16-13B).
         (1) aVR: Augmented vector right-side.
         (2) aVL: Augmented vector left-side.
         (3) aVF: Augmented vector foot (left).
      c. Limb lead electrodes are applied to the patient's extremities.

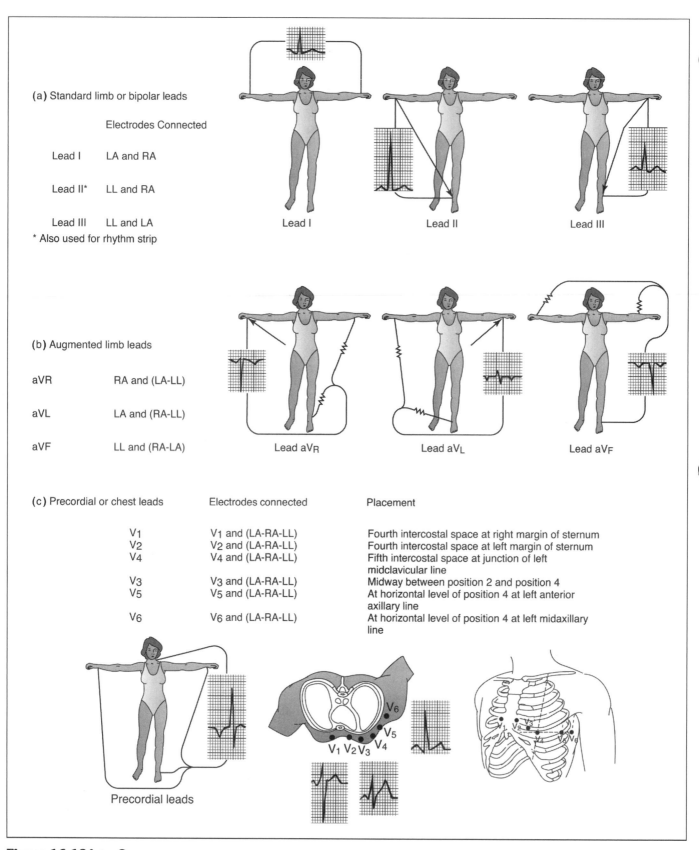

(a) Standard limb or bipolar leads

Electrodes Connected

Lead I   LA and RA

Lead II*   LL and RA

Lead III   LL and LA
* Also used for rhythm strip

Lead I   Lead II   Lead III

(b) Augmented limb leads

aVR   RA and (LA-LL)

aVL   LA and (RA-LL)

aVF   LL and (RA-LA)

Lead aV$_R$ Lead aV$_L$ Lead aV$_F$

(c) Precordial or chest leads

	Electrodes connected	Placement
V$_1$	V$_1$ and (LA-RA-LL)	Fourth intercostal space at right margin of sternum
V$_2$	V$_2$ and (LA-RA-LL)	Fourth intercostal space at left margin of sternum
V$_4$	V$_4$ and (LA-RA-LL)	Fifth intercostal space at junction of left midclavicular line
V$_3$	V$_3$ and (LA-RA-LL)	Midway between position 2 and position 4
V$_5$	V$_5$ and (LA-RA-LL)	At horizontal level of position 4 at left anterior axillary line
V$_6$	V$_6$ and (LA-RA-LL)	At horizontal level of position 4 at left midaxillary line

Precordial leads

Figure 16-13A to C

Lead types, connections, and placement: (a) Standard limb or bipolar leads, (b) Augmented limb leads, (c) Precordial or chest leads.
Delmar/Cengage Learning.

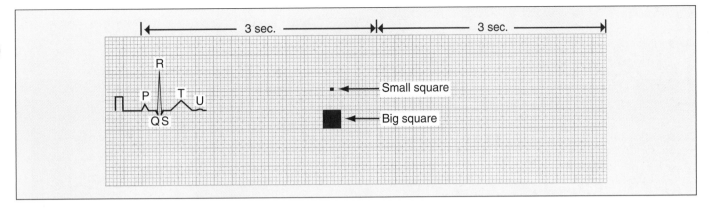

Figure 16-14A

ECG paper indicating the sizes of squares and a cardiac cycle. Delmar/Cengage Learning.

6. Precordial (chest) leads (see Figure 16-13C).
   a. Six unipolar chest leads that require a combination of electrodes from the extremities to represent one pole (at the posterior heart).
   b. The positive electrode is then attached to the anterior chest in six specified locations.
   c. The precordial leads provide points of reference across the chest wall. They differentiate right-sided and left-heart events.
   d. Lead V_1: Electrode is placed at the fourth intercostal space just to the right of the sternum.
   e. Lead V_2: Fourth intercostal space just to the left of the sternum.
   f. Lead V_4: Electrode is placed at the left midclavicular line in the fifth intercostal space.
   g. Lead V_3: Electrode is placed at the line midway between leads V_2 and V_4.
   h. Lead V_5: Electrode is placed at the anterior left axillary line at the same level as V_4.
   i. Lead V_6: Electrode is placed at the left midaxillary line at the same level as lead V_4.
7. Each of the 12 leads has a unique individual axis. Any lead may be used to monitor cardiac activity for the occurrence of arrhythmias.
8. The most important leads in relation to the anatomy of the heart are:
   a. V_1, AVR: Right side of heart.
   b. V_2, V_3, V_4: Transition between right and left sides of heart.
   c. V_5, V_6, I, AVL: Left side of heart.
   d. II, III, AVF: Inferior heart.
9. The area of pathology shown on the ECG can be localized by analyzing tracings from different leads. For example, if an infarct shows up on leads II, III, and AVF only, it is located in the inferior aspect of the heart.
D. Electrocardiograph (Figure 16-14A and B)
   1. ECG paper: The ECG presents a visible record of the heart's electrical activity by means of a heated stylus that traces the activity on a continuously

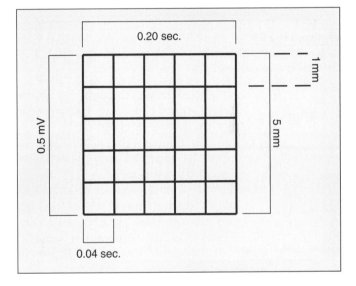

Figure 16-14B

Section of ECG paper enlarged. Delmar/Cengage Learning.

moving strip of special heat-sensitive paper (see Figures 16-15A and B).
   a. Composed of 1 mm squares where every fifth line is darkened creating large blocks of five small blocks high and five wide.
   b. Cardiac voltage is measured on the vertical scale and time on the horizontal.
   c. Horizontally, each large block represents 0.2 seconds; whereas vertically it represents 0.5 millivolts of electricity.
   d. The paper moves through the ECG machine at the rate of 1 inch per second (standard setting).
2. ECG control panel
   a. Main power switch: Turns the instrument on and off.
   b. Record switch: Controls amplifier and paper drive.
      (1) Amp off: Places instruments in standby mode. In some models it is the STOP button.

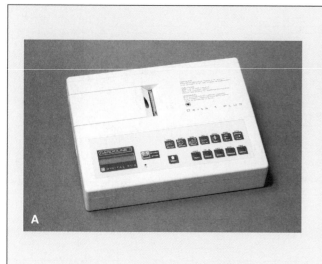

Figure 16-15A

Single-channel 12-lead electrocardiograph machine.
Delmar/Cengage Learning.

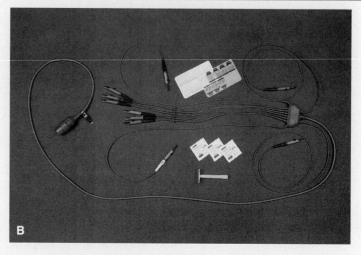

Figure 16-15B

Supplies for a single-channel 12-lead electrocardiograph.
Delmar/Cengage Learning.

(2) Amp on: Activates the amplifier so the stylus can react to heart beat. In some models, it is the RUN button.

(3) Run 25: Engages the paper drive to move the paper 25 mm (1 inch) per second. Standard speed.

(4) Run 50: Doubles paper drive speed, moves paper 50 mm (2 inches) per second. Used to show detail of wave configuration on patients with tachycardia.

c. Sensitivity control: Regulates output of amplifier.

(1) One-half: Produces a 5-mm deflection. Used when the machine is picking up high electrical voltage; adjusts for abnormally large peaks and valleys of waves.

(2) 1: 10 mm deflection (standard setting).

(3) 2: 20 mm deflection. Used when the machine is picking up low electrical voltage; adjusts for abnormally small peaks and valleys of waves.

d. Standard (STD) button: Manual check of instrument calibration.

e. Standardization adjustment knob: Adjusts the deflection to the proper height when the STD button is pushed.

f. Stylus control knob: Moves stylus so recording will be in the center of the strip.

g. Lead selector: Changes the leads to be recorded (older models).

h. Stylus heat control: Raises or lowers the heat in the tip of the stylus.

i. Marker button: Allows for manual identification of the different leads being recorded

(older models). Marking codes uses dashes and dots:

(1) Lead I: .
(2) Lead II: . .
(3) Lead III: . . .
(4) AVR: –
(5) AVL: – –
(6) AVF: – – –
(7) V_1:   –   .
(8) V_2:   –   . .
(9) V_3:   –   . . .
(10) V_4:   –   . . . .
(11) V_5:   –   . . . . .
(12) V_6:   –   . . . . . .

3. Procedure

a. Patient preparation

(1) Have the patient assume a relaxed supine position and advise the patient to remain still.

(2) Place the sensors as marked on the fleshy parts of the limbs, not the ankles or wrist. If electrolyte gel is used, squeeze a dab at each site and place the suction bulbs on the gel.

(3) Connect the lead cables to the proper sensors so that the connector is pointing toward the patient's feet.

(4) Ensure that the lead cables follow the contour of the body, avoiding large loops and crossed cables.

b. ECG recording

(1) Turn on main power switch. Warm-up may be required.

(2) Standardize the instrument: Digital units do not require standardization.

(a) Set the lead selector switch to STD (standard) and the sensitivity control switch to 1.

(b) Press the STD button. The stylus should be deflected 1 cm (10 mm or two large squares).

(c) If not, turn the standardization adjustment knob and repeat until it is calibrated.

(3) Automatic models will record and mark the entire ECG at the touch of a button.

c. Turn off the instrument, remove the sensors and wipe away any electrolyte gel from the patient.

4. Artifact: Defects on the electrocardiogram not caused by the electrical activity of the heart (see Figure 16-16).

a. Somatic tremor: Often produced by muscle movement of the patient, such as in Parkinson's disease.

b. AC (alternating current) interference: Standard source for electrical power present in electrical equipment and wires. Improper grounding of nearby electrical equipment, concealed electrical wiring, lead cables being crossed, or dirty electrodes.

c. Wandering baseline: Electrodes applied too loosely or tightly, too little gel, tension on lead wires, skin creams or lotions where electrodes are applied, excessive hair, or dirty electrodes.

E. Diagnostic ECG

1. Rhythm: Regularity may be determined using calipers or any device that can be marked to show a fixed interval for comparison.

2. Cardiac rate

a. Each large block on the ECG paper represents 0.20 second, 300 large blocks represent 1 minute (0.20 × 300 = 60 seconds). If rhythm is regular, count the large blocks between two R waves and divide 300 by this figure.

b. Count the complexes in a 6-inch strip (30 large blocks) and multiply by 10 (useful for irregular rhythms).

3. Myocardial infarction (MI)

a. The provider can locate the damage by noting which leads show indicative changes.

b. About 15% of infarcts show no changes on the initial tracing. ECG changes evolve later in hours or days as tissue damage changes electrical impulse conduction pathways.

c. Elevation of the ST segment followed by T wave inversion, which in turn is followed by a large Q wave (wider than one small block, or larger than one-third the QRS complex height). As the infarct heals, the Q wave may remain as the only sign of an old infarction.

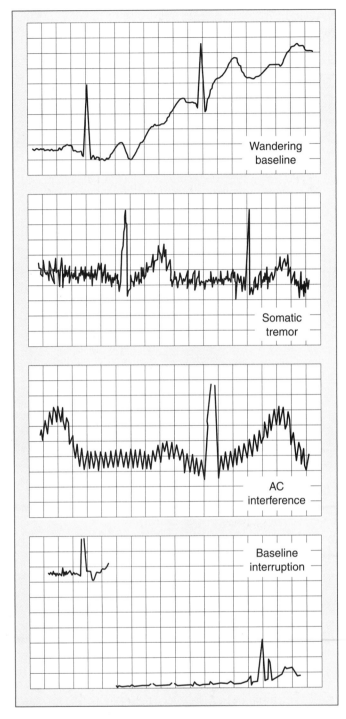

Figure 16-16

ECG readings caused by artifact. Delmar/Cengage Learning.

4. Sinus arrhythmias (see Figures 16-17A and B).

a. The P wave, the PR interval, and the QRS complex are of normal configuration. The difference lies in the regularity and rate of the impulses.

b. All complexes are normal, but the heart rhythm is irregular. The rate increases with inspiration, and decreases with expiration. This irregularity is common in children and may occur in

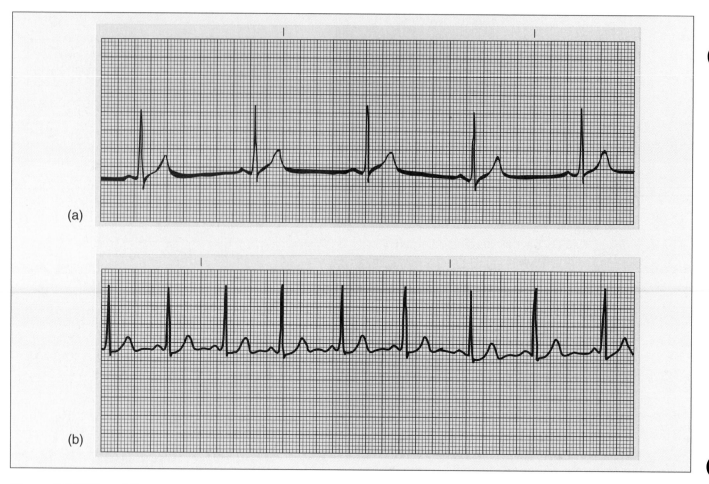

(a)

(b)

Figure 16-17A and B

(a) Heart rate shown is 50 bpm, known as sinus bradycardia because it is less than 60 bpm. (b) Sinus tachycardia is a heart rate faster than 100 bpm. Delmar/Cengage Learning.

adults relative to certain respiratory patterns. It does not decrease cardiac output and does not lead to more serious arrhythmias.

c. Sinus tachycardia: Heart rate is more than 100. Caused by excessive sympathetic nerve stimulation, physical activity, anxiety, and fever, or a compensatory response to decreased cardiac output.

d. Sinus bradycardia: Heart rate below 60. Seen in well-trained athletes, in patients on digitalis, propranolol (Inderal), and morphine. A significant slowing may cause a decrease in cardiac output that can lead to cerebral or coronary insufficiency.

e. Sinus block: A beat is not transmitted out of the SA node. No P, QRS, or T wave is present at the cycle interval for one or more beats.

f. Sinus arrest: The SA node fails to send out an impulse for a period of time.

5. Atrial arrhythmias (see Figures 16-17C to E).
   a. Portions of atrial tissue may become excitable and initiate impulses. These ectopic foci

will control the heartbeat as they occur at a rate faster than impulses from the SA node.

b. Premature atrial contraction (PAC): A beat initiated by an ectopic atrial focus appearing early in the cycle, before the next expected sinus beat. The P wave may be superimposed on the preceding T wave. Frequent PACs may be warnings of more serious atrial arrhythmias and may be treated with quinidine.

c. Paroxysmal atrial tachycardia (PAT): An abrupt episode of tachycardia with the heart rate usually between 140 and 250 beats per minute, averaging about 170.
   (1) The patient frequently complains of a sudden pounding or fluttering in the chest associated with weakness or breathlessness.
   (2) The fast rate stresses the heart and increases its need for oxygen.
   (3) Tachycardia may also diminish cardiac output because of the shortened ventricular filling time.

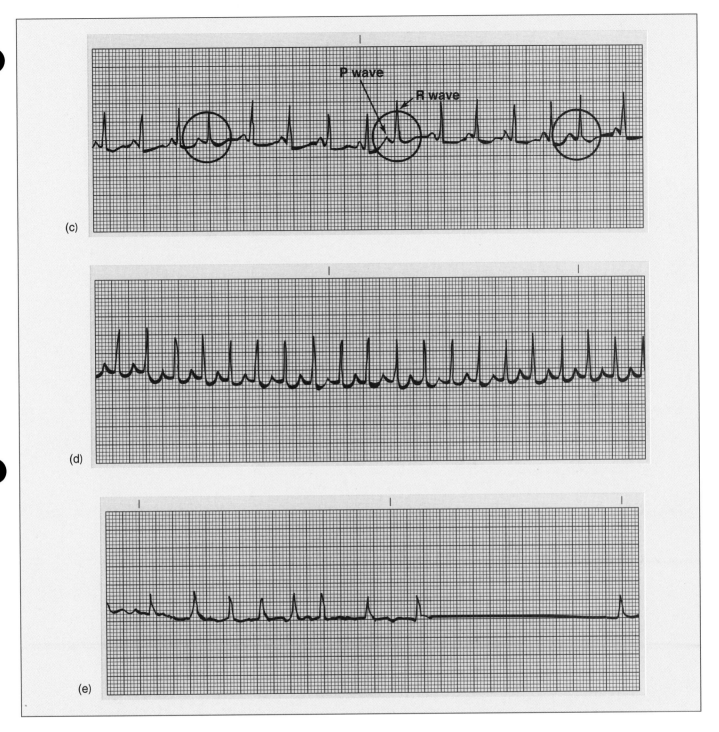

Figure 16-17C to E

Atrial arrhythmias: (c) Premature atrial contractions (PAC), (d) Paroxysmal atrial tachycardia (PAT), (e) Atrial fibrillation. Delmar/Cengage Learning.

(4) Treatment: Stimulation of the vagus nerve, which slows the heart rate. Measures that stimulate the vagus nerve include vomiting, stimulating the anal sphincter, and applying pressure to the eyeball.

d. Atrial flutter: The impulses are coming so rapidly, the AV node cannot accept and conduct each one, and therefore some degree of block-

age occurs at the node. A fast cardiac rate is relatively ineffectual and may lead to congestive heart failure. The quickest way to slow a very fast flutter is by electrocardioversion. By using low voltage, depolarization of all heart tissue is accomplished with the electrical energy of the defibrillator paddles. Cardioversion permits the sinus node to gain control.

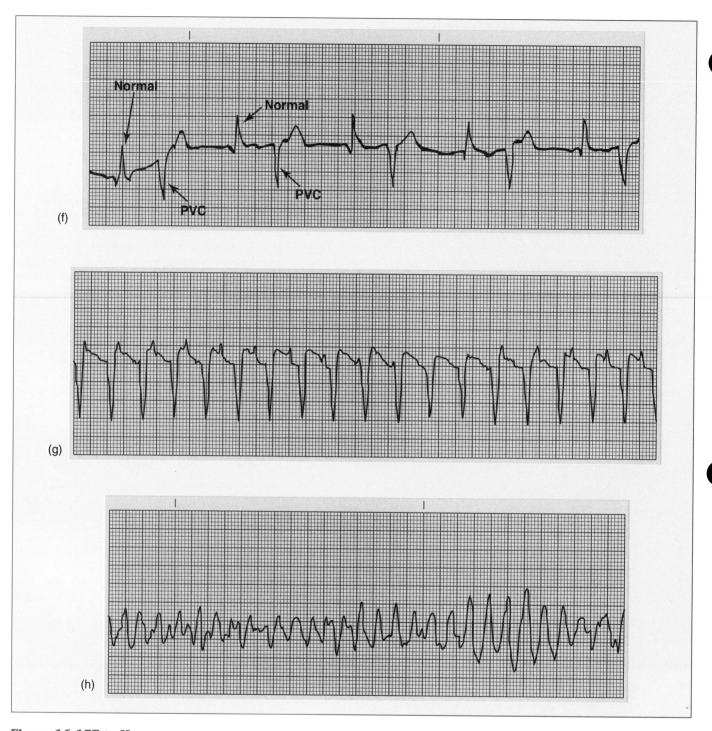

Figure 16-17F to H

Ventricular arrhythmias: (f) Premature ventricular contractions (PVC), (g) Ventricular tachycardia, (h) Ventricular fibrillation. Delmar/ Cengage Learning.

e. Atrial fibrillation: A very fast atrial rate rising from many ectopic foci. The total atrial configuration may resemble a wavy baseline or almost straight line. This occurs in enlarged atrial chambers often impaired by arteriosclerotic heart disease, scar tissue from surgery, or infections such as rheumatic fever.

6. Junctional (AV nodal) arrhythmias

a. AV node functions to receive the impulse, delay it for an instant, and then conduct it to the ventricular pathway.

b. When an impulse arises in the junctional area, it will activate the atria through retrograde (backward) conduction, causing the P wave to be inverted (downward in leads where the P would normally be upright).

c. AV block: The AV node is diseased and has difficulty conducting the P waves into the ventricles. The most common causes are arteriosclerosis and myocardial infarction. Scarring, inflammation, or edema prevents or slows transmission of the electrical impulse by the AV node.

7. Ventricular arrhythmias (see Figures 16-17F to H).

a. Ventricular arrhythmias may diminish the ability of the heart to function as a pump. Without adequate blood flow, all body organs deteriorate.

b. Premature ventricular contraction (PVCs): Occur in most myocardial infarction patients. They are also seen in normal persons, and may be caused by smoking, coffee, or alcohol.

(1) Originate in the ventricles below the AV node, showing a bizarre QRS configuration.

(2) Characteristics of PVCs

(a) Usually occur early in the cycle.

(b) Are not usually preceded by a P wave.

(c) Have a wide and distorted QRS.

(d) Have a large looping ST segment opposite in direction to that of the QRS.

(e) The interval between the R waves before and after the PVC is twice the normal R-R interval.

c. Ventricular tachycardia: Series of multiple (three or more), consecutive PVCs occurring at a rate usually between 150 and 200 beats per minute. Ventricular tachycardia is very dangerous because it leads to reduced cardiac output and, many times, to ventricular fibrillation.

d. Ventricular fibrillation: Numerous ectopic foci in the ventricles are firing erratically. Thus, there is no effective contraction of the cardiac musculature, and the patient has no pulse. Death is imminent without prompt treatment.

8. Artificial pacemaker: Unit that generates a pulse to stimulate the myocardium to produce a ventricular contraction when the sinus pacemaker activity malfunctions or the heart does not maintain a sufficiently rapid rate.

XI. PULMONARY FUNCTION TESTS (PFTS)

A. General

1. PFTs are diagnostic tests used to assess the health of the respiratory system, principally the lungs.

2. Indications

a. Evaluate signs and symptoms of lung disease.

b. Assess the progression of lung disease.

c. Monitor the effectiveness of therapy.

d. Screen patients at risk of pulmonary disease, e.g., smokers, and occupational exposure.

e. Monitor potential toxicity of drugs or chemicals, e.g., amiodarone, beryllium.

3. PFT terms (see Figure 16-18)

a. TV: Tidal volume; volume of air that is inhaled and exhaled with each at-rest breath.

b. ERV: Expiratory reserve volume; maximum volume of air that can be exhaled during the end-expiratory tidal position.

c. IRV: Inspiratory reserve volume; maximum volume of air than can be inhaled from the end-inspiratory tidal position.

d. IC: Inspiratory capacity; maximum volume of air that can be inhaled from tidal volume end-expiratory level (= IRV + TV).

e. RV: Residual volume; volume of air that remains in the lungs after maximal exhalation.

f. FRC: Functional residual capacity; volume of air in the lungs following a tidal volume exhalation (= ERV + RV).

g. FVC: Forced vital capacity; total volume that can be forcefully expired from a maximum inspiratory effort.

h. FET: Forced expiratory time; amount of time (in seconds) the patient exhales during the FVC maneuver.

i. FEV_1: Forced expiratory volume in one second; volume of air forcibly expired from a maximum inspiratory effort in the first second.

j. PEF: Peak expiratory flow; highest forced expiratory flow (L/second).

k. VC: Vital capacity; maximum volume of air that can be exhaled starting from maximum inspiration.

l. TLC: Total lung capacity; total volume of air in the lungs at full inhalation (= IC + FRC + IRV + TV + ERV + RV).

B. Spirometry

1. Measures air movement in and out of the lungs during selected respiratory maneuvers.

2. Used to determine the speed and volume of air that can be inhaled and exhaled.

3. All volumes are measures in liters.

4. The respiratory cycle is composed of lung volumes and lung capacities.

5. A lung capacity is the sum of two or more volumes.

6. Forced vital capacity (FVC)

a. Patient inhales as deeply as possible.

b. Then the patient exhales as long and as forcefully as possible.

c. The volume of air exhaled in this manner is the FVC.

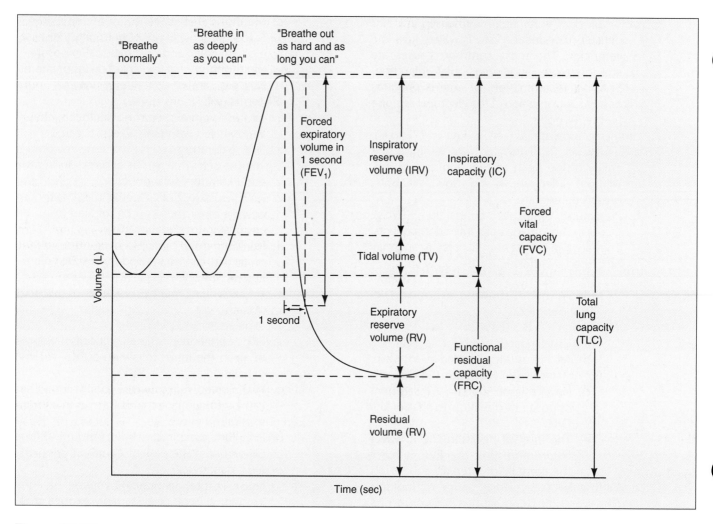

Figure 16-18

Lung volumes and capacities. Delmar/Cengage Learning

7. Forced expiratory volume in one second (FEV₁)
   a. The volume of air exhaled during the first second of the FVC maneuver.
   b. Tends to be lower in diseases that obstruct the airway, e.g., asthma or emphysema.
8. FEV₁/FVC Ratio: Used to determine if the PFT pattern is obstructive, restrictive, or normal.
C. Diffusing capacity (DLCO—diffusing lung capacity to transfer carbon monoxide)
   1. Measures the ability of the lungs to transfer gas.
   2. Lung diffusion is most efficient when the alveolar-capillary surface area for gas transfer is high and the blood is able to accept the gas.
   3. Diffusing capacity is decreased in the following conditions:
      a. Anemia and other conditions that minimizes the ability of the blood to accept and bind the gas.
      b. Emphysema, pulmonary embolism and other conditions that decrease the surface area of the alveolar-capillary membrane.

   c. Pulmonary fibrosis and other conditions that alter the membrane's thickness or permeability.
4. Carbon monoxide is used because it is more soluble in blood than in lung tissue.
5. Ideally, the volume of gas entering the blood should be limited by the lung's ability to transfer it.
D. Residual volume (RV)
   1. Represents the volume of air that remains in the lungs after exhaling as long and hard as possible.
   2. Cannot be measured by spirometry—requires specialized testing.
   3. Commonly called a static lung volume, RV and total lung capacity enhance the diagnostic value of spirometry.
E. Total lung capacity (TLC)
   1. Represents the total volume of air in the lungs at full inhalation.
   2. Like RV it cannot be measured by spirometry—requires specialized testing.

3. Is the sum of all volume compartments in liters: IC + FRC + TV + ERV + RV.

F. PFT Interpretation

1. Normal results—called predicted values—are based on the patient's age, sex, and height.

2. The predicted values for a 6-foot-tall 80-year-old man would be lower than that of a 6-foot-tall 50-year-old man.

3. The FVC maneuver is considered acceptable if there is a rapid increase in airflow at the start of exhalation.

4. A complete maneuver requires at least 6 seconds of exhalation ending with a plateau in flow, i.e., no further air is being exhaled.

5. In a proper FVC maneuver, flow rates should peak near the start of exhalation and should decline through the end of exhalation.

6. The test should be repeated at least three times and all three FEV_1 and FVC measurements should be within 200 mL of each other.

7. The test with the greatest sum of the FEV_1 and FVC measures is reported.

8. The results may vary if patients do not give their best effort.

G. Spirometry procedure

1. Wash hands; assemble equipment; identify patient, explain procedure.

2. Have the patient assume a comfortable standing or sitting position.

3. Instruct the patient to make a tight seal with his lips around the mouthpiece.

4. Instruct the patient to inhale as deeply as possible and then exhale as hard and as long as possible.

5. Coach the patient to blow, blow, blow as hard as he can—to keep blowing...until the patient can exhale no longer.

6. Wash hands; record results; stow equipment.

XII. PULSE OXIMETRY

A. A noninvasive method to monitor the oxygenation of arterial hemoglobin.

B. A sensor is placed on a fingertip, on an earlobe, or on an infant's foot.

C. The sensor emits infrared light that is passed from one side to the other.

D. A photo detector measures the amount of light absorbed by arterial hemoglobin.

E. Because of the difference in absorbance between oxygen-bound (bright red) and oxygen unbound (dark red) hemoglobin, the oximeter measures the level of oxygen saturation—the percent of hemoglobin molecules bound with oxygen molecules.

F. It is useful in the diagnosis and evaluation of respiratory and cardiac function.

G. A reading of less then 95% indicates hypoxemia; however, a reading less than 85% usually results in cyanosis.

H. Procedure

1. Wash hands; assemble equipment; identify patient, explain procedure.

2. Select a site for the sensor—typically, the finger tip—and clean with alcohol wipe. Remove nail polish if necessary.

3. Clip the sensor onto the fingertip; the sensor may need to be covered with gauze and tape so room lighting does not interfere with the measurements.

4. Connect the sensor cable to the oximeter. Turn on oximeter; adjust volume of pulse tone. Set alarms for extreme readings as warranted.

5. Inform the physician if readings are below 95%.

6. Wash hands; document procedure; charge and stow oximeter.

XII. DIAGNOSTIC IMAGING

A. Introduction

1. X-radiation: High energy, invisible electromagnetic waves that have the ability to penetrate body structures and leave an image on X-ray sensitive film.

2. Discovered in 1895 by a German physicist, Wilhelm Konrad Roentgen.

3. Common imaging technologies

a. Radiology: The medical specialty that deals with the diagnostic and therapeutic use of ionizing radiation.

(1) X-ray: Diagnostic screening film using ionizing radiation.

(2) Cinefluorography/Fluoroscopy: Motion picture X-rays.

(3) Mammography: X-ray of the breast.

b. Tomography: Radiographic viewing of cross-sections, slices, or planes of the body. Computed axial tomography (CAT) provides three-dimensional, cross-sectional images.

c. Nuclear medicine: Introduces radioactive material into the body where it will emmit gamma rays, creating images that can be recorded by special equipment.

d. Magnetic resonance imaging (MRI): Uses a magnetic field to create images.

e. Ultrasound: Uses sound waves to create an image.

4. Functions

a. To reveal position and presence of foreign bodies. To reveal the position and presence of fractures and abnormalities.

b. To reveal radiopaque substances that are purposely introduced enabling the viewing of tissues on developed film.

c. To allow for fluoroscopy that detects size, shape, and movement.

d. To ionize pathological cells.

e. To allow for perception of depth by stereo-radiography.

5. Primary waves: X-ray that passes directly out of the tube.

6. Secondary waves: X-ray that strikes an object and bounce off.

B. X-ray machine, equipment, and materials (see Figure 16-19)

1. Table: Platform that supports the body to afford X-ray penetration. It contains grids and tray for bucky film placement.

2. X-ray tube: Glass vacuum tube such as a Coolidge tube that produces and transmits the X-radiation.

3. Collimator: Boxlike apparatus below the tube that permits adjustment of the area of the X-ray beam that penetrates the body part and strikes the film. The shutter window must be coned to the proper film size.

4. Control panel: Allows for the control of X-ray emissions. Regulates the machine. Located behind a lead lined wall for protection of operator.

a. Main switch: Turns machine on and off.

b. MA (milliampere) setting: 25, 50, 100, 200, and 300. The amount of radiation that will be emitted from the tube.

c. Time switch: Goes from 0.1 to 2 seconds. The number of seconds the patient is exposed to the radiation.

d. MaS (milliampere—second): MA × time; this controls the quantity and duration of radiation exposure.

e. KVP (kilovolts peak) setting: Adjusted from 20 to 120. The penetrating power of the X-ray beam as determined by density of the body part being X-rayed.

f. Bucky switch: It is only used when bucky technique is utilized.

g. Exposure switch: Takes the X-ray and is always away from the machine.

5. High-voltage generator: Supplies the power needed to generate x-radiation.

6. Grid

a. Absorbs scattered (secondary) radiation caused when rays strike objects such as bone.

b. Helps prevent blurring of film.

c. Composed of numerous lead strips alternating with radiolucent strips.

d. Placed between patient and film to reduce secondary wave interferance.

7. Potter-Bucky diaphragm (Bucky). Framelike apparatus situated under the table that holds the grid above the film.

a. When the machine is activated, the bucky moves the grid to blur the lines that would be created by the lead strips.

b. Used when thicker body parts (>10 cm) are being radiographed.

8. Cassette: Device for holding X-ray film that protects it from light.

9. Intensifying screens: Special plates within the cassette that help obtain images in shorter period of time, reducing the amount of exposure to the patient.

10. Radiographic film

a. Coated with a special material that is sensitive to X-ray energy. Visible record of the x-radiation that struck the film.

b. Film areas that received x-radiation will appear black or shades of gray; whereas, areas that did not will appear white. The more dense the material being radiographed the lighter the image on X-ray film.

c. Radiopaque: Dense substances or structures that absorb x-radiation and prevent it from striking the film making the structure appear white on film.

d. Radiolucent: Low density substances or structures that do not absorb x-radiation and allow it to strike the film making the structure appear gray or black.

11. View box: Lighted screen for the viewing of X-ray film.

12. Positioning devices: Sandbags and sponges that assist in immobilizing body parts.

13. Contrast media: Radiopaque substances that increase the density of low-density structures such as soft tissues to permit radiographic imaging.

a. Barium sulfate: Commonly used to delineate the countours of the gastrointestinal tract.

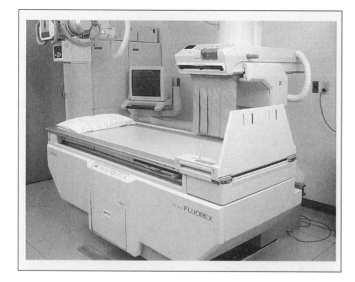

Figure 16-19

X-ray machine. Delmar/Cengage Learning.

b. Iodine: Commonly used to visualize blood vessels, urinary tract, and spinal cord.

C. X-ray adjustments
1. Technique chart: Control panel settings are established on a chart based on the particular position and body part being exposed.
2. Focal film distance (FFD): The distance from the X-ray tube to the table; 40 inches is standard FFD.
3. Caliper: Measures, in centimeters, the thickness of the body part to be exposed.

D. Radiation safety
1. Hazards
   a. Cumulative effect: The more often the exposure and the larger the body part exposed, the greater the risk.
   b. Exposure may injure body cells, especially immature cells, gametes, and the developing fetus.
   c. Exposure to eyes may cause cataract development.
   d. Acute radiation syndrome: High radiation exposure during a short period of time may cause nausea, vomiting, diarrhea, infections, and hair loss.
   e. Somatic effects of radiation: High radiation exposure over a long period of time may cause cancer, genetic defects and mutations, sterility, and shortened life span.
2. Precautions
   a. Use appropriate equipment and good technique to avoid unnecessary retakes.
   b. Establish a routine maintenance and repair schedule including the performance of radiation leak checks.
   c. Prevent exposure to gonads: Especially in children, adolescents, and pregnant females.
   d. Prevent exposure to unborn fetus: Always ask women of childbearing age if they are pregnant. If so, perform X-rays only after approved by a healthcare provider.
   e. Provide a lead barrier or apron to the patient.
   f. Strictly adhere to all safety rules
      (1) Use a lead apron.
      (2) Use a shield and gloves.
      (3) Wear a dosimeter: X-ray badge that contains material that is sensitive to radiation exposure. The badge is periodically checked to measure one's radiation exposure level.

E. Patient positions
1. AP (Anteroposterior): The rays enter the anterior and exit the posterior surfaces before striking the film.
2. PA (Posteroanterior): The rays enter the posterior and exit the anterior surfaces before striking the film.
3. Lateral: The rays pass from one side to the other side before striking the film.
   a. Right lateral: Rays enter left side and exit the right side before striking the film.
   b. Left lateral: Rays enter right side and exit the left side before striking the film.
4. Oblique: The x-radiation passes through the body at an angle between the horizontal and vertical planes.
5. The body part nearest the film provides the greatest detail.

F. X-ray studies
1. Angiogram: Contrast medium injected through a catheter to detect presence of cardiovascular disease. Nothing by mouth (NPO) 4 to 5 hours before X-ray.
2. Angiocardiogram: Similar to angiogram with catheter being introduced into the heart.
3. Arteriogram: Similar to angiogram; specifically studies the condition of an artery.
4. Barium enema: Contrast medium instilled in the colon to visualize the lower intestinal tract.
   a. Also called lower GI Series. Procedure lasts approximately 1 hour.
   b. No milk products. Laxative and Fleet's enema administered before X-ray. Nothing by mouth (NPO) after midnight.
5. Barium meal: Also called upper GI. Contrast medium administered orally to visualize stomach and esophagus.
6. Bronchogram: Contrast medium instilled through the trachea and into the bronchial tree. Detects cancer and other lung disorders.
7. Cholecystogram: Contrast medium in tablet form ingested the evening before the test. Gallbladder is then observed. A light, low-fat dinner is allowed the evening before.
8. Hysterosalpingogram: Contrast medium injected into the fallopian tubes; patency of tubes as well as diseases of uterus is determined.
9. KUB (kidney, ureter and bladder): Basic flat plate of the abdomen.
10. Intravenous pyelogram (IVP): Contrast medium injected IV to observe pathway of dye as it is excreted. Outline of ureter and bladder is observed.
    a. Films taken at intervals requiring approximately 2 hours.
    b. Laxative the evening before. Liquid diet evening before. NPO after midnight.
11. Lymphangiogram: Contrast medium injected into lymphatic vessel to visualize the system.
12. Mammogram: Survey films of the breast from three angles.
13. Myelogram: Contrast medium injected into the subarachnoid space of the spinal column. Patient remains in supine position with no pillow for 12 hours following procedure.

14. Pneumoarthrogram: Air injected into the articular capsule of a joint to determine condition of joint.
15. Pneumoencephalogram: Contrast medium of air or gas injected into subarachnoid space of the brain using lumbar puncture. Spinal fluid must be removed first. Usually a hospital procedure.

XIII. PHYSICAL THERAPY

A. Introduction
1. The physical therapist is an allied health professional who has completed at least a 4 year baccalaureate program in physical therapy and has received a state license.
2. A physician specialist is called a physiatrist.
3. The objective of physical therapy is to relieve pain, increase or improve circulation, increase or restore muscular function, improve strength, range of motion, or joint mobility.
4. Physical therapy may require the use of physical and mechanical agents such as massage, exercise, hot or cold application, electricity or diathermy, to diagnose, treat, and prevent neuromuscular disease.
5. Physical therapy procedures are often recommended for the following conditions commonly encountered in the medical office:
   a. Arthritis: To increase circulation and maintain mobility.
   b. Cardiovascular disease: To restore strength and increase circulation.
   c. Cerebral palsy: To maintain mobility.
   d. Cerebral vascular accident (CVA or stroke): To restore function and strength.
   e. Low back pain: To relieve discomfort and maintain mobility.
   f. Muscle spasm: To relax the musculature and relieve pain.
   g. Muscle disease and injuries: To maintain mobility, restore function, and prevent deformity.
   h. Skin disorders: To promote healing, reduce inflammation, and kill microorganisms.
6. The provider may prescribe a program of physical therapy for a patient and then expect the physical therapist to implement the mechanics of the program, or the provider may refer the patient for evaluation and treatment relying on the physical therapist's judgment.
7. Chiropractic: Approach that emphasizes the diagnosis and treatment of diseases and disorders by manipulating the musculoskeletal system, especially the spine, under the theory that health is mediated via the nervous system.
8. Massage therapy: Approach that uses the manipulation of soft and connective tissues to restore health and function.
9. Acupuncture: Technique of inserting fine needles into specific points on the body to relieve pain and restore health by affecting the path of energy forces.
10. Acupressure: Similar to acupuncture except pressure is applied to points on the body.

B. Heat therapy (thermotherapy)
1. Purpose
   a. Heat functions to relieve pain, congestion, muscle spasms, and inflammation. Heat promotes muscle relaxation and is often used for the relief of pain due to overexertion of muscle tissue.
   b. Reduce edema: Heat increases blood supply, which functions to increase the absorption of fluid from the tissues through the lymphatic system.
2. Local effects of heat
   a. The local effects of heat application include dilation of blood vessels, resulting in increased blood supply to the area, and increased tissue metabolism.
   b. Expedient provision of nutrients and oxygen and elimination of wastes and toxins.
   c. Physiologically, heat applications promote healing; however, prolonged exposure (>1 hour) produces secondary antagonistic effects that reverse the healing process: blood vessels constrict, and blood supply to the area decreases.
3. Precautions
   a. Extreme caution should be used in applying heat on affected body parts of very young children to avoid burning.
   b. Elderly patients should be observed carefully for low tolerance to heat and subsequent burning.
   c. Soaking or immersion should occur in water temperatures between 105° and 115°F.
4. Infrared therapy: Administered by heat lamp.
   a. Surface heat is transmitted through the skin to a depth of 5 to 10 mm.
   b. Placing the heat lamp at a distance of 2 to 4 feet from the area is generally recommended to avoid burning the skin.
   c. Exposure time is usually 15 to 20 minutes.
5. Diathermy
   a. A form of heat therapy in which the area to be treated requires deep heat penetration rather than superficial exposure.
   b. Diathermy creates an electrical field that heats the tissue and increases circulation.
   c. Commonly used in the treatment of muscular injuries and inflammatory joint disease.
   d. Three basic diathermic approaches
      (1) Microwave: Electromagnetic radiation is directed to the tissues.

(2) Shortwave: High-frequency electric current is directed to the tissues.

(3) Ultrasound: High-frequency sound waves are directed to the tissues.

e. Because of enormous heat generation, it is vitally important to adhere to recommended dosage and time allowances.

6. Ultrasound

a. High-frequency sound waves, above the frequency of sound waves audible by the human ear, that can be used therapeutically as a deep-heating agent for the soft tissues of the body.

b. Physiologically, ultrasound reduces edema, breaks up exudates and precipitates, increases cellular metabolism, relieves pain, and produces micromassage.

c. Commonly used to treat sprains, strains, joint contractures, neuritis, arthritis, edema, synovitis, scar tissue, bursitis, varicosities, osteoarthritis, and dislocations.

d. Ultrasound should never be used over the eyeball, over malignant tumors, directly over the spinal cord, over the heart or brain, over reproductive organs, over a pregnant uterus, over areas of impaired sensation, or inadequate circulation.

e. The applicator head is firmly placed on the patient's skin surface and is slowly and steadily moved over the treatment area, which allows the sound waves to penetrate the patient's soft tissues.

f. As the sound waves travel through the tissues, part of the waves are absorbed by the tissues and transformed into heat. This produces a vigorous deep heating in the soft tissues of the body.

g. A micromassage effect is also produced by the mechanical vibration of the sound waves as they pass through the tissues.

h. Air is a poor conductor of sound; therefore, a coupling agent must be used with ultrasound treatments to increase conductivity. Coupling agents include mineral oil and commercial products such as Soni-Gel.

i. The coupling agent must be at room temperature and must be applied liberally to the treatment area of the patient's skin.

j. Water may also be used as a coupling agent because it is a good conductor of sound. In this method, both the patient's skin surface to be treated and the applicator head are completely submerged under water.

k. Ultrasound dosage is expressed in watt-minutes. Watt refers to the intensity of the sound waves ordered by the provider and minutes refers to the duration of the treatment.

7. Paraffin wax hand bath

a. A dry hand is immersed in melted wax and quickly lifted out.

b. Paraffin wax baths are usually prescribed for patients with arthritis to relieve pain, increase circulation, and reduce stiffness.

c. The wax is usually melted and heated to 126°F (52°C) and mixed with mineral oil in a proportionate amount (usually 7 to 1).

8. Procedures

a. Hot water bag application

(1) Wash hands; identify patient; explain procedure.

(2) Fill the water bag one-third to one-half full with water, 115° to 125°F (46° to 52°C).

(3) Expel excess air and fasten the top; dry the outside of the bag and ensure no leakage.

(4) Place the bag in a protective covering and apply to the affected body part for the time prescribed; ensure that the bag feels warm but not uncomfortable.

(5) Change the water as needed to maintain a stable temperature.

(6) Clean up; make a chart entry to include application method, temperature, location, duration patient reaction, date, and time.

b. Hot soak application

(1) Wash hands; identify patient; explain procedure.

(2) Fill a basin half full with warmed soaking solution, 105° to 110°F (41° to 44°C).

(3) Slowly immerse the patient's body part into the solution; keep immersed for the time prescribed.

(4) As the solution cools, gradually remove and replace with warm solution.

(5) Gently dry the body part; clean up; make a chart entry to include application method, temperature, location, duration, patient reaction, date, and time.

c. Hot compress application

(1) Wash hands; identify patient; explain procedure.

(2) Fill a basin half full with warmed solution, 105° to 110° F (41° to 44° C); immerse a washcloth or gauze squares.

(3) Wring out the compress of any excess solution; lightly apply it to the affected part.

(4) Replace with new compresses every 2 to 3 minutes for the time prescribed.

(5) Periodically check the solution temperature and add hot water as needed.

(6) Gently dry the body part; clean up; make a chart entry to include application method, temperature, location, duration, patient reaction, date, and time.

C. Cold therapy (cryotherapy)
  1. Purpose
    a. Prevents edema by constricting blood vessels and reduces fluid leakage into the tissues.
    b. Often applied immediately after direct trauma such as a bruise, sprain, muscle strain, or fracture.
    c. Temporarily relieves pain by retarding stimulation of the nerve receptors.
    d. Retards the movement of blood and tissue fluids in the affected area, resulting in less pressure against nerve receptors, and therefore less pain.
  2. Local effects of cold
    a. Produces vascular constriction leading to decreased blood supply to the area, decreased tissue metabolism, decreased oxygen, and reduced accumulation of waste.
    b. Prolonged cold applications (>1 hour) has an antagonistic secondary effect: blood vessels dilate and there is an increase in tissue metabolism.
  3. Procedures
    a. Ice bag application
      (1) Wash hands; identify patient; explain procedure.
      (2) Fill the bag one-half to two-thirds full with ice chips; expel excess air and fasten top; dry bag and place in protective covering.
      (3) Apply the bag to the affected part for the prescribed time.
      (4) Periodically check the skin for extreme palor, numbness, or mottled blue appearance and report to the physician immediately.
      (5) Clean up; make a chart entry to include application method, temperature, location, duration, patient reaction, date, and time.
    b. Cold compress application
      (1) Wash hands; identify patient; explain procedure.
      (2) Place ice cubes and some water in a basin; immerse a washcloth or gauze squares.
      (3) Wring out the compress of any excess solution; lightly apply it to the affected part.
      (4) Replace with new compresses every 2 to 3 minutes for the time prescribed.
      (5) Add ice as needed to keep solution cold.

(6) Gently dry the body part; clean up; make a chart entry to include application method, temperature, location, duration, patient reaction, date, and time.

D. Hydrotherapy
  1. External water applications for therapeutic purposes, especially for relaxation, increased circulation, and improved mobility.
  2. Three common modalities
    a. Whirlpool: Provides moist heat along with a gentle massage action.
    b. Contrast baths: employs two different containers of water: One hot and the other cold. The patient is required to move the affected body part quickly from the hot to the cold and then back to the hot bath.
    c. Underwater exercise: This is often prescribed in cases of joint injuries, burns, or arthritis, or exercise conditions that require the buoyant effect of water.

E. Ultraviolet (UV) therapy
  1. Ultraviolet rays are rays beyond the violet end of the visible spectrum. They are produced by the sun and by sunlamps.
  2. Although producing very little heat, they can cause tanning on the skin or a sunburn.
  3. UV light is capable of killing bacteria and other microorganisms and activates the formation of vitamin D.
  4. Used to treat acne, psoriasis, pressure sores, and wound infections.
  5. UV rays stimulate epithelial cell growth, cause capillary hyperemia, and increases cellular metabolism and vascular engorgement, which increases the skin's defenses against bacterial infections.
  6. Before receiving UV treatment, the patient's sensitivity is determined by exposing different areas of the patient's skin to different dosages of the rays for different time periods. The following day the patient returns so that the response can be evaluated and the proper dosage determined.
  7. The patient must never be left unattended while being exposed to UV radiation.

F. Joint mobility
  1. Goniometry: The process of measuring joint mobility. It helps establish a base level of limited mobility caused by disease or injury, thus helping to monitor the success of treatment or the progress of disease.
  2. The goniometer is a simple 360-degree protractor with a movable pointer arm.
  3. Muscle testing
    a. Range of motion tests: Testing that is focused on muscle flexibility and resilience.
    b. Strength tests: Testing to establish the force with which a muscle or muscle group can act.

c. Task skill tests: Testing the person's capacity to carry out certain important activities.

G. Exercise therapy
1. Exercise therapy is the use of body motion to achieve an improvement of a particular function.
2. Exertherapy, or "PT exercise," is a modality used to help patients regain body function, improve their ability to perform important motor functions, or to return to their usual occupations.
3. Therapeutic methods
   a. Active-voluntary mobility: Self-directed exercises.
   b. Passive-involuntary mobility: Body parts are moved by external force.
   c. Aided mobility: Voluntary mobility with conductive aids, such as a therapy pool.
   d. Active resistance: Voluntary mobility with counterpressure.
   e. Range of motion: Active or passive joint mobility.
4. Because the process of exertherapy is dynamic, the dosage (repetition frequency) must constantly be adjusted as the patient gets stronger.

H. Massage: The manipulation of external body tissues, is one of the oldest known methods to promote healing.
1. Three basic approaches
   a. Stroking: Most common method employing the systematic movement of the hand across the skin.
   b. Compression: Squeezing, pressing, or kneading of soft tissues.
   c. Percussion: Alternating thumping of the skin with various parts of the hand.
2. Guidelines for massage
   a. The patient must be relaxed.
   b. A lubricating cream or oil should be used.
   c. Pressure is transmitted through relaxed muscles. Tense muscles impair effective massage.

I. Electrotherapy
1. Employs the use of electricity to stimulate muscles or other body tissues.
2. Electrodiagnosis: Use of electrical stimulation to study nerve conduction and muscle action potentials to identify neuromuscular disorders.
3. Electromyography: Process of measuring the electrical activity in a muscle as a result of nerve conduction. A needle electrode is introduced into a muscle belly to study muscle action potentials. It will also measure the general electrical excitability of the muscle cells.
4. Electrical threshold: Used to test the reaction time of a muscle to a shot of electricity. Measures the amount of electricity required to generate a muscle reaction. The results obtained are compared with normal levels.

5. Nerve conduction studies are performed to test the speed with which the nerve conducts electrical impulses.
6. Galvanic current: Steady, low-voltage direct current (DC).
   a. Galvanic and faradic current is used for muscle stimulation, particularly to retrain patients who have developed nerve injuries.
   b. Galvanic stimulation can be used just to maintain the contractility of the muscle while awaiting nerve regeneration.
   c. If a nerve does not conduct stimuli, galvanic current (direct current) is the only thing that can be used to stimulate a muscle.
7. Faradic current: Low-voltage alternating current (AC).
   a. Faradic current will not stimulate a muscle if the nerve supplying it cannot conduct an electrical impulse.
   b. Faradic current is used mainly for the stimulation of weak muscles that have a normal nerve supply.
   c. This current causes contractions, which in turn increases blood supply to the muscle and thus helps the muscle gain strength.

J. Traction
1. Pulling or stretching action applied to the musculoskeletal system to ensure proper alignment of bones following injury or disease, or to correct or prevent deformities.
2. Traction can be accomplished manually (using the hand to exert a pull), or by means of appliances, weights, or weighted pads applied to the sides of limbs.

K. Casts
1. Material used to immobilized fractured limbs to facilitate healing.
2. Common types: Plaster, plastic, fiberglass, and inflatable air casts.
3. Short arm cast (SAC): Fractures of forearm and wrist. Extends from fingers to just below the elbow.
4. Long arm cast (LAC): Fractures of upper arm. Extends from fingers to axilla, with elbow slightly bent.
5. Short leg cast (SLC): Extends from below the knee to the toes; may include a rubber walking heel.
6. Long leg cast (LLC): Extends from the thigh to the toes; may include a rubber walking heel.
7. Plaster cast application
   a. Wash hands, assemble equipment, identify the patient, explain procedure.
   b. Position the patient and align the body part as directed by the physician.
   c. Don gloves and drape the area.
   d. Clean and dry the area to be cast; document any skin lesions, aberrations, or discolorations.

e. Pad bony prominences.
f. Prepare the correct size stockinette for the area.
g. Provide the correct width of Webril (cotton strips).
h. Immerse the plaster roll in warm water for 5 seconds. Remove and squeeze excess water.
i. Assist the physician with the application as directed.
j. Reassure patient as needed.
k. After the cast is applied, provide cast care and follow-up instructions.
l. Clean up, remove gloves, wash hands, document procedure.

8. Cast removal
a. Wash hands, assemble equipment, identify the patient, explain procedure.
b. Position the patient and drape the area.
c. Assist the physician with the removal as directed.
d. Reassure patient as needed.
e. After the cast is removed, provide follow-up instructions.
f. Clean up, remove gloves, wash hands, document procedure.

L. Mobility-assisting devices
1. Crutches (see Figure 16-20)
a. Wood or tubular aluminum devices that serve as walking aids by transferring weight from the legs to the arms.
(1) Axillary crutch: Consists of a shoulder rest and hand grip that extends from the ground to the patient's axillary region. Commonly used by patients requiring temporary ambulatory assistance.
(2) Lofstrand crutch: Consists of a cuff and hand grip that extends from the ground to the patient's forearm. Commonly used by patients afflicted with cerebral palsy or paraplegia.
b. Axillary crutch measurement
(1) Direct the patient to stand erect; position the crutches with the tips 2 inches in front of and 6 inches to the side of each foot.
(2) Adjust the crutch length so that the shoulder rests are 2 inches below the axilla.
(3) Adjust the handgrips so that the patient's elbows are flexed approximately 30 degrees.
(4) Check to ensure that there is a two-fingerwidth clearance between the shoulder rests and the patient's axilla when standing erect; if not, readjust as described above.
c. Crutch gaits (see Figure 16-21)
(1) Four-point gait: Patient must be able to bear weight on both legs. Commonly used for muscle weakness or poor coordination.
(a) Move right crutch forward.
(b) Move left foot to the level of the left crutch.
(c) Move left crutch forward.
(d) Move right foot to the level of the right crutch.
(e) Repeat.
(2) Three-point gait: Used when patients cannot bear weight on one leg as seen in trauma, surgery, or amputation.
(a) Move both crutches and weak leg forward.
(b) Move the strong leg forward while balancing on both crutches.
(c) Repeat.
(3) Two-point gait: Similar to four-point gait, but faster requiring greater coordination.
(a) Move right crutch and left foot forward simultaneously.
(b) Move left crutch and right foot forward simultaneously.
(c) Repeat.
(4) Swing gait: Used for patients with severe lower extremity disabilities such as paralysis or leg braces.
(a) Move both crutches forward.
(b) Lift both legs off the floor and swing them past the crutches.
(c) Repeat.

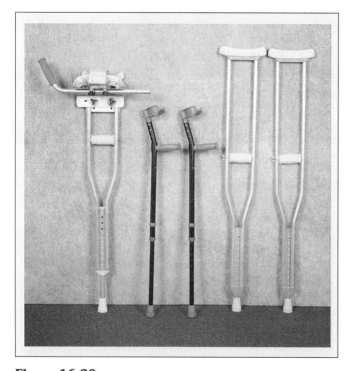

Figure 16-20

Types of crutches. Delmar/Cengage Learning.

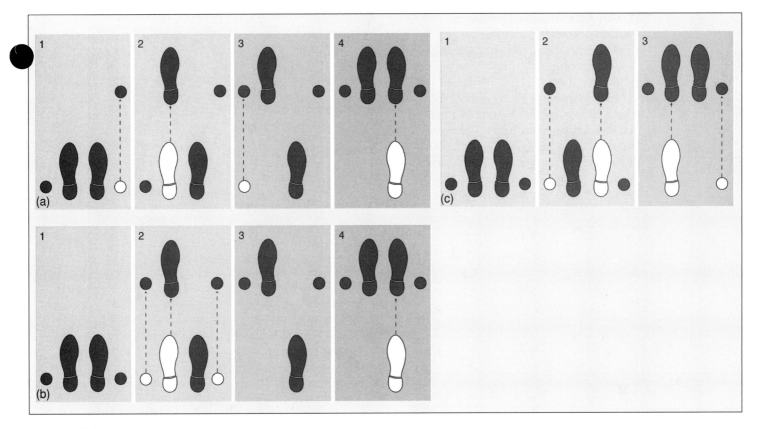

Figure 16-21

Crutch gaits. (a) Four point gait, (b) Three point gait, (c) Two point gait. Delmar/Cengage Learning.

d. Navigating stairs: Place both crutches under one arm and balance the body between the pair of crutches and the handrail.

e. Navigating obstructions: Obstructions such as curbs or steps without handrails can be approached by placing the lead crutch either up (ascending) or down (descending) and then twisting and elevating (or lowering) the body simultaneously.

f. Single crutch: Patients for whom one crutch is prescribed should be advised to carry the crutch on the side of the strong leg, not the weak leg.

2. Cane: Wood or aluminum pole with a handle or handgrip that provides balance or support to patients who have a weakness on one side of the body (see Figure 16-22).

a. Standard cane: Cane having only one contact point on the floor to provide minimal support.

b. Tripod cane: Cane having three contact points on the floor to provide greater stability.

c. Quad cane: Cane having four contact points on the floor.

d. The cane should be measured so that the handle is level with the greater trochanter with an elbow flexion of 25 to 30 degrees.

e. Patient instruction
   (1) Hold the cane on the strong side of the body with the tip 6 inches to the side of the foot.
   (2) Move the cane forward about 12 inches.

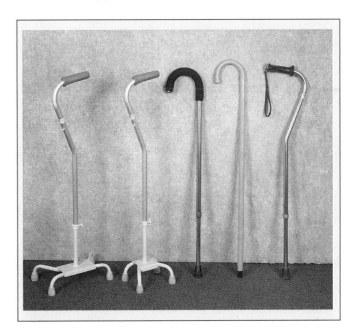

Figure 16-22

Cane types. Delmar/Cengage Learning.

(3) Move the weak leg forward to the level of the cane.

(4) Move the strong leg ahead of the weak leg and cane.

(5) Repeat.

3. Walker: Aluminum frame consisting of two handgrips and four squarely placed legs that provides optimum balance for patients experiencing weakness or balance problems (see Figure 16-23).

   a. Pick up the walker and move it forward 6 inches.

   b. Move the right foot then the left foot forward to the walker.

   c. Repeat.

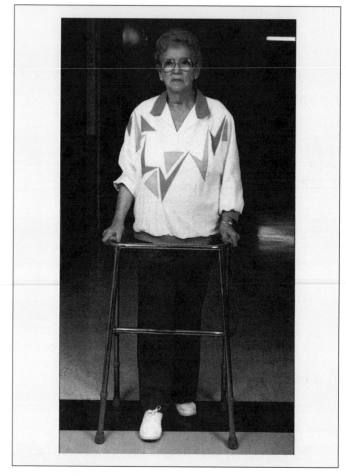

Figure 16-23

Walker. Delmar/Cengage Learning.

CHAPTER 17

Surgical Care

I. INTRODUCTION

A. Minor surgery is defined as a surgical procedure that does not require general anesthesia; e.g., debridement, suturing of lacerations, and removal of skin growths.

B. Infection control measures

1. Sanitization: Process of cleaning or freeing materials, especially instruments, from dirt. Requires scrubbing materials with brushes and detergents.
   a. Detergents: Wetting agents that mechanically remove bacteria, emulsify fats and oils, as well as dissolve high protein substances such as blood.
   b. Ultrasound: Instruments may be placed in an ultrasonic bath containing a detergent solution. The ultrasonic bath is a device that passes sound waves through the liquid causing vibration that loosens contaminants, blood, and dirt.
   c. Antiseptics (germicides): Agents of sanitization used on the skin.

2. Disinfection: Process of removing infectious material from selected objects, but not necessarily their spores.
   a. Chemical: Surface germicides used on inanimate materials that are sensitive to heat.
   b. Soap: Mechanically removes some infectious material such as bacteria, but does not generally destroy them unless it contains a germicide.
   c. Alcohol: Isopropyl alcohol is commonly used on skin because it has some germicidal properties; iodine sometimes added for strength.
   d. Acids: Phenol is an excellent germicidal.
   e. Alkalies: 10% sodium hypochlorite (bleach) is commonly used on laboratory surfaces and selected equipment.
   f. Formaldehyde: 5% formalin is effective but requires thorough rinsing with water.
   g. Ultraviolet radiation: Ultraviolet light has a germicidal effect on surfaces and airborne microbes, but has no penetrating power.
   h. Desiccation: Drying inhibits bacterial growth and is commonly used as a preservative; spores are highly resistant.
   i. Boiling: Kills most bacteria, except some spore-forming bacteria and viruses.

3. Sterilization: Complete destruction of all microorganisms or infectious agents and their spores.
   a. Chemical: Agents such as glutaraldehyde may be used for heat-sensitive material, but must be submerged for extended periods.
   b. Steam under pressure (autoclave): Most common and effective means of sterilization.
   c. Gas: Special sterilization chamber that uses a sterilizing gas and sometimes pressure.

II. SURGICAL INSTRUMENTS

A. Precision instruments designed for use in operative procedures.

B. Cutting and dissecting instruments (see Figure 17-1A to I)

1. Scalpel: Surgical knives used to make incisions. They may be either disposable or reusable with several shapes and sizes of blades and handles designed for making specific types of incisions.
2. Surgical scissors
   a. Used primarily to cut tissue and sutures. Scissor blades touch precisely at the tips and are either curved or straight.
   b. Blade point combinations include sharp-sharp, blunt-blunt, or sharp-blunt.
3. Bandage scissor: Consists of a knobby tip that is used to slide under bandages for cutting the dressing without injuring the skin.
4. Suture scissors: Consists of a hook or beak near the tip to get under and sever the suture.

C. Forceps: Instruments designed to grasp or clamp down objects or tissue (see Figure 17-2A to L).

1. The tips are either straight or curved with a variety of types of serrations or teeth and different lengths and sizes to meet special needs.
2. The handle clamps together by means of a ratchet near the handle to prevent slipping and serves to hold the forcep closed without using the hands.

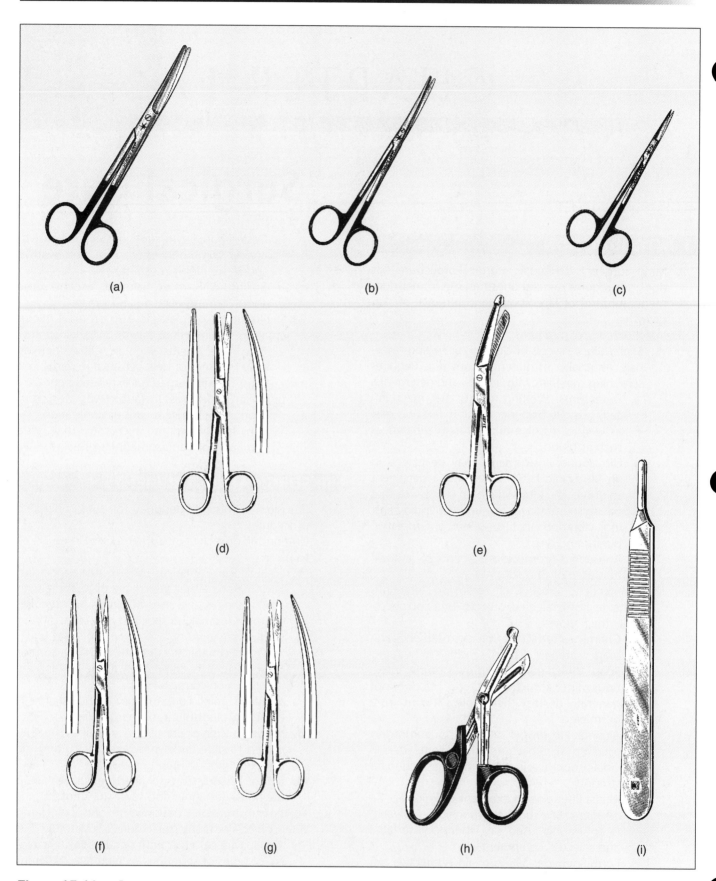

Figure 17-1A to I

Cutting and dissecting instruments: (a) Mayo scissors, (b) Metzenbaum scissors, (c) Iris scissors, (d) Blunt-blunt scissors, (e) Bandage scissors, (f) Sharp-sharp scissors, (g) Sharp-blunt scissors, (h) Utility scissors, (i) Scalpel handle. Courtesy of Jarit Surgical Instruments.

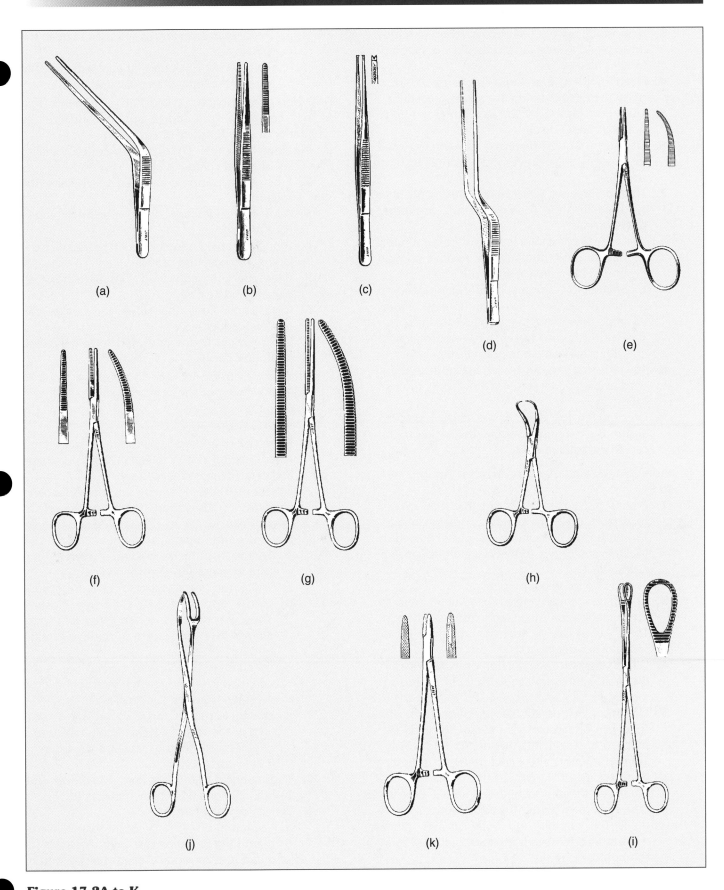

Figure 17-2A to K

Forceps: (a) Angular thumb forceps, (b) Plain thumb forceps, (c) Tissue thumb forceps, (d) Bayonette thumb forceps, (e) Mosquito hemostatic forceps, (f) Kelly hemostatic forceps, (g) Rochester-Pean hemostatic forceps, (h) Towel forceps, (i) Sponge forceps, (j) Sterilizer (transfer) forceps, (k) Needle holder. Courtesy of Jarit Surgical Instruments.

3. Hemostatic forceps (hemostats): Used to tightly grasp blood vessels to stop the flow of blood or to hold tissue.
4. Needle holder: Hemostatlike forcep used to firmly grasp the needle during a suturing procedure.
5. Tissue forceps: Have clawlike teeth at the tip to grasp and hold tissue.
6. Sterilizer (transfer) forceps: Large forceps used to remove sterile objects from containers and sterilizers.
7. Thumb forceps: Tweezerlike instruments that are used to grasp tissue, dressings, and other sterile objects.
   a. Lucae bayonet forceps: A crooked thumb forcep used primarily to remove foreign bodies from the ear and nose.
   b. Splinter forceps: Fine, sharply pointed thumb forcep designed to grasp foreign bodies imbedded in the skin or under the nails.
   c. Tissue (thumb) forceps: Tweezerlike forcep with clawlike teeth to grasp tissue.
8. Towel forceps (clamps): Forceplike instrument used as clamps to secure cloth drapes to each other.
9. Dressing forceps: Used to hold gauze in place to absorb discharge or to apply medication to the cervix and vaginal walls.

D. Probing and dilating instruments (see Figure 17-3A to K)
1. Probes: Instruments used to enter body cavities to explore cavities, wounds, or foreign bodies. The ends may be bulbous, straight or curved to facilitate conformity to the shape of the canal or cavity.
2. Sounds: Long, slender probes.
3. Applicators: Long-handled instruments used to apply medication by twisting cotton at the top. These can usually be inserted through an endoscope or speculum.
4. Directors: Instruments, often grooved, used to guide the direction and depth of a surgical incision.
5. Obturator: Instrument that fits inside a scope or speculum and protrudes forward to guide the scope or speculum into the canal or body cavity. Some obturators also puncture tissue for insertion (trocar).
6. Trocar: A sharply pointed instrument that fits into a cannula (sheath) used to puncture and guide the cannula into body cavities. Once the trocar is removed, it allows fluids to drain through the cannula.
7. Speculum: An instrument having two blades that when extended widens an orifice or cavity.
   a. Vaginal speculum: Instrument used for opening and exposing the interior of the vaginal canal for proper visualization.

b. Nasal speculum: Instrument used to open the nares.
c. Ear speculum: Cone-shaped plastic tip that directs the light of an otoscope.

E. Endoscopes: Hollow, cylindrical instruments that may contain a light source used to visualize the interior of a body orifice or cavity.
1. Sigmoidoscope: Endoscope used to visualize the sigmoid colon.
2. Proctoscope: Endoscope used to visualize the rectum.
3. Anoscope: Endoscope used to visualize the superficial rectum.
4. Bronchoscope: Endoscope used to visualize the larynx, trachea, and bronchi.
5. Otoscope: Endoscope used to visualize the external and middle ear.
6. Cystoscope: Endoscope used to visualize the urinary bladder.
7. Laparoscope: Endoscope used to visualize the peritoneal cavity.

F. Retractors: Instruments used to pull back tissue to facilitate viewing of the operative site (see Figures 17-4A to O).

G. Specialized instruments
1. Fingernail drill: Used to perforate an injured nail when a blood clot or infection makes drainage and pressure release necessary.
2. Extractors: Used to remove substances (such as comedos, or blackheads) from the superficial layer of skin.
3. Ear, nose, and throat instruments
   a. Snares: Instruments holding a sharp cutting wire loop used to remove polyps.
   b. "Alligator" forceps are so termed because of the appearance of their jaw closure. These forceps are inserted through a speculum in the ear or nose to remove foreign bodies.
   c. Ear curettes: Handle with a metal loop at the end used to scrape accumulated or impacted cerumen from the ear canal.
   d. Laryngeal mirror: Small round mirror situated at the end of a long handle similar to a dental mirror used to visualize the pharynx and larynx.
4. Biopsy punch: Instrument used to remove tissue for examination and detection of cancer.
5. Gynecologic instruments
   a. Uterine curette: Sharp, spoon-shaped instrument used to scrape cells from the cervix for a Pap test, to remove minor polyps, and to obtain secretion samples for testing.
   b. Uterine sounds: Used to dilate the cervix to facilitate insertion of a uterine curette.
   c. Uterine tenaculum: Forceplike instrument used to grasp cervical or vaginal tissue.

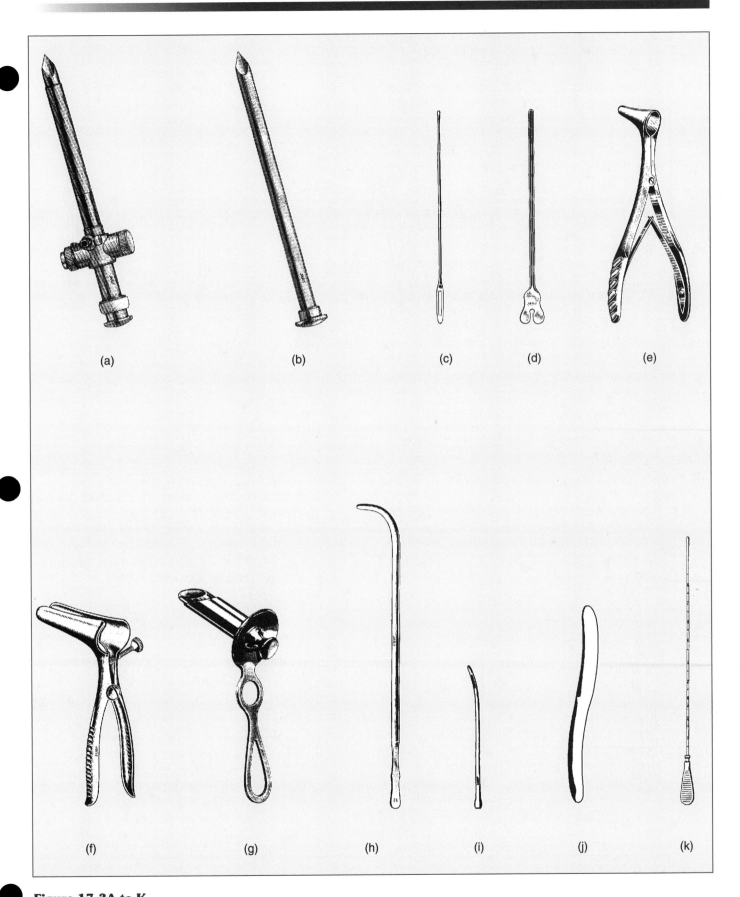

Figure 17-3A to K

Probing and dilating instruments: (a) Cannula and trocar, (b) Trocar, (c) Probe, (d) Director, (e) Nasal speculum, (f) Rectal speculum, (g) Anoscope with obturator, (h) Urethral sound, (i) Urethral dilator, (j) Uterine dilator, (k) Sims uterine sound. Courtesy of Jarit Surgical Instruments.

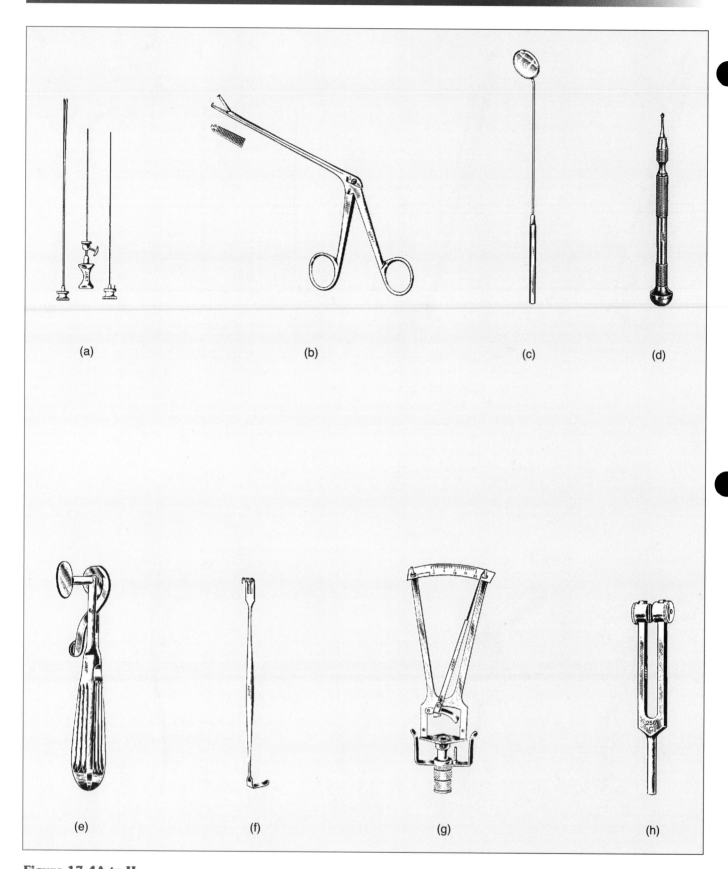

(a)

(b)

(c)

(d)

(e)

(f)

(g)

(h)

Figure 17-4A to H

Specialty instruments: (a) Biopsy needle, (b) Alligator forceps, (c) Laryngeal mirror, (d) Nail drill, (e) Ring cutter, (f) Retractor, (g) Tonometer, (h) Tuning fork. Courtesy of Jarit Surgical Instruments.

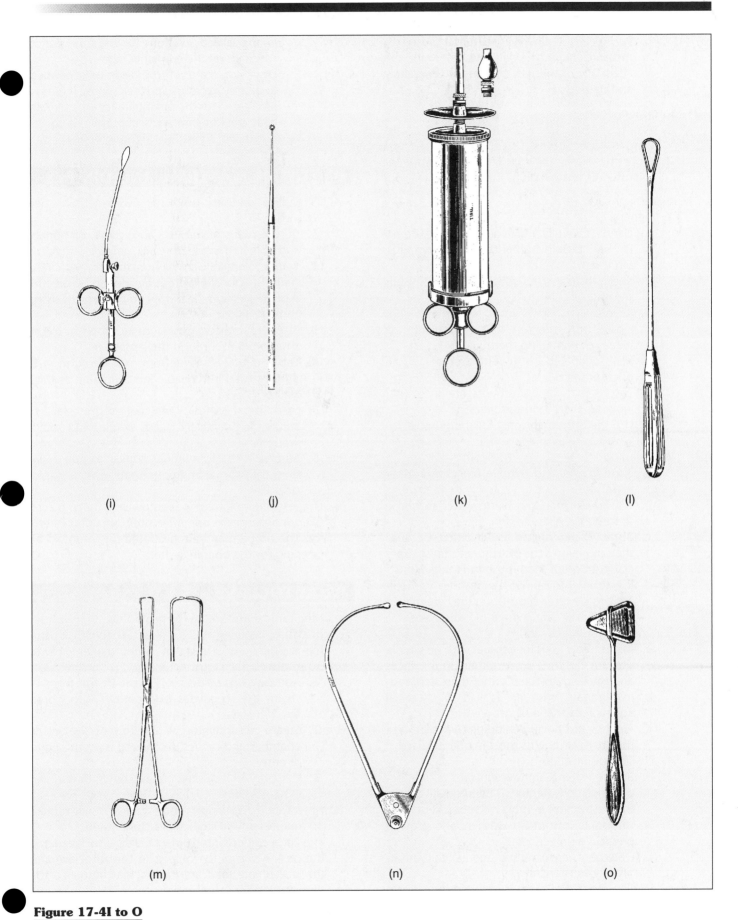

(i) (j) (k) (l)

(m) (n) (o)

Figure 17-4I to O

*Specialty instruments: (i) Ear snare, (j) Ear curette, (k) Ear syringe, (l) Uterine curette, (m) Uterine tenaculum, (n) Pelvimeter,
(o) Percussion hammer.* Courtesy of Jarit Surgical Instruments.

d. Pelvimeter: Caliperlike instrument used to measure the female pelvis to determine the adequacy of the pelvic basin for pregnancy and delivery.

H. Surgical needles
   1. Abscess needle: Used to withdraw fluid or pus from a cyst or abscess.
   2. Biopsy needle: Used to obtain a core of tissue for microscopic examination.

I. Instrument care
   1. General
      a. Handle carefully and avoid dropping them.
      b. Do not stack instruments to avoid entangling them.
      c. Keep instruments with differing finishes separate.
      d. Keep sharp and delicate instruments separated from the rest to avoid dulling the blades or damaging them.
      e. Keep ratcheted instruments (forceps) in an open position.
      f. Ensure that all instruments are in proper working order before sterilizing.
      g. Use the instrument only for the purpose for which it is designed.
   2. Cleaning
      a. Rinse in water to remove blood and other secretions.
      b. Wash with soap and warm water and rinse thoroughly. Allow to dry.
      c. Abrasive detergents are avoided because their use injures the instrument's finish. Special instrument soap is used to inhibit rust.
      d. If instruments cannot be cleansed immediately following a procedure, they are placed in a solution containing a blood solvent.
   3. Chemical disinfection
      a. Instruments used for contact with nonsterile sites such as the skin or natural body orifices are usually disinfected rather than sterilized.
      b. Instruments must be soaked in chemical agents for varying lengths.
      c. Alcohol and povidone-iodine (Betadine) are the chemical agents most frequently used.
   4. Physical disinfection
      a. Boiling water is a physical means of disinfection; boiling water for 15 minutes will ensure the destruction of most microbes.
      b. Ultrasonic instrument washers also provide physical disinfection.
      c. Detergents are "wetting agents" that emulsify oily substances.
   5. Sterilization: Sterilization is required for surgical instruments that come in contact with internal tissue.
      a. Chemical sterilization methods used for heat-sensitive materials include immersion

in specialized solutions for the time period specified on the container label.
      b. Dry ovens are used to provide sufficient heat to destroy microbes and their spores. It is most often used for those supplies for which moist heat would be impractical or damaging.
      c. Autoclave: Moist heat under pressure.

III. SUTURE MATERIAL AND DRAPES

A. Threadlike material used to sew together open wounds.
   1. Suture material may be absorbable or nonabsorbable and made from silk, catgut, or nylon.
   2. Gauge: Available in varying thicknesses called gauges. Choice of gauge depends on the wound size and location, and the type of tissue to be repaired.
   3. Sizes are registered in gauge numbers from the smallest, 6-0, through the largest, 6.
   4. Facial sutures range from 6-0 through 4-0. Sutures used in movable joints may be as thick as 0 or 1.
   5. Steri-Strips: Adhesive material used in place of sutures for relatively clean, simple, and minor wounds.
   6. Staples: Metallic material, similar to paper staples, that approximates wounds using a stapler device.

B. Drapes: Sterile cloths or paper toweling that is placed over or around the operative site to maintain sterility. The drape may be fenestrated, i.e., contain an opening for the operative site.

IV. AUTOCLAVE

A. Mechanical apparatus for providing steam under pressure, usually at 250° F at 20 to 30 lbs/in^2, for a specified length of time, usually 15 to 30 minutes. (see Figure 17-5)
   1. Autoclaves provide moist heat in the form of steam that circulates in a pattern throughout the autoclave.
   2. Steam accumulates at the top of the inside chamber and moves downward from the point of entry.
   3. Cool, dry air is pushed out and down through an exhaust drain.

B. Unwrapped instruments and supplies usually require 30 minutes at 250° to achieve sterilization.

C. The composition of the object being autoclaved and the positioning of the objects in the autoclave and the size of the load are factors that influence the time required for sterilization.

D. Some instruments and supplies to be autoclaved require special wrapping and positioning techniques. Instruments are wrapped following the cleansing and drying procedure.

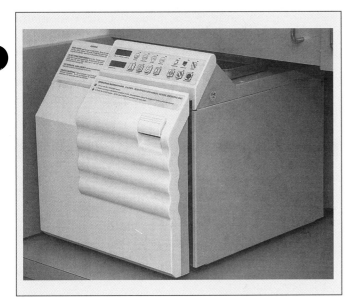

Figure 17-5

Autoclave. Delmar/Cengage Learning.

E. Materials such as clean muslin, cotton, disposable paper packages, or plastic-like materials are used to wrap items for sterilization. The material must be penetrable by steam but strong enough to resist tearing and keep contaminants out.

F. Hinged instruments are opened to allow steam to penetrate all surfaces.

G. Items to be wrapped are placed in the center of the wrap diagonal to the wrapper. A sterilization indicator should be placed in the middle of the pack; when the pack is opened following the sterilization procedure, the indicator will be a different color if sterilization of the pack interior has occurred. The bottom and side corners of the wrap are placed over the object, with a small tab of each corner turned to allow grasping the corner without contaminating the object when the package is opened following sterilization. The top corner of the wrap is placed around the object and secured with autoclave tape. Autoclave tape can be marked to identify the contents and date of sterilization; additionally, autoclave tape will display black striations when exposed to steam, but this in itself does not ensure that sterilization of the package contents has occurred. After securing with autoclave tape, the pack should be snug so that instruments do not fall from the package, but loose enough to permit steam to circulate.

H. Packs should be no larger than 12 × 12 × 20 inches and spaced at least 1 to 3 inches from each other and the chamber.

I. Packs containing layers of fabric such as dressing or drapes should be placed vertically.

J. Hard goods should be placed below soft goods.

K. Instruments for immediate use or those that are kept readily available can be sterilized in trays without being wrapped separately. Usually, a plastic-type wrap or muslin toweling is placed under the instruments. Following the sterilization procedure, the lid is placed on the tray and the instruments are ready for use.

L. A sterilization indicator should be used to determine whether the proper time and temperature for sterilization was achieved.

M. Instruments and utensils should be spaced so as not to touch one another.

N. When possible, utensils and glassware should be inverted.

O. Solutions: Liquids that can withstand heat under pressure without degradation may be autoclaved. Solutions are usually placed in a glass container with the cap loosened or a gauze plug inserted in the opening to allow the steam to circulate.

P. After the sterilization cycle is complete, the autoclave should be opened slightly for venting and to facilitate drying.

Q. When items are dried, they can be removed with clean, dry hands if wrapped. If unwrapped, sterile forceps or sterile gloves are required.

R. Storing objects removed from the autoclave
   1. A clean, dry storage area is required to keep sterilized items from becoming contaminated.
   2. The storage area should be closed to prevent dust accumulation.
   3. Shelf life is dependent on the type of wrapper/package material used, but is usually four weeks. The product manufacturer provides shelf-life data. Storage beyond the shelf life necessitates resterilization.

S. Autoclave procedure
   1. Thoroughly sanitize articles to be sterilized; wrap the articles; mark each pack with its contents, date, and preparer's initials.
   2. Check the autoclave water level; add distilled water if necessary.
   3. Properly place the sterilization indicators in the autoclave; properly load the autoclave.
   4. Close the autoclave door securely; turn on the autoclave.
   5. When the autoclave reaches the desired temperature (250° to 270° F) and pressure (20 to 30 lb/in²), set the timer for the desired sterilization time.
   6. After the autoclave has completed its sterilization cycle, vent the chamber if not done automatically.
   7. Open the autoclave door slightly 5 to 20 minutes to dry the contents.
   8. Turn off the autoclave and remove the sterilized items; check the sterilization indicators to ensure sterilization has occurred.
   9. Store the articles in a clean, dustproof area.

V. PATIENT PREPARATION

A. Patient positioning: Have the patient disrobe sufficiently to facilitate the operative procedure, and as well as adopt a comfortable position to minimize unnecessary movement.

B. Skin preparation
 1. Because skin cannot be sterilized, the objective of presurgical skin preparation is to remove as many microorganisms as possible to reduce the likelihood of infection.
 2. The area is usually shaved because bacteria cling to hair. A wet shave is preferred to reduce cuts and scrapes. The hair should first be shaved in the direction of growth for greater comfort and perhaps against the direction of growth for more complete removal.
 3. Procedure
    a. Wash hands; don gloves; identify the patient; explain the procedure.
    b. Drape the site with two towels far enough from each other to extend past the surgical field.
    c. Soak sterile gauze in a detergent solution, and cleanse the site in a circular motion from the center outward, passing over each area only once.
    d. Use new gauze for each pass until thoroughly cleansed; rinse with sterile water and pat dry.
    e. Resoap and wet shave if required; rinse with sterile water and pat dry.
    f. Resoap, rinse, and dry again.
    g. Apply an antibacterial solution to the skin (such as Betadine) using an applicator in a circular pattern described previously; if the provider is not ready to proceed, cover with a sterile towel.

C. Local anesthesia
 1. Before the surgical procedure, the provider usually administers an anesthetic agent by injecting it at the surgical site to prevent the sensation of pain.
 2. Xylocaine (lidocaine hydrochloride) is commonly used.
 3. Some procedures require the use of epinephrine to enhance the anesthetic effect as well as prevent vascular absorption of the anesthetic. The epinephrine may also minimize bleeding at the surgical site.
 4. The anesthesia usually takes effect in 5 to 15 minutes.
 5. The provider may inject the anesthetic prior to donning sterile gloves; if so, the MA loads the syringe with the prescribed amount and recaps the needle.
 6. If, however, the provider dons sterile gloves, the MA must hand the provider a sterile needle and syringe if not already contained in the sterile surgical pack. The MA must then select the prescribed vial of anesthetic (the outside of the vial is unsterile), wipe the stopper with alcohol, and hold it in a position that will allow the provider to insert the needle to draw the proper amount.

VI. ASEPSIS

A. General
 1. The major objective in surgical asepsis is to free the surgical site of all microbes and their spores.
 2. Clean must always come in contact with clean.
 3. Unclean must always come in contact with unclean.
 4. Sterile must always come in contact with sterile.

B. Handwashing
 1. Appropriate handwashing is the most important defense against disease transmission.
 2. Use a surgical scrub containing chlorhexidine.
 3. Proper handwashing requires a wetting agent, friction, and running water.
 4. Procedure
    a. Remove all jewelry except wedding bands.
    b. Turn on the water faucet. Allow your hands to get completely wet; apply soap from a dispenser and lather while keeping the fingers pointed downward.
    c. Rub, using friction, between fingers and over hands for 30 seconds.
    d. Rinse so that the water flows from the wrist downward to the fingertips.
    e. Apply soap and scrub for an additional 15 seconds; rinse as before; inspect for cleanliness.
    f. Dry hands with a paper towel; turn faucet off with the paper towel.

C. Surgical scrub: Same as handwashing except:
 1. Use a sterile scrub brush to scrub the hands and fingers, and work toward the elbow. Allow 5 minutes for each hand.
 2. Raise the hands, bending the arms at the elbows, and pass under running water to rinse, starting with the fingers.
 3. Glove immediately.

D. Using sterile gloves: Sterile gloves are used whenever the patient needs to be protected from all microorganisms or whenever the medical assistant is required to handle sterile equipment and supplies while maintaining their sterility (see Figures 17-6A to F).
 1. Select proper glove size and inspect package for tears.
 2. Open outer wrapper according to package directions and discard.
 3. Open the inner package by completely grasping the folded edges and pulling firmly.

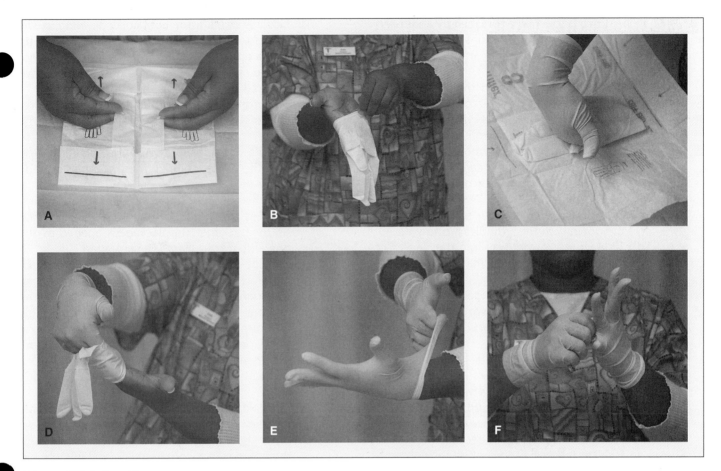

Figure 17-6 A to F

Donning sterile gloves. Delmar/Cengage Learning.

4. Place inner wrapper on a flat, clean surface with labeled cuffed edges toward worker.
5. Perform surgical scrub.
6. With the nondominant hand, lift the glove for the dominant hand by the folded edge of the cuffed end, keeping it well away from the body and objects.
7. Keeping the gloves above the waist, put the glove on; if the fingers or thumb fail to insert into the appropriate glove fingers, do not adjust until after the second glove is on.
8. Pick up the second glove by placing the gloved fingers under the cuff, avoiding touching the exposed end.
9. Insert second hand, straightening cuffs by touching only the outside of the gloves to adjust the fingers of the first hand if necessary.
10. Once the sterile gloves are on, keep them above the waist and away from the body.
11. Remove the gloves if they become contaminated or are torn.
12. Following the completion of the procedure, remove the gloves by pulling them down and off from the cuff so the outside of the glove is not touched.

E. Surgical gowns
1. If the MA touches the outside of the gown while donning it, the gown is contaminated and discarded.
2. The MA is to touch only the inside of the gown while putting it on.
3. Surgical gowns are folded with the inside facing the MA. This method of folding facilitates picking up and donning the gown without touching the outside surface.
4. The MA's scrubbed hands and arms are contaminated if she allows them to fall below waist level or to touch her body. The MA keeps hands and arms above the waist, away from the body, and at an angle of about 20 to 30 degrees above the elbows.
5. After donning the surgical gown, the only parts of the gown that are considered sterile are the sleeves (except for the axillary area) and the front from waist level to a few inches below the neck opening.

6. If the gown is touched or brushed by an unsterile object, the gown is then considered contaminated and discarded.
7. Gowning procedure:
   a. With one hand, pick up the entire folded gown from the wrapper by grasping the gown through all layers, being careful to touch only the exposed top layer.
   b. Hold the gown near the gown's neck, and allow it to unfold, being careful that it does not touch either your body or other unsterile objects.
   c. Grasp the inside shoulder seams and open the gown with the armholes facing you.
   d. Slide your arms partway into the sleeves of the gown, keeping your hands at shoulder level away from the body.
   e. With the assistance of another, slide your arms further into the gown sleeves keeping them inside the sleeve and not protruding from the cuff.
   f. Have an assistant position and adjust the gown over your shoulders by grasping the inside surface of the gown at the shoulder seams. The assistant's hands are in contact with only the inside surface of the gown.
   g. The assistant secures the back and neck with a Velcro tab or ties preventing the contaminated surfaces at the back of the gown from coming into contact with the front of the gown.
8. Gown removal
   a. After the assistant unties the neck and back ties, grasp the gown at the shoulders and pull the gown forward and down over the arms and gloved hands.
   b. Holding the arms away from the body, fold the gown so that the outside of the gown is folded in; discard it into the linen hamper.
F. Aseptic handling of instruments and supplies: The objective is to keep the instruments and supplies free from contamination.
   1. Sterile forceps are used to handle sterile instruments and supplies when sterile gloves are not worn. The handle of the forceps is nonsterile; the tips are sterile.
      a. Lift the transfer forceps out of the container without touching the sides of the container.
      b. Tap the blades of the forceps together to expel excess solution or touch them to a sterile gauze.
      c. Grasp the sterile object with the tip of the forcep facing down and transfer it to the sterile field or to the provider's gloved hand.
      d Replace the transfer forcep into the container without touching the sides of the container.

2. Lids removed from containers housing sterile instruments and supplies are always face up when placed on the counter surface. Lids not placed on the counter surface are held face down to avoid breathing into the inside of the lid.
3. Pouring sterile solution from a bottle requires opening the lid carefully to avoid touching the inside, pouring well above the receptacle to avoid touching the rim of the sterile receptacle with the bottle. Solution must not splash on the sterile field.
4. Commercially packaged sterile instruments and supplies are opened by using the flaps provided on the package. The package is opened in one movement by pulling the flaps apart.
5. Do not reach over the sterile field. Approximately 1 inch around the edge of the wrap is considered contaminated. If equipment in the package has to be handed to a gloved individual or dropped onto a sterile field, it is best to move the package contents with the transfer forceps.
6. Ointments must be placed on a sterile gauze pad with a sterile cotton-tipped swab or tongue blade.
7. A sterile tray must be covered with a sterile towel if it is not to be used immediately.
8. When there is any break in the above techniques, the entire field is contaminated and must be set up again. When there is any doubt about the sterility of an object, it must be replaced.

VII. COMMON MINOR SURGERY PROCEDURES

A. Incision and drainage (I&D)
   1. Usually performed to remove an abscess, a collection of pus in a cavity surrounded by inflamed tissue.
   2. If the abscess does not rupture and drain naturally, the provider may have to incise the infective site to allow drainage.
   3. A local anesthetic is usually administered followed by an incision made with a scalpel.
   4. A rubber penrose drain or a gauze wick is inserted into the wound separating the edges of the wound to facilitate drainage of the exudate. The exudate should be considered infectious and handled accordingly.
   5. Items placed on the sterile field
      a. Antiseptic solution.
      b. Sterile swabs or cotton balls.
      c. Fenestrated drape.
      d. Needle and syringe.
      e. Scalpel.
      f. Surgical scissors.
      g. Hemostatic forceps.
      h. Tissue forceps.

     i. Thumb forceps.

     j. Sterile 4" × 4" gauze.

  6. Items not placed on the sterile field:

     a. Sterile gloves.

     b. Local anesthetic.

     c. Alcohol wipe.

     d. Rubber penrose drain.

     e. Iodoform packing material.

     f. Surgical tape.

B. Laceration repair

  1. Performed to close up a traumatic or surgical wound for proper healing with minimal scarring.

  2. The MA usually cleans the wound before the provider examines it for possible debridement of dead or damaged tissue.

  3. Items placed on the sterile field:

     a. Antiseptic solution.

     b. Sterile swabs or cotton balls.

     c. Fenestrated drape.

     d. Needle and syringe.

     e. Scalpel.

     f. Surgical scissors.

     g. Hemostatic forceps.

     h. Needle holder

     i. Tissue forceps.

     j. Thumb forceps.

     k. Suture.

     l. Sterile 4" × 4" gauze.

  4. Items not placed on the sterile field:

     a. Sterile gloves.

     b. Local anesthetic.

     c. Alcohol wipe.

     d. Antibiotic ointment.

     e. Surgical tape.

C. Cyst removal

  1. Performed to remove a sebaceous cyst, a thin, closed capsule containing sebaceous gland secretions. This is often done before it becomes infected; if it is infected, however, the provider will perform an I&D before removing it.

  2. After anesthetizing the area, the provider will make an incision and remove the cyst, followed by suturing the surgical incision.

  3. The cyst will be placed in a specimen container with formalin and sent to a pathologist for examination, in a biohazard transport bag.

  4. Items placed on the sterile field:

     a. Antiseptic solution.

     b. Sterile swabs or cotton balls.

     c. Fenestrated drape.

     d. Needle and syringe.

     e. Scalpel.

     f. Surgical scissors.

     g. Hemostatic forceps.

     h. Needle holder.

     i. Tissue forceps.

     j. Thumb forceps.

     k. Suture.

     l. Sterile 4" × 4" gauze.

  5. Items not placed on the sterile field:

     a. Sterile gloves.

     b. Local anesthetic.

     c. Alcohol wipe.

     d. Antibiotic ointment.

     e. Specimen container and lab request form.

     f. Surgical tape.

D. Ingrown toenail resection

  1. Performed to remove an ingrown toenail to relieve pain and discomfort. The edge of the toenail grows deeply into the nail groove, often caused by pressure such as that from tight shoes.

  2. Usually the MA will soak the patient's foot in an antibacterial solution for 10 to 15 minutes to reduce the likelihood of infection and to soften the nail bed.

  3. The provider anesthetizes the area and surgically removes a wedge of the nail using toenail scissors.

  4. Items placed on the sterile field:

     a. Antiseptic solution.

     b. Sterile swabs or cotton balls.

     c. Fenestrated drape.

     d. Needle and syringe.

     e. Toenail scissors.

     f. Surgical scissors.

     g. Hemostatic forceps.

     h. Sterile 4" × 4" gauze.

  5. Items not placed on the sterile field:

     a. Sterile gloves.

     b. Local anesthetic.

     c. Alcohol wipe.

     d. Surgical tape.

VIII. POSTOPERATIVE CARE

A. Wound types

  1. A wound is any interruption in the continuity of internal or external soft tissues. A closed wound is an injury that occurs but the skin remains intact.

  2. Wounds are classified as superficial when the injury does not extend beyond the subcutaneous layer.

  3. Deep wounds are those that extend beyond the subcutaneous layer.

  4. A puncture wound is a hole made with a thin, sharp instrument and is an example of a deep wound.

B. The healing process

  1. Wound repair is classified according to how the healing process occurs. Classification depends on the nature of the wound, the amount of tissue lost or removed, and the potential for infection.

2. First intention (primary union or closure): When wounds such as sutured surgical incisions heal, there is minimal tissue damage and scarring.

3. Second intention (granulation or indirect union): The wound edges are not sutured or approximated. The body's repair of these wounds is slower and produces more scarring.

4. Third intention: A surgical wound becomes infected and requires reopening of the initial wound. These wounds take longer to heal and produce much scar tissue.

5. The body's ability to heal after surgery or trauma depends on adequate circulation and normal clotting time, good general health, and proper intake of essential nutrients.

C. Wound cleansing

  1. Using an antiseptic solution, proceed from a clean to a contaminated area.

  2. Use one swab or gauze pad per stroke when circular motions cannot be used.

  3. If a drain is present, clean around it after the suture is cleansed.

D. Dressings

  1. Sterile cover placed over a wound to prevent contamination and injury, control bleeding, and absorb blood and secretions.

  2. Procedure

    a. Assemble equipment: Sterile gloves, sterile dressing, bandage scissors, and bandage materials.

    b. Plan the dressing and cut the adhesive tape.

    c. Wash hands using surgical aseptic technique.

    d. Using aseptic technique, open the dressing packages and create a sterile field; don sterile gloves.

    e. Apply the amount of dressing needed. For absorption, several layers of sterile gauze dressing squares are required. Gloved fingers touch only sterile gauze squares, not the skin or wound.

    f. Secure the dressing with a bandage that wraps and conforms to the body contour. Apply tape to the bandage to hold it in place.

E. Bandage application

  1. Bandages differ from dressings in that they are nonsterile long strips ranging from 1 to 6 or more inches in width. The purposes of the bandage are to:

    a. Splint and/or protect an injured tissue.

    b. Maintain pressure over an area.

    c. Aid in circulation of an extremity.

    d. Hold a sterile dressing in place.

  2. Procedure

    a. Start at the distal end of the body part, progressing proximally, rolling the gauze without stretching or pulling.

    b. If the bandage is applied too tightly, it can impair circulation and neurological function. Therefore, it is important to keep the distal body part accessible to visual inspection.

    c. At the first sign of cyanosis of the extremity or a complaint of numbness, the bandage must be removed immediately.

F. Suture/staple removal

  1. Identify patient, wash hands, open suture/staple removal kit.

  2. Don sterile gloves.

  3. Sutures: Using thumb forceps, grasp suture knot and gently pull toward suture line so as to exert the least amount of pressure on the suture line. Holding the knot with the forceps, cut one side of the suture as close to the skin as possible using a suture removal scissors. Gently pull the suture from the skin.

  4. Staples: Gently insert the jaw of the staple remover under the staple. Gently squeeze the staple remover handle until the staple bends upward and is released from the skin.

  5. Remove all sutures/staples ensuring the same number have been removed that were applied, as noted in the chart. Place sutures/staples on gauze or tissue to make a final count.

  6. Apply antibiotic ointment and dressing as ordered.

  7. Remove gloves and properly dispose of used materials.

  8. Wash hands, provide post-procedure instructions, document procedure.

G. Patient instructions: Patient should be instructed to immediately report:

  1. Excess bleeding.

  2. Fever.

  3. Swelling redness, or streaking around the surgical site.

  4. A dislodged drain.

  5. The patient should be instructed to keep all dressings clean and dry.

H. Medical assistant's role

  1. Prepare the room.

  2. Assemble and set up the equipment.

  3. Verify completion of operative consent forms.

  4. Prepare the patient.

  5. Adjust the lighting.

  6. Assist the provider during the procedure.

  7. Apply dressings as ordered.

  8. Reinforce postprocedure instructions.

  9. Properly dispose of used supplies.

  10. Prepare the room for the next patient.

CHAPTER 18

Pharmacology and Drug Therapy

I. INTRODUCTION

A. General
1. Pharmacology: Science that deals with the study of drugs, their nature, origin, properties, uses, and actions.
2. Drug: Any substance other than food that causes a change in body structure or function.
3. Uses of drugs
   a. Therapeutic: To treat a disease or condition, to relieve symptoms of disease, or to replace a necessary body substance.
   b. Prophylactic: To prevent disease.
   c. Diagnostic: To diagnose an illness.
4. Sources of drugs
   a. Synthetic: Artificially prepared substances that do not exist naturally, using various chemicals and techniques; e.g., prednisone.
   b. Plant: Naturally occurring substance obtained from plants such as berries, bark, leaves, or resin; e.g., digitalis.
   c. Mineral: Naturally occurring substance obtained from the earth or soil; e.g., potassium chloride.
   d. Animal: Substances obtained from glands, organs, and tissues of animals; e.g., insulin.
5. Nomenclature
   a. Chemical name: A drug's chemical formula that identifies its molecular structure; e.g., 4-dimethyl-amino 1,4,4a,5,5a,6,11. . . .
   b. Generic name: Shorter, common name that is a contraction of its chemical formula (not capitalized); e.g., tetracycline.
   c. Trade (brand) name: Special copyrighted name given to a drug by the manufacturer (capitalized); e.g., Achromycin.

B. Drug reference
1. Physician's Desk Reference (PDR)
   a. Commonly used reference that provides information such as use, precautions, indications, warnings, and dosages on commercially available pharmaceuticals.
   b. Organization: The PDR is organized to allow easy access to pertinent information. Sections within the text include information surrounding manufacturers; drug categories and classifications; trade, generic, and chemical names; color pictures of selected drugs; description and use of drugs; list of discontinued drugs; diagnostic drug Information; list of Poison Control Centers, as well as emergency phone numbers.
2. Product insert: A folded sheet of paper in the drug container. The information is usually very similar to that found in the PDR.
3. United States Pharmacopoeia/National Formulary (USP/NF): Both are published every 5 years. The drugs listed in the USP have met specific government standards and bear the initials USP.
4. Desk Reference for Nonprescription Drugs: Similar to the PDR for OTC medications.

C. Forms of drugs
1. Liquid preparations
   a. Syrup: A drug dissolved in sugar, water and flavoring; e.g., syrup of ipecac.
   b. Solution: Liquid preparation containing one or more substances (solutes) that are dissolved in a substance (solvent); e.g., epinephrine solution.
   c. Suspension: A drug that is not evenly dissolved in a liquid and must be shaken before administration; e.g., amoxicillin.
   d. Emulsion: A mixture of oil or fat and water that requires shaking before administration; e.g., cod liver oil.
   e. Tincture: A drug dissolved in an alcohol solution; e.g., tincture of iodine.
   f. Elixir: A drug dissolved in a solution of water, alcohol, and sugar; e.g., terpin hydrate elixir.
   g. Lotion: A nongreasy, aqueous preparation containing suspended particles used for topical applications; e.g., calamine lotion.
   h. Liniment: A drug mixed with soap, oil, alcohol, or water and applied topically, producing a feeling of heat; e.g., camphor liniment.
   i. Aerosol: A suspension of drugs administered in a spray form; e.g., epinephrine inhalant.
   j. Spirit (essence): A drug combined with an alcoholic solution that evaporates into a vapor; e.g., aromatic spirit of ammonia.

2. Solid preparations

a. Capsule: A liquid or powdered drug in a gelatin capsule; e.g., Benadryl capsules.

b. Gelcap: A gelatin-coated capsule.

c. Spansule: A granulated drug enclosed in a capsule so that medication is released at various times after administration; e.g., Contac.

d. Tablet: Powdered medication pressed into a round disc shape. Some tablets are scored for ease in breaking in half. Tablets may also be enteric-coated so that they do not dissolve until reaching the intestines; e.g., aspirin.

e. Caplet: Oblong tablet.

f. Geltab: Gelatin-coated tablet.

g. Suppository: A cone-shaped drug mixed with a firm base such as cocoa butter and made to dissolve when inserted into a body cavity such as the rectum, vagina, or urethra; e.g., glycerin suppository.

h. Ointment: A semisolid drug preparation usually having a fatty or greasy material for topical application; e.g., Vitamin A&D Ointment.

i. Troche (Lozenge): A small medicinal disc, containing a candy base, to be held in the mouth until it dissolves to relieve local irritation and coughing; e.g., Sucrets throat lozenges.

3. Transdermal (patch): Application of patch for the delivery of drug(s) across the skin and into systemic circulation.

D. Pharmaceutical regulation and control

1. General

a. Federal Comprehensive Drug Abuse Prevention and Control Act of 1970 (Controlled Substances Act [CSA]): Legislation designed to control dispensation of potentially abused drugs. Divides drugs into five schedules based on abuse potential and medical usefulness.

(1) Schedule I: Drugs with high potential for abuse and no acceptable medical use; limited to research with proper governmental approval; e.g., LSD, heroin, marijuana.

(2) Schedule II: Drugs are accepted for medical use, but have a high physical and/or psychological potential for dependency and abuse. This is the most closely regulated schedule of drugs because of the abuse potential. Requires a written prescription with no refills permitted. In emergency situations, the prescription may be phoned in to a pharmacy; however, the DEA requires the prescriber to supply a written prescription to the pharmacy within 72 hours of the phone order. If a written prescription is not received within the allotted time, the pharmacy is mandated to report the prescriber to the DEA. Examples of drugs in this schedule are morphine, barbiturates, and amphetamines.

(3) Schedule III: Drugs with moderate abuse potential requiring a prescription. Limited to five refills within a 6-month period; e.g., drug preparations with small amounts of schedule II drugs, such as Tylenol #3 with codeine.

(4) Schedule IV: Drugs with low abuse potential. Limited to five refills within a 6-month period; e.g., phenobarbital, Darvon, Valium.

(5) Schedule V: Drugs with low abuse potential. They may be purchased OTC (over the counter) depending on state laws; e.g., Drixoral, Actifed, Novahistine, Contac.

b. Federal Food, Drug, and Cosmetic Act: Legislation that allows the Food and Drug Administration (FDA) the power to protect the public by requiring rigid standards before commercial availability of drugs.

c. Drug Enforcement Agency (DEA): As a Branch of the Department of Justice, the DEA is responsible for controlling narcotic and dangerous drug abuse, drug diversion, and illegal sale.

2. Pharmaceutical transactions

a. Terminology

(1) Prescribe: A written order (prescription) for medication is completed by a health care provider; a pharmacist prepares the medication and sells it to the patient.

(2) Administer: A medication dose is taken by the patient during the visit.

(3) Dispense: A medication is given to the patient for a fee which is subsequently taken at home.

b. All providers who prescribe, administer, or dispense controlled substances must register with the DEA using form DEA-224.

c. Registered providers will receive a DEA registration number and a Controlled Substances Registration Certificate, which is valid for three years.

d. DEA registration renewal form DEA-224a will be sent 60 days before current registration expiration. If not received within 45 days of expiration, it is the provider's responsibility to notify the DEA.

e. Providers who dispense controlled substances must maintain a record of each transaction.

f. Administration of controlled substances requires a record if the patient is charged for the drug.

3. Inventory
   a. Schedule II inventories must be made every 2 years at the time of registration. Records must always be available for inspection and must account for all drugs dispensed. The records must be kept for a minimum of 2 years.
   b. Schedule II information must include: The patient's name and address; date of administration; medication name, dosage, and route; method of dispensing; and indication for the drug. This specific record keeping is required only when the provider administers or dispenses a scheduled drug in the office.
   c. Prescriptions: Giving the patient a completed prescription does not require the above records. The provider records all prescribed drugs in the patient record.
   d. All inventory records require the provider's name, address, DEA registration number, date of inventory, and the signature of the person taking the inventory.
   e. Schedule II drug orders from suppliers must be made using Federal Triplicate Order Form DEA-222.
4. Security
   a. Storage: Controlled substances must be stored separately from other drugs and securely locked with restricted access.
   b. Theft or loss of inventory: Requires immediate notification of the DEA field office and local police, as well as completion of the Report of Theft of Loss of Controlled Substances Form DEA-106.
   c. Damage: Or contamination of controlled substances requires DEA notification and completion of disposal form DEA-41.
   d. Disposal of drugs: The DEA regulates the disposal of controlled substances in order to help eliminate the routing of legitimate controlled substances into the illegal market. Additionally, many states have declared all drugs to be regulated medical waste that must be tracked and documented for disposal. Check state requirements before disposing of any drug.
E. Dependency and abuse
   1. Dependence: Inability to control the use of a drug that has an abuse potential.
      a. Psychological dependence: Emotional state of craving a drug for its desired effect.
      b. Physical dependence: Physiological adaptation to a drug that causes physical disturbances during periods of prolonged abstinence.

2. Abuse: Any use of drugs that cause physical, psychological, legal, economic, or social harm to the user.
3. Common signs and symptoms
   a. Changes in school or work performance/attendance.
   b. Changes in appearance; especially dishevelment.
   c. Changes in attitude and mood.
   d. Weight loss and unusual odors.
   e. Withdrawal from family and friends.
   f. Association with substance abusers.
   g. Unusual behavior or mannerisms.
   h. Defensiveness.
4. Withdrawal symptoms
   a. Malaise, lethargy, nausea, vomiting.
   b. Anxiety, diaphoresis, and pupillary dilation.
   c. Muscle contractions, pain, and chills.
   d. Hyperpnea, tachypnea, hypertension, delirium tremens.
   e. Irritability, agitation.
F. Pharmacokinetics: The study of drug movement through the body.
   1. Absorption: The process by which drugs enter the circulation.
   2. Distribution: The process by which circulating drugs are transported to cellular and tissue sites of action.
   3. Localization: The accumulation of drugs at the tissue site whereby its intended effect occurs.
   4. Metabolism: After drugs have been used by the body, their by-products must be converted to harmless substances for eventual elimination.
   5. Excretion: The process by which the body eliminates a drug's metabolites.
G. Miscellaneous pharmacological terms
   1. Cumulative effect: Repeated doses of a drug may build up or accumulate in the body.
   2. Idiosyncrasy: A response to a drug that is unique to the individual.
   3. Synergism (potentiation): Drug action in which the effect of using two drugs together is greater than the sum of the effects of using each one alone.
   4. Side effect (adverse reaction): Toxic effect or undesirable results other than for which the drug was intended.
   5. Toxicity: Harmful effects of a drug.
   6. Antagonism: Interaction of two or more drugs causing a change in the expected effect of each drug. Together they produce a lesser effect than is expected from either drug alone.
   7. Tolerance: Capacity for enduring a specified amount of a drug without adverse effect; demonstrating a decreased sensitivity to subsequent doses of a drug; progressive decrease in the effectiveness of a drug.

II. PRESCRIPTIONS

A. Order written by provider for dispensing of a drug. It is a legal document giving directions to the pharmacist for filling the prescription.

B. Parts of a prescription (see Figure 18-1)
1. Provider information: Name, address, phone number, DEA number.
2. Date: Date prescription was written.
3. Patient information: Name, address, phone number, age for children.
4. Superscription: Describes the symbol Rx (fr. L. *recipe*) meaning "take thou."
5. Inscription: Name of the drug, form, and strength.
6. Subscription: Number of doses dispensed and special preparation instructions to the pharmacist.
7. Signature: Sig. (fr. L. *signetur*) meaning write on label. Patient instructions for taking medication.
8. Refill information: If permitted, the number allowed.
9. Provider's signature: Handwritten.

C. Pharmacological acronyms and abbreviations
1. Forms of drugs
   a. aq: water
   b. caps: capsules
   c. elix: elixir
   d. emul: emulsion
   e. fl/fld: fluid
   f. lin: liniment
   g. pulv: pulvis, powder
   h. sol: solution

   i. supp: suppository
   j. syr: syrup
   k. tab: tablet
   l. tinct, tr: tincture
   m. ung: unguentum, ointment
2. Routes of administration
   a. ID: intradermal
   b. IM: intramuscular
   c. IV: intravenous
   d. po: per os, by mouth
   e. top: topical
   f. subl: under the tongue
   g. SQ/SC: subcutaneous
   h. vag: vaginally
   i. ophth: instill in eyes
   j. otic: instill in ears
   k. inj: injection
   l. R: rectally
   m. AD: auris dextra, right ear
   n. AS: auris sinistra, left ear
   o. AU: auris unitas, both ears
   p. OD: oculus dextra, right eye
   q. OS: oculus sinistra, left eye
   r. OU: oculus unitas, both eyes
3. Dosage times
   a. $\bar{a}$:   ante, before
   b. ac: ante cibos, before meals
   c. ad lib: ad libitum, as desired
   d. bid: bis in die, twice daily
   e. d: dies, day
   f. h: horae, hour
   g. hs: hora somni, hour of sleep
   h. noc/noct: nocte, night
   i. $\bar{p}$:   post, after
   j. pc: post cibos, after meals
   k. prn: pro re nata, as needed
   l. q: quaque, every
   m. qd: quaque diem, every day
   n. qh: quaque hora, every hour
   o. q2h: every two hours
   p. q3h: every three hours
   q. qhs: every hour of sleep
   r. qid: quater in die, four times a day
   s. qod: every other day
   t. tid: ter in die, three times a day
4. Miscellaneous directions
   a. $\overline{aa}$:   ana, of each
   b. $\bar{c}$:   cum, with
   c. dil: dilute
   d. D/C: discontinue
   e. npo: nulla per os, nothing by mouth
   f. per: by, with
   g. qs: quantity sufficient
   h. Rx: take, take thou
   i. $\bar{s}$:   sine, without
   j. $\overline{ss}$:   semisse, one half
   k. stat: statim, immediately

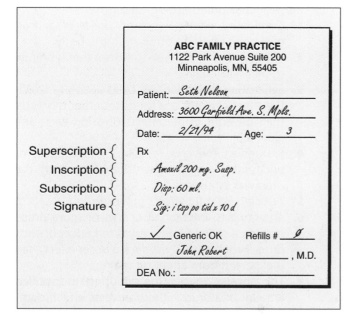

ABC FAMILY PRACTICE
1122 Park Avenue Suite 200
Minneapolis, MN, 55405

Patient: *Seth Nelson*

Address: *3600 Garfield Ave. S. Mpls.*

Date: *2/21/94*   Age: *3*

Superscription { Rx

Inscription {   *Amoxil 200 mg. Susp.*

Subscription { *Disp: 60 ml.*

Signature {   *Sig: i tsp po tid x 10 d*

___✓___ Generic OK   Refills # *∅*

___*John Robert*___ , M.D.

DEA No.: _____

Figure 18-1

Parts of a prescription. Delmar/Cengage Learning.

5. Prescription numerals

a. i: 1
b. ii: 2
c. iii: 3
d. iv: 4
e. v: 5
f. vi: 6
g. vii: 7
h. viii: 8
i. ix: 9
j. x: 10
k. L: 50
l. C: 100
m. D: 500
n. M: 1,000

6. Measurements

a. cc/cm^3: cubic centimeter
b. dr: dram
c. g/gm: gram
d. gr: grain
e. gt, gtt: guttae, gt drop, gtt drops
f. kg: kilogram
g. l: liter
h. m/min: minim
i. mEq: milliequivalent
j. mg: milligram
k. ml: milliliter
l. oz: ounce
m. pt: pint
n. tsp/t: teaspoon
o. tbsp/T: tablespoon
p. U: units

D. The Joint Commission "Do Not Use" List

1. To ensure patient safety, the Joint Commission requires that the following abbreviations and acronyms not be used in handwritten or free-text computer entry orders and medication related documentation.

2. U: Mistaken for zero (0), four (4), or "cc." Instead, write "unit."

3. IU: Mistaken for intravenous (IV) or ten (10). Instead, write "international unit."

4. Q.D., QD, q.d., qd: Mistaken for each other. Instead, write daily.

5. Q.O.D., QOD, q.o.d., qod: Periods and O's mistaken as "I." Instead, write "every other day."

6. Trailing zero: Do not use a trailing zero, e.g. 10.0 mg, as often the decimal point is missing or illegible. Instead, write 10 mg.

7. lack of leading zero: E.g. .5 mg. Because the decimal point may not be seen, use a leading zero, e.g. 0.5 mg.

8. MS: Can mean morphine sulfate or magnesium sulfate. The chemical abbreviations can also be confused, MSO4, MgSO4. Instead, write "morphine sulfate," or "magnesium sulfate."

III. DRUG CLASSIFICATIONS

A. Anti-infectives: Prevents or treats infections.

1. Antibiotic: Bactericides that prevent or treat bacterial infections by inhibiting their growth.
a. Penicillin: Amoxil, Augmentin.
b. Cephalosporin: Keflex, Ceclor.
c. Tetracycline: Achromycin, Vibramycin.
d. Erythromycin: Erythrocin, Ilotycin.

2. Antifungal: Prevents or treats fungal infections.
a. Amphotericin: Fungizone.
b. Griseofulvin: Fulvicin.
c. Nystatin: Mycostatin.
d. Miconazole: Monostat.
e. Fluconazole: Diflucan.

3. Antiviral: Prevents or treats viral infections.
a. Acyclovir sodium: Zovirax.
b. Zidovudine (AZT): Retrovir.
c. Idoxuridine: Herplex.

4. Antiparasitic: Prevents or treats parasitic infections.
a. Mebendazole: Vermox. Antihelmintic used to treat parasitic roundworm infections.
b. Niclosamide: Niclocide. Antihelmintic used to treat tapeworm infections.
c. Lindane: Kwell. Antilousing used to treat lice and scabies.

5. Sulfonamides (sulfa drugs): Prevent or treat bacterial infections by inhibiting their growth.
a. Sulfamethoxazole: Bactrim.
b. Sulfisoxazole: Gantrisin.

B. Dermatological agents

1. Emollient: Soothes skin and mucous membranes; e.g., petrolatum, lanolin.

2. Astringent: Prevents tissue weepage and secretions; e.g., phenol, aluminum hydroxide.

3. Keratolytic: Causes sloughing of hardened skin; e.g., benzoic acid, Resorcinol.

4. Anesthetic: Causes local numbing and loss of sensation; e.g., lidocaine, Novocaine.

5. Antiacneic: Prevents or treats acne vulgaris; e.g., Retin-A, Accutane.

6. Antiseptic: Kills or prevents growth of infectious agents; e.g., Betadine, Zephiran.

C. Respiratory agents

1. Antitussive: Cough suppressant; e.g., Robitussin, Sorbutuss.

2. Antihistamine: Relieves allergic symptoms and reduces mucus secretions; e.g., Benadryl, Actifed, Allegra, Claritin.

3. Bronchodilator: Opens or dilates the bronchi; e.g., epinephrine, aminophylline.

4. Decongestant: Relieves local congestion of the upper respiratory tract; e.g., Naldecon, Dimetapp.

5. Expectorant: Liquifies mucus in bronchi and helps to expel phlegm; e.g., Benylin Expectorant, Ru-Tuss Expectorant, Terpin Hydrate.

D. Cardiovascular agents
 1. Antiarrhythmic: Regulates heart rate and rhythm; e.g., Inderal, Pronestyl.
 2. Anticoagulant: Slows, inhibits blood clotting; e.g., Coumadin, heparin sodium.
 3. Antihypertensive: Lowers blood pressure; e.g., Aldomet, Lopressor, Tenormin.
 4. Inotropic (cardiotonic): increases heart contractility; e.g., Digitalis, digoxin.
 5. Hematinic: Increases blood iron levels; e.g., Feosol, Imferon.
 6. Vasoconstrictor: Constricts blood vessels and raises blood pressure; e.g., Adrenalin, Levophed.
 7. Vasodilator: Dilates blood vessels and lowers blood pressure; e.g., Nitroglycerin, Apresoline.
E. Central nervous system agents
 1. CNS stimulant: Increases brain and spinal cord functions or body activity such as amphetamines; e.g., Ritalin, Benzedrine.
 2. CNS depressant: Decreases brain and spinal cord functions or body activity; e.g., secobarbital, amobarbital.
 3. Analgesics: Relieves pain.
    a. Narcotic agents: Highly addictive analgesics; e.g., morphine, codeine, Demerol.
    b. Non-narcotic: Tylenol, aspirin, ibuprofen.
 4. Antipyretic: Reduces fever; e.g., aspirin, Tylenol.
 5. Antidepressant: Relieves depression; a mood elevator; e.g., Elavil, Tofranil.
 6. Anticonvulsant: Controls seizures and epilepsy; e.g., Dilantin, Mesantoin.
 7. Sedative: Produces a state of relaxation; e.g., Nembutal, Seconal, phenobarbital.
 8. Hypnotic: Induces sleep; e.g., Dalmane, Halcion, Noludar.
 9. Tranquilizer: Reduces anxiety, produces a calming effect; e.g., Valium, Librium, Thorazine.
F. Autonomic nervous system agents
 1. Adrenergic (sympathomimetic): Stimulates the sympathetic nervous system; e.g., epinephrine, Neo-Synephrine.
 2. Antiadrenergic (sympatholytic): Depresses the sympathetic nervous system; e.g., Aldomet, Inderal.
 3. Cholinergic (parasympathomimetic): Stimulates the parasympathetic nervous system; e.g., Eserine, Tensilon.
 4. Anticholinergic (parasympatholytic): Depresses the parasympathetic nervous system; e.g., Valpin, Librax.
G. Gastrointestinal agents
 1. Antacid: Neutralizes stomach acid; e.g., Gelusil, Maalox, Mylanta.
 2. Antisecretory: Inhibits gastric secretions, especially hydrochloric acid; e.g., Tagamet, Zantac.
 3. Antiemetic: Prevents nausea and vomiting; e.g., Tigan, Compazine.

 4. Antidiarrheal: Stops diarrhea; e.g., Lomotil, Kaopectate.
 5. Cathartic: Relieves constipation, promotes bowel movements, softens stool; e.g., methylcellulose, Metamucil.
 6. Emetic: Induces vomiting; e.g., syrup of ipecac, apomorphine hydrochloride.
 7. Antispasmotic: Prevents or relieves spasms of the GI tract; e.g., Donnatal, Combid.
H. Endocrine agents: Hormonal agents
 1. Thyroid agents: Synthroid (agent used for supplementation for patients with hypothyroidism), Proloid (agent used to suppress thyroid function for patients with hyperthyroidism).
 2. Adrenal agents: Cortisone, prednisone.
 3. Pancreatic agents: Insulin, Glucotrol, Diabeta.
 4. Ovarian agents: Premarin, Theelin.
 5. Contraceptive: Lo/Ovral, Ovulen.
I. Urinary agents
 1. Urinary antiseptic: Inhibits the growth of urinary microorganisms; e.g., Furodantin, NegGram.
 2. Urinary analgesic: Relieves dysuria; e.g., Pyridium, Thiosulfil-A Forte, Trac Tabs.
 3. Diuretic: Increases urinary output; e.g., Lasix, Dyazide, Hygroton, Diuril.
J. Antineoplastic agents: Inhibits the growth of malignant cells; e.g., Chlorambucil USP, Myleran, Alkeran, Taxol.
K. Musculoskeletal agents
 1. Antiarthritic: Relieves joint inflammation; e.g., Motrin, Celebrex, Mobic.
 2. Antigout: Relieves gouty arthritis; e.g., Benemid, Colbenemid, Lopurin, Zyloprim.
 3. Anti-inflammatory: Relieves redness and swelling; e.g., Kenalog cream, Clinoril.
 4. Muscle relaxant: Relaxes muscles; e.g., Robaxin, Soma, Parafon Forte, Flexeril.

IV. COMMONLY PRESCRIBED PHARMACEUTICALS (INCLUDES 50 MOST COMMON DRUGS)

A. Cardiovascular
 1. Antianginal: Relieves angina (chest pain).
    a. Norvasc (amlodipine)
       (1) Indication: Angina pectoris, hypertension.
       (2) Contraindication: Hypersensitivity.
       (3) Adverse reaction: Vertigo, headache, weakness, edema.
    b. Cardizem (diltiazem): Vasodilator.
       (1) Indication: Angina pectoris
       (2) Contraindication: Hypersensitivity, hypotension, kidney/liver disease.
       (3) Adverse reaction: Allergic symptoms, vertigo, edema, GI upset, insomnia.
    c. Inderal (propanolol): Antiarrhythmic, antimigraine, antihypertensive.

(1) Indication: Angina pectoris, hypertension, migraine, arrhythmia.
(2) Contraindication: Asthma, diabetes mellitus, heart disease.
(3) Adverse reaction: Fatigue, bradycardia, hypotension.

d. Calan (verapamil): Antihypertensive, antiarrhythmic
(1) Indication: Angina pectoris, hypertension, arrhythmia.
(2) Contraindication: Heart disease, hypotension.
(3) Adverse reaction: Pulmonary edema, GI upset, vertigo, bradycardia.

e. Nitroquick (nitroglycerin): Antihypertensive
(1) Indication: Angina pectoris, hypertension.
(2) Contraindication: Anemia, intracranial pressure.
(3) Adverse reaction: Weakness, headache, tachycardia, syncope.

2. Lanoxin (digoxin): Antiarrhythmic, cardiotonic.
a. Indication: Congestive heart failure, atrial fibrillation, paroxysmal atrial tachycardia.
b. Contraindication: Ventricular fibrillation, kidney disease, pulmonary disease, hypothyroidism.
c. Adverse reaction: Vertigo, weakness, headache, GI upset, blurred vision, hallucination.

3. Coreg (carvedilol)
a. Indication: Heart failure, high blood pressure, angina pain, and cardiomyopathy.
b. Contraindication: Hypersensitivity, AV block, sick sinus syndrome or severe bradycardia, bronchial disease, liver disease.
c. Adverse reaction: Dizziness, sleepiness or sleeplessness, diarrhea, abdominal pain, slow heartbeat, dizziness when rising from a sitting or lying position, swelling of the hands or feet, sore throat, breathing difficulties, tiredness, back pain, urinary infection, and viral infection.

4. Digitek (digoxin)
a. Indication: Congestive heart failure (CHF) and other heart conditions involving a very rapid heartbeat.
b. Contraindication: Ventricular fibrillation, sick sinus syndrome, AV block.
c. Adverse reaction: Dizziness, headache, nausea, diarrhea, appetite loss, and apathy.

5. Antihypertensive
a. Vasotec (enalapril)
(1) Indication: Hypertension.
(2) Contraindication: Hypersensitivity.
(3) Adverse reaction: Vertigo, fatigue, headache, GI upset, syncope, chest pain, insomnia.
b. Altace (ramipril)
(1) Indication: Hypertension.

(2) Contraindication: Hypersensitivity.
(3) Adverse reaction: Dizziness, headache, nausea.

c. Zestril (lisonopril)
(1) Indication: Hypertension.
(2) Contraindication: Angioedema.
(3) Adverse reaction: Hypotension, neutropenia, agranulocytosis.

d. Tenormin (atenolol): Antianginal.
(1) Indication: Hypertension, angina pectoris.
(2) Contraindication: Bradycardia, heart disease.
(3) Adverse reaction: Fatigue, bradycardia, GI upset, hypotension.

e. Lopressor (metoprolol): Antianginal, antiarrhythmic.
(1) Indication: Hypertension.
(2) Contraindication: Heart disease, hypotension.
(3) Adverse reaction: Allergic symptoms, bradycardia, fatigue, vertigo, gastric disorders.

f. Hytrin (terazosin hydrochloride)
(1) Indication: Hypertension.
(2) Contraindication: None known.
(3) Adverse reaction: Asthenia, blurred vision, vertigo, nausea.

g. Monopril (fosinopril sodium)
(1) Indication: Hypertension, adjunct therapy for heart failure.
(2) Contraindication: Hypersensitivity.
(3) Adverse reaction: Headache, elevated liver enzymes, fatigue, cough.

h. Cozaar (losartan potassium)
(1) Indication: Hypertension; nephropathy in type 2 diabetes.
(2) Contraindication: Hypersensitivity, pregnant.
(3) Adverse reaction: Respiratory infection, heartburn, stuffy nose, sleeplessness, diarrhea.

i. Diovan (valsartan)
(1) Indication: Hypertension, heart failure; and treatment following heart attack.
(2) Contraindication: Hypersensitivity, pregnancy.
(3) Adverse reaction: Dizziness, sleeplessness, headache, fatigue, diarrhea, upset stomach, heartburn, abdominal pain.

j. Diovan HCT (valsartan + hydrochlorothiazide)
(1) Indication: Hypertension, heart failure; and treatment following heart attack.
(2) Contraindication: Hypersensitivity, pregnancy.
(3) Adverse reaction: Dizziness, sleeplessness, headache, fatigue, diarrhea, upset stomach, heartburn, abdominal pain.

k. Lotrel (amlodipine + benazepril hydrochloride)
      (1) Indication: Hypertension.
      (2) Contraindication: Hypersensitivity, pregnant.
      (3) Adverse reaction: Cough, headache, dizziness, and swelling.
   l. Toprol XL (metoprolol)
      (1) Indication: Hypertension, angina pectoris, abnormal heart rhythms, prevention of second heart attack, migraine, tremors, side effects of antipsychotic drugs, congestive heart failure, and bleeding from the esophagus.
      (2) Contraindicaion: Hypersensitivity,asthma, very slow heart rate, or heart block.
      (3) Adverse reaction: Impotence, unusual tiredness or weakness, slow heartbeat, heart failure, dizziness, breathing difficulties, bronchospasm, depression, confusion, anxiety, nervousness, sleeplessness, disorientation, short-term memory loss, emotional instability, cold hands and feet, constipation, diarrhea, nausea, vomiting, upset stomach, increased sweating, urinary difficulties, cramps, blurred.

B. Cholesterol-reducing agents
   1. Pravachol (pravastatin)
      a. Indication: Hypercholesterolemia.
      b. Contraindication: Hypersensitivity, acute liver disease.
      c. Adverse reaction: Elevated liver enzymes, mild gastrointestinal disturbances.
   2. Lipitor (atorvastatin)
      a. Indication: Hypercholesterolemia.
      b. Contraindication: Hypersensitivity, acute liver disease.
      c. Adverse reaction: Infections, mild gastrointestinal disturbances.
   3. Tricor (fenofibrate)
      a. Indication: High blood cholesterol and/or triglycerides, syndrome X.
      b. Contraindication: Hypersensitivity, liver or severe kidney disease.
      c. Adverse reaction: Abnormal liver function, abdominal pain, and respiratory disorders.
   4. Crestor (rosuvastatin calcium)
      a. Indication: High blood levels of cholesterol, low-density lipoprotein (LDL) cholesterol, and triglycerides; also prescribed for atherosclerosis, diabetes-related blood-fat problems, preventing heart attacks and strokes, and reducing the risk for cardiac bypass surgery.
      b. Contraindication: Hypersensitivity, liver disease.
      c. Adverse reaction: Sore throat and headache, diarrhea, and upset stomach.

   5. Vytorin (ezetimibe + simvastatin)
      a. Indication: High cholesterol, high LDL cholesterol, high triglycerides, and low HDL cholesterol, homozygous familial hypercholesterolemia and homozygous sitosterolemia.
      b. Contraindication: Hypersensitivity, liver disease or elevated liver enzymes.
      c. Adverse reaction: Headache, back pain, joint pain, and abdominal pain.
C. Hematological
   1. Coumadin (warfarin sodium): Anticoagulant.
      a. Indication: Pulmonary emboli, thrombosis, ASHD.
      b. Contraindication: Hemorrhagic disorders, pregnancy, liver/kidney disease, vitamin K deficiency.
      c. Adverse reaction: Hemorrhage, GI upset, allergic symptoms.
   2. Plavix (clopidogrel): Inhibits platelet aggregation.
      a. Indication: Reduction of atherosclerotic events such as stroke and heart attacks.
      b. Contraindication: Hypersensitivity, acute (pathological) bleeding.
      c. Adverse reaction: Gastrointestinal hemorrhage.
D. Central nervous system
   1. Sedative
      a. Restoril (temazepam): Hypnotic.
         (1) Indication: Insomnia.
         (2) Contraindication: Pregnancy.
         (3) Adverse reaction: Drowsiness, headache, fatigue.
      b. Ambien (zolpidem tartrate): Hypnotic.
         (1) Indication: Insomnia.
         (2) Contraindication: Hypersensitivity, liver disease, kidney disease, severe depression, severe lung disease, sleep apnea, drunkenness.
         (3) Adverse reaction: Drowsiness, headache, fatigue.
   2. Antianxiety
      a. Paxil (paroxetine)
         (1) Indication: Social anxiety disorders, panic disorders, obsessive-compulsive disorders, depressive disorders.
         (2) Contraindication: Not to be used with concurrent monoamine oxidase inhibitors (MAOIs).
         (3) Adverse reaction: Nausea, drowsiness.
      b. Xanax (alprazolam)
         (1) Indication: Anxiety and tension.
         (2) Contraindication: Glaucoma, psychoses, breast-feeding.
         (3) Adverse reaction: GI upset, drowsiness, tachycardia, confusion, hostility, weight gain/loss.

3. Antidepressant

    a. Prozac (fluoxetine hydrochloride)
        (1) Indication: Depression.
        (2) Contraindication: Unknown.
        (3) Adverse reaction: Nervousness, anxiety, insomnia, weight loss, decreased concentration.

    b. Zoloft (sertraline hydrochloride)
        (1) Indication: Depression.
        (2) Contraindication: Unknown.
        (3) Adverse reaction: GI upset, vertigo, insomnia.

    c. Celexa (citalopram)
        (1) Indication: Depression.
        (2) Contraindication: Not to be used concurrently with MAOIs.
        (3) Adverse reaction: Nausea, dry mouth, dizziness, insomnia.

    d. Wellbutrin (bupropion HCl)
        (1) Indication: Depression.
        (2) Contraindication: Seizure disorders, not to be used concurrently with MAOIs.
        (3) Adverse reaction: Rash.

    e. Cymbalta (duloxetine)
        (1) Indication: Major depressive disorder, generalized anxiety disorder, and the management of pain related to diabetes. It is also used to treat fibromyalgia and stress urinary incontinence.
        (2) Contraindication: Hypersensitivity, narrow-angle glaucoma, mania, or hypomania.
        (3) Adverse reaction: Nausea, dry mouth, constipation, loss of appetite, headache, dizziness, fatigue, and sleeplessness, diarrhea, tiredness.

    f. Lexapro (escitalopram oxylate)
        (1) Indication: Depression, bulimic binge-eating and vomiting, obsessive-compulsive disorder (OCD), social anxiety disorder, generalized anxiety disorder, panic disorder, migraine, hot flashes, post-traumatic stress disorder (PTSD), Reynaud phenomenon, and borderline personality disorder.
        (2) Contraindication: Hypersensitivity.
        (3) Adverse reaction: Headache, anxiety, nervousness, sleeplessness, drowsiness, tiredness, weakness, sexual dysfunction, tremors, sweating, dizziness, lightheadedness, dry mouth, upset or irritated stomach, appetite loss or increase, nausea, vomiting, diarrhea, gas, rash, weight loss or gain, electric-shock sensations, increased sweating, increased yawning, tinnitus, abnormal dreams, difficulty concentrating, acne, hair loss, dry skin, dizziness or fainting when rising suddenly from a sitting or lying position and itching.

    g. Effexor XR (venlafaxine)
        (1) Indication: Major depressive disorder, generalized anxiety disorder, and the management of pain related to diabetes. It is also used to treat fibromyalgia and stress urinary incontinence
        (2) Contraindication: Hypersensitivity, narrow-angle glaucoma, mania, or hypomania.
        (3) Adverse reaction: Nausea, dry mouth, constipation, loss of appetite, headache, dizziness, fatigue, and sleeplessness, diarrhea, tiredness.

4. Dilantin (phenytoin): Anticonvulsant.
    a. Indication: Grand mal seizure disorders, epilepsy.
    b. Contraindication: Hypersensitivity.
    c. Adverse reaction: Slurred speech, decreased coordination, nystagmus, blurred vision.

5. Lyrica (pregabalin)
    a. Indication: Anticonvulsant, pain reliever.
    b. Contraindication: Hypersensitivity.
    c. Adverse reaction: Dizziness, tiredness, dry mouth, loss of muscular coordination, swelling in the arms or legs, blurred or double vision, weight gain, and loss of concentration.

6. Risperdal (risperidone)
    a. Indication: Psychotic disorders and schizophrenia, bipolar disorders, symptoms of Alzheimer's disease and treatment resistant depression.
    b. Contraindication: Hypersensitivity.
    c. Adverse reaction: Sleepiness, sleeplessness, agitation, anxiety, uncontrolled movements, headache, nasal stuffiness and irritation.

7. Seroquel (quetiapine)
    a. Indication: Psychotic disorders, bipolar disorder, and schizophrenia.
    b. Contraindication: Hypersensitivity.
    c. Adverse reaction: Dizziness, headache, agitation, upset stomach, tiredness, sleepiness, dizziness or fainting when rising from a sitting or lying position, abdominal pain, weight gain and dry mouth.

8. Topamax (topiramate)
    a. Indication: Partial onset seizures, tonic-clonic seizures, cluster headaches, migraine prevention, infantile spasms, and Lennox-Gastaut syndrome, alcohol dependence, bipolar disorder, bulimia, and obesity.
    b. Contraindication: Hypersensitivity.

c. Adverse reaction: Tiredness or fatigue, slow reflexes and thought processes, difficulty concentrating, speech or language problems, especially word finding; dizziness, weakness, poor muscle coordination, tingling in the hands or feet, tremors, nervousness, insomnia, depression, nausea, loss of appetite, respiratory infections, sensitivity to the sun and visual disturbances, including double vision.

E. Antimicrobial

1. Cipro (ciprofloxacin)
   a. Indication: Urinary tract infection (UTI), upper respiratory infection (URI), bone/joint infections.
   b. Contraindication: Hypersensitivity.
   c. Adverse reaction: GI upset, headache, vertigo, oral candidiasis.
2. Keflex (cephalexin)
   a. Indication: Bronchitis, cystitis, skin infections.
   b. Contraindication: Hypersensitivity.
   c. Adverse reaction: GI upset, allergic symptoms.
3. Diflucan (fluconazole): Antifungal.
   a. Indication: Candidiasis.
   b. Contraindication: Hypersensitivity.
   c. Adverse reaction: Headache, abdominal pain.
4. Cefzil (cefprozil)
   a. Indication: Upper and lower respiratory infections from *Streptococcus;* skin and skin structure infections from *Staphylococcus.*
   b. Contraindication: Allergy to cephalosporins.
   c. Adverse reaction: Gastrointestinal disturbances, elevated liver enzymes, rash.
5. Zithromax (azithromycin)
   a. Indication: Moderate infections.
   b. Contraindication: Hypersensitivity.
   c. Adverse reaction: GI disturbances, abdominal pain.
6. Biaxin (clarithromycin)
   a. Indication: URI, skin infections.
   b. Contraindication: Hypersensitivity.
   c. Adverse reaction: GI upset, headache.
7. Amoxil, Polymox, Trimox, Augmentin (amoxicillin)
   a. Indication: Ear, nose, and throat (ENT); genitourinary (GU); soft-tissue infections.
   b. Contraindication: Mononucleosis.
   c. Adverse reaction: GI upset, allergic symptoms.
8. Macrobid (nitrofurantoin)
   a. Indication: UTI.
   b. Contraindication: Significant renal impairment.
   c. Adverse reaction: Pulmonary reaction, chest pain, dyspnea.
9. Bactrim (trimethoprim and sulfamethoxazole)
   a. Indication: UTI, URI, otitis media.
   b. Contraindication: Pregnancy, breast-feeding.
   c. Adverse reaction: GI upset, pancytopenia.
10. Doxycycline
    a. Indication: Fevers caused by rickettsiae infections (such as Rocky Mountain spotted fever) and chlamydial infections.
    b. Contraindication: Hypersensitivity to tetracycline.
    c. Adverse reaction: Anorexia, nausea, vomiting, diarrhea.
11. Veetids (penicillin V)
    a. Indication: URI and rheumatic fever prophylaxis.
    b. Contraindication: Kidney disease, asthma.
    c. Adverse reaction: GI upset, allergic symptoms.
12. Levaquin (levofloxacin)
    a. Indication: Infections of the lower respiratory system, sinuses, urinary tract, skin, bone and joints, lungs, and prostate; also for sexually transmitted diseases, prostatitis, infectious diarrhea, bronchitis, pneumonia, typhoid fever, and anthrax.
    b. Contraindication: Hypersensitivity.
    c. Adverse reaction: Nausea, vomiting and diarrhea.
13. Valtrex (valacyclovir)
    a. Indication: Herpes zoster (shingles), recurrent genital herpes, and herpes labialis (cold sores).
    b. Contraindication: Hypersensitivity, HIV or a compromised immune system.
    c. Adverse reaction: Headache, diarrhea, dizziness, weakness, constipation, abdominal pain, appetite loss, nausea, and vomiting.
14. Zetia (ezetimibe)
    a. Indication: Herpes zoster (shingles), recurrent genital herpes, and herpes labialis (cold sores).
    b. Contraindication: Hypersensitivity, HIV or a compromised immune system.
    c. Adverse reaction: Headache, diarrhea, dizziness, weakness, constipation, abdominal pain, appetite loss, nausea, and vomiting.

F. Antiulcer

1. Zantac (ranitidine)
   a. Indication: Gastric/duodenal ulcer, esophageal reflux.
   b. Contraindication: Liver disease.
   c. Adverse reaction: GI upset, allergic symptoms, pancytopenia.
2. Nexium (esomeprazole)
   a. Indication: Gastroesophageal reflux disease (GERD), erosive esophagitis.
   b. Contraindication: Hypersensitivity.
   c. Adverse reaction: Headache, diarrhea.

3. Prevacid (lansoprazole)
   a. Indication: Duodenal ulcer.
   b. Contraindication: Hypersensitivity to any penicillin.
   c. Adverse reaction: Diarrhea, nausea.
4. Prilosec (omeprazole)
   a. Indication: Duodenal ulcer.
   b. Contraindication: Hypersensitivity.
   c. Adverse reaction: Headache, GI upset, vertigo.
5. Protonix (pantoprazole sodium)
   a. Indication: Stomach or duodenal ulcers, gastroesophageal reflux disease (GERD), and conditions in which there is an excess of stomach acid; also used to treat and maintain healing of ulcers of the esophagus.
   b. Contraindication: Hypersensitivity.
   c. Adverse reaction: Headache, diarrhea, nausea, gas, abdominal pain, constipation, and dry mouth.
G. Respiratory
   1. Bronchodilator
      a. Theo-Dur, Theophylline (aminophylline)
         (1) Indication: Asthma, emphysema, bronchospasm.
         (2) Contraindication: Peptic ulcers, seizure disorders.
         (3) Adverse reaction: Tachycardia, hypotension.
      b. Ventolin, Proventil (albuterol)
         (1) Indication: Bronchospasm.
         (2) Contraindication: Hypersensitivity.
         (3) Adverse reaction: GI upset, tremors, headache, drowsiness.
      c. Singulair (montelukast sodium)
         (1) Indication: Prophylaxis and chronic treatment of asthma.
         (2) Contraindication: Hypersensitivity.
         (3) Adverse reaction: Headache, abdominal pain, flulike symptoms.
      d. Advair Diskus (salmeterol + fluticasone)
         (1) Indication: Asthma and bronchospasm.
         (2) Contraindication: Hypersensitivity, cardiovascular disease, high blood pressure, stroke or seizure, thyroid disease, prostate disease, or glaucoma.
         (3) Adverse reaction: Heart palpitations, rapid heartbeat, tremors, cough, dizziness and fainting, shakiness, nervousness, tension, headache, diarrhea, heartburn or upset stomach, dry or sore and irritated throat, respiratory infections, and nasal or sinus conditions.
      e. ProAir HFA (albuterol)
         (1) Indication: Bronchospasm associated with asthma or other obstructive pulmonary diseases, or induced by exercise.

      (2) Contraindication: Hypersensitivity.
      (3) Adverse reaction: Worsening of asthma, ear infection, URI, stuffy nose, dizziness, headache, nausea, vomiting, and muscle cramps.
   2. Antihistamines
      a. Seldane (terfenadine)
         (1) Indication: Rhinitis, allergies.
         (2) Contraindication: Hypersensitivity.
         (3) Adverse reaction: None noted to date.
      b. Allegra (fexofenadine)
         (1) Indication: Allergic rhinitis, urticaria (hives).
         (2) Contraindication: Hypersensitivity.
         (3) Adverse reaction: Viral infection, drowsiness.
      c. Zyrtec (cetirizine)
         (1) Indication: Allergic rhinitis.
         (2) Contraindication: Hypersensitivity.
         (3) Adverse reaction: Fatigue, dry mouth.
      d. Nasonex (mometasone furoate monohydrate)
         (1) Indication: Rhinitis associated with seasonal or chronic allergy and other causes; also used to prevent recurrence of nasal polyps.
         (2) Contraindication: Hypersensitivity.
         (3) Adverse reaction: Mild irritation of the nose, nasal passages, and throat; burning, stinging, dryness, and headache.
   3. Hydrocodone: Antitussive.
      a. Indication: Dry, nonproductive cough.
      b. Contraindication: Hypersensitivity.
      c. Adverse reaction: Drowsiness, GI upset, respiratory depression, addiction.
H. Contraceptive
   1. Ortho Tri-cyclen (norgestimate/ethinyl estradiol)
      a. Indication: Contraception.
      b. Contraindication: Thromboembolic disorders, cardiovascular disease (CVD), coronary artery disease (CAD), breast carcinoma, endometrial carcinoma, genital bleeding, liver disease/carcinoma.
      c. Adverse reaction: GI upsets, menstrual irregularities, edema, breast enlargement/tenderness, weight change.
   2. Ortho Evra (norelgestromin and ethinyl estradiol)
      a. Indication: Transdermal contraception.
      b. Contraindication: Thromboembolic disorders, CVD, CAD, breast carcinoma, endometrial carcinoma, genital bleeding, liver disease/carcinoma.
      c. Adverse reaction: Nausea and vomiting, application site reaction, headache, breast symptoms, emotional lability.

3. Ortho-Novum (norethindrone/estradiol)
   a. Indication: Contraception.
   b. Contraindication: Thrombophlebitis, pregnancy, genital bleeding, CAD, CVD.
   c. Adverse reaction: GI upset, menstrual irregularities, edema, breast enlargement.
4. Yasmin 28 (intermediate-dose progestin + intermediate-dose estrogen + no androgen activity [single-phase combination])
   a. Indication: Prevention of pregnancy, endometriosis, excessive menstruation, and cyclic withdrawal bleeding.
   b. Contraindication: Hypersensitivity, pregnant, blood clots, stroke, blood-coagulation disorder, cancer of the breast, sex organs or liver, heavy smokers.
   c. Adverse reaction: Nausea, bloating, high blood pressure, migraine, excess cervical mucous, skin discoloration, colon polyps, water retention, swelling, breast fullness or tenderness, breakthrough bleeding, tiredness, acne, depression.

I. Analgesic and anti-inflammatory
1. Acetaminophen with codeine: Antipyretic.
   a. Indication: Mild to moderately severe pain.
   b. Contraindication: Head injuries, abdominal conditions.
   c. Adverse reaction: Vertigo, GI upset, shortness of breath (SOB).
2. Naproxen: Anti-inflammatory.
   a. Indication: Arthritis, dysmenorrhea.
   b. Contraindication: Asthma, pregnancy, breastfeeding, peptic ulcers.
   c. Adverse reaction: GI upset, allergic symptoms, vertigo, headache, drowsiness.
3. Ibuprofen: Anti-inflammatory.
   a. Indication: Pain, arthritis, dysmenorrhea.
   b. Contraindication: Asthma, pregnancy, breastfeeding, peptic ulcers.
   c. Adverse reaction: GI upset and bleeding, vertigo, headache, tinnitus, edema, anorexia.
4. Celebrex (celecoxib)
   a. Indication: Anti-inflammatory for pain associated with arthritis.
   b. Contraindication: Hypersensitivity.
   c. Adverse reaction: Dyspepsia, diarrhea, nausea.
5. Percocet (oxycodone/acetaminophen)
   a. Indication: Analgesic and antipyretic for moderate to moderately severe pain.
   b. Contraindication: Hypersensitivity.
   c. Adverse reaction: Dizziness, sedation, nausea and vomiting.
6. Mobic (meloxicam)
   a. Indication: Anti-inflammatory for use in osteoarthritis and primary dysmenorrhea.
   b. Contraindication: Liver/kidney disease, bleeding disorders, alcoholism.
   c. Adverse reaction: Abdominal pain, muscle cramps, mouth ulcers, tinnitus.
7. Ultracet (tramadol/acetaminophen)
   a. Indication: Analgesic for acute pain (short-term use).
   b. Contraindication: Hypersensitivity.
   c. Adverse reaction: Constipation, drowsiness, increased sweating.

J. Diuretic
1. Triamterene/hydrochlorothiazide: Antihypertensive.
   a. Indication: Edema, hypertension.
   b. Contraindication: Kidney disease, potassium supplements.
   c. Adverse reaction: GI upset, vertigo, insomnia, SOB, depression, anxiety.
2. Furosemide: Antihypertensive.
   a. Indication: Edema, hypertension.
   b. Contraindication: Anuria.
   c. Adverse reaction: Electrolyte imbalances, hypotension, GI upset.

K. Hormone
1. Premarin (estrogen)
   a. Indication: Osteoporosis, atrophic vaginitis, breast engorgement, prostate cancer.
   b. Contraindication: Pregnancy, breast cancer, thrombophlebitis.
   c. Adverse reaction: GI upset, vertigo, menstrual irregularities, vaginal candidiasis, edema.
2. Synthroid/Levoxyl (levothyroxine)
   a. Indication: Hypothyroidism, cretinism, myxedema.
   b. Contraindication: Heart disease, liver disease, hypertension, adrenal insufficiency.
   c. Adverse reaction: GI upset, insomnia, tremor, tachycardia, hypertension, cramps.
3. Humulin (insulin): Hypoglycemic.
   a. Indication: Diabetes mellitus.
   b. Contraindication: Hypersensitivity.
   c. Adverse reaction: Allergic symptoms, erythema, edema, tachycardia, drowsiness.
4. Micronase, Diabeta (glyburide): Hypoglycemic.
   a. Indication: Non–insulin-dependent (type 2) DM.
   b. Contraindication: Insulin-dependent (type 1) diabetes mellitus (DM).
   c. Adverse reaction: GI upset, allergy symptoms.
5. Prempro (conjugated estrogens/medroxyprogesterone acetate)
   a. Indication: Postmenopausal therapy.
   b. Contraindication: Suspected/known pregnancy, genital bleeding, breast cancer, estrogen-dependent neoplasms, history of thromboembolic disorders.
   c. Adverse reaction: Headache, breast pain, infection.

6. Proscar (finasteride)
   a. Indication: Symptomatic benign prostatic hypertrophy (BPH).
   b. Contraindication: Hypersensitivity.
   c. Adverse reaction: Impotence, decreased libido.
7. Glucophage (metformin): Hypoglycemic.
   a. Indication: Non–insulin-dependent diabetes mellitus (NIDDM), type 2.
   b. Contraindication: Renal disease, congestive heart failure, hypersensitivity.
   c. Adverse reaction: Diarrhea, nausea, vomiting.
8. Glucotrol (glipizide): Hypoglycemic.
   a. Indication: Non–insulin-dependent diabetes mellitus (NIDDM), type 2.
   b. Contraindication: Hypersensitivity, diabetic ketoacidosis.
   c. Adverse reaction: Nausea, diarrhea.
9. Actos (pioglitazone hydrochloride)
   a. Indication: Treats type 2 diabetes
   b. Contraindication: Hypersensitivity, liver disease.
   c. Adverse reaction: URI, headaches, sinus irritation, muscle aches and sore throat.
10. Avandia (rosiglitazone maleate)
   a. Indication: Type 2 diabetes
   b. Contraindication: Hypersensitivity, liver disease.
   c. Adverse reaction: URI, accidental injuries, and headache.
11. Lantus (insulin glargine)
   a. Indication: Types 1 and 2 diabetes, gestational diabetes, hyperkalemia, and for severe complications of diabetes such as ketoacidosis or diabetic coma.
   b. Contraindication: None.
   c. Adverse reaction: Low blood sugar, weight gain, low blood potassium.

L. Mineral and vitamin supplement
   1. Klor-Con (potassium chloride)
      a. Indication: Hypokalemia.
      b. Contraindication: Hyperkalemia, kidney disease.
      c. Adverse reaction: GI disorders.
   2. Feosol (ferrous sulfate): Hematinic.
      a. Indication: Iron deficiency anemia.
      b. Contraindication: Tetracycline antibiotic treatment.
      c. Adverse reaction: GI upset, black stool.
   3. Mephyton (phytonadione [vitamin K])
      a. Indication: Coagulation disorders.
      b. Contraindication: Hypersensitivity.
      c. Adverse reaction: GI upset, allergy symptoms, arrhythmia, hypotension.
   4. Fosamax (alendronate)
      a. Indication: Treatment of osteoporosis.
      b. Contraindication: Esophageal abnormalities, inability to stand or sit upright for 30 minutes, hypersensitivity.
      c. Adverse reaction: GI disturbances, muscle and/or joint pain.

M. Musculoskeletal
   1. Carisoprodol
      a. Indication: Muscle spasms and pain.
      b. Contraindication: Hypersensitivity.
      c. Adverse reaction: Dizziness, vertigo, headache, hypotension.
   2. Flexeril (cyclobenzaprine hydrochloride)
      a. Indication: Muscle spasms and pain.
      b. Contraindication: Heart disease, hyperthyroidism.
      c. Adverse reaction: Vertigo, tachycardia, drowsiness.
   3. Actonel (risedronate sodium)
      a. Indication: Prevention and treatment of osteoporosis.
      b. Contraindication: Hypersensitivity, kidney disease, stomach or intestinal disease.
      c. Adverse reaction: Headache, diarrhea, abdominal pain, rash, severe joint pain, chest pain, dizziness.

N. Retin-A (tretinoin): Antiacneic.
   1. Indication: Acne vulgaris.
   2. Contraindication: Hypersensitivity.
   3. Adverse reaction: Irregular pigmentation, blistering, photosensitivity.

O. Timoptic (timolol maleate): Antiglaucomic.
   1. Indication: Elevated intraocular pressure, glaucoma.
   2. Contraindication: Asthma, chronic obstructive pulmonary disease (COPD), heart disease.
   3. Adverse reaction: Headache, fatigue, bradycardia, anorexia, hypotension, syncope.

P. Miscellaneous medications
   1. Prednisone
      a. Indication: Endocrine, rheumatic, collagen, and dermatological disorders (severe).
      b. Contraindication: Hypersensitivity.
      c. Adverse reaction: Fluid and electrolyte disturbances, musculoskeletal disorders, gastrointestinal involvements, increased dermatological conditions such as bruising and slowed wound healing.
   2. Viagra (sildenafil citrate)
      a. Indication: Treatment of erectile dysfunction.
      b. Contraindication: Hypersensitivity.
      c. Adverse reaction: Headache, flushing, dyspepsia.
   3. Detrol LA (tolterodine)
      a. Indication: Overactive bladder.
      b. Contraindication: Urinary or gastric retention, uncontrolled narrow-angle glaucoma.
      c. Adverse reaction: Dry mouth, headache, fatigue.
   4. Imitrex (sumatriptan succinate)
      a. Indication: Migraine headache.

   b. Contraindication: Angina of any type, cerebrovascular syndromes, peripheral vascular disease.

   c. Adverse reaction: Atypical sensations, chest pain or pressure.

5. Meclizine

   a. Indication: Antiemetic, treatment of motion sickness.

   b. Contraindication: Hypersensitivity.

   c. Adverse reaction: Drowsiness, dry mouth, blurred vision.

6. Allopurinol

   a. Indication: Primary or secondary gout.

   b. Contraindication: Previous reaction of any type to this drug.

   c. Adverse reaction: Skin rash.

7. Aricept (donepezil hydrochloride)

   a. Indication: Alzheimer's dementia.

   b. Contraindication: Hypersensitivity.

   c. Adverse reaction: Nausea, vomiting, diarrhea.

8. Procrit (erythropoietin)

   a. Indication: Anemia associated with decreased erythropoietin secretion by the kidneys.

   b. Contraindication: None.

   c. Adverse reaction: Hypertension.

9. Adderall XR (dextroamphetamine sulfate)

   a. Indication: Attention-deficit hyperactivity disorder (ADHD) and narcolepsy (uncontrollable desire to sleep).

   b. Contraindication: Hypersensitivity, heart disease, heart defect, high blood pressure, liver or kidney disease, tics or Tourette's syndrome, seizures or abnormal brain wave tests, thyroid disease, glaucoma or a history of drug abuse.

   c. Adverse reaction: Heart palpitations, restlessness, overstimulation, dizziness, sleeplessness, increased blood pressure, rapid heartbeat, upper abdominal pain, and weight loss.

10. Concerta (methylphenidate)

   a. Indication: Attention-deficit hyperactivity disorder (ADHD); also prescribed for psychological, educational, or social disorders, narcolepsy; and mild depression in the elderly. It's also used in cancer treatment and stroke recovery and for treating hiccups after anesthesia.

   b. Contraindication: Hypersensitivity, glaucoma or other visual problems, a seizure disorder, severe depression, tics or Tourette's syndrome, drug dependence, alcoholism, high blood pressure.

   c. Adverse reaction: Nervousness, inability to sleep.

11. Chantix (varenicline)

   a. Indication: Smoking cessation.

   b. Contraindication: Hypersensitivity, kidney disease, diarrhea

   c. Adverse reaction: mild or moderate nausea, headache, sleeplessness, abnormal dreaming, vomiting, abdominal pain, gas, constipation, dry mouth, loss of taste.

12. Flomax (tamsulosin)

   a. Indication: Benign prostatic hyperplasia (BPH)

   b. Contraindication: Hypersensitivity.

   c. Adverse reaction: Dizziness, weakness and headache.

Q. Immunizations

1. Diphtheria tetanus acellular pertussis vaccine (DTaP)

   a. Contains toxoids of diphtheria and tetanus combined with pertussis antigen.

   b. Five doses, 0.5 ml-IM, administered between age 2 months to 6 years.

   c. Do not administer after 7th birthday.

2. Adult tetanus diphtheria (Td) vaccine

   a. Seven years through adult. Every 10 years for life.

   b. For severe wounds, administer booster if last immunization was more than five years ago; otherwise within 10 years for clean minor wounds.

3. *Haemophilus influenzae type B* (HIB)

   a. Contains an inactivated (killed) influenza virus grown in chick embryo tissue.

   b. Four doses administered between 2 months and 18 months. Doses may change from year to year; follow instructions.

   c. Administered seasonally for high-risk groups such as the elderly and those with chronic illness.

4. Inactivated polio vaccine (IPV)

   a. Three doses administered between 2 to 18 months.

   b. IPV, 0.5 ml, administered SC.

5. Hepatitis B vaccine (Hep B)

   a. Contains hepatitis B virus.

   b. Three doses between birth to 18 months.

6. Measles, mumps, rubella (MMR)

   a. Contains attenuated measles, mumps, and rubella (German measles) virus.

   b. One to two doses, 0.5 mL-subcutaneously, between 12 months and 12 years.

7. Rotavirus (RV)

   a. Contains live rotavirus.

   b. Three doses administered orally.

8. Pneumococcal conjugate vaccine (PCV)

   a. Contains seven strains of pneumococcal bacteria responsible for the most severe infections among children.

   b. Four doses given between 2 to 15 months.

9. Influenza vaccine: Administer annually to children aged 6 months through 18 years.

10. Varicella

   a. Virus that causes chickenpox.

   b. Two doses administered between 12 months and 6 years.

11. Hepatitis A vaccine (Hep A)
    a. Contains hepatitis A virus.
    b. Two doses administered between 12 and 24 months.
12. Schedule
    a. Birth: Hep B
       2 months: DTaP(1), IPV(1), HIB(1), Hep B(2), RV(1), PVC(1)
    b. 4 months: DTaP(2), IPV(2), HIB(2), Hep B(3), RV(2), PCV (2)
    c. 6 months: DTaP(3), HIB(3), RV(3), PCV(3)
    d. 12 months: Hep A (1). Immunization catch-up period.
    e. 15 months: DTaP(4), IPV(3), HIB(3), PCV(4), MMR(1), Varicella(1).
    f. 18 months: Hep A(2). Immunization catch-up period.
    g. 4 to 6 years: DTaP(5), IPV(4), MMR(2), Varicella (2)
13. Storage: Follow the manufacturer's instructions. Vaccines may require refrigeration, freezing, or protection from light or other environmental elements.
14. Documentation: A record of immunizations shall be maintained in the patient medical chart to include the following:
    a. Date of administration.
    b. Vaccine administered.
    c. Name of manufacturer.
    d. Lot number and expiration date.
    e. Site and route of administration.
    f. Name, address, and title of administering provider.

V. DOSAGE CALCULATIONS

A. Metric system: The metric system is a system of weights and measures based on multiples of ten.
  1. Basic units of measure
     a. Gram (g): Unit of weight used to measure solids.
     b. Liter (L): Unit of volume used to measure liquids.
     c. Meter (m): Unit of linear measure used to measure length or distance.
  2. Metric prefixes
     a. mega: One million   1000000.0
     b. kilo: One thousand   1000.0
     c. hecto: One hundred   100.0
     d. deka: Ten   10.0
     e. unit
        (g/m/L): one   1.0
     f. deci: One tenth   0.1
     g. centi: One hundredth   0.01
     h. milli: One thousandth   0.001
     i. micro: One millionth   0.000001

B. Metric conversions
  1. Changing from larger to smaller units
     a. Multiplication method: Multiply by the number of smaller units contained in the larger unit.
        (1) For example: Convert 5 liters to milliliters.
            (a) 1 L = 1000 mL.
            (b) 5 L × 1000 mL = 5000 mL.
        (2) For example: Convert 15 milliliters to microliters.
            (a) 1 mL = 1000 mcL.
            (b) 15 mL × 1000 mcL = 15000 mcL.
     b. Decimal point method: Move the decimal point to the right the number of places equal to the number of zeros found in the smaller equivalent unit.
        (1) For example: Convert 5 grams to decigrams.
            (a) 1 g = 10 dg. The decigram equivalent has one zero.
            (b) 5.0 g moving the decimal point one place to the right equals 50 dg.
        (2) For example: Convert 2 kilometers into centimeters.
            (a) 1 km = 100,000 cm. The centimeter equivalent has five zeros.
            (b) 2.0 km moving the decimal point five places to the right equals 200,000 cm.
  2. Changing from smaller to larger units
     a. Division method: Divide by the number of smaller units contained in the larger unit.
        (1) For example: Convert 500 milliliters to liters.
            (a) 1 L = 1000 mL.
            (b) 500 mL ÷ 1000 = 0.5 L.
        (2) For example: Convert 850 centigrams to grams.
            (a) 1 g = 100 cg.
            (b) 850 cg ÷ 100 = 8.5 g.
     b. Decimal point method: Move the decimal point to the left the number of places equal to the number of zeros found in the smaller equivalent unit.
        (1) For example: Convert 250 milligrams to grams.
            (a) 1 g = 1000 mg. The milligram equivalent has three zeros.
            (b) 250.0 mg moving the decimal point three places to the left equals 0.25 g.
        (2) For example: Convert 25 deciliters to liters.
            (a) 1 L = 10 dL. The deciliter equivalent has one zero.
            (b) 25.0 dL moving the decimal point one place to the left equals 2.5 L.

C. English: Metric conversions
  1. Changing pounds to kilograms: Divide by 2.2.
     a. For example: Convert 36 pounds to kilograms. $36 \div 2.2 = 16.4$ kg.
     b. For example: Convert 150 pounds to kilograms. $150 \div 2.2 = 68.2$ kg.
  2. Changing kilograms to pounds: Multiply by 2.2.
     a. For example: Convert 70 kilograms to pounds. $70 \times 2.2 = 154$ lb.
     b. For example: Convert 85 kilograms to pounds. $85 \times 2.2 = 187$ lb.
  3. Common household equivalents
     a. 1 teaspoon = 60 drops = 5 milliliters
     b. 1 tablespoon = 3 teaspoons = 15 milliliters
     c. 2 tablespoons = 1 fluid ounce = 30 milliliters
     d. 1 cup = 8 fluid ounces = 240 milliliters
     e. 16 ounces = 1 pound
D. Dosage calculation
  1. Adult dosage
     a. Formula: (Dosage Ordered ÷ Available Strength) × Dosage form = Dosage given
        (1) Dosage ordered: The amount of medication the provider requests to be administered.
        (2) Available strength: The available concentration of medication.
            (a) 500 mg/mL: 500 mg of the medication is contained in 1 mL of liquid.
            (b) 325 mg/5 mL: 325 mg of the medication is contained in 5 mL of liquid.
            (c) 0.5 g/capsule: 0.5 g of the medication is contained in 1 capsule.
        (3) Dosage form: The amount of liquid or number of pills that contain the unit dosage.
            (a) 500 mg/mL: The dosage form is 1 mL.
            (b) 325 mg/5 mL: the dosage form is 5 mL.
            (c) 0.5 g/capsule: The dosage form is 1 capsule.
        (4) Dosage given: The actual amount of the medication available given to the patient to satisfy the provider's medication order.
     b. For example: Provider orders 500 mg Tylenol. Available strength is 250 mg/capsule.
        (1) $(500 \div 250) \times 1$ capsule.
        (2) $(2) \times 1$ capsule = 2 capsules given.
     c. For example: Provider orders 300 mg Demoral. Available strength is 200 mg/mL.
        (1) $(300 \div 200) \times 1$ mL.
        (2) $(1.5) \times 1$ mL = 1.5 mL given.
     d. For example: Provider orders 100 mg Augmentin. Available strength is 500 mg/5 mL.
        (1) $(100 \div 500) \times 5$ mL.
        (2) $(0.2) \times 5$ mL = 1 mL given.
     e. For example: Provider orders 250 mg Amoxil. Available strength is 0.5 g/4 mL.
        (1) Convert 0.5 grams to milligrams.
            (a) 1 g = 1000 mg.
            (b) $0.5 \text{ g} \times 1000 = 500$ mg (500 mg/4 mL).
        (2) $(250 \div 500) \times 4$ mL.
        (3) $(0.5) \times 4$ mL = 2 mL given.
  2. Pediatric dosage
     a. Young's rule: Used for children under 12 based on age.
        (1) Formula: Child's age ÷ (child's age + 12) × average adult dose.
        (2) For example: Five-year-old child; average adult dose is 250 mg Tylenol.
            (a) $5 \div (5 + 12) \times 250$
            (b) $(5 \div 17) \times 250$
            (c) $(0.29) \times 250 = 73$ mg given.
     b. Clark's rule: Used for children under 12 based on weight (in lb), or older children who are small for age.
        (1) Formula: (Child's weight ÷ 150) × average adult dose.
        (2) For example: 65-pound child; average adult dose is 250 mg Tylenol.
            (a) $(65 \div 150) \times 250$
            (b) $(0.43) \times 250 = 108$ mg given.
     c. Fried's rule: Used for infants and children under 2 based on age in months.
        (1) Formula: (Infant's age ÷ 150) × average adult dose.
        (2) For example: Fourteen-month-old child; average adult dose is 250 mg Tylenol.
            (a) $(14 \div 150) \times 250$
            (b) $(0.093) \times 250 = 23$ mg given.

VI. MEDICATION ADMINISTRATION

A. Routes of administration
  1. Oral: Drug is given by mouth and swallowed.
  2. Buccal: Drug is placed between gum and cheek and allowed to dissolve.
  3. Sublingual: Drug is placed beneath the tongue and allowed to dissolve.
  4. Inhalation: Drug is inhaled into the lungs by means of a nebulizer.
  5. Rectal: Drug is inserted into the rectum and absorbed.
  6. Vaginal: Drug is inserted into or applied to the vagina.
  7. Topical: Drug is externally applied to the skin or mucous membranes. This includes eye, ear, and nasal instillations.
  8. Transdermal patch: Drug, in a patch form, that is applied to the skin and is absorbed.

9. Parenteral: Drug is given by injection through a needle.
   a. Intradermal: Injected into the upper layers of the skin, under the epidermis and into the dermis.
      (1) Absorption is very slow, and drug action is local rather than systemic.
      (2) Sites: Injected in any area lacking visible, superficial vessels, usually the forearm.
   b. Subcutaneous: Injected into the adipose tissue under the skin.
      (1) Injected into fatty tissue. A maximum of 2 mL of solution can be given to an adult in this manner.
      (2) This route is used when a more prolonged absorption is desired.
      (3) Sites: Upper arms, thighs, and abdomen.
   c. Intramuscular: Injected into a body muscle.
      (1) This route of injection is second only to intravenous injection in rate of absorption.
      (2) A maximum of 5 mL of solution is recommended for injection into a large muscle mass.
      (3) Solution for injection that would be irritating to subcutaneous tissue. Thick medications are usually given intramuscularly because they are less painful. Antibiotics, for example, are commonly given intramuscularly.
      (4) Sites: Deltoid, gluteus medius, ventrogluteal region, and vastus lateralis (primarily infants).
   d. Intravenous: Injected into a vein. Has the fastest absorption rate; usually not performed by MAs.
B. Administration guidelines
   1. Six rights of administration
      a. Right documentation.
      b. Right patient.
      c. Right drug.
      d. Right dose.
      e. Right route.
      f. Right time.
   2. Safety guidelines
      a. Read label: Read the label three times when preparing medication.
         (1) Before it is removed from the shelf or storage area.
         (2) Before pouring the medication.
         (3) Before placing back in storage.
      b. Missing label: Do not use drug if label is missing or difficult to read.
      c. Drug information: Know about the drug before administering. Check the PDR or other reference sources.
      d. Preparation: Prepare in a well-lighted area with no distractions. Never leave medication unattended in patient rooms.
      e. Appearance: Do not use medications that have changed color, turned cloudy, or developed unusual odors or that have sediment at the bottom.
      f. Expiration: Check all expiration dates before using. Never administer an expired drug.
      g. Mixing: Never return medication to a container or transfer medication from one container to another.
      h. Identify patient: Verify the patient's identity before administration.
      i. Medication allergies: Make sure patient is not allergic to medication before administration.
      j. Observation of patient: Observe the patient for any unusual reactions; report unusual observations immediately.
      k. Record information: Record the correct information in the patient's chart immediately after administration. Record date, time, drug, dosage, route, any reactions, and your initials.
      l. Organization of drugs: Organize drugs according to classification, type, form, or in alphabetical order.
      m. Emergency drug tray: Keep emergency drug tray in an accessible area. Keep tray well supplied with drugs and items according to the provider's preference.
         (1) Activated charcoal: Given to absorb or inactivate ingested poisons or drug overdoses.
         (2) Amytal (amobarbital): Barbiturate used as a sedative.
         (3) Benadryl: Antihistamine used to relieve allergic symptoms and anaphylaxis.
         (4) Atropine: Anticholinergic, bronchodilator.
         (5) Dextrose: Sugar solution to treat insulin shock.
         (6) Valium (diazepam): Muscle relaxant, anticonvulsant.
         (7) Lanoxin (digoxin): Antiarrhythmic, as well as treatment of SOB.
         (8) Adrenalin (epinephrine): Bronchodilator, vasoconstrictor.
         (9) Lasix (furosemide): Used to treat pulmonary edema.
         (10) Glucagon: Antihypoglycemic used to treat insulin overdose.
         (11) Ipecac syrup: Emetic for ingested poisons.
         (12) Isuprel (isoproterenol hydrochloride): Bronchodilator.
         (13) Lidocaine: Antiarrhythmic, anesthetic, and antidote for digitalis overdose.
         (14) Aramine (metaraminol): Anticholinergic used to treat shock.

3. General considerations

   a. Age: Infants, children, and the elderly usually require smaller dosages.

   b. Weight: Smaller or lighter patients also require smaller dosages.

   c. Gender: Average woman usually requires less medication than the average man because of differences in body size.

   d. Drug tolerance: Patient who has taken a drug for an extended amount of time usually requires larger dosages to obtain optimum results.

   e. Physical or emotional condition: Depressed patients or patients in severe pain may require larger dosages.

   f. Route of administration: Parenterally administered drugs are absorbed faster than oral, and usually require smaller dosages.

   g. Time of administration: Most drugs are absorbed more rapidly on an empty stomach. Irritating drugs are usually taken after or with meals.

4. Allergic reactions

   a. Sign and symptoms

     (1) Mild reactions will cause a rash, rhinitis, or pruritus.

     (2) Anaphylactic reaction: Severe allergic reaction that may occur suddenly and death may occur without emergency intervention.

       (a) Initially, sneezing, edema, and pruritus.

       (b) Eventually dyspnea, cyanosis, decrease in blood pressure.

       (c) Weakness, thready pulse, convulsions, shock and unconsciousness. Possible coma and death.

   b. Prevention

     (1) Monitor: Stay with the patient after administration of a drug, especially after allergy skin testing or injections.

     (2) Observe: For any of the signs and symptoms of an allergic reaction.

     (3) Notify: Tell the provider immediately.

     (4) Be prepared: Be ready to access the emergency drug tray and provide assistance or emergency treatment.

C. Equipment and materials

  1. Parts of a syringe (see Figures 18-2A and B)

   a. Barrel: Cylindrical portion that holds the medication. Most are calibrated in cubic centimeters and minims.

   b. Flange: The rim at the end of the barrel which aids in depressing the plunger and prevents rolling on a flat surface.

   c. Plunger: Fits inside the barrel and draws medication in and out of the syringe.

   d. Tip: The point at the end of the barrel where the needle is attached. It may be a Luer-Lok or plain tip.

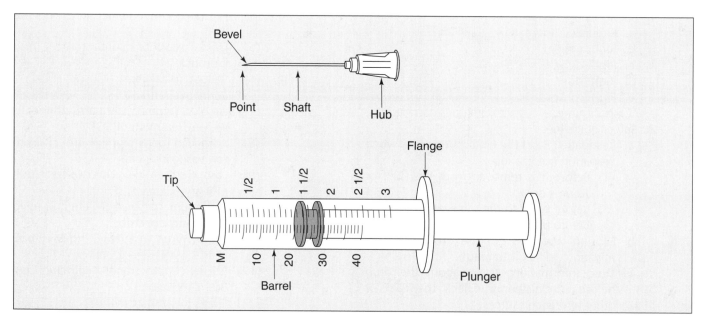

Figure 18-2A

Parts of a syringe and needle. Delmar/Cengage Learning.

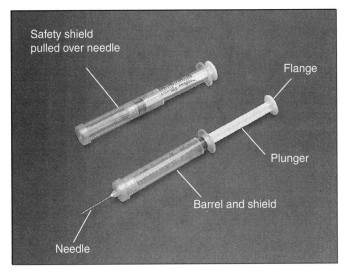

Safety shield pulled over needle

Flange

Plunger

Barrel and shield

Needle

Figure 18-2B

A type of safety syringe. Delmar/Cengage Learning.

2. Syringe variations (see Figure 18-3)
   a. Barrels of syringes are most commonly calibrated in 2 mL, 3 mL, 5 mL, and 10 mL volumes. They may be nondisposable glass, or disposable plastic.
      (1) Intradermal: Use a 1 mL tuberculin syringe.
      (2) Subcutaneous: Use a 2 to 5 mL syringe.
      (3) Intramuscular: Use a 3 to 5 mL syringe.
      (4) Insulin: Use a syringe that is calibrated to the concentration of the type of insulin prescribed.
   b. Insulin syringe: Calibrated in units per cubic centimeter (U40, U80, and U100). The syringe used **MUST** correspond to the insulin concentration prescribed.

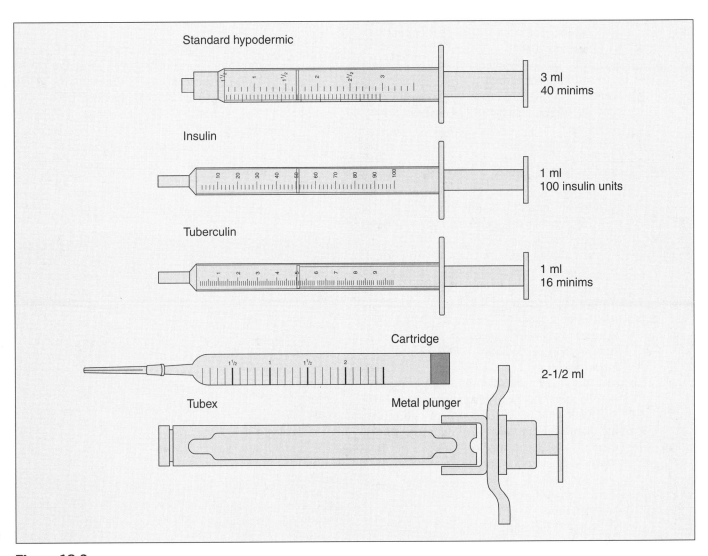

Standard hypodermic

3 ml
40 minims

Insulin

1 ml
100 insulin units

Tuberculin

1 ml
16 minims

Cartridge

Tubex

Metal plunger

2-1/2 ml

Figure 18-3

Syringe types. Delmar/Cengage Learning.

c. Tuberculin syringe: Calibrated in fine increments up to 1 mL; each increment represents 0.1 mL.

d. Tubex/Carpuject syringe: Closed injection system using a reusable metal or plastic syringe frame that holds a disposable medication cartridge-needle unit.

3. Parts of a needle

a. Hub: Needle part that fits on the syringe tip.

b. Cannula (shaft): Length of the needle that is inserted into body tissue.

c. Point: Sharp end of needle shaft.

d. Bevel: Slant of needle point.

e. Lumen: Inside diameter of the needle.

4. Needle size

a. Gauge (G): The smaller the gauge of the needle, the larger the lumen or inside diameter of the needle. Gauges may vary from 13 G to 27 G.

   (1) Intradermal: 26 to 27 G.

   (2) Subcutaneous: 25 to 26 G.

   (3) Intramuscular: 21 to 23 G.

   (4) Aqueous solutions: Use a needle with a small lumen.

   (5) Oily or thick solutions: Use a needle with a large lumen.

b. Length: Length may range from one-quarter inch to 6 inch. The length varies according to its use.

   (1) Intradermal: One-quarter to three-eighths in.

   (2) Subcutaneous: One-half to five-eighths in.

   (3) Intramuscular: one-half to 2 in.

      (a) Normal adults: Use a 1- to 1.5-inch needle.

      (b) Obese patients: Use a 1.5- to 2-inch needle.

      (c) Pediatric and thin patients: Use a 0.5- to 1-inch needle.

5. Containers and diluents (see Figure 18-4)

a. Diluent: Use sterile water or bacteriostatic normal saline as a diluent when reconstituting medications.

b. Vial: Single or multiple dose bottles with rubber stoppers that hold injectable medication.

c. Ampule: Small glass container for injectable medication that requires the stem to be broken to collect the medication. The needle must be changed before administering the injection.

D. Administration procedures

1. Oral medications

a. Wash hands; identify the patient; verify correct medication.

b. Pour pills into bottle cap before transferring them to a medicine cup; do not touch pills.

c. Holding the medicine cup at eye level, pour liquids away from the label (to prevent staining) into the medicine cup; wipe bottle neck before replacing cap.

d. Multiple medications are administered in the following order:

   (1) Tablets, capsules, and spansules with liquid.

   (2) Liquid medication diluted with water.

   (3) Cough medications (undiluted).

   (4) Sublingual medications.

e. Remain with the patient to ensure all medication has been taken; record in patient's chart.

2. Ophthalmic medications

a. Allow ophthalmic medications to warm to room temperature as needed; verify by comparing the order with the medication label.

b. Wash hands and don gloves; identify the patient; explain procedure.

c. Have the patient tilt back head; gently pull down lower eyelid and ask the patient to look up.

d. Release the indicated number of drops on the inner portion of lower lid at the center without touching the dropper to any tissue.

e. Ask the patient to lightly close the eye for several minutes.

f. Record procedure noting the medication, dosage, and eye medicated; clean up.

3. Otic medications

a. Wash hands and don gloves; identify the patient; explain procedure; verify by comparing order with medication label.

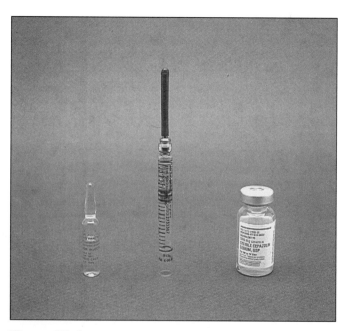

Figure 18-4

From L-R: Ampule, cartridge, and vial. Delmar/Cengage Learning.

b. Have patient assume a sitting or lying position; ask patient to tilt head back and to the side.

c. Position the ear to straighten the ear canal; expel the number of drops indicated without touching the dropper to tissue.

d. Ask the patient to remain in this position for a few minutes; place a wick (cotton plug) in the ear canal as warranted; record procedure noting the medication used, dosage, and the ear medicated.

4. Charging syringe

a. Ampule

   (1) Tap any medication localized above the neck down to the bottom.

   (2) Cleanse the ampule neck with alcohol. Break open the ampule by using a bending motion at the neck of the ampule; a clean gauze should be held over the neck area and the motion should direct the area of breaking away from the body. These measures direct any small shards of glass away from the body.

   (3) Insert a filter needle into the upright ampule and withdraw a little more medication than is needed by drawing back the plunger; allow any bubbles to float to the top of the syringe; lightly tapping the syringe will hasten this process; expel the extra medication withdrawn to the proper quantity; recap the needle.

   (4) Remove the needle and replace with a new, sterile needle before giving the injection.

b. Vial

   (1) Wipe the rubber stopper with alcohol.

   (2) Draw air into the syringe equal to the volume of medication that will be taken from the vial.

   (3) Insert the needle into the upright vial above the medication level; expel the air.

   (4) Turn the vial upside down while the needle is still inserted; position the needle point below the medication level; pulling back on the plunger, slowly withdraw a little more medication than needed.

   (5) Allow any bubbles present to float to the top of the syringe; lightly tapping the syringe may hasten this process; expel the extra medication withdrawn to the proper quantity; withdraw the needle and recap.

5. Intradermal injection (see Figure 18-5)

a. Wash hands; properly charge a tuberculin syringe verifying correct medication; adhere to standard precautions; identify the patient; verify any known allergies.

b. Locate a site having no visible blood vessels; cleanse with alcohol.

c. Pull the skin taut with nondominant hand; at a 15-degree angle, insert the needle, bevel up, just below the skin surface approximately one-eighth inch; turn the needle 180 degrees so the bevel is facing down if desired.

d. Slowly inject the medication until a visible wheal appears; withdraw needle and dispose in a sharps container.

e. Gently place gauze over the injection site; do not press or massage; observe patient for any allergic reactions; clean up; wash hands; record in patient's chart.

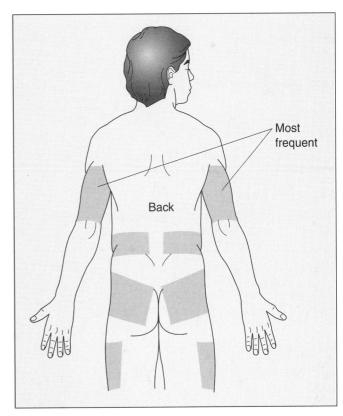

Figure 18-6

Subcutaneous injection sites. Delmar/Cengage Learning.

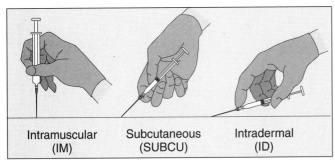

Figure 18-5

Angles of injection. Delmar/Cengage Learning.

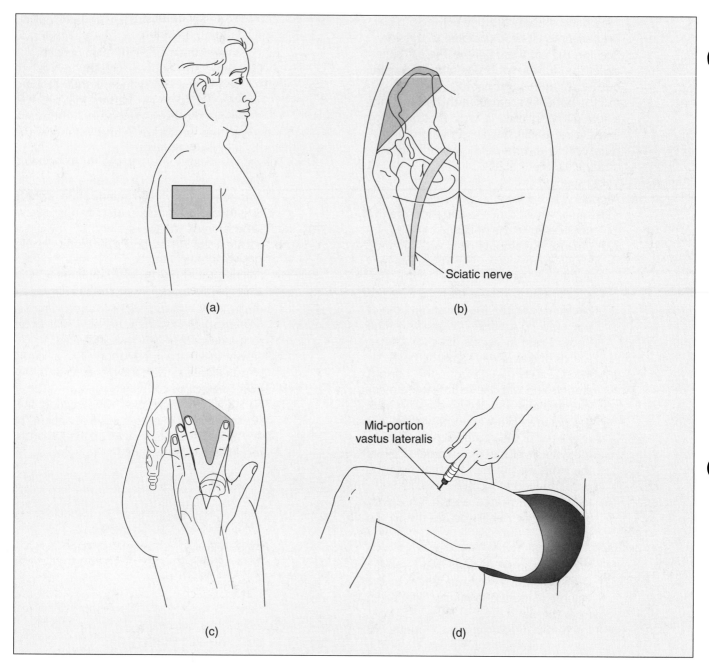

Figure 18-7A to D

Intramuscular injection sites: (a) Deltoid, (b) Gluteus medius, (c) Ventrogluteal, (d) Vastus lateralis. Delmar/Cengage Learning.

6. Subcutaneous and intramuscular injection
   a. Wash hands; properly charge a syringe verifying correct medication; adhere to standard precautions; identify the patient; verify any known allergies.
   b. Locate the injection site; cleanse with alcohol.
   c. Inserting the needle
      (1) Subcutaneous (see Figures 18-5 and 18-6)
         (a) With the nondominant hand, pinch the skin forming a raised skinfold; at a 45-degree angle, quickly insert the needle, bevel up, to its hub.
         (b) Using the nondominant hand, release the skinfold and pull back the plunger slightly to ensure no blood enters the syringe.
      (2) Intramuscular (see Figures 18-5 and 18-7A to D)
         (a) With the nondominant hand, pinch a large portion of muscle, or pull skin taut; at a 90-degree angle, insert the needle to its hub.
         (b) Using the nondominant hand, release the musclefold, and pull back the plunger slightly to ensure no blood enters the syringe.
      (3) If blood is aspirated, you have punctured a blood vessel.
      (4) Usually, the needle and syringe is withdrawn and discarded and a new syringe with fresh medication is prepared.
      (5) Some medications, however, are very expensive; the provider may request that the needle be reinserted in an adjacent area. Follow clinic protocol.
   d. Slowly depress the plunger to release the medication; withdraw the needle and dispose in sharps container.
   e. Gently press gauze over the injection site; observe patient for any allergic reactions; clean up; wash hands; record in patient's chart.

VII. INTRAVENOUS THERAPY

A. Role of the MA varies according to state law and organizational policies.
B. Provides long-term access for the infusion of medications, fluids, electrolytes, blood products, and nutritional supplements.
C. Advantages
   1. Immediate distribution and absorption.
   2. Does not require GI processing.
D. Disadvantages
   1. Patient discomfort.
   2. Infiltration: IV fluid can escape into the surrounding tissues.

3. Thrombosis may occur.
4. Potential for an embolism.
5. Increased chance of infection.
6. Possible hyperhydration.

E. Common IV solution forms
   1. Crystalloid: Those that contain crystallized compounds, e.g., electrolyte solutions.
   2. Colloid: Those that are glutinous (thick, sticky).
F. Common IV infusates
   1. D5W: 5% dextrose in water, a rehydrating solution.
   2. Normal saline solution (NSS): 0.9% sodium chloride (NaCl).
G. Equipment and materials
   1. IV bag containing appropriate solution.
   2. Infiltration set
      a. Piercing pin: Used to spike the bag.
      b. Drip chamber: Used to control the fluid flow.
      c. Clamp: Used to close or adjust fluid flow.
      d. Injection port: Used to inject medication.
H. IV order information
   1. Name of patient; date and time of day.
   2. Infusate name.
   3. Route of administration.
   4. Infusion volume.
   5. Infusate dosage.
   6. Rate of infusion.
   7. Duration of infusion.
   8. Physician's signature.
I. IV Administration procedure
   1. Prepare infusion bag and administration set
      a. Close the clamp on the tubing.
      b. Spike the bag with the piercing pin.
      c. Squeeze drip chamber to begin the flow of fluid into the tubing.
      d. Release the clamp and allow the fluid to flow through the rest of the tubing until a few drops flow out into a trash can. The line is now primed.
      e. Re-clamp the tubing. It is ready to be attached to the cannula.
   2. Wash hands; don gloves; verify correct medication; adhere to standard precautions; identify the patient; verify any known allergies.
   3. Apply tourniquet.
   4. Select a vein and clean site.
   5. Access the vein.
   6. Thread the cannula into the vessel.
   7. Remove the needle and dispose in sharps container.
   8. Attach the primed line to the cannula.
   9. Secure and cover the IV site with dressings and tape.
   10. Observe for any allergic reactions.
   11. Remove gloves, wash hands, document the procedure.

CHAPTER 19

First Aid and Cardiopulmonary Resuscitation

I. INTRODUCTION

A. First aid is the immediate care given to an injured or suddenly ill person.

B. Emergency action steps

  1. Survey the scene: Quickly observe the scene surrounding the victim to determine the following:

    a. Safety

      (1) Determine if the scene is safe for you to proceed. Do not put yourself in unnecessary danger: you are of no use as a rescuer if you too become a victim.

      (2) If you can safely get to the victim, determine if it is safe to remain while you render first aid. Do not move the victim unless the scene poses an immediate danger.

    b. Incident

      (1) Determine what happened. If the victim is conscious, ask questions.

      (2) Look for physical clues that may indicate what happened.

      (3) Look to see if the victim has a medical alert tag at the neck or wrist that would provide a clue as to the victim's condition.

    c. Other victims: Observe to locate any other victims, especially unconscious ones who may go unnoticed.

    d. Bystanders

      (1) Check to see if anyone knows what happened or is acquainted with any of the victims; ask questions.

      (2) Assign tasks to bystanders such as calling for emergency medical services (EMS), providing emotional support, and treatment assistance.

  2. Primary victim survey: Carefully observe the victim for life-threatening conditions.

    a. Check for responsiveness: Gently tap the victim and ask, "Are you OK?" If the person is conscious, ask if you can be of assistance. If unconscious or delirious, proceed as described below.

    b. Assess ABCs

      (1) Airway

        (a) Determine if the victim has an open airway.

        (b) Perform the head-tilt/chin-lift to ensure the airway is open.

      (2) Breathing: Determine if the victim is moving or breathing.

        (a) Look for the chest to rise and fall, listen for breathing sounds, and feel for air emanating from the mouth and nose.

        (b) If the victim is not breathing, you must perform artificial respiration.

      (3) Circulation

        (a) Determine if the heart is beating.

          (i) If the victim is breathing, the heart is circulating blood.

          (ii) Check the carotid pulse for a beat.

          (iii) If no pulse is palpated, you must perform cardiopulmonary resuscitation (CPR).

        (b) Determine if the victim is bleeding.

          (i) Observe the entire body for wet, blood-soaked clothing.

          (ii) Severe bleeding will generally spurt from the wound.

    c. Complete the primary survey before rendering first aid. Life-threatening conditions such as breathlessness, pulselessness, and severe bleeding must be attended to first before less serious conditions are addressed.

  3. Activate the emergency medical services system (EMS).

    a. If possible, assign two bystanders to phone the local EMS (911) while you stay with the victim(s); otherwise, make the call yourself.

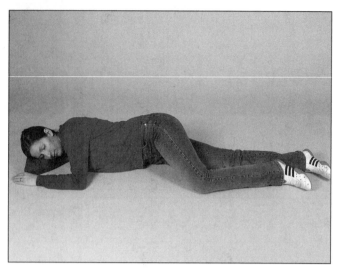

Figure 19-1

Recovery position. Delmar/Cengage Learning.

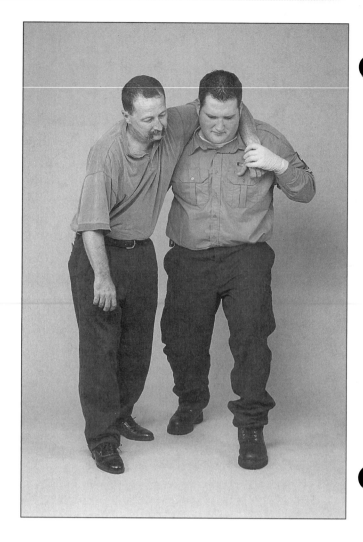

Figure 19-2

Walking assist. Delmar/Cengage Learning.

b. If you are alone and have to leave the victim for any reason, e.g., call for help, place the victim in a recovery position (see Figure 19-1). The recovery position will keep the airway open and clear if he vomits.

c. Information provided to EMS:

    (1) Location of the emergency: Address and major cross streets.

    (2) Phone number calling from.

    (3) Caller's name.

    (4) Description of the situation.

    (5) Number and condition of the victims.

    (6) Description of the help being rendered.

d. Allow the EMS dispatcher to hang up first in case more information or instructions are required.

4. Secondary victim survey

    a. Once any life-threatening conditions have been stabilized, carefully check the victim for other problems that are not an immediate threat but could become serious if uncorrected.

    b. Interview the victim and bystanders to determine the details of the situation and potential problems.

    c. Assess vital signs and examine the victim from head to toe.

C. Do not provide care beyond the scope of your abilities or training.

II. EMERGENCY MOVES

A. Walking assist (see Figure 19-2)

    1. Used with a conscious person.

    2. Place the victim's arm across your shoulders and hold it in place with one hand.

3. Support the victim with your other hand around the victim's waist.

4. If a second rescuer is present, the victim can be further supported in the same fashion on the other side.

5. Not to be used if the victim has a suspected head, neck, or back injury.

B. Pack-strap carry (see Figure 19-3A and B)

    1. Used with both conscious and unconscious victims.

    2. Have the victim stand or ask a second rescuer to support the victim.

    3. Position yourself with your back to the victim so that your shoulders fit into the victim's axillae.

    4. Cross the victim's arms in front of you and grasp the victim's wrists.

    5. Lean forward and pull the victim up onto your back.

    6. Stand up and walk to safety.

    7. Not to be used if the victim has a suspected head, neck, or back injury.

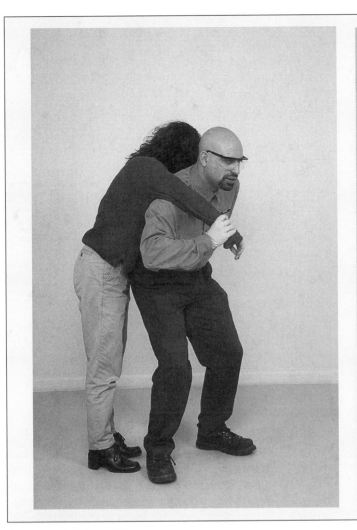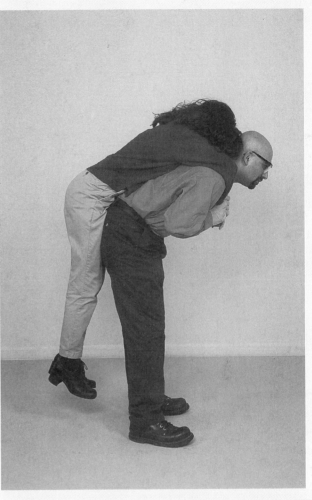

Figure 19-3A and B

Pack-strap carry. Delmar/Cengage Learning.

C. Two-person seat carry (see Figure 19-4)
    1. Used for conscious victims who are not seriously injured.
    2. Put one arm behind the victim's thighs and the other across the victim's back.
    3. Interlock your arms with those of a second rescuer behind the victim's legs and across her back.
    4. Lift the victim with the rescuers' arms forming a cradle.
D. Blanket drag (see Figure 19-5)
    1. Keep the victim between you and the blanket.
    2. Gather half the blanket and place it against the victim's side.
    3. Roll the victim as a unit toward you.
    4. Reach over and place the blanket so that it will be positioned under the victim.
    5. Roll the victim onto the blanket.
    6. Gather the blanket at the head and drag the victim to safety.

E. Clothes drag (see Figure 19-6)
    1. Used on victims with suspected spinal injuries.
    2. Grasp the victim's clothes at the collar and shoulders, while supporting the victim's head.
    3. Keeping your body low, pull the victim to safety.
F. Foot drag
    1. If the victim is large, grasp each ankle and pull the victim to safety.
    2. Do not use this technique if the victim's head will be injured by rough ground.

III. ARTIFICIAL RESPIRATION: RESCUE BREATHING

A. Method of breathing air into someone's lungs whose breathing has ceased.
B. Common causes of breathing emergencies
    1. Obstruction.
    2. Drugs and poisons.

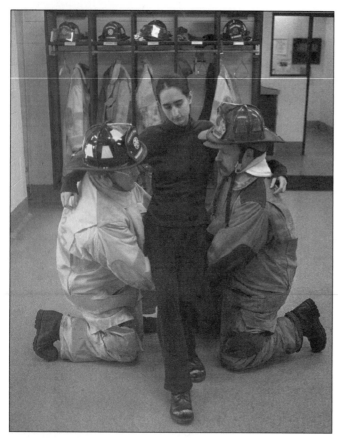

Figure 19-4

Seat carry. Delmar/Cengage Learning.

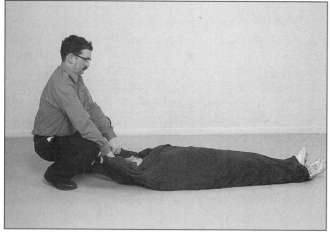

Figure 19-5

Blanket drag. Delmar/Cengage Learning.

3. Chest injuries.
4. Near-drowning.
5. Electrocution.
6. Burns and smoke inhalation.
7. Asthma.
8. Allergic reactions.
9. Shock.

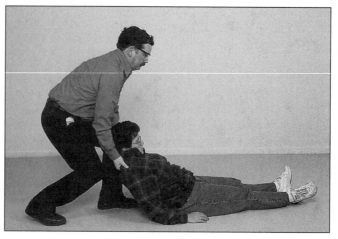

Figure 19-6

Clothing drag. Delmar/Cengage Learning.

C. First aid: Adult
   1. Check for responsiveness: Tap the victim and ask, "Are you OK?"
   2. If unresponsive, yell for help.
   3. Roll victim onto back if necessary.
   4. Open the airway by tilting the head back.
   5. Look, listen, and feel for breathing.
   6. If the victim is not breathing, and if no face mask or shield is available for use, pinch the victim's nostrils shut, seal your mouth around the victim's and give two slow breaths, each breath lasting 1 second, just enough to cause the chest to rise.
   7. Check the carotid pulse for 5 to 10 seconds and check for severe bleeding.
   8. If there is a pulse but no breathing, continue giving a breath every 5 seconds.
   9. If the victim is both breathless and pulseless, administer CPR (discussed later).
D. Child: Same as the adult except a ventilation is given every 3 seconds.
E. Infant: Same as the adult except your mouth should be sealed over both the infant's mouth and nose, a ventilation is given every 3 seconds, and the brachial artery is palpated.
F. Special situations
   1. Gastric distension: Excessive air entering the stomach, causing it to bulge, thereby decreasing the capacity of the lungs to receive air. Caused by:
      a. Excessive ventilations.
      b. Improper head-tilt.
      c. Giving ventilations too quickly.
   2. Vomiting: Sometimes unconscious victims may vomit. Turn the victim's head and body to one side, wipe the vomitus out of the victim's mouth, and continue ventilating.
   3. Mouth-to-nose ventilations: In the event the victim's mouth or jaw is injured or cannot be

opened, keep the victim's mouth closed as you tilt the head and ventilate through the nose.

4. Mouth-to-stoma ventilations: Treat the stoma as you would the victim's mouth, but do not tilt the head back.

5. Suspected neck or spinal injury: Minimize head movement by lifting the chin at the jaw below the ears to open the airway.

G. Airway obstruction (see Figure 19-7)
 1. The airway becomes blocked by foreign bodies, fluids, or the back of the tongue.
 2. Partial obstruction: The victim can usually cough and perhaps wheeze or speak between breaths; stay with the victim, but do not interfere with any attempts to cough up the object.
 3. Complete obstruction: A partial obstruction can progress to a complete obstruction. The victim will be unable to speak, cough, or breathe.
 4. First aid: Adult
    a. Conscious victim:
       (1) Ask the victim, "Are you choking?"
       (2) If so, indicate that you can help.
       (3) Stand behind the victim and wrap your arms around the victim's waist (see Figure 19-9).
       (4) Make a fist with one hand and place thumb side against the victim's midabdomen just above the navel, well below the xyphoid process.

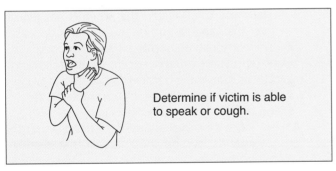

Figure 19-7

Patient with blocked airway. Delmar/Cengage Learning.

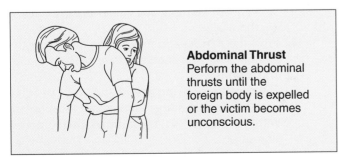

Abdominal Thrust
Perform the abdominal thrusts until the foreign body is expelled or the victim becomes unconscious.

Figure 19-8

Performing abdominal thrusts. Delmar/Cengage Learning.

(5) Grasp the fist with the other hand and quickly press the fist into the abdomen with an upward motion.
(6) Repeat the thrust until the object is dislodged or the victim becomes unconscious.

b. Unconscious victim
   (1) If just arriving on the scene proceed through the emergency action steps.
   (2) Roll victim onto back if necessary.
   (3) Open airway via head-tilt/chin-lift.
   (4) Check for breathlessness for 10 seconds or less.
   (5) If the victim is not breathing, give two ventilations.
   (6) If the lungs do not ventilate, reposition the head and try two breaths again. If the lungs still do not ventilate, assume an obstruction.
   (7) Locate the correct hand position for chest compressions as used in CPR.
   (8) Perform chest compressions—a depth of 2 inches 30 times in 18 seconds.
   (9) Observe for a foreign object—if seen, remove it with your finger.
   (10) Give two breaths. If the chest does not rise—no air is entering the lungs, repeat the cycles of chest compressions, foreign object check, and rescue breaths until:
        (a) The object is removed and air enters the lungs.
        (b) The victim begins breathing.
        (c) EMS personnel arrive and take over.
        (d) You are too exhausted to continue.
        (e) The scene become unsafe.
   (11) If the chest rises—air is entering the lungs, check the pulse for 10 seconds or less.
   (12) Care for the conditions discovered.
   (13) In an unconscious adult, you may detect an irregular, gasping or shallow breath known as agonal breathing; because it is abnormal, begin CPR immediately.

c. Chest compressions
   Perform the compression at the center of the chest at least 2 inches above the xyphoid process.

5. First aid: Child
   a. Conscious victim: Same as adult.
   b. Unconscious victim: Same as adult except only one hand is used to give the chest compressions to a depth of about 1.5 inches.

6. First aid: Infant
   a. Conscious victim

(1) Call for help.

(2) Holding the infant face down, supporting the head lower than the body, deliver five back blows between the shoulder blades using the heel of one hand.

(3) Turn the infant over and administer five chest compressions, 0.5 to 1 inch in depth, at the center of the chest above the xyphoid process using your middle and ring fingers.

(4) Repeat until the infant can either breathe independently or becomes unconscious.

b. Unconscious victim

(1) Attempt to ventilate the infant twice.

(2) If no air is entering the lungs, turn the infant over as described above and give five back blows.

(3) Administer five chest thrusts as described above.

(4) Grasp the infant's tongue and lower jaw, open the mouth and visually inspect the airway. If you observe a foreign body, carefully remove it.

(5) Regardless of finding a foreign object or not, give a ventilation.

(6) Repeat the sequence until air enters the lungs, then proceed with CPR measures.

IV. CARDIOPULMONARY RESUSCITATION

A. Adult CPR

1. Carry out the emergency action steps.

2. Check for responsiveness: Gently tap the victim and ask, "Are you OK?"

3. If unconscious or unresponsive, call for help.

4. Perform head-tilt/chin-lift to ensure the airway is open.

5. Look, listen, and feel for breathing for no more than 10 seconds.

6. If the victim is not breathing, give two ventilations.

a. If the chest fails to rise, reposition the head and attempt to ventilate again.

b. If still no air is entering the lungs, assume that a foreign body airway obstruction (FBAO) exists and begin the sequence for an obstructed airway on an unconscious victim described earlier.

7. If there are no signs of life (movement or breathing), begin 15 chest compressions:

a. Landmark the compression site.

(1) As you kneel next to the victim's chest, use the middle and index finger of the hand nearer the victim's legs and locate the lower rib cage; slide your fingers up to the notch at the lower end of the breastbone.

(2) Place the middle finger over the notch and index finger next to it.

(3) Place the heel of the other hand on the victim's sternum next to the index finger.

(4) Place the hand that located the notch over the hand resting on the chest, keeping the fingers off the victim's chest.

b. Position your shoulder directly over the hand placement, with arms straight and elbows locked.

c. Using your upper body weight, compress the sternum 1.5 to 2 inches at a rate of 30 compressions in about 18 seconds.

d. Count aloud 1 and 2 and 3 and 4 and 5 . . . and so on to 30, making the compressions on the count.

e. The compression and release should be of equal duration and the hands should not lose contact with the chest; if so, re-landmark.

8. Quickly move to the victim's head, tilt and give two ventilations.

9. Continue the cycles of 30 compressions and two ventilations.

10. Recheck pulse and breathing every few minutes.

11. If both are absent, give two ventilations and resume the cycle of 30 compressions followed by two ventilations.

B. Child CPR: Same as adult except for the following:

1. Only one hand is used to compress the chest. The hand that located the notch is not placed over the hand resting on the sternum.

2. The compression depth is 1 to 1.5 inches.

C. Infant CPR: Same as adult except for the following:

1. The brachial pulse is palpated to assess circulation.

2. The compression to ventilation ratio is 30:2.

3. Landmark the compression site.

a. Place the index finger of the hand nearer the infant's legs on the chest so that it covers both nipples.

b. Draw the fingers back to the center of the chest midway between the infant's nipples.

c. Lift the index and little finger up so that just the middle and ring finger is resting on the infant's sternum one finger-breadth below the nipples.

4. With the middle and ring finger, compress the sternum 0.5 to 1 inch at a rate of 30 in about 18 seconds.

6. The compression and release should be of equal duration and the fingers should not lose contact with the chest; if so, re-landmark the compression site.

7. Without losing contact with the chest, use the other hand to tilt the head, form a seal over the

infant's mouth and nose with your mouth and ventilate once just enough to cause the chest to rise.

8. Administer repeated cycles of 30 compressions followed by two ventilations.

9. Recheck the brachial pulse and breathing 5 to 10 seconds or less.

10. If both are absent, give two ventilations and resume the cycle of 30 compressions followed by two ventilations.

11. Recheck pulse and breathing every few minutes.

D. Discontinuing CPR: You may stop CPR efforts under the following conditions:
   1. The victim recovers.
   2. You are relieved by someone having equal or superior skill.
   3. Members of the EMS arrive and take over.
   4. You are too physically exhausted to continue.
   5. An AED becomes available and ready to use.
   6. The scene becomes unsafe.

E. Automated external defibrillator (AED) (see Figure 19-9)
   1. Most people experiencing sudden cardiac arrest require an electric shock to the heart to temporarily stop the arrhythmia so that it may begin a normal rhythm.
   2. An AED is an instrument that is designed to assess the need for and deliver the appropriate shock to the heart muscle to that end.
   3. Most AEDs are operated as follows:
      a. Turn on the AED.
      b. Wipe the victim's chest dry.
      c. Apply the pads to the bare chest: Place one pad on the upper right chest and the other on the lower left side (see Figure 19-10).
      d. Plug the connector into the AED if necessary.
      e. Allow the AED to assess the heart rhythm—If prompted by the AED, push the button marked "analyze."
      f. Advise all by standers to stand clear and not to touch the victim.
      g. If prompted by the AED, deliver a shock by pushing the button indicated.
      h. If the AED indicates "no shock advised," you may have to continue CPR.
      i. In such cases, leave the AED attached and continue CPR for 5 cycles, about 2 minutes.
   4. For a child the same steps apply, except for the following:
      a. Use pediatric AED pads
      b. Make sure the pads are not touching—you may have to place one pad on the child's chest and the other on the back.
   5. AED precautions:
      a. Do not touch the victim while the AED is analyzing—doing so will cause interference.

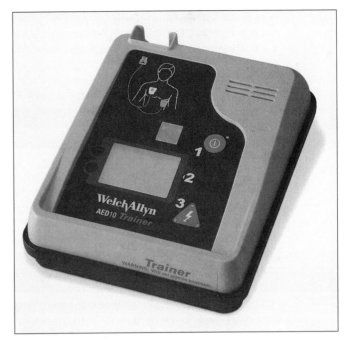

Figure 19-9

Automated external defibrillator (AED). Courtesy of Welch-Allyn.

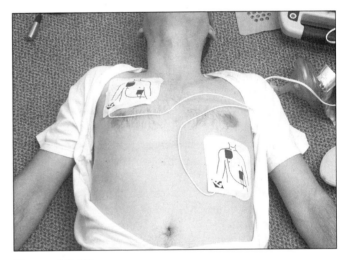

Figure 19-10

Electrode placement for AED pads. Delmar/Cengage Learning.

   b. Do not touch the victim during defibrillation.
   c. Before shocking the victim, ensure no one is in contact with the victim or the equipment.
   d. Do not use alcohol to dry the victim's chest—it is flammable.
   e. Do not defibrillate in the presence of flammable materials, including oxygen.
   f. Do not use an AED in a moving vehicle—may cause interference.
   g. Do not use an AED on a victim who is in contact with water—move away from water source.

h. Do not use adult AED pads on children under age 8 or less than 55 pounds unless pediatric pads are not available—protocols may differ and should be followed.

i. Do not use an AED on a victim wearing any kind of patch on the chest, e.g., nitroglycerin; remove patches before attaching the AED.

j. Do not use a cellular phone or radio within 6 feet of AED—may cause interference.

6. Wet conditions: After removing the victim from water, dry the victim's chest before applying the AED. Shelter the victim from rain and dry the victim as much as possible.

7. Implantable devices: E.g., pacemakers and implantable cardioverter defibrillator (ICD) are often located below the right clavicle and make a visible protrusion. If you observe or know the victim has such a device, do not place the pads over the device—adjust the pads away from the device. Follow the procedure as described earlier.

V. SECONDARY SURVEY

A. Purpose: Carefully check the victim for conditions that are not immediately life-threatening, but could become so if not attended to.

B. The secondary survey is performed on a conscious person. If unconscious, however, the ABCs are monitored until the EMS arrives.

C. Interview the victim and bystanders.
   1. Provides clues as to what to look for while you complete the secondary survey.
   2. Identify yourself as a trained first aid provider and acquire consent from the victim to render first aid.
   3. Ask for the victim's name. Address the victim by name and ask how he or she feels, if and where there is any pain, and if there are any past medical problems, allergies and/or medications.
   4. Ask any bystanders what they saw and what they know about the victim.

D. Assess vital signs.
   1. Check breathing: Normally, breathing should be effortless and quiet.
      a. Normal rate: 12 to 20 per minute.
      b. Abnormal breathing includes:
         (1) Gasping for air.
         (2) Noisy such as whistling, crowing, and gurgling sounds.
         (3) Abnormally fast or slow breathing.
         (4) Painful.
   2. Check pulse.
      a. Normal: 60 to 100 per minute, strong, and regular.
      b. Abnormal pulse includes:
         (1) Irregular.

         (2) Weak, hard to find.
         (3) Abnormally fast or slow.
      c. If the victim is breathing, the heart is beating; however, there may not be a pulse in the injured area.
   3. Check skin appearance and temperature.
      a. Assess to see if the skin is pale, red, or bluish.
      b. Check to see if it feels hot to the touch.
   4. Check blood pressure if you have access to a sphygmomanometer and stethoscope.

E. Perform a head-to-toe exam: Note any pain, discomfort, or immobility.
   1. Inform the victim that you are about to perform an exam.
   2. Ask the victim to remain still and do not move any area that is experiencing pain or discomfort, especially if you suspect a head, neck, or back injury.
   3. Observe for any bleeding, cuts, bruises, or deformities.
   4. Examine the ears, nose, and mouth for blood or any fluid discharge.
   5. Examine the neck and ask the victim to slowly move the head from side to side.
   6. Examine the shoulders and ask the victim to shrug shoulders.
   7. Examine the chest and abdomen and ask the victim to take a deep breath and blow air out.
   8. Examine the arms and ask the victim to move hands and fingers and bend each arm.
   9. Examine hips and legs and ask the victim to move each foot, toes, ankle, and bend each leg.
   10. If the victim can move body parts without pain or discomfort and is not dizzy:
      a. Have the victim sit up and rest.
      b. If no further difficulty is noted, have the victim slowly stand.
      c. Determine if further care is needed.
      d. If pain or dizziness is present:
         (1) Assess and monitor ABCs.
         (2) Have victim assume most comfortable position.
         (3) Maintain normal body temperature.
         (4) Reassure victim.
         (5) Call EMS.

VI. SHOCK

A. Physiological response to sudden illness and injury that is characterized by inadequate peripheral circulation that deprives vital organs and tissues of oxygen-rich blood. Untreated, shock progresses to coma and death.
   1. Hypovolemic shock: Shock caused by sudden blood or body fluid loss.
   2. Respiratory shock: Shock caused by insufficient blood oxygen.

3. Psychogenic shock (syncope): Shock caused by sudden mental trauma.
4. Cardiogenic shock: Shock caused by inadequate heart function.
5. Septic shock: Shock caused by systemic infection.
6. Anaphylactic shock: Shock caused by a severe allergic reaction.
7. Neurogenic shock: Shock caused by trauma to the brain or spinal cord, or neurotoxins as in some snake and spider bites.

B. Signs and symptoms
1. Restlessness and irritability.
2. Tachycardia, tachypnea.
3. Pale to cyanotic, cool, moist skin.
4. Nausea and vomiting.
5. Polydipsia.
6. Loss of consciousness.

C. First aid
1. Carry out the emergency action steps.
2. Assess and monitor ABCs.
3. If no head or neck, leg, or hip injuries are suspected, elevate the victim's legs approximately 12 inches; otherwise, have the victim lay flat while awaiting for EMS.
4. If vomiting occurs, place the victim on her side to avoid aspiration into the lungs.
5. If dyspneic, have victim assume a reclining position.
6. Keep the victim from becoming chilled by covering with a blanket, but do not overheat.
7. Do not give anything to eat or drink.
8. Ensure activation of EMS.

VII. HEMORRHAGE

A. Internal or external bleeding from arteries, veins, or capillaries.
B. External bleeding is often discovered during the primary survey; however, internal bleeding may go unnoticed until the secondary survey.
C. Signs and symptoms
1. External hemorrhage
   a. Arterial bleeding: Blood appears bright red and usually spurts from the wound; life threatening.
   b. Venous bleeding: Blood appears dark red or maroon and flows steadily from the wound.
   c. Capillary bleeding: Blood appears medium red and flows slowly or oozes from the wound.
2. Internal hemorrhage
   a. Bruising or discoloration in the injured area.
   b. Swollen, tender, or hard soft tissue such as in the abdomen.
   c. Anxiety or restlessness.
   d. Tachycardia and tachypnea.
   e. Shock.

D. First aid
1. Activate EMS.
2. External hemorrhage
   a. Cover the wound with a dressing and apply direct pressure or a pressure bandage.
   b. If fracture is not suspected, elevate the injured part above the level of the heart.
   c. If the dressing becomes saturated with blood, add more dressings; do not remove blood-soaked dressings.
   d. If bleeding continues, apply pressure at a pressure point.
   e. Tourniquet: Applied as a last resort.
   f. Treat for shock if necessary.
3. Internal bleeding
   a. Ensure immediate activation of EMS.
   b. Have victim assume most comfortable position.
   c. Assess and monitor ABCs.
   d. Maintain normal body temperature.
   e. Provide reassurance; care for other conditions.
   f. Treat for shock if necessary.

VIII. MYOCARDIAL INFARCTION

A. Blockage of circulation to the heart muscle often attributable to cardiovascular disease.
B. Signs and symptoms
1. Chest pain
   a. Intense pressure, squeezing, or tightness at the center of the chest.
   b. Pain may radiate to either shoulder, arm, neck, or lower jaw.
   c. Symptoms need not be severe to warrant a cardiac emergency.
2. Diaphoresis.
3. Nausea.
4. Shortness of breath.
5. Weakness.

C. First aid
1. Have the victim stop whatever activity brought on the attack and sit or lie down in a comfortable position.
2. Loosen restrictive clothing.
3. Conduct a secondary survey.
   a. If the victim has been treated for angina, check to see if nitroglycerin is available.
   b. If so, administer the nitroglycerin.
   c. Ensure that no more than three doses have been taken in the last 15 minutes.
   d. If the pain is simple angina, the pain should momentarily dissipate.
   e. If there is no pain relief after 10 minutes, activate the EMS; if necessary, transport the victim to the nearest emergency room.

4. Treat for shock if required.
5. Be prepared to administer CPR if the victim undergoes cardiac or respiratory arrest.

IX. CEREBROVASCULAR ACCIDENT ([CVA] STROKE)

A. Interruption of blood flow to the brain often caused by occlusion, arterial rupture, or arterial compression resulting in partial or complete brain damage.
B. Signs and symptoms
   1. Weakness or numbness of the face, arm, or leg, often on one side of the body.
   2. Difficulty speaking or understanding speech.
   3. Blurred vision.
   4. Unequal pupils.
   5. Vertigo, confusion, and tinnitus.
   6. Severe headache, nausea and vomiting.
   7. Loss of bladder or bowel control, as well as unconsciousness.
C. First aid
   1. Assess and monitor ABCs.
   2. Activate EMS.
   3. Have victim assume most comfortable position.
   4. Give nothing to eat or drink.
   5. If victim is drooling or having difficulty swallowing, place the victim on one side to help drain fluids to maintain an open airway.
   6. Treat for shock if necessary.

X. SEIZURES

A. Convulsive muscular contractions caused by a head injury, fever, sudden illness, or epilepsy.
B. Signs and symptoms
   1. May be preceded by an aura, i.e., unusual sensation such as hallucinations, strange sound, taste, or smell. The victim may have time to warn bystanders before the attack.
   2. Sudden unresponsiveness, as in day-dreaming, or unconsciousness.
   3. Uncontrollable muscular contractions.
C. First aid
   1. If the victim has epilepsy, it is usually unnecessary to activate EMS unless:
      a. The seizure lasts longer than 5 minutes.
      b. Another seizure begins subsequent to the first.
      c. The victim fails to regain consciousness after the seizure is over.
   2. Activate EMS if the victim is:
      a. Pregnant.
      b. Diabetic.
      c. Injured.
      d. In water.
      e. Seizure follows a sudden rise in body temperature.

3. Do not restrain or hold the victim during the seizure.
4. Do not put anything in the victim's mouth.
5. Protect the victim from injury by removing objects such as furniture.
6. Maintain an open airway and protect the head from injury by placing padding under and around the head.
7. After the seizure is over, the victim will be drowsy and disoriented.
8. Have the victim rest while you perform a secondary survey to identify and treat any injuries.
9. Reassure the victim and stay until the victim is fully conscious or EMS arrives.

XI. BURNS

A. Injuries resulting from exposure to heat, chemicals, electricity, or radiation.
B. Classified according to source and depth of injury.
C. Signs and symptoms
   1. First degree
      a. Involves the epidermal layer only.
      b. Appears red and dry, and perhaps mildly swollen.
      c. Pain and discomfort.
   2. Second degree
      a. Involves the epidermis and upper dermis.
      b. Appears red with blisters and swelling.
      c. Pain and discomfort.
   3. Third degree
      a. Involves the epidermis, dermis, and subcutaneous layers.
      b. Appears brown or charred with deeper tissue taking on a whitish appearance.
      c. May or may not be painful depending on degree of nerve damage.
D. First aid
   1. Activate EMS immediately for the following:
      a. Burn victim has trouble breathing.
      b. Burns that cover more than one body part.
      c. Burns on the head, neck, hands, feet, or genitals.
      d. Second- or third-degree burns to a child or elderly person.
      e. Burns resulting from chemicals, explosions, or electricity.
   2. Heat burns
      a. Cool the burned area with cool water, except for third-degree burns.
      b. Cover the burned area with the most sterile material available without exerting any pressure on the burn.
      c. Treat for shock if necessary.
   3. Chemical burns
      a. Remove contaminated clothing.
      b. Flush with copious amounts of water.

   c. Lime and phosphorus must be brushed away before flushing with water.

   d. Monitor ABCs.

   e. Treat for shock if necessary.

4. Electrical burns

   a. Ensure that all electrical power sources are turned off.

   b. Carry out primary survey; assess ABCs.

   c. Activate EMS.

   d. Often an electrical burn will occur at point of entrance and exit of electrical current.

   e. Cover burns with the most sterile material available.

   f. Electrocution can cause cardiac and respiratory arrest, so be prepared to administer CPR or defibrillation.

   g. Immediately seek advance medical care.

XII. THERMAL INJURIES

A. Thermal injuries include heat stroke, heat exhaustion, heat cramps, hypothermia, and frostbite.

B. Heat stroke: Severe heat exposure that interferes with the body's heat regulating system; life threatening.

   1. Signs and symptoms

     a. Dry, hot, red skin.

     b. Elevated body temperature.

     c. Weak tachycardia.

     d. Shallow tachypnea.

     e. Delirium or unconsciousness.

   2. First aid

     a. Activate EMS.

     b. Transport victim to a cool place and place in the recovery position.

     c. Quickly cool the victim by immersing in a cool bath, or wrap cool, wet sheets around the body Ice packs may be placed on the victims wrists, ankles, groin, axilla, and neck to cool the large blood vessels. Do not apply rubbing alcohol.

     d. If conscious, give small amounts of cool water to drink.

     e. Treat for shock if necessary.

C. Heat exhaustion: Heat-induced shock as a result of sudden fluid loss.

   1. Signs and symptoms

     a. Same as that for shock.

     b. Untreated heat exhaustion can progress to heat stroke.

     c. Refusing water, vomiting, and changes in consciousness signal a worsening condition.

   2. First aid

     a. Activate EMS.

     b. Transport victim to a cool place.

     c. Treat for shock.

     d. If the victim is conscious, give small amounts of water to drink.

D. Heat cramps: Muscular pain and spasms occurring subsequent to heavy exertion often resulting from fluid and sodium loss.

   1. Signs and symptoms: Muscle spasms of the legs and abdominal muscles.

   2. First aid

     a. Transport victim to a cool place.

     b. Give the victim small amounts of water to drink. Do not give salt tablets or salt water as this can worsen the condition.

     c. Lightly stretch and massage the affected muscles.

E. Hypothermia: Sudden decrease in body temperature due to exposure to cold.

   1. Stages

     a. Shivering.

     b. Apathy.

     c. Loss of consciousness.

     d. Bradycardia and bradypnea.

     e. Death.

   2. Signs and symptoms

     a. Shivering.

     b. Vertigo.

     c. Numbness.

     d. Confusion.

     e. Weakness.

     f. Impaired vision.

     g. Drowsiness.

   3. First aid

     a. Activate EMS.

     b. Transport victim out of the cold and change into dry clothing.

     c. Warm the body slowly.

     d. Unless fully conscious, give nothing to eat or drink.

     e. Monitor ABCs.

F. Frostbite: Formation of ice crystals in body tissues resulting from exposure to cold.

   1. Signs and symptoms

     a. Initially, the skin will appear slightly flushed and be somewhat painful.

     b. After time, the skin will appear white or grayish yellow and then eventually grayish blue. The pain may eventually subside.

     c. The affected part will feel cold and numb.

     d. Moderate frostbite may cause blistering.

     e. Untreated frostbite may develop into gangrene.

   2. First aid

     a. Transport victim to a warm place.

     b. Place affected parts in warm, but not hot water until normal color returns and it feels warm.

     c. Do not rub or massage the affected area Do not break any blister.

     d. Place dry, sterile gauze between toes or fingers after warming, and gently bandage.

XIII. DIABETIC EMERGENCIES

A. Diabetes mellitus is a metabolic condition characterized by a decrease or lack of insulin production resulting in improper glucose metabolism.

B. Insulin shock (hypoglycemia): Caused by an excessive amount of insulin with a subsequent decrease in the availability of glucose.
   1. Signs and symptoms
      a. Vertigo.
      b. Drowsiness.
      c. Confusion.
      d. Tachycardia, tachypnea.
      e. Slurred speech.
   2. First aid
      a. If conscious, give the victim something containing sugar such as candy, soda pop, or orange juice.
      b. Treat for shock if necessary.
      c. Activate EMS.

C. Diabetic coma (hyperglycemia/ketoacidosis): Caused by reduced amount of insulin coupled by increased levels of blood glucose.
   1. Signs and symptoms
      a. Similar to insulin shock.
      b. Sweet, fruity odor on breath.
   2. First aid
      a. If conscious, administer fluids.
      b. Activate EMS.
      c. Treat for shock if necessary.

D. If you are uncertain as to whether the victim is suffering from insulin shock or diabetic coma, always administer sugar to avoid brain damage. It will help a victim of insulin shock and have no appreciable harmful effect on diabetic coma.

XIV. SYNCOPE (FAINTING)

A. Transient loss of consciousness resulting from inadequate blood flow to the brain.

B. First aid
   1. If the victim feels faint but is still conscious, instruct the victim to sit down and place the head between the knees.
   2. Place your hand on the back of the victim's head and instruct the victim to push the head up against your hand as you exert mild pressure preventing the head from coming all the way up. This will force blood to the brain.
   3. If victims are unconscious, place them in the supine position with legs elevated.
   4. Monitor ABCs.

XV. ORTHOPEDIC INJURIES

A. Musculoskeletal injuries to the bones, muscles, ligaments, and tendons such as fractures, dislocations, sprains, and strains.

B. Definitions
   1. Fracture: Break or crack in a bone.
      a. Simple (closed) fracture: A fracture with no external wound caused by the bone.
      b. Compound (open) fracture: A fracture where the bone extrudes from the skin.
      c. Greenstick fracture: An incomplete break as when a soft twig is bent.
      d. Comminuted fracture: A fracture that shatters or creates bone fragments.
      e. Impacted fracture: A fracture in which one broken end is forced into the other.
      f. Transverse fracture: A straight break across the bone.
      g. Spiral fracture: A break caused by a twisting force creating an "S"-shaped fracture.
   2. Dislocation: A bone is separated or displaced from its normal position at a joint.
   3. Sprain: Stretching or tearing of ligaments within a joint.
   4. Strain: Stretching or tearing of muscle or tendons.

C. Signs and symptoms
   1. Pain.
   2. Swelling.
   3. Deformity.
   4. Discoloration or bruising.
   5. Abnormal function.

D. First aid
   1. Because it is often difficult to distinguish among orthopedic injuries, treat all such injuries as you would a fracture.
   2. Activate EMS if necessary.
   3. Immobilize and prevent further injury by splinting the injured limb.
      a. Splint the injury in the position you find it.
      b. Apply the splint so that it immobilizes the fractured bone and joints above and below it.
         (1) Use any available material that is rigid or can be made to be rigid.
         (2) If no splinting material is available, splint the injured part to another part of the body.
   4. Check pulse near the injured area before and after splinting.
   5. Apply a cold pack to a closed injury.
   6. Elevate the affected area.
   7. Monitor ABCs and treat for shock if necessary.
   8. RICE (acrostic memory cue):
      a. Rest—do not move or straighten the injured area.
      b. Immobilize—stabilize the injured area in the position found. Splint only if the victim must be moved and does not cause more pain.
      c. Cold—Apply an ice pack with a thin barrier between the skin and ice pack for 20 minutes, remove it for 20 minutes, and then reapply for 20 minutes as needed.

d. Elevate—if causing no additional pain, raise the injured area.

E. Head, neck, and spinal injuries
1. These injuries can be very serious and paralysis can result if handled improperly.
2. Traumatic injuries such as falls, motor vehicle accidents, and sports-related injuries pose a high probability for head, neck, and spinal injuries.
3. If the victim has sustained a head injury, a spinal injury should always be assumed.
4. When to suspect a head, neck, or back injury:
   a. Victim was involved in a motor vehicle crash.
   b. Injured from a fall greater than standing height.
   c. Complains of neck or back pain.
   d. Tingling or weakness in the extremities.
   e. Is not fully alert.
   f. Appears to be intoxicated.
   g. Appears to be frail or over age 65.
5. First aid
   a. Stabilize the victim's head in the position it is found.
   b. Do not move the victim unless the scene is unsafe.
   c. If you must leave or move the victim, move the victim onto his side while keeping the head, neck, and back in a straight line by placing him in a modified high arm in endangered spine (HAINES) position.
   d. Continue to stabilize the head; activate EMS; monitor ABCs; treat for shock if necessary.

XVI. POISONING

A. Poison is any substance that causes illness, injury, or death when introduced into the body.
B. Ingested poisons
1. Signs and symptoms
   a. Nausea and vomiting.
   b. Diarrhea.
   c. Chest and abdominal pain.
   d. Dyspnea.
   e. Diaphoresis.
   f. Loss of consciousness.
   g. Seizure.
   h. Burn injuries around the mouth.
   i. Opened or spilled containers, overturned or damaged plants.
2. First aid
   a. Assess ABCs and treat accordingly.
   b. Activate EMS.
   c. Contact the National Poison Control Center at 800–222–1222. Attempt to determine and describe poisonous agent. Follow PCC instructions.

d. Treat for shock if necessary and monitor ABCs.
e. Save open containers, poisonous agents, and vomitus for definitive identification of poisonous agent.
f. If the person becomes violent or threatening, retreat to safety until EMS arrives.

C. Inhaled poisons
1. Signs and symptoms
   a. Vertigo.
   b. Headache.
   c. Dyspnea.
   d. Cyanosis.
   e. Loss of consciousness.
2. First aid
   a. Survey the scene: If safe to enter, remove the victim from poisonous agent.
   b. Assess ABCs and treat accordingly.
   c. Activate EMS.
   d. Contact PCC and follow their instructions.
   e. Treat for shock if necessary and monitor ABCs.

D. Absorbed poisons
1. Poisonous plants, e.g. poison ivy, oak, and sumac.
2. Signs and symptoms
   a. Skin reactions.
   b. Pruritus.
   c. Irritation.
   d. Abnormal breathing and pulse changes.
   e. Headache.
3. First aid
   a. Assess ABCs and treat accordingly.
   b. Remove victim from source of poison.
   c. Remove contaminated clothing. Wash exposed clothing and hands throughly with soap and water.
   d. Flush affected area with copious amount of water.
   e. Place a paste of baking soda and water on the areas several times a day.
   f. Calamine and/or benedryl lotion may be helpful.
   g. Treat for shock if necessary and monitor ABCs.

E. Injected poisons: See bites and stings.

XVII. BITES AND STINGS

A. Human and animal bites
1. As the mouths of humans and animals are teeming with bacteria, there is a high risk for infection.
2. First aid
   a. Without endangering yourself, separate the victim from the animal; do not attempt to capture the animal.

b. If the wound is not bleeding heavily, wash it with soap and water.

c. Control any bleeding; apply an antibiotic ointment, dressing, and bandage.

d. Seek medical care if infection ensues.

e. If the wound is bleeding heavily, take measures to control bleeding; activate EMS.

f. If the animal is suspected of having rabies, activate EMS, the police, and animal control.

B. Insect and arachnid bites and stings

1. First aid for tick bites

a. Grasp the tick with a splinter forceps as close to the skin as possible pulling it off firmly but slowly.

b. Do not attempt to burn off the tick or apply oil or jelly.

c. If you cannot remove the tick or the mouth parts are still embedded in the skin, seek medical attention.

d. Once the tick is removed, wash the area with soap and water; apply an antibiotic ointment; seek medical attention if infection ensues.

2. First aid for insect sting

a. If the stinger is still in the skin, remove it by scraping it away with a credit card or similar material; do not use forceps because this may inject more venom.

b. Wash the area with soap and water, cover and apply a cold pack to reduce swelling and pain.

c. Watch the victim for anaphylaxis (an allergic reaction).

3. Signs and symptoms of anaphylaxis:

a. Affected area may swell and become red

b. Urticaria

c. Pruritus

d. Erythema

e. Weakness

f. Nausea

g. Vomiting

h. Cramps

i. Vertigo

j. Dyspnea

k. Hypotension

l. Shock

4. Auto-injectors (EpiPen):

a. Contains a preloaded dose of 0.15 to 0.3 mg. of epinephrine.

b. Uses a spring-loaded plunger that when activated injects the epinephrine.

c. Forcefully pushing the auto-injector against the skin activates the plunger.

d. Should be used on the victim's deltoid or vastus lateralis.

e. Keep the injector in place for 10 seconds to allow the medication to fully discharge.

f. Assist the victim as necessary to use the auto-injector.

g. Activate EMS.

C. Snakebites

1. Poisonous snakes indigenous to the United States are the rattlesnake, cotton-mouth, copperhead, and coral snake.

2. Signs and symptoms

a. Discoloration, bruising, pain, and swelling at the site.

b. Two fang marks.

c. Tachycardia.

d. Weakness.

e. Nausea and vomiting.

f. Dyspnea.

g. Convulsions and paralysis.

h. Shock, if treatment is delayed.

3. First aid

a. Remove the victim from the snake's presence.

b. Wash the wound and immobilize the area where bitten. Try to keep the area lower than the heart, if possible.

c. Activate EMS.

d. Do not apply ice to the wound.

e. Do not cut or supply suction to the wound.

f. Do not apply a tourniquet.

g. Transport the victim as quickly as possible.

h. Monitor ABCs and treat accordingly; treat for shock if necessary.

D. Marine-life sting:

1. E.g. jelly fish, sea anemone, or Portuguese man-of-war.

a. Remove the victim from the water.

b. Activate EMS

c. Soak the injured part in vinegar as soon as possible. Rubbing alcohol or baking soda may also be used.

d. Do not rub the wound or apply fresh water or ammonia.

2. E.g. stingray, sea urchin, or spiny fish.

a. Flush the wound with water.

b. Keep the injured part still.

c. Soak the affected area in water that is as hot as the victim can tolerate for 30 minutes.

d. If hot water is unavailable, pack in hot sand.

e. Then clean the wound and apply a bandage.

f. Observe for infection and check with a provider to determine the need for a tetanus shot.

XVIII. SEVERED BODY PART

A. Call 911 or local emergency number.

B. Locate the body part and wrap it in the cleanest material available.

C. Place the wrapped body part in a plastic bag.

D. Keep the bagged body part cold by placing it on ice, but do not freeze.

E. Ensure body part accompanies the victim to the hospital because surgeons may be able to reattach it.

XIX. EMBEDDED OBJECTS

A. If a knife or other object is embedded in a wound, do not remove it.

B. Place several dressings around the object to immobilize it.

C. Bandage the dressings in place around the object.

D. Splinters
   1. If in the eye—do not remove it—activate EMS.
   2. If on the surface of skin, can be removed with tweezers.
   3. Wash area with soap and water.
   4. Rinse areas with cold tap water for 5 minutes.
   5. After drying the areas, apply an antibiotic ointment and cover.

XX. NOSE INJURIES

A. Control bleeding by having the victim sit with head slightly forward while pinching the nostrils together for 10 minutes.

B. Activate EMS if bleeding persists.

XXI. MOUTH INJURIES

A. Ensure the victim is able to breathe.

B. If head, neck, or back injury is not suspected, have victim assume a seated position with the head tilted slightly forward to allow drainage of blood.

C. If this position is not possible, place the victim in the recovery position.

D. Tooth injuries
   1. Knocked out teeth should be saved and bleeding controlled.
   2. Victim should seek dental care in an hour or less to reinsert the tooth.
   3. Rinse out the mouth with water.
   4. Place a piece of rolled sterile dressing in the tooth cavity and have the victim gently bite down to maintain pressure.
   5. Place the tooth in milk or cool water.
   6. Handle the tooth by the crown, not the root.

XXII. THORACIC INJURIES

A. Rib fractures
   1. Have the victim assume a position that is most comfortable for breathing.
   2. You may support the injured area by binding the victim's upper arm to the chest on the injured side.

   3. You can use a pillow or rolled blanket to support and immobilize the area.
   4. Monitor ABCs and treat for shock if necessary.

B. Pneumothorax (sucking chest wound)
   1. Cover the wound with a large occlusive dressing, i.e., plastic wrap or bag.
   2. Tape the dressing in place, leaving one corner loose—prevents air from entering the wound and permits air to escape during exhalation.
   3. Activate EMS—treat for shock.

XXIII. ABDOMINAL INJURIES

A. Always suspect an abdominal injury in a victim who has multiple injuries.

B. Signs and symptoms
   1. Severe pain.
   2. Hematoma.
   3. Hemorrhage.
   4. Nausea.
   5. Vomiting.
   6. Weakness.
   7. Polydipsia.
   8. Protruding organs.
   9. Rigid abdominal muscles.
   10. Shock.

C. Treatment
   1. Activate EMS.
   2. Use gloves or other barriers.
   3. Position victim on back with knees bent if doing so does not cause pain.
   4. Do not apply pressure or push protruding organs back in the wound.
   5. Remove clothing from around the wound.
   6. Apply moist (e.g., warm tap water), sterile dressings loosely over the wound.
   7. Cover dressings loosely with plastic wrap if available.

XXIV. EMERGENCY CHILDBIRTH

A. Childbirth is a natural process, so complications typically do not arise.

B. Activate EMS.

C. Report woman's name, age, due date, duration of labor pains, number of live births.

D. Quietly talk to her to help her remain calm.

E. Place layers of newspaper covered with linen, towels, or blankets under her.

F. Control the scene for privacy.

G. Position the woman on her back with knees bent and legs spread apart.

H. Allow her to deliver the baby.

I. Catch the baby, who will be slippery—avoid dropping.

J. Keep the baby warm by placing it on the mother's stomach and covering.

XXV. CRIME SCENES

A. Activate EMS and remain at a safe distance until the scene is secured.
B. Do not enter the scene of a suicide.
C. If a victim refuses care or threatens you, withdraw.

XXVI. CRASH CART

A. A cart containing equipment, supplies, and medications used to treat sundry medical emergencies.
B. Typically includes the following materials:
  1. Sphygmomanometer.
  2. Tape.
  3. Alcohol wipes.
  4. Scissors.
  5. Forceps.
  6. Bandage materials.
  7. Dressing materials.
  8. Defibrillator.
  9. Intravenous materials.
  10. Syringes and needles.
  11. Personal protective equipment.
  12. Stethoscope.
  13. Constriction band.
  14. Ambu bag.
  15. Bulb aspirator.
  16. Oxygen delivery materials.
C. Review crash tray medications in Chapter 18.

XXVII. RESCUES

A. General considerations:
  1. If there is no immediate danger, administer first aid at the scene, do not move the victim, and await arrival of EMS.
B. If the scene poses a danger to either you or the victim, move the victim to safety while minimizing further injury to the victim.
C. First aid considerations
  1. Provide support to the victim's neck and back.
  2. Avoid bending or twisting the victim.
  3. Drag a victim to safety while keeping the body straight; do not move the victim sideways.
  4. Lift from the knees, not with your back.

CHAPTER 20

Clinical Laboratory Science

I. INTRODUCTION

A. Laboratory organization
  1. Laboratory departments: Depending on the size and complexity of the facility, the clinical laboratory may be organized into the following departments:
     a. Hematology: Blood components are studied such as cell counts, hematocrit, hemoglobin, differential, and coagulation factors.
     b. Immunohematology (bloodbank): Blood components are analyzed for transfusion therapy.
     c. Chemistry: Body fluids and substances are analyzed for the presence and quantity of chemicals such as glucose, potassium, enzymes, etc.
     d. Serology: Serum and other body fluids are examined to detect disease through antigen-antibody reactions.
     e. Microbiology: The study and identification of pathogenic microorganisms. May be further divided into the following departments:
        (1) Bacteriology: Study and identify pathogenic bacteria.
        (2) Parasitology: Study and identify human parasites.
        (3) Virology: Study and identify pathogenic viruses.
     f. Cytology/histology: Gross and microscopic examination of cells and tissues to diagnose disease.
  2. Laboratory personnel
     a. Pathologist: A physician (M.D. or D.O.) who has completed a pathology residency.
     b. Medical technologist: A laboratory technician who has usually completed at least a bachelor's degree.
     c. Medical laboratory technician: A laboratory technician who has completed 1 or 2 years of training.
B. OSHA standards: see Chapter 14.

C. Laboratory safety
  1. Emergency protocol
     a. Clearly posted evacuation routes.
     b. Emergency phone numbers close at hand: Fire department, police department, poison control center, local emergency room, 911 or local emergency medical service network.
     c. Well-stocked, accessible first aid kit.
  2. Safety equipment
     a. Eyewash station: Special sink used to flush out hazardous substances from the eyes.
     b. Fire extinguisher: Carbon dioxide canister used to extinguish fires.
     c. Fire blanket: Specially treated material used to smother clothing that catches fire.
     d. Hoods: A specially enclosed and ventilated workbench used when working with caustic or volatile substances such as acids, alkalies, and gaseous materials.
  3. Safety guidelines
     a. General
        (1) Wear sturdy shoes; avoid open toe/heel and high-heel shoes.
        (2) Lab coats should be worn at all times while in the laboratory and removed before leaving.
        (3) Control hair, keep nails trimmed, and minimize the amount of jewelry worn.
        (4) Dispose of broken glassware immediately in a puncture-resistant container.
        (5) Observe the hazard identification system developed by the National Fire Protection Association:
           (a) Diamond shape divided into four smaller diamonds.
           (b) Top: Red. Indicates a flammability hazard.
           (c) Right: Yellow. Indicates a chemical reactivity hazard.
           (d) Left: Blue. Indicates a health hazard.
           (e) Bottom: White. Indicates a special hazard such as radiation.

(f) Numerical hazard designation from 0 to 4 is printed over each diamond: 0 means no hazard, 4 means very hazardous.
  b. Chemical (reagent) hazards
   (1) Work under a hood when using flammable or volatile substances.
   (2) Store flammable and volatile substances in a well-ventilated area.
   (3) Do not pipette by mouth; use mechanical suction.
   (4) Chemical spills should be flushed with copious amounts of water.
   (5) Close all reagent containers when not in use.
   (6) Label all reagent containers as described by OSHA including date of preparation, expiration date, and preparer's initials.
   (7) When preparing solutions, slowly pour acids into water, not vice versa.
   (8) Wear goggles when working with caustic materials.
  c. Electrical hazards
   (1) Ground all electrical equipment using three-pronged plugs.
   (2) Avoid the use of extension cords and multiple outlet adapters.
   (3) Keep all electrical cords in good repair.
   (4) Unplug electrical equipment during maintenance and repair.
   (5) Properly label high-voltage equipment.
  d. Biological hazards
   (1) Adhere to standard precautions.
   (2) Wash hands after handling potentially infectious materials, after removing gloves, and before leaving the laboratory.
   (3) Do not eat, drink, smoke, apply cosmetics or lip balm, or handle contact lenses in the laboratory.
   (4) Do not store food or drink in the same area or container as blood or infectious material.
   (5) Some laboratory reagents are derived from human blood and are potentially infectious; treat them with the same care as patient samples by adhering to standard precautions.
   (6) Wear gloves when handling blood or infectious material.
   (7) Wear a face shield when infectious splashes are likely.
   (8) Dispose of contaminated sharps in a puncture-proof container.
   (9) Do not recap, shear, or bend contaminated needles.
   (10) Decontaminate work surfaces and spills using a disinfectant such as 10% bleach solution.
   (11) Cap all tubes before centrifuging.
   (12) Dispose of all contaminated nonsharp material in a clearly labeled biohazard waste container.
D. Clinical Laboratory Improvement Amendments (CLIA) of 1988:
  1. General
   a. Legislation intended to regulate the testing of human specimens for the purpose of diagnosis, prevention, or treatment of diseases and disorders.
   b. The Centers for Medicare and Medicaid Services (CMS) and the Centers for Disease Control and Prevention (CDC) collectively enforce CLIA regulations at the federal level.
   c. Compliance with CLIA is required to receive Medicare/Medicaid reimbursement.
   d. States can develop their own standards if they minimally meet the federal standards.
   e. CLIA is divided into three main standard provisions
    (1) Personnel standards: Identifies the qualification requirements of those directing or performing laboratory tests according to complexity level.
    (2) Testing standards: Identifies the tests that fall in three levels of testing complexity.
    (3) Quality assurance standards: Identifies the QA requirements for qualified laboratories.
  2. Personnel standards
   a. Laboratory director or technical consultant:
    (1) Highly complex testing laboratories: Typically a pathologist (MD/DO) or doctorate-trained laboratory scientist.
    (2) Moderately complex testing laboratories: A master's-trained laboratory scientist with at least 1 year of experience or a bachelor's-trained laboratory scientist with at least 2 years of experience.
   b. Clinical consultant: Typically requires MD/DO, PhD, or for moderately complex laboratories, the same qualification as a laboratory director.
   c. Technical supervisor: Same as laboratory director, or a bachelor's-trained laboratory scientist with at least 4 years of specialty experience. Need not be on site daily, but must be available.
   d. General supervisor: Moderately complex laboratories only; associate degree with at least 2 years of experience. Must be on site

if lesser trained personnel are performing tests.

   e. Testing personnel
      (1) Highly complex: At least an associate degree in laboratory science.
      (2) Moderately complex: High school graduates with training and experience under the direction of a general supervisor.

3. Testing standards: Based on test complexity and the risks associated with reporting erroneous results. These factors depend on the level of training, experience, knowledge, and independent judgment required to accurately perform the test.
   a. Waived tests: Are not subject to personnel requirements or quality assurance requirements.
      (1) Chemistry/serology: Fecal occult blood, ASO slide card agglutination, cholesterol screens, urine pregnancy, visual color ovulation tests, monospot tests, semen analysis, glucose.
      (2) Urinalysis: Includes reagent strip or tablet tests.
      (3) Hematology: Spun microhematocrits, ESR, non-automated sickle cell screens, whole blood clotting time, hemoglobin.
      (4) Microbiology: Gram stain, specimen inoculation, rapid Group A strep tests.
   b. Moderately complex tests (level I)
      (1) Chemistry/serology: Cholesterol, BUN, creatinine, uric acid, glucose, electrolytes.
      (2) Hematology: WBC, RBC, platelets, differentials.
      (3) Microbiology: Microorganism identification.
   c. Highly complex tests (level II and III): All others not identified above.

4. Quality assurance standards: Applies to moderately and highly complex laboratories only.
   a. Written policies and standards: Formal written laboratory policies and procedures.
   b. Personnel training and safety: Documentation of ongoing personnel education, training, and safety program.
   c. Procedure manual: Formal written specimen collection, processing, and testing procedures.
   d. Instrument maintenance: Documentation of periodic cleaning, maintenance, repair, and service checks.
   e. Quality control: Documented QC procedures and results.
   f. Proficiency testing: Contract with an approved proficiency testing service to monitor laboratory performance.
   g. Laboratory inspection: Laboratory specialists authorized by CMS will perform an inspection of facilities and documents and prepare a report of their findings.
   h. Record maintenance: Documentation of all activities described above.

E. Glassware (see Figures 20-1A to C)
   1. Containers and receivers: Used to hold, transfer, or mix liquids; not well suited for precise measurements.
      a. Beaker: Wide, straight-sided, cylindrical vessel used for general reagent preparation.
      b. Erlenmeyer flask: Round, triangular, or cone-shaped vessel used for general reagent preparation.
      c. Bottle: Plastic or glass vessel with a lid used for general reagent storage.
      d. Test tube: Small, narrow, cylindrical vessel with a rounded bottom used for mixing small quantities or to prepare chemical reactions.
      e. Cuvette: Precision glass or plastic test tube having a cylindrical, or rectangular shape. Used for photometric procedures allowing light to pass through the cuvette without any distortion.
   2. Volumetric glassware: Precision-made glassware calibrated to measure quantities with a high degree of accuracy.
      a. Volumetric flask: Vessel with a bulb-shaped base and a long cylindrical neck containing an etched line. Each flask is calibrated to contain (TC) one volume when filled to the etched line.
      b. Graduated cylinder: Long, cylindrical vessel that can measure multiple volumes when a high degree of accuracy is not required; usually calibrated to deliver (TD) or transfer a specific volume.

F. Instrumentation
   1. Centrifuge: Instrument that uses centrifugal force via high-speed spinning action to force solids and heavy material to the bottom of a test tube. Often used to separate plasma or serum from the cells of whole blood.
   2. Spectrophotometer: Precision instrument used to measure the quantity of a substance in solution based on the amount of light that passes through it or the degree of color change when mixed with diagnostic reagents.
   3. Balance/scale: Instrument used to weigh materials.

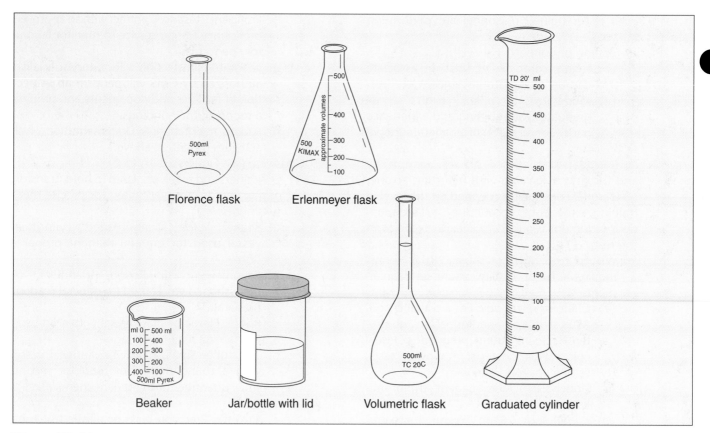

Figure 20-1A

Lab glassware. Delmar/Cengage Learning.

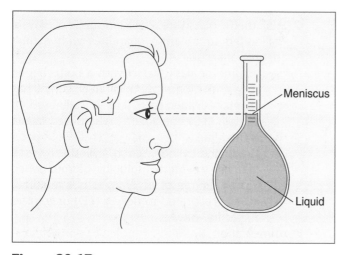

Figure 20-1B

Adjustment of meniscus. Delmar/Cengage Learning.

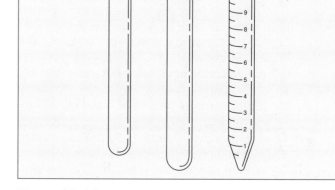

Figure 20-1C

Test tubes. Delmar/Cengage Learning.

II. SPECIMEN COLLECTION AND PROCESSING

A. Urine
  1. Urine is normally a sterile fluid.
  2. Ideally, urine should be analyzed within 30 minutes of collection; however, urine may sit up to 1 hour before analysis without preservation.
  3. If refrigerated, urine may be preserved for 24 hours. However, any specimen refrigerated must be allowed to come to room temperature and to be well mixed before testing, for accurate results.
  4. Chemical preservatives may be used; however, all interfere with at least one urine component.

5. The first morning void is often the specimen of choice as it is usually more concentrated.
6. Midstream specimen: Used for routine urinalysis (UA).
   a. The patient is instructed to retract the foreskin or labia before urinating.
   b. Begin passing the first portion in the toilet, collect the midportion in a clean, dry container, and pass the remaining portion in the toilet.
   c. Properly label the specimen container and transport to the laboratory.
7. Clean-catch specimen: Used for urine culture.
   a. Instruct the patient to thoroughly cleanse the glans penis or urethral orifice with a mild antiseptic solution using sterile gauze or prepackaged cleansing pads.
   b. Collect in a sterile container using the midstream approach.
8. Twenty-four–hour specimen: Used to measure urine volume and quantitative chemical analysis.
   a. This specimen requires a preservative as well as refrigeration between collections.
   b. The patient is instructed to pass the first morning void of the first day into the toilet.
   c. The patient collects all subsequent urinations including the first morning void of the second day.
9. If both a urine culture and urinalysis (UA) are ordered, always perform the culture first to avoid contamination and then the UA.

B. Blood
1. Components: If blood is prevented from clotting, centrifuged or allowed to settle, three distinct layers can be observed (see Figure 20-2).
   a. Plasma: Liquid, uppermost layer. Comprises about 55% of whole blood.
   b. Buffy coat: Thin, middle, whitish-gray layer composed of white blood cells (WBCs) and platelets (plts) or thrombocytes. Comprises about 1% of whole blood.
   c. Red blood cells (RBCs): Bottom, dark red layer composed of packed RBCs. Comprises about 44% of whole blood.
2. Plasma: Liquid portion of unclotted blood. Contains inactivated coagulation factors.
3. Serum: Liquid portion of clotted blood. Contains no coagulation factors as they have been bound to the RBCs in a clot formation.
4. Normally, serum or plasma appears a transparent yellow color.
   a. Hemolysis: The serum or plasma will appear pink to red because of the release of hemoglobin from destroyed RBCs.
   b. Lipemia: The serum or plasma will appear cloudy to opaque or milky due to the presence of fat. Often seen after a patient has eaten a meal.
   c. Icterus (jaundice): The serum or plasma appears brownish-yellow as a result of hyperbilirubinemia.
   d. Certain assays should not be performed on hemolyzed, lipemic, or icteric specimens, especially photometric procedures and chemistry assays.
5. Blood collection tubes: Vacuum tubes that have various color stoppers depending on the assay to be performed (see Figures 20-3A and B).
   a. Common tubes and additives
      (1) Bright yellow top: Serum.
         (a) Usually contains no additive.
         (b) Sterile interior; used for bacteriological studies.
      (2) Plain red top: Serum or clot tube.
         (a) Contains no additive. Must sit for 15 minutes to allow blood to clot before centrifugation.
         (b) Commonly used for chemistry and serological assays.

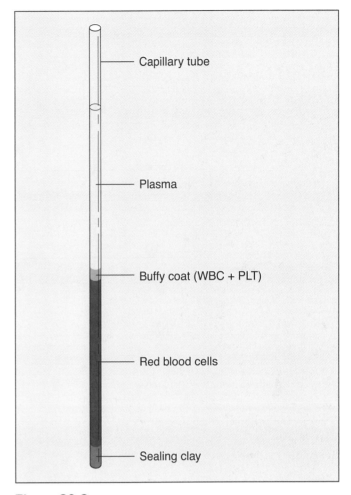

Figure 20-2

Layers of anticoagulated blood. Delmar/Cengage Learning.

The image labels, top to bottom: Capillary tube, Plasma, Buffy coat (WBC + PLT), Red blood cells, Sealing clay

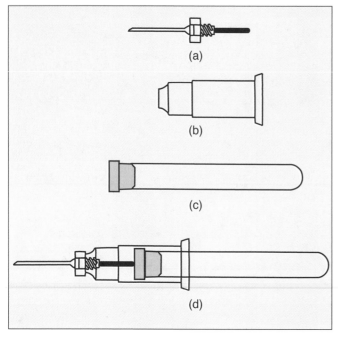

Figure 20-3A

Vacuum tube blood set: (a) Needle, (b) Needle holder, (c) Vacuum tube, (d) Assembled unit. Delmar/Cengage Learning.

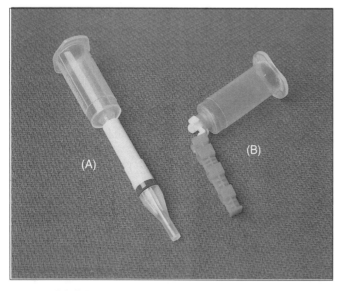

Figure 20-3B

Safety tube holders: (a) Safety needle and holder, (b) Locking cover. Delmar/Cengage Learning.

(3) Speckled/camouflage top: Serum; stopper has a blend of red and black color.
  (a) Contains a silicon gel that upon centrifugation creates a barrier between the clotted cells and serum.
  (b) Commonly used for chemistry and serological assays.
(4) Lavender top: Plasma.

(a) Contains the anticoagulant ethylenediaminetetraacetic acid (EDTA) which inactivates calcium to prevent clotting.
(b) Commonly used in the hematology department to perform cell counts.
(c) Blood sample must be mixed well upon collection to prevent clotting.
(5) Light blue top: Plasma.
  (a) Contains the anticoagulant sodium citrate, which inactivates calcium.
  (b) Commonly used in the hematology department to perform coagulation assays.
(6) Green top: Plasma.
  (a) Contains the anticoagulant sodium heparin.
  (b) Commonly used in the chemistry department for stat or emergency chemistry assays.
  (c) Since the blood is automatically anticoagulated, the 15-minute clotting time is avoided, allowing immediate centrifugation and testing of the plasma.
(7) Gray top: Plasma.
  (a) Contains the anticoagulant sodium fluoride.
  (b) Commonly used in the chemistry department for glucose and alcohol assays as sodium fluoride prevents glycolysis.
b. Recommended order of draw
  (1) Yellow: Blood cultures, reduces any chance of microbial contamination.
  (2) Red: Plain tubes, other additives can contaminate and alter test results.
  (3) Light blue: Sodium citrate, prevents tissue thromboplastin contamination.
  (4) Speckled or Gold (dark yellow)/serum separator tubes (SSTs): Order of draw will help to eliminate contamination from additives such as sodium citrate. These tubes have a silica particle coating to accelerate clotting and may interfere with anticoagulated tubes if drawn out of proper order.
  (5) Green: heparin. Heparin can affect coagulation tests and also interfere with collection of serum specimens, although this anticoagulant causes the least interference with other tests except coagulation studies.
  (6) Lavender: EDTA. This anticoagulant elevates sodium and potassium levels if carried over into other tubes, plus decreasing iron and calcium levels. It can

also increase protime (prothrombin) and partial thromboplastin time results if carried over into the light blue top tube.

(7) Gray: oxalate/fluoride. This tube should come after any hematological tubes because oxalate can damage membranes of cells, resulting in abnormal red blood cell morphology.

(8) Any additional tubes may then be drawn.

6. If serum is to be analyzed, the blood must be allowed to clot for 15 minutes before centrifugation; otherwise, fibrin clot formation will interfere with the testing procedure.

7. Once centrifuged, the plasma or serum should be immediately removed from the cells to avoid biochemical degeneration.

8. Serum or plasma may be left at room temperature, refrigerated, or frozen depending on the analysis.

   a. Serum and plasma freeze in layers with different concentration, and for this reason these specimens must be well mixed before they are used in chemical determinations.

   b. Whole blood, however, cannot be frozen as hemolysis will result.

9. Capillary puncture

   a. Identify the patient.

   b. Observe standard precautions; wash hands.

   c. Select the puncture site (see Figure 20-4A); usually the upper side of the finger; cleanse with 70% isopropyl alcohol and allow to dry.

   d. Using either an autolet or safety lancet, quickly puncture the skin; set the autolet aside or dispose of the lancet in a sharps container (see Figure 20-4B).

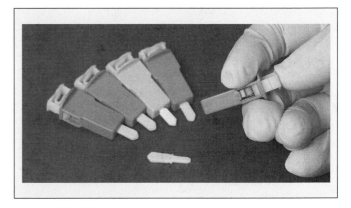

Figure 20-4B

Microtainer brand safety lancet. Delmar/Cengage Learning.

   e. Gently press the finger near the puncture site and wipe away the first drop of blood.

   f. Collect the blood using the appropriate container.

   g. Firmly apply pressure to the puncture wound using gauze.

   h. Label specimen; clean up; wash hands.

10. Venipuncture (phlebotomy) (see Figure 20-5)

   a. Identify the patient.

   b. Observe standard precautions; wash hands.

   c. Apply a tourniquet to upper arm to cause distension of a vein.

   d. Observe/palpate for vein; release tourniquet.

   e. Assemble needed materials.

   f. Cleanse the venipuncture site with 70% isopropyl alcohol and allow to dry; apply tourniquet.

   g. Anchor the vein below the venipuncture site and insert the needle, bevel facing up, into the vein at a 15-degree angle.

   h. Insert the vacuum tube into the barrel; as the blood fills the tube, release the tourniquet.

   i. After collection is completed, gently, without pressure, place a sterile gauze on the puncture site. Quickly withdraw the needle and then apply pressure on the gauze; instruct the patient to continue applying pressure on the puncture wound, keeping the arm straight.

   j. Dispose of the needle in a sharps container; label the specimen; clean up; wash hands.

11. Blood culture: discussed later in this chapter

C. Extravascular fluids: Body fluids occurring outside the vascular system.

   1. Most body fluids appear similar to serum or plasma. The body fluid source must, therefore, be identified on the test request form.

   2. Common assays

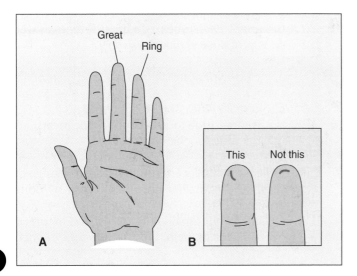

Figure 20-4A

Capillary blood collection sites. Delmar/Cengage Learning.

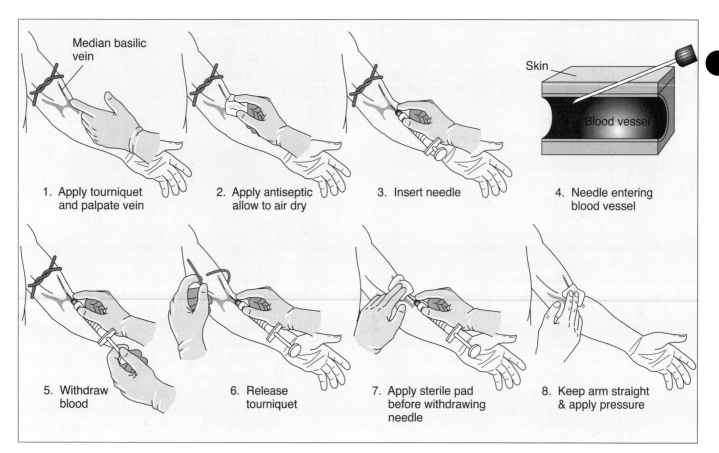

Figure 20-5

Venipuncture procedure. Delmar/Cengage Learning.

1. Apply tourniquet and palpate vein
2. Apply antiseptic allow to air dry
3. Insert needle
4. Needle entering blood vessel
5. Withdraw blood
6. Release tourniquet
7. Apply sterile pad before withdrawing needle
8. Keep arm straight & apply pressure

a. Protein: Performed in the chemistry laboratory.

b. Cell counts: An anticoagulant may be required such as heparin or EDTA. Performed in hematology.

c. Glucose: Sodium fluoride may be required to prevent glycolysis. Performed in a chemistry laboratory.

d. Culture: Performed in microbiology.

3. Cerebral spinal fluid (CSF): Fluid that bathes the spinal cord and brain.

a. Normally, CSF appears clear and colorless.

b. CSF is collected in three tubes about 1 mL each through lumbar puncture between L3, 4, or 5.

c. Tube 1: Tube of choice for culture. Performed in microbiology laboratory. Bacterial contamination is minimized; the longer a needle remains in a puncture wound the greater the likelihood is of contamination.

d. Tube 2: Usually sent to chemistry laboratory for glucose and protein analysis.

e. Tube 3: Tube of choice for cell counts; sent to hematology laboratory. If performed on tube 1, a traumatic tap may cause a falsely elevated cell count.

4. Synovial fluid: Fluid that lines and lubricates the joints.

a. Normally, appears yellow and viscous.

b. Usually collected in two tubes via joint puncture.

c. Tube 1: Should contain heparin for cell counts, crystal analysis, and culture.

d. Tube 2: Plain tube to observe clotting, as well as protein and glucose analysis.

5. Serous fluids

a. Includes pericardial, pleural, and peritoneal fluid.

b. Normally, they appear light yellow.

c. Lavender tube for cell counts and smears.

d. Gray tube for chemistry assays.

D. Feces

1. Collection: Collect feces in a clean plastic or cardboard container uncontaminated by urine or water.

2. Occult blood: Small amount of feces is spread over a guaiac card to detect any hidden blood.

3. Fecal fat: Performed in the chemistry laboratory for fat quantification. Usually requires three samples collected over 3 days.

4. Fecal leukocytes: Performed in the hematology department; a smear is prepared and immersed in Wright's stain for the detection of WBCs.
5. Fecal culture: Discussed later this chapter.
6. Ova and parasites (O&P): Discussed later in this chapter.

E. Sputum
1. Phlegm or secretions of the trachea and bronchi.
2. The patient is asked to cough deeply first thing in the morning into a wide-mouthed container for culture.
3. Nasal and salivary secretions should be avoided.

F. Secretions: Discussed later in this chapter.
1. Genital.
2. Wound.
3. Throat.

G. Chain of custody
1. Specimens that may be introduced into evidence in a court of law require special handling.
2. A record, or chain of custody form must be maintained of all persons who handle the specimen from collection to reporting of results.
3. The specimen must be securely locked to prevent tampering or contamination.
4. To be admissible, the collection, handling, processing, and testing of the specimen must be of indisputable quality and accuracy.

III. QUALITY ASSURANCE (QA)

A. General
1. QA, collectively, denotes the policies, procedures, and activities required to ensure that patient care is delivered appropriately and with high quality.
2. QA in the laboratory requires that test data be accurate and reliable reflecting the true status of the patient so that medical practitioners may rely on the data in making informed patient care decisions.

B. Regulations
1. The Joint Commission, formerly JCAHO: A voluntary accrediting agency that sets forth policy and procedural standards to safeguard the quality and appropriateness of patient care.
2. Clinical Laboratory Improvement Act of 1988 (CLIA): Legislation enforced by the Centers for Medicaid and Medicare Services (CMS) mandating that any facility that performs clinical laboratory procedures must develop and implement a quality assurance program including documentation of QA activities.

C. Major QA components
1. Assay request: The request for laboratory testing must be legible, free from contamination and include the date of request, patient's name, identification number, diagnosis, specimen source, and the test(s) to be done.
2. Patient identification: The patient must be properly identified to ensure the correct specimen is collected from the correct patient.
3. Specimen collection: The medical assistant must properly collect the specimen in keeping with established standards. The test result is no better than the quality of the specimen on which the test is performed.
4. Specimen identification: The specimen must be clearly labeled at the time it is collected by the person collecting it with much the same information found on the test request form. Additionally, the date and time of collection and the collector's initials should be written on the label.
5. Specimen transportation: The specimen must be transported to the laboratory in a timely fashion to avoid biochemical degeneration. The time the specimen is received should be noted on the request form to monitor turnaround time of test completion and reporting.
6. Specimen processing: The specimen must be handled properly to avoid contamination, degeneration, or loss, and to prepare it for testing.
7. Assay protocol: A laboratory procedure manual should be available and followed when performing all laboratory assays.
8. Quality control: Formal, documented methods of monitoring performance of laboratory personnel, instruments, reagents, products, and equipment to ensure accuracy and precision of assay data. Examples include:
   a. Periodic scheduling of preventive maintenance, cleaning, and repair of equipment and instruments.
   b. Use of temperature charts to monitor performance of refrigerators and incubators.
   c. Proficiency testing to monitor technician effectiveness.
   d. Performing statistical analyses of assay data to monitor accuracy and precision.
   e. Reagents should be stored in the proper containers and at the correct temperatures. When first opened, the MA should mark the container with date opened, date of expiration, and her initials.

D. Quality control concepts
1. Accuracy: Closeness of a test result to the truth.
2. Precision: Repeatedly getting the same test result on the same sample.
3. Standard: A solution that contains a known exact quantity of a substance. Commonly used to calibrate an instrument as a measure of accuracy.

4. Control: A solution that has the same or similar qualities as the specimen which contains a known quantitative range of a substance.
   a. Commonly tested along with each group of patient samples as a measure of accuracy and precision.
   b. Many quality control programs require a low, normal, and high control. This practice monitors an instrument's accuracy and precision along a range of assay concentrations.

E. Quality control methods
   1. Instrument calibration
      a. Standards should be used to calibrate a laboratory instrument at the beginning of every shift.
      b. Calibration should also be performed after equipment maintenance, repair, or periods of inoperation.
      c. Standard solutions generally have a small margin of variance. A glucose standard for example may contain 150 +/− 2 mg/dL of glucose. This means that if the instrument on repeated trials provides results between 148 to 152 mg/dL, it has been successfully calibrated.
   2. Controlled runs
      a. Each group of specimens tested (batch) must include controls.
      b. If the controls are within the accepted test range, the accuracy of the results obtained from each patient sample in the batch is reasonably ensured.
      c. If, however, the control samples are outside the accepted test range (out of control), the patient test results are invalid and, therefore, test results will not be reported to the physician until the controls are within range.
   3. Duplicate testing
      a. A patient sample from each batch may be randomly selected for a repeat test to monitor precision.
      b. It is a prudent practice to repeat all patient sample tests that are abnormal, even if the batch is in control.
   4. Control charting: The results of all controls run with each batch should be plotted on a quality control chart such as a Levey-Jennings chart.

F. Levey-Jennings chart
   1. A quality control chart that plots the daily controls of each assay performed in a laboratory.
   2. In order to prepare the Levey-Jennings chart, the mean and standard deviations of a control must be known. This information is usually provided by the control manufacturer.
   3. Generally, it is expected the control values to fall between +/− 2s 95% of the time.

4. When running a batch of assays, if the controls fall between +/− 2s, the tests are considered in control and can be reported to the provider.
5. Outside that range and the controls must be repeated, the instrument recalibrated and serviced, or whatever is necessary to bring the test in control.
6. It is expected that control variation will occur equally above and below the mean.
   a. Trend: Gradual movement of six consecutive control values in one direction.
   b. Shift: Six or more consecutive control values above or below the mean.

IV. MICROSCOPY

A. General
   1. A microscope is a precision magnifying glass.
   2. Resolution: Measures how small and close objects can be and still be recognizable. The naked eye can resolve two dots 0.25 mm apart from each other. Any closer and the two dots appear to be one dot.
   3. Magnification: The compound light microscope consists of two lenses, the objective and ocular. The total magnification observed is the product of the power of both lenses.
      a. 10× means the lense will magnify the image of the object being observed ten times its true diameter.
      b. 10× ocular and 40× objective will yield a total magnification of 400 times the object's true diameter.
   4. Because of the manner in which light passes through the microscope, the image will appear upside down and reversed.

B. Microscope parts (see Figure 20-6A)
   1. Framework: Comprises the following:
      a. Base: Firm, wide, often horseshoe-shaped portion that supports the microscope.
      b. Arm: Structure that supports the lenses and focus knobs.
      c. Stage: Horizontal platform that supports the object being observed. The stage-clip holds the object firmly on the stage.
   2. Illumination system: Adjustment of the components of the illumination system will permit optimal viewing of the specimen.
      a. Light source: Consists of a lightbulb housed in the base that illuminates the object. A control knob (rheostat) is usually available to regulate the intensity of light.
      b. Condenser: Lense situated over the light source that can be adjusted up or down to direct and focus the light on the object being observed.

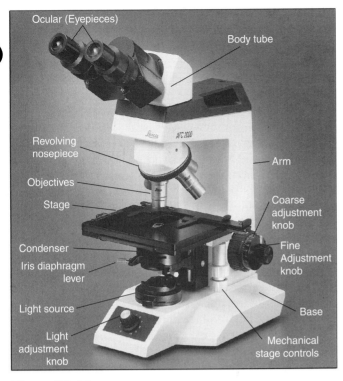

Figure 20-6A

Parts of a microscope. Delmar/Cengage Learning.

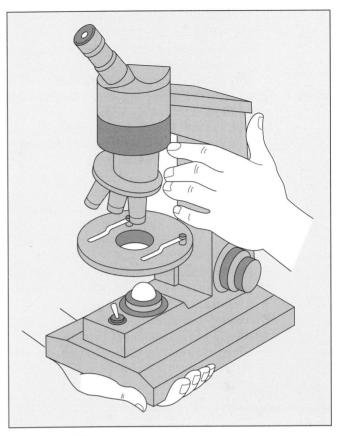

Figure 20-6B

Carrying the microscope. Delmar/Cengage Learning.

c. Iris diaphragm: A shutter mechanism situated on the bottom of the condenser that can be opened and closed to regulate the amount of light passing through the object.
3. Magnification system
   a. Ocular: A monocular or binocular eyepiece that contains a lens to magnify the image formed by the objective lenses.
   b. Objectives: Most microscopes contain three objective lenses mounted on a revolving nosepiece for quick change of objective magnification powers.
      (1) Low power: Usually 10× lense. Used for initial focusing.
      (2) High dry: Usually 40× lense. Used to study wet preparations, urinary sediment, and cellular specimens.
      (3) Oil immersion: Usually 100× lense. Requires the use of immersion oil to prevent refraction of light at such high power. Used to study nuclear and cytoplasmic detail as well as bacterial specimens.
4. Adjustment system
   a. Body tube: Allows the pathway of light between the objectives and oculars.
   b. Coarse adjustment: Large focusing knob that moves the stage up and down for rapid focusing.

c. Fine adjustment: Smaller focusing knob for slight movement of the stage to afford precise focusing.
C. Care and maintenance
   1. Transport the microscope with one hand under the base and the other hand grasping the arm (see Figure 20-6B).
   2. Lenses should be cleaned with lenspaper only. Other materials will scratch the soft lenses.
   3. After use, immediately wipe away immersion oil with lenspaper.
   4. When not in use, the objective should be turned to 10×, the stage brought to its lowest level, and covered.

V. URINALYSIS

A. General
   1. Review the urinary system in Chapter 5.
   2. Urine composition
      a. Water: Comprises 95% of urine.
      b. Dissolved solids: Comprises 5%.
         (1) Urea: Principal end-product of protein metabolism.
         (2) Sodium and potassium: Salt.
         (3) Uric acid: End product of purine metabolism.

(4) Creatinine: Waste product related to muscle mass.

(5) Ammonium: End product of protein metabolism.

(6) Phosphate and sulfate: Minerals.

3. Urinalysis (UA) is the physical, chemical, and microscopic examination of urine. As a diagnostic tool, it provides information regarding the state of the kidney and urinary tract, as well as metabolic and systemic disorders.

4. Decomposition: Urine should be examined when fresh, ideally within 30 minutes of collection. If not refrigerated or preserved, urine will decompose and lose its diagnostic value.

a. Primarily involves bacterial growth, which reproduce rapidly at room temperature.

b. Phosphates and urates may precipitate out of solution.

c. Urine pH becomes alkaline.

d. Cellular components such as WBC, RBC, casts, and epithelium disintegrate.

e. Sugar decomposes and acetone evaporates.

f. Bilirubin and urobilinogen oxidize.

5. Urine collection

a. The first morning void is often the specimen of choice as it is usually more concentrated.

b. Midstream specimen: Used for routine UA.

(1) The patient is instructed to retract the foreskin or labia before urinating.

(2) Begin passing the first portion in the toilet, collect the midportion in a clean dry container, and pass the remaining portion in the toilet.

(3) Properly label the specimen container and transport to the laboratory.

c. Clean-catch specimen: Used for urine culture.

(1) Instruct the patient to thoroughly cleanse the glans penis or urethral orifice with a mild antiseptic solution using sterile gauze or prepackaged cleansing pads.

(2) Collect in a sterile container using the midstream approach.

d. 24-hour specimen: Used to measure urine volume and for quantitative chemical analysis.

(1) This specimen requires a preservative as well as refrigeration.

(2) The patient is instructed to pass the first morning void into the toilet of the first day.

(3) The patient collects all subsequent urinations including the first morning void of the second day.

B. Physical examination

1. Color

a. Normal urine color is yellow, mainly comprising three pigments: urochrome, uroerythrin, and urobilin.

b. Pale (straw colored): Suggests a dilute urine and may be associated with diabetes mellitus or diabetes insipidus.

c. Dark yellow (brown-red or amber): Suggests a concentrated urine often seen in dehydration and fever.

d. Yellow-brown, green-brown (beer brown): Suggests the presence of bilirubin and may form a yellow foam when shaken. Often will turn green on standing as a result of bilirubin oxidation.

e. Bright orange: Often seen in patients taking Pyridium, a urinary analgesic. Interferes with reagent strip tests.

f. Red: A clear red urine suggests the presence of hemoglobin (hemoglobinuria) resulting from intravascular hemolysis. A cloudy red appearance usually results from the presence of RBCs causing hematuria.

g. Dark red-brown (cola colored): Suggests the presence of myoglobin, a form of hemoglobin in muscle tissue that is toxic to the kidneys, and is often associated with muscle injury.

h. Dark brown or black: Suggests the presence of melanin or homogentisic acid if the urine is colorless when voided and becomes brown or black on standing. Melanin is a pigment that when found in urine is associated with melanoma, a tumor. Homogentisic acid is associated with an inborn error of metabolism of tyrosine.

i. Colors such as pink, blue, green may result from vitamins, certain foods, dyes, and chemicals.

2. Transparency

a. Normally, freshly voided urine is clear, but becomes cloudy when allowed to stand.

b. Hazy: Small amounts of solid particles in solution that make the urine appear less than clear; however, print is not distorted when viewed through the urine.

c. Cloudy: Particulate matter concentration is such that it is difficult to view print through the urine.

d. Turbid: Urine does not allow any light to pass through; it is impossible to view print through the urine.

e. Normal constituents causing cloudiness: Mucus, epithelial cells, certain crystals, spermatozoa, and external substances such as powders, and antiseptics.

f. Pathological constituents causing cloudiness: Certain crystals, WBCs, RBCs, pus, epithelial cells, fat, and casts.

3. Specific gravity (SG)

a. Measures the weight of a solution as compared to the weight of an equal volume of water.

b. Normal urine SG is 1.005 to 1.030.

c. Normal urine is a little heavier than water because of the presence of dissolved solids; therefore, the SG of urine indirectly measures the urinary concentration of dissolved solids.

d. Except in certain diseases, SG often varies inversely with urinary volume. For example, with low urinary volume, the urine is concentrated, yielding a high SG; whereas, with high urine volume, the urine is dilute yielding a low SG.

   (1) Diabetes mellitus: Characterized by high urinary volume and SG often resulting from dissolved glucose.

   (2) Glomerulonephritis: Characterized by low urinary volume and SG resulting from the kidney's inability to excrete water or concentrate the urinary waste.

   (3) Diabetes insipidus: Characterized by high urinary volume and low SG.

e. Refractometer: A device that measures the refractive index of a solution, which is correlated to SG (see Figure 20-7).

f. Reagent strip: A color change on a reagent strip pad corresponds to a specific gravity level as indicated on a color chart affixed to the reagent bottle.

g. Quality control (QC): All laboratory instruments require periodic quality control assessment to monitor accuracy and precision.

   (1) Water: Deionized water should read 1.000 in the refractometer or the reagent strip.

   (2) Potassium sulfate (K_2SO_4): 20.29 grams of K_2SO_4 dissolved in 1 liter of deionized water should measure 1.015.

4. Miscellaneous physical characteristics: Routinely not performed on UA.

a. Foam: The presence and color of foam may be noted.

   (1) Normally, urine will form scant, white foam when shaken.

   (2) Increased protein: Creates a large amount of white foam appearing similar to beaten egg white when shaken.

   (3) Increased bilirubin: Creates a large amount of yellow foam when shaken.

b. Volume: Occasionally volume is also noted.

   (1) Normally, average 24-hour urine output is 1200 to 1500 mL; however, it can range from 600 to 2000 mL.

   (2) Quantitative tests generally require measuring total urinary volume in 24 hours.

c. Odor: Occasionally odor may be noted.

   (1) Normally, urine has a faintly aromatic odor.

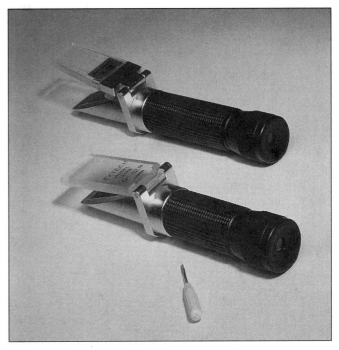

Figure 20-7

Refractometer. Delmar/Cengage Learning.

   (2) Bacterial growth: Causes an ammonia odor because of the breakdown of urea.

   (3) Ketones: Causes a sweet or fruity odor.

   (4) Errors in amino acid metabolism: May smell like sweaty feet, maple syrup, cabbage, and rotten fish, to name a few.

   (5) Foodstuff: May cause an odor; e.g., asparagus.

5. Procedure

a. Observe the urine for color and transparency, as well as others as requested; record the findings.

b. Perform specific gravity.

   (1) Refractometer

      (a) Clean prism; calibrate (QC) the refractometer; clean prism; close coverplate.

      (b) Using a pipette, apply a drop of urine to the exposed portion of the prism.

      (c) Hold the refractometer up to a light source or in the lighted stand.

      (d) Look into the eyepiece, focus, read, and record the point where the dark field crosses the scale.

      (e) Clean up.

C. Chemical examination

  1. Chemical constituents are qualitatively or semi-quantitatively determined using reagent strips that cause a color change in the presence of the substance being tested for.

2. pH
   a. Measures the hydrogen ion concentration that determines the acidity (sourness) or alkalinity (bitterness) of urine.
   b. Normal: The kidney functions to eliminate excess acid; therefore, it is normally 5 to 7.
   c. Bacterial growth will cause the urine to become more alkaline, which may cause abnormal constituents to degenerate.
   d. Alkaline urine: Usually indicates urinary tract infection (UTI).
   e. Crystals: Certain crystals form in acid (<7) urine; whereas, others form in alkaline urine (>7). Urine pH is required for crystal identification.
3. Protein
   a. The presence of protein is significant for renal diseases.
   b. Proteinuria: Usually results from glomerular damage, tubular damage, or excess hemoglobin, myoglobin, or immunoglobulins.
   c. Low levels of protein may normally be seen after excessive exercise or exposure to cold.
   d. Casts: Casts, which will be discussed later, are highly correlated to proteinuria.
   e. False-positive: High pH may cause a false-positive protein.
4. Blood
   a. The distinction between hemoglobin, myoglobin and intact RBCs is of high diagnostic value.
   b. Hematuria: RBCs in the urine may be caused by a variety of kidney diseases, including hemorrhage anywhere along the urinary tract.
   c. Hemoglobinuria: Free hemoglobin in the urine is often due to intravascular hemolysis caused by hemolytic anemia, transfusion reactions, and severe infections.
   d. Myoglobinuria: Myoglobin in the urine is often caused by muscle injury, excessive unaccustomed exercise, and beating or crushing injuries. Excessive myoglobinuria damages the kidney and may cause anuria.
   e. False-negative: Vitamin C may cause a false-negative test.
5. Nitrite: Certain bacteria convert nitrate, a normal component of urine, to nitrite. The presence of nitrite, therefore, suggests possible UTI.
6. Leukocyte esterase
   a. Measures the presence of an enzyme commonly found in WBCs.
   b. The presence of leukocyte esterase suggests the presence of WBCs which may indicate a UTI.
7. Glucose
   a. Normally, glucose filtered through the glomerulus is reabsorbed in the tubule.
   b. Glycosuria: High glucose concentrations will spill into the urine, suggesting diabetes mellitus; however, large intakes of sugar, emotional strain, exercise, pregnancy, meningitis, hypothyroidism, adrenal tumors, and some brain injuries may also cause glycosuria.
   c. Galactosuria: High galactose levels may cause permanent physical and mental retardation in children; for this reason a specific test for galactose should be done for early detection.
   d. False-negative: May be caused by vitamin C or tetracycline.
8. Ketones: Ketones such as acetone are the by-product of incomplete fat metabolism commonly seen in diabetes mellitus and starvation, in which the body, lacking a glucose source, must resort to braking down fat for energy.
9. Bilirubin
   a. A byproduct of RBC destruction, it is a component of bile, a substance that aids in the digestion of fats that is ultimately excreted in feces.
   b. Bilirubinuria: High levels of bilirubin may be seen during liver disease or bile duct obstruction.
10. Urobilinogen: Is the result of the reduction of bilirubin in the intestine and will be seen in most conditions causing bilirubinuria, including hemolytic anemia, pernicious anemia, and malaria.
11. Procedure
    a. Using well-mixed, uncentrifuged urine, completely immerse the reagent strip into the urine for not longer than 1 second.
    b. Draw the strip out of the urine, and keep it in a horizontal position to avoid cross contamination among reagent pads.
    c. Read each reagent pad at the time indicated on the bottle or product insert.
    d. Compare each pad to the color chart supplied by the manufacturer.
    e. Record the results in the units dictated by each particular laboratory.
    f. Clean up.
D. Microscopic examination
   1. Urine is microscopically examined under low power (10×) and high dry (40×) for the presence of abnormal constituents such as cells and bacteria (see Figures 20-8A to R).
   2. Erythrocytes
      a. Normal: 0 to 2 RBCs per high power field (HPF). More than that indicates hematuria.
      b. Small, clear, biconcave to spherical-shaped cells.
      c. Highly correlated to positive blood.

3. Leukocytes
   a. Normal: 0 to 5 WBCs/HPF. More than that suggests inflammation, pyuria, or infection.
   b. About two to three times the size of RBC, they are round with a grainy appearance.
   c. Highly correlated to positive leukoesterase and positive nitrite.

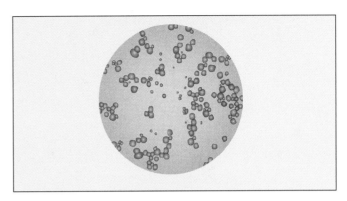

Figure 20-8E

Yeast buds in urine sediment. Delmar/Cengage Learning.

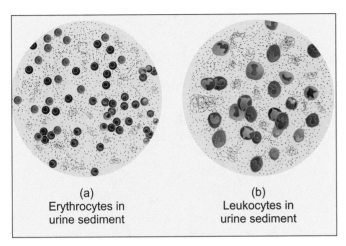

(a)
Erythrocytes in
urine sediment

(b)
Leukocytes in
urine sediment

Figure 20-8A and B

(a) Erythrocytes in urine sediment, (b) Leukocytes in urine sediment. Delmar/Cengage Learning.

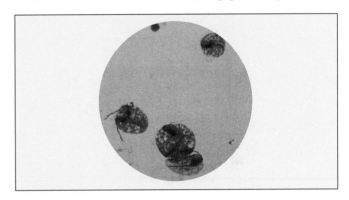

Figure 20-8F

Trichomonas vaginalis in urine sediment. Delmar/Cengage Learning.

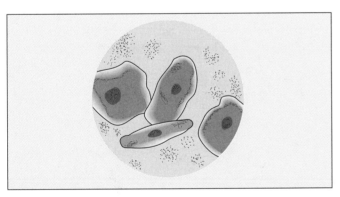

Figure 20-8C

Squamous epithelial cells. Delmar/Cengage Learning.

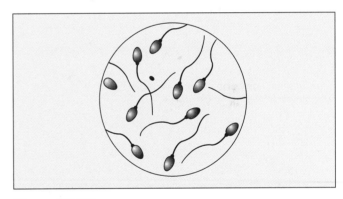

Figure 20-8G

Spermatozoa in urine sediment. Delmar/Cengage Learning.

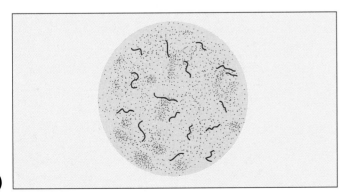

Figure 20-8D

Bacteria in urine sediment. Delmar/Cengage Learning.

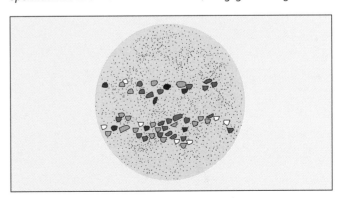

Figure 20-8H

Amorphous deposits in urine sediment. Delmar/Cengage Learning.

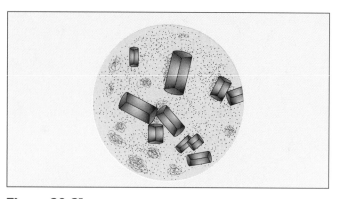

Figure 20-8I

Triple phosphate crystals in urine sediment. Delmar/Cengage Learning.

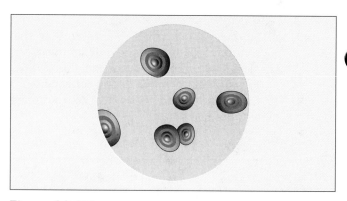

Figure 20-8M

Leucine crystals in urine sediment. Delmar/Cengage Learning.

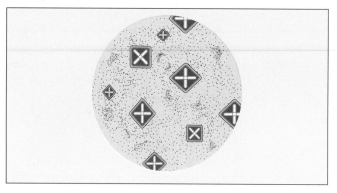

Figure 20-8J

Calcium oxalate crystals in urine sediment. Delmar/Cengage Learning.

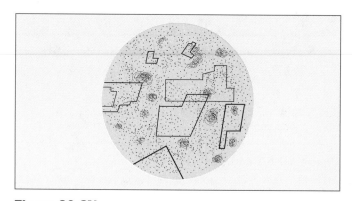

Figure 20-8N

Cholesterol crystals in urine sediment. Delmar/Cengage Learning.

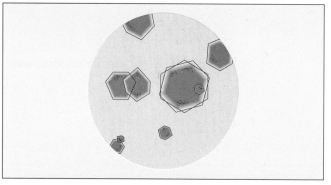

Figure 20-8K

Cystine crystals in urine sediment. Delmar/Cengage Learning.

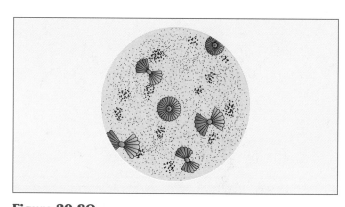

Figure 20-8O

Sulfonamide crystals in urine sediment. Delmar/Cengage Learning.

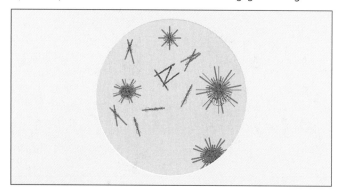

Figure 20-8L

Tyrosine crystals in urine sediment. Delmar/Cengage Learning.

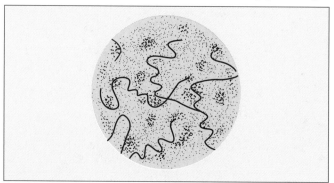

Figure 20-8P

Mucus threads in urine sediment. Delmar/Cengage Learning.

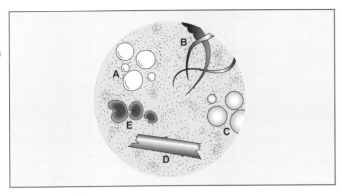

Figure 20-8Q

Common artifacts in urine sediment: (a) Air bubbles, (b) Fibers, (c) Oil droplets, (d) Hair, (e) Starch granules. Delmar/Cengage Learning.

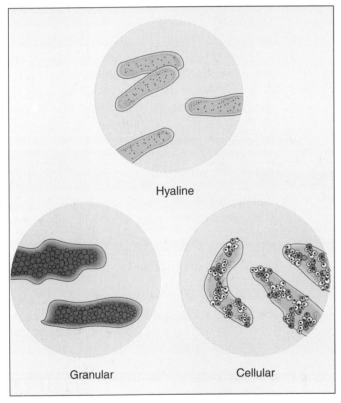

Hyaline

Granular   Cellular

Figure 20-8R

Casts. Delmar/Cengage Learning.

4. Epithelial cells
   a. Squamous epithelial cells
      (1) Normal: Generally not clinically significant unless in large quantities/HPF.
      (2) Large cells that contain a nucleus about the size of a WBC.
   b. Renal epithelial cells
      (1) Normal: None/HPF. Their presence indicates renal tubule destruction.
      (2) Round, grainy appearing cells about twice the size of a WBC, or four to five times larger than a RBC.

5. Bacteria
   a. Normal: A few may be seen/HPF. More than this usually indicates UTI.
   b. Cocci appear as tiny grains; rods appear similar to tiny hair slivers.
6. Yeast
   a. Normal: None/HPF. More than this indicates a yeast infection (*Candida albicans*).
   b. Appear as oval to round, clear bodies often confused with RBCs. There is often considerable size variation with buds or hyphae.
7. Mucus: Appear as wavy threadlike structures in the background.
8. *Trichomonas vaginalis*
   a. Normal: None/HPF. One or more indicates vaginal infection.
   b. Appear similar to a large WBC with a flagella (whipping tail).
9. Spermatozoa: Appear as a small, oval body with a tail. Reported in males only; considered a contaminant in females.
10. Casts
    a. Normal: 0 to 2 hyaline per low power field (LPF).
    b. Structures that are formed within the tubules of the nephron indicating a temporary blockage.
    c. The material that forms the cast solidifies in the tubule and may include WBCs, RBCs, epithelial cells, fat globules, and bacteria.
    d. They appear as cylindrical bodies of uniform diameter, about seven to eight times wider than a RBC, have parallel sides and rounded ends, and are several times longer than wide.
    e. Highly correlated to positive protein.
    f. Types
       (1) Hyaline: Colorless, homogenous, semi-transparent, delicate-appearing casts composed of protein. Usually found in acidic urine.
       (2) Cellular casts: Unless morphologically distinguishable, report out as cellular casts.
       (3) Fatty cast: Contain fat globules.
       (4) RBC cast: Casts that contain orange-yellow matter.
       (5) WBC cast: Contain WBC nuclei.
       (6) Granular cast: Contain sandlike granules resulting from WBC disintegration.
       (7) Waxy cast: Yellowish, wide, hard-appearing cast often having irregularly broken ends and fissures along the sides. Felt to be the final stage in cellular cast disintegration, and imply renal failure.
11. Crystals
    a. Normal acidic urine crystals
       (1) Amorphous urate: Composed of sodium salt of uric acid. They have variable mor-

phology, but typically appear as sand deposits.

   (2) Uric acid: Morphology is variable, but typically appear lemon-shaped, barrel-shaped, and rosette-shaped.
   (3) Calcium oxalate: Look similar to square crystals containing a refractive "X" shape. Common constituent of kidney stones.

b. Normal alkaline urine crystals
   (1) Amorphous phosphate: Commonly causes turbidity; appears similar to amorphous urates.
   (2) Triple phosphate: Have a coffin-lid shape.
   (3) Calcium phosphate: Appear as flat plates or rosettes.

c. Abnormal crystals: All are found in acidic urine.
   (1) Cystine: Appear as hexagonal plates that often overlap with each other.
   (2) Tyrosine: Appear as fine needles arranged in sheaves.
   (3) Leucine: Yellow, oily-appearing spheres containing radial and concentric lines.
   (4) Cholesterol: Large, flat, hexagonal plates with one or more notched corners often associated with fatty casts.
   (5) Sulfonamide: Large needles in sheaves or rosettes.

12. Artifact: Structures or contaminants that have no clinical significance.
   a. Threads: Cotton, wool, wood fibers, hair fibers.
   b. Diaper fibers: Found in disposables are troublesome as they appear similar to waxy casts.
   c. Scratches: Scratches in the glass slide or coverslip.
   d. Droplets: Oil or starch.
   e. Glass particles.

13. Procedure
   a. Centrifuge 10 to 12 mL of well-mixed urine for 5 minutes.
   b. Decant the supernatant leaving approximately 1 mL of urine in the centrifuge tube.
   c. Gently shake the tube to resuspend the sediment.
   d. Place one drop of urine sediment on a glass slide and coverslip.
   e. Observe 10 separate fields (LPF) under the microscope using $10\times$. Observe for the presence of casts and report the average number of casts seen.
   f. Observe 10 separate fields (HPF) using $40\times$. Observe for the presence of the other elements and report the average numbers of

observed elements only. Elements not seen are generally not reported unless requested to do so.

g. Reporting protocol
   (1) Casts, abnormal crystals, RBCs, and WBCs: Use ranges such as 0 to 3, 3 to 5, 5 to 10, 10 to 25, 25 to 50, 50 to 100, too numerous to count (TNTC).
   (2) Epithelial cells, normal crystals, bacteria, yeast, and *Trichomonas:* Use terms such as "few," "moderate," "many," and "packed."
   (3) Sperm (males only) and mucus: Use the term present.

VI. IMMUNOLOGY AND SEROLOGY

A. General
   1. Immunology: Study of immunity.
   2. Serology: In vitro study of serum to detect disease by evaluating antigen-antibody reactions.
   3. In vivo: Activities that occur within the body.
   4. In vitro: Activities that occur outside the body usually in a laboratory apparatus such as a test tube.
   5. Sensitivity: The ability of a test to demonstrate a positive result when the substance being tested is present.
   6. Specificity: The ability of a test to demonstrate a negative result when the substance being tested is absent and not cross-react with other substances.
   7. False-negative: A test yields a negative result even though the substance being tested is present.
   8. False-positive: A test yields a positive result even though the substance being tested is absent.
   9. Titer: Relative concentration of antibody per unit volume of serum.

B. Immunity
   1. Immune system: Coordinated body defense system that recognizes, attacks, and eliminates harmful foreign substances. It recognizes self from nonself.
   2. Nonspecific immunity
      a. Mechanical and chemical barriers: Skin, mucous membranes, and body fluids.
      b. Inflammation: Local response to injury, irritation, or invasion of pathogens.
         (1) Vasodilation: The vessels in the area dilate increasing circulation causing heat and redness.
         (2) Edema: Blood vessel permeability increases and allows plasma to leak into the tissue spaces. This causes swelling, which puts pressure on nerve endings creating pain.
         (3) Phagocytosis: Increased circulation brings about WBC, principally neutrophils and

macrophages (monocytes), to the area to phagocytose the pathogens.

    (4) Repair: Destroyed pathogens and WBCs are absorbed and filtered through the lymphatic system with simultaneous regeneration of tissue.

    (5) Suppuration: If the inflammatory response is insufficient, the destroyed pathogens and WBCs will collect and form pus and subsequently, infection.

  c. Natural killer cells: Lymphocytes that destroy tumor cells and cells invaded by viruses by damaging plasma membranes creating cytolysis.

  d. Interferon: Cellular production of proteins that attack viruses.

  e. Complement: Group of enzymes that lyse foreign cells when activated by specific or nonspecific immune processes.

3. Specific immunity

  a. Cellular immunity: T cell–mediated immunity.

    (1) Lymphocytic T cells produced in the bone marrow migrate to the thymus to be processed for antigenic responsiveness.

    (2) While in the thymus, the T cells develop binding sites on their surfaces that are specific to a particular antigen.

    (3) The T cell is released into circulation at the site of the antigen so that the antigen can bind to the T cell, thereby sensitizing it to form several subsets of T cells.

    (4) Killer T cells: Release lymphotoxin to destroy the antigen.

    (5) Helper T cells: Assists B cells to destroy antigens.

    (6) Suppressor T cells: Discontinue the immune response when the threat is overcome.

  b. Humoral immunity: Antibody mediated immunity.

    (1) Lymphocytic B cells, once sensitized by an antigen, form two subsets of itself.

      (a) Plasma cells: Activated B cells that synthesize and secrete antibodies.

      (b) Memory B cells: Inactivated B cells that remain in lymphatic tissue as a reserve antibody source. If subsequently exposed to the antigen, the memory B cell will become a plasma cell and produce antibodies.

    (2) Complement: Collection of 20 protein compounds found in plasma.

      (a) When activated, begins a chemical reaction (cascade) that bores a hole in the antigenic cell creating an influx of fluid thereby causing cytolysis.

    (b) Some cause vasodilation in the affected area.

    (c) Others enhance phagocytosis.

C. Immunogens (antigens [Ag])

  1. Any molecular substance that, when introduced into the body, elicits an immune response.

  2. Most antigens are proteins or large polysaccharides.

  3. Most antigens are foreign to the body and is interpreted by the body as a threat.

D. Immunoglobulins (antibodies [Ab])

  1. Proteins called immunoglobulins (Ig) secreted by activated B cells (plasma cells).

  2. Substances produced in response to antigenic stimulation to defend against the antigen.

  3. Structure (see Figure 20-9)

    a. Consists of two light and two heavy polypeptide chains bound by disulfide bonds

    b. Has two antigen-binding sites and two complement-binding sites.

    c. Has a Y-shaped appearance.

  4. Classes

    a. IgG: Composed of one antibody molecule (monomer) representing 75% of all circulating antibodies. Produced in response to secondary exposure to an antigen.

    b. IgM: Composed of five antibody molecules (pentamer) bound by a J-ring. B cells synthesize them in response to primary exposure to an antigen. Synthesized at birth.

    c. IgA: Composed of two antibody molecules (dimer) bound by a J-ring. Found in mucous membranes, saliva, and tears. Responds to sinobronchial infections.

    d. IgE: Is associated with allergies.

    e. IgD: Monomer found in blood, function unknown.

  5. Function: Recognizes and destroys foreign substances (antigens).

    a. Transforms toxic antigens into harmless substances.

    b. Agglutinates antigens to make them large enough for cells to phagocytose them.

    c. Binding to the antigen may alter the shape of the antigen allowing complement to bind to it.

E. In vitro antigen-antibody reactions

  1. Antigen-antibody complex: Antibodies combine with antigens and are held together by weak chemical bonds.

  2. Precipitation: The process by which an antigen-antibody complex visibly settles out of solution.

  3. Agglutination

    a. A precipitation method that creates a visible clumping reaction.

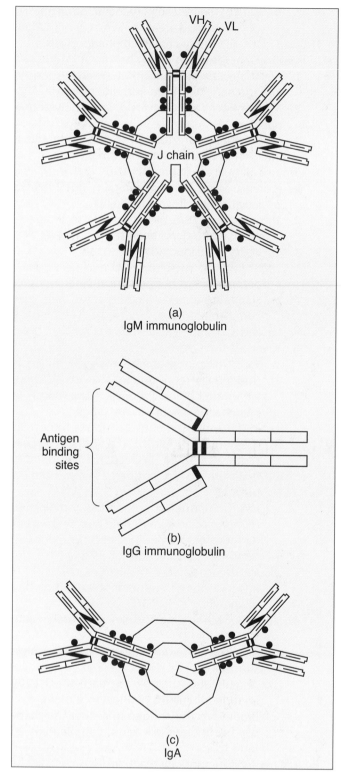

Figure 20-9

Antibody structure. Delmar/Cengage Learning.

b. Usually involves particles such as blood cells, bacteria, or, more commonly, specs of latex that have an antigen embedded on them.

c. Sensitization: Serum antibodies become sensitive to the antigen and attach to it forming an antigen-antibody complex.

d. Lattice formation: The antigen-antibody complexes when in close proximity begin attaching to each other forming visible clumps of matter.

e. Visible agglutination will occur when the proportion of antigens and antibodies are optimal.

  (1) Prozone effect: Ag-Ab reaction failure caused by an excessive concentration of antibody. Antibodies bind to all of the antigenic sites leaving no room for the Ag-Ab complexes to bind with each other.

  (2) Postzone effect: Ag-Ab reaction failure due to an excessive concentrations of antigen. A few antigens bind up most of the antibodies leaving the majority of antigens unbound.

F. Infectious mononucleosis (IM)

  1. A self-limiting disease caused by the Epstein-Barr virus characterized by fever, malaise, lethargy, pharyngitis, and lymphadenomegaly.

  2. The body produces heterophil antibodies in response to IM.

  3. Heterophil: Name given to a group of antigens that are common to a number of unrelated animal species.

  4. Serological tests for IM such as Monospot are designed to detect the heterophil antibody.

G. *Streptococcus* screen

  1. Group A, beta hemolytic streptococcus such as *Streptococcus pyogenes* causes pharyngitis (strep throat), rheumatic fever, and impetigo.

  2. Strep screening tests typically detect either the antigenic cellular wall of the bacteria or the antibody, antistreptolysin O (ASO), produced against the toxic enzyme, streptolysin O, that causes hemolysis.

  3. Depending on the method used, cytomegalovirus, leukemia, and Hodgkin's disease may cause a false-positive result.

H. Rheumatoid factor (RF)

  1. Rheumatoid arthritis (RA) is a systemic disease characterized by swelling and painful joints accompanied by cartilage and muscular atrophy.

  2. Most persons afflicted with RA exhibit in both blood and synovial fluid the presence of a reactive group of proteins, or autoantibodies known collectively as rheumatoid factor.

  3. Depending on the method used, lupus erythematosus, hepatitis, tuberculosis, and syphilis may cause a false-positive result.

I. Human chorionic gonadotropin (hCG)
   1. hCG is a hormone produced by the placenta shortly after implantation of the fertilized ovum.
   2. hCG tests usually use agglutination inhibition to detect hCG in urine.
   3. The first morning void is the specimen of choice as it contains the highest concentration of hCG.
   4. Depending on the method used, hematuria and proteinuria may cause a false-positive result.
J. Luteinizing hormone (LH)
   1. A hormone produced by the anterior pituitary.
   2. An acute rise in LH in women (the LH surge) triggers ovulation.
   3. In men, LH stimulates the production of testosterone.
   4. LH (ovulation) kits are available to predict ovulation for reproductive control.
K. Blood groups
   1. ABO group
      a. Four blood groups may be expressed by the presence or absence of two antigens, A or B.
         (1) Group A: The A antigen is present on the RBC.
         (2) Group B: The B antigen is present on the RBC.
         (3) Group AB: Both the A and B antigens are present.
         (4) Group O: Neither A nor B antigen is present.
      b. Two antisera, anti-A and anti-B, are used to identify the ABO group.
      c. The patient's blood cells are added to both antisera; the presence of agglutination indicates which antigens are present on the RBCs and hence the ABO group.
   2. Rh group
      a. Two major Rh groups, Rh$^+$ and Rh$^-$, are determined by the presence or absence of the Rh antigen.
      b. Anti-Rh antisera is mixed with the patient's blood; agglutination represents Rh$^+$, no agglutination represents Rh$^-$.
      c. Eighty-five percent of the population is Rh$^+$, 15% is Rh$^-$.
   3. Universal donor: Group O, Rh$^-$ blood, having no antigens, can generally be donated to group A, B, and AB, Rh$^+$ or Rh$^-$ individuals.
   4. Universal receiver: Group AB, Rh$^+$ individuals, having all three antigens, can generally receive A, B, AB, or O, as well as Rh$^+$ or Rh$^-$ blood.
   5. Erythroblastosis fetalis (hemolytic disease of the newborn [HDN])
      a. HDN, a potentially fatal hemolytic disease, may occur when an Rh$^-$ mother is pregnant with an Rh$^+$ fetus.
      b. During the first such pregnancy, the fetal Rh$^+$ blood, which is foreign to the Rh$^-$ mother, sensitizes the mother's immune system.
      c. This sensitization stimulates the production of IgM antibodies. IgM, a pentamer, is too large to cross the placental barrier to destroy the foreign fetal blood, so HDN generally does not occur during the first pregnancy.
      d. Subsequent pregnancies, however, will stimulate the production of IgG antibodies that can cross the placental barrier to seek out and destroy fetal RBCs causing severe hemolysis. If untreated, the unborn fetus may develop jaundice or brain damage, or may die.
      e. To prevent production of anti-Rh antibodies, all Rh$^-$ mothers are given Rhogam (Rh$_o$ gammaglobulin) within 72 hours of giving birth or termination of pregnancy.
L. Miscellaneous immunoassays
   1. Syphilis serology assays: Antibody tests for the detection of *Treponema pallidum,* the spirochete that causes syphilis.
      a. Rapid plasma reagin (RPR).
      b. Venereal Disease Research Laboratory (VDRL).
   2. Antinuclear antibodies (ANA): Antibody test for systemic lupus erythematosus (SLE).

VII. CLINICAL CHEMISTRY

A. Carbohydrates
   1. Glucose
      a. Simple sugar ($C_6H_{12}O_6$) generated from the digestion of carbohydrates providing energy to cells and tissue.
      b. Excess glucose is stored as glycogen in the liver for later use.
      c. The pancreas produces two hormones that regulate blood glucose levels.
         (1) Glucagon: Converts glycogen into glucose when needed, thereby increasing blood glucose levels.
         (2) Insulin: Facilitates the transport of glucose into the cells, thereby reducing blood glucose levels.
      d. As glucose in the blood increases after a meal, glucose metabolism tests should be done on fasting blood specimens or on specimens drawn 2 hours after a meal (postprandial).
      e. Fasting blood sugar (FBS): A blood glucose test is drawn before eating.
      f. When unhemolyzed serum or plasma is separated from the cells, the glucose concentration is generally stable for up to 8 hours at room temperature, and up to 72 hours at 4° Celsius.
      g. Cerebrospinal fluids are frequently contaminated with bacteria or WBCs that may cause

the breakdown of glucose. Thus, cerebro-spinal fluids should be analyzed for glucose without delay.

   h. Fasting blood glucose concentration should normally be less than 105 mg/dL and the blood glucose taken 2 hours after a meal should normally be less than 120 mg/dL.

     (1) FBS that is greater than or equal to 140 mg/dL on more than one occasion is diagnostic for diabetes mellitus.

     (2) FBS 2-hours postprandial that is greater than or equal to 200 mg/dL on two occasions indicates diabetes mellitus.

   i. Normal range

     (1) Serum: 70 to 105 mg/dL.

     (2) CSF: 40 to 70 mg/dL.

2. Glucose tolerance test (GTT)

   a. Measures the body's ability to respond appropriately to a heavy load of glucose. The degree and timing of the rising and falling of the blood glucose concentration after administration of glucose indicates how well the person can respond.

   b. The test begins with the patient in a fasting state, and blood is sampled and tested as a baseline control.

   c. Glucose is then administered, by either ingestion (glucola) or injection, and samples are obtained at timed intervals.

   d. Urine specimens may also be tested at fasting and time intervals that coincide with the blood sampling.

   e. Usually samples are taken at intervals of 30, 60, 120, and 180 minutes.

3. Lipids

   a. Cholesterol

     (1) Fatty compound metabolized from carbohydrates and fats that helps form cellular membranes, myelin sheath, and the production of sex hormones, vitamin D, and bile.

     (2) High-density lipoproteins (HDL) produced by the liver help transport cholesterol through the watery environment of blood, thereby preventing atherosclerosis.

     (3) Low-density and very low-density lipoproteins (LDL, VLDL) permit the development of atherosclerosis.

     (4) Normal range: Serum: Less than 200 mg/dL.

   b. Triglycerides

     (1) A group of fatty acids that are the principal lipids in blood.

     (2) They bind to lipoproteins forming HDL, LDL, and VLDL.

     (3) Normal range: Serum: 50 to 150 mg/dL.

B. Electrolytes

   1. General

     a. These substances are the major ions in the body. Changes in the concentration of one electrolyte is almost always accompanied by changes in the concentration of one or more of the others.

     b. Electrolytes are substances that form or exist as ions or charged particles when dissolved in water. Other electrolytes include calcium, magnesium, sulfate, and phosphate.

     c. Cation: Positively charged ion; an element that has more protons than electrons.

     d. Anion: Negatively charged ion; an element that has more electrons than protons.

     e. The electrolytes are the major charged particles present in the extracellular fluid.

       (1) The chief anions are chloride (Cl^-) and bicarbonate (HCO_3^-).

       (2) The chief cations are sodium (Na^+) and potassium (K^+).

     f. It is essential that the positively charged particles balance, or electrically neutralize, the negatively charged particles. When this balance is not achieved, electrolyte imbalance occurs. This is extremely dangerous for the patient and can be fatal.

     g. Electrical neutrality is maintained at all times in the body fluids. This means that the sum of all the cations (positively charged particles) equals the sum of all the anions (negatively charged particles).

     h. Functions: Maintenance of water in the various body compartments, maintenance of pH, activity of blood coagulation and enzyme cofactors, control of neuromuscular excitability, and involvement in oxidation-reduction reactions.

     i. The kidneys and the lungs are the organs that furnish the most control over electrolyte concentration.

   2. Sodium (Na^+)

     a. Major extracellular cation. It is important in maintaining osmotic pressure and in electrolyte balance.

     b. Associated with the levels of chloride and bicarbonate ion, and for this reason it has a major role in maintaining the acid-base balance of the body cells.

     c. A low serum sodium level is called hyponatremia and a high one is called hypernatremia.

     d. Normal value: 136 to 146 mmol/L serum.

   3. Potassium (K^+)

     a. The major intracellular cation that has an important influence on the muscle activity of the heart.

b. Because potassium is largely excreted by the kidney, it becomes elevated in kidney failure and shock.

c. Like sodium, potassium is influenced by the presence of the adrenocortical hormones and is associated with acid-base balance.

d. An elevated potassium level in serum is called hyperkalemia and a decreased level is called hypokalemia.

e. Even in potassium deficiency, the kidney continues to excrete potassium. The body has no effective mechanism to protect itself from excessive loss of potassium, so a regular daily intake of potassium is essential.

f. Normal value: 3.5 to 5.5 mmol/L serum.

4. Chloride (Cl^-)

a. The major extracellular anion is the major anion that counterbalances the major cation, sodium, to maintain the electrical neutrality of the body fluids.

b. Chloride has two main functions in the body: it is important in determining the osmotic pressure, which controls the distribution of water between cells, plasma, and interstitial fluid, and it is important in maintaining the acid-base balance.

c. Chloride also plays an important role in the buffering action when oxygen and carbon dioxide exchange in the red blood cells. This activity is known as chloride shift.

d. The chief extracellular anions are chloride and bicarbonate, and there is a reciprocal relationship between them; that is, when there is a decrease in the amount of one, there is an increase in the amount of the other.

e. Normal value: 98 to 106 mmol/L serum.

5. Bicarbonate (HCO_3^-)

a. Major extracellular anion.

b. Plasma or serum CO_2 is used to measure bicarbonate since about 90% of all the HCO_3^- in serum is in the form of carbon dioxide.

c. Normal value: 21 to 31 mmol/L serum.

C. Nitrogenous compounds

1. Blood urea nitrogen (BUN)

a. Urea (NH_2CONH_2) is the chief component of nonprotein nitrogen (NPN) in the blood.

b. Urea is a waste product of protein metabolism that is removed from the blood in the kidneys. Accumulation of urea in the blood above a certain amount may indicate a flaw in the filtering system of the kidneys.

c. The liver is the sole site of urea formation. As protein breakdown occurs, ammonia is formed in increased amounts. This potentially toxic substance is removed in the liver, where the ammonia combines with other amino acids and is finally converted to urea.

d. Abnormally high urea is called uremia. Decreased levels are usually not clinically significant, unless liver damage is suspected.

e. Normal value: 7 to 18 mg/dL serum.

2. Creatinine

a. Creatinine in the blood is a product of creatine metabolism in the muscles. Its formation is constant and has a direct relationship to muscle mass. Its concentration varies, therefore, with age and gender.

b. Creatinine is freely filtered by the glomeruli of the kidney and is not reabsorbed under normal circumstances.

c. The constancy of concentration and excretion makes creatinine a good measure of renal function, especially of glomerular filtration.

d. The concentration of creatinine is not affected by dietary intake, amount of dehydration in the body, or protein metabolism, which makes the assay a more reliable screening index of renal function than the BUN assay.

e. Normal value: 0.7 to 1.5 mg/dL serum.

3. Uric acid

a. By-product of purine and nucleic acid metabolism that is excreted in the urine.

b. Normal blood uric acid levels derive partly from normal muscle tissue breakdown and food metabolism.

c. Hyperuricemia: Increased serum uric acid resulting from renal disorders, gout, leukemia, and anemia.

d. Normal value: 4 to 6 mg/dL.

D. Proteins

1. Total protein

a. A group of amino acid chains found in the blood.

b. Normal range: 6.0 to 8.5 g/dL.

2. Albumin:

a. Principal plasma protein.

b. Normal range: 3.5 to 5.0 g/dL.

3. Myoglobin

a. Primary oxygen-carrying pigment of muscle tissue.

b. Nonspecific test for muscle injury.

c. Normal range: 0 to 85 ng/mL.

4. Troponin

a. Complex of three proteins integral to muscle contraction.

b. Subtypes I and T are specific to cardiac muscle.

c. Normal range: 0 to 0.2 ng/mL.

5. Hemoglobin A1C (Glycosylated or glycated hemoglobin)

a. A form of hemoglobin used to identify the average plasma glucose over prolonged periods of time.

b. In the normal 120-day life span of the red blood cell, glucose molecules join hemoglobin, forming glycated hemoglobin. Those with poorly controlled diabetes show an increased glycated hemoglobin.

c. The HbA1C level is proportional to average blood glucose concentration over the previous four weeks to three months.

d. Normal range: 4%–5.9%.

6. C-reactive protein (CRP)

a. A protein produced by the liver. The level of CRP rises during systemic inflammation.

b. The assay reveals nonspecific, general inflammation and may be elevated with inflammatory diseases like rheumatoid arthritis, lupus, or vasculitis.

c. Also used to evaluate anti-inflammatory treatment.

d. Normale range: Generally, there is no CRP detectable in the blood.

E. Bilirubin

1. Bilirubin is derived from the heme of hemoglobin, arising from the breakdown of aged red cells.

2. Unconjugated (indirect) bilirubin: It is transported to the liver as a complex with albumin and is not water soluble.

3. Conjugated (direct) bilirubin: In the liver cells, this bilirubin is conjugated with glucuronide and is made water soluble. In this form, it enters the bile fluid for transport to the small intestine. In the small intestine, most of the conjugated bilirubin is converted to urobilinogens.

4. An increased serum bilirubin concentration may indicate increased destruction (hemolysis) of RBCs, impaired excretory function of liver cells, or obstruction of the bile flow.

5. In obstructive jaundice there is an increase in total bilirubin; however, this is primarily in the form of conjugated bilirubin—measured as "direct" bilirubin—giving an increased value for direct bilirubin.

6. With liver damage such as viral hepatitis, both the unconjugated bilirubin increase, and total, direct, and indirect fractions are elevated.

7. The blood should be drawn when the patient is in a fasting state to avoid alimentary lipemia. Exposure of serum to heat and light, espcially that of wavelengths at the lower end of the visible region, results in oxidation of bilirubin.

8. Normal value: 0.1 to 1.0 mg/dL.

F. Enzymes

1. General

a. Enzymes are biological catalysts. They regulate (increase or decrease) the speed of biochemical reactions without being used up themselves.

b. The particular substances on which enzymes act are called substrates. The new substance formed as a result of the enzyme activity is called the end-product.

c. The measurement of enzymes present in serum and body fluids is expressed in terms of activity units, or international units (IU). This unit is the amount of the enzyme that will catalyze the reaction of 1 mmol of substrate per minute.

d. Enzymes end with the suffix "-ase."

e. All serum enzymes originate in the cells. Some enzymes are found in many tissues while others are unique to specific organs or tissues. It is these differences that enable differential testing to indicate the presence of some enzymes that are specific to certain tissues.

f. The increased enzyme value is related to an increased rate of release of the enzyme from the tissues. In diseases where there is increased necrosis of the tissues, as in liver, heart and pancreatic diseases, clinical enzyme tests are of diagnostic value.

2. Aspartate aminotransferase (AST)

a. In viral hepatitis and other necrotic liver diseases, serum AST levels are elevated even before clinical signs and symptoms appear. Levels may reach 100 times the upper reference limit although 20- to 50-fold elevations are more usual.

b. AST levels rise after a myocardial infarction. There is a relatively high concentration of AST in heart muscle. These AST levels do not usually rise until 6 to 8 hours after the onset of chest pain.

c. Hemolyzed samples are not acceptable, as there is a high level of AST in red cells.

d. Normal value: 8 to 20 IU/L serum.

3. Alanine aminotransferase (ALT)

a. High levels are seen in the disorders previously described under AST, although ALT is a more liver-specific enzyme.

b. ALT increases are rarely seen unless the liver parenchyma is diseased.

c. Normal value: 0 to 35 IU/L.

4. Lactate dehydrogenase (LDH)

a. LDH is present in all cells of the body.

b. Serum LDH is increased in liver, heart, skeletal, and kidney disease and in some hematopoietic and neoplastic diseases.

c. The assay should be performed on fresh serum, as storage in the refrigerator will result in loss of some of the enzyme activity. Frozen specimens are totally unacceptable.

d. Hemolyzed specimens should not be used.

e. Normal value: 50 to 150 IU/L.

5. Creatine phosphokinase (CK)
   a. A cytoplasmic mitochondrial enyzme. It is found in very high concentrations in skeletal and heart muscle and appreciable amounts are found in the brain.
   b. CK assays are most useful in the diagnosis of myocardial infarction and muscle disease.
   c. In diseases affecting skeletal muscle, serum CK is greatly increased. In muscular dystrophy, levels of up to 50 times the upper reference value can be seen.
   d. Following a myocardial infarction, total CK begins to rise within 4 to 6 hours and peaks within 18 to 30 hours. It rapidly returns to normal by the third day.
   e. Serum is the blood specimen of choice. Anticoagulants other than heparin should not be used.
   f. The CK in the serum is light sensitive so the specimen should be stored in the dark.
   g. CK-MB: Heart-related isoenzyme of CK. Peaks in 12-20 hours after MI. Returns to normal within 24-48 hours. Often ordered when Troponin is not available.
   h. Normal value: 25 to 130 IU/L serum.
6. Alkaline phosphatase
   a. Alkaline phosphatase is present in high concentration in the bone and in somewhat lower concentration in the liver.
   b. Serum alkaline phosphatase activity is increased in bone and liver disease.
   c. Serum or heparinized plasma can be tested; gross hemolysis should be avoided.
   d. Normal value: 30 to 120 IU/L.
7. Acid phosphatase
   a. The largest source of acid phosphatase is the prostatic tissue of the male.
   b. Metastatic carcinoma of the prostate gland produces very high serum acid phosphatase levels.
   c. Normal value: 0 to 0.8 IU/L.
8. Amylase
   a. Amylase is formed in the pancreas. Increased amounts of pancreatic amylase are found in the blood during the early stage of acute pancreatitis.
   b. Amylase catalyzes the hydrolysis of starch into simpler molecules, with maltose as the end product.
   c. Amylase is also secreted by the salivary glands and is present in saliva.
   d. All the common anticoagulants, except heparin, inhibit the activity of this enzyme. The test for amylase activity should therefore be performed only on serum or on heparinized plasma.
   e. Normal value: 0 to 130 IU/L serum.

9. Lipase
   a. Lipase, which is found in the pancreas, hydrolyzes fats into fatty acids and glycerol.
   b. Increased amounts of this enzyme indicate disease and inflammation of the pancreas (pancreatitis).
   c. Lipase is not present in salivary glands so this test is more specific for pancreatic involvement than the amylase test described above.
   d. Normal value: 0 to 160 IU/L.
G. Minerals
   1. Calcium (Ca^{++})
      a. Fifth most abundant body element found mainly in bone tissue.
      b. Required for bone development, transmission of nerve impulses, muscle contraction, coagulation, and cardiac function.
      c. Hypercalcemia causes muscle weakness, lethargy, and coma.
      d. Hypocalcemia causes seizures.
      e. Normal value: 9 to 11 mg/dL.
   2. Phosphorus (P)
      a. Essential for the metabolism of protein, calcium, and glucose.
      b. Phosphorus in phosphate form (PO_4^-) acts as an anion.
      c. Normal value: 3 to 5 mg/dL.
   3. Magnesium (Mg)
      a. Second most abundant intracellular cation essential to enzyme activity, muscle action, nerve impulse transmission, and calcium regulation.
      b. Normal value: 1.6 to 2.6 mg/dL.
H. Common chemistry panels
   1. Basic metabolic panel (BMP)
      a. Glucose.
      b. Electrolytes.
      c. Blood urea nitrogen (BUN).
      d. Creatinine.
      e. Calcium.
   2. Comprehensive metabolic panel (CMP)
      a. BMP, plus the following:
      b. Albumin.
      c. Total protein.
      d. ALP.
      e. ALT (SGPT).
      f. AST (SGOT).
      g. Bilirubin.
   3. Renal profile
      a. Blood urea nitrogen (BUN).
      b. Creatinine.
      c. Uric acid.
      d. Calcium.
      e. Phosphorus.
      f. Electrolytes.
      g. Total protein.
      h. Albumin.

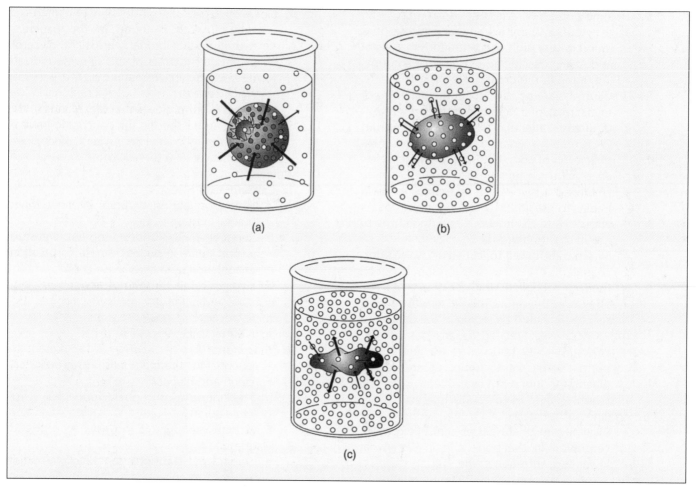

Figure 20-10

Tonicity: (a) Hypotonic solution (fresh water), (b) Isotonic solution (human blood serum), (c) Hypertonic solution (seawater). Delmar/Cengage Learning.

4. Liver panel (LFT, liver function tests)
   a. Alkaline phosphatase (ALP).
   b. Total protein.
   c. Albumin.
   d. Bilirubin.
   e. Aspartate aminotransferase (AST).
   f. Alanine aminotransferase (ALT).
5. Lipid profile
   a. Cholesterol: Total, HDL, and LDL.
   b. Triglycerides.
6. Cardiac panel
   a. Troponin.
   b. CK.
   c. CK-MB.
   d. Myoglobin.

VIII. HEMATOLOGY

A. Hematology is the scientific study of blood and blood-forming tissues.
B. The total volume of blood in an average adult is about 6 L, or 7% to 8% of body weight.

C. Blood constituents
   1. Plasma: Comprises about 55% of the blood.
      a. Water: Comprises about 90% of plasma.
      b. Solutes: The remaining 10% are proteins (albumin, globulin, fibrinogen), carbohydrates, vitamins, hormones, enzymes, lipids, and salts.
   2. Formed elements: Comprises about 45% of blood.
      a. Erythrocytes: Red blood cells (RBCs).
      b. Leukocytes: White blood cells (WBCs).
      c. Thrombocytes: Platelets (plt).
D. Anticoagulated blood that is allowed to settle or is centrifuged will develop three distinct layers:
   1. Packed RBCs: Dark red bottom layer (45%).
   2. Buffy coat: Thin whitish layer of WBCs and plts (1%).
   3. Plasma: Yellow liquid, upper layer (54%).
E. Function: As part of the circulatory system, blood transports nutrients, waste products, and agents of defense to selected tissues.
F. Hematological assays: Laboratory tests measure cellular number or concentration, the distribution of various types of cells, and structural or biochemical abnormalities.

G. Hematological diseases are not uncommon, and many diseases may show signs or symptoms of a hematological nature.

H. Osmotic pressure: The difference in concentration between solutions on either side of a cell membrane (see Figure 20-10).
1. Isotonic: A solution that has an equal concentration of solute inside and outside the cell such as blood cells.
2. Hypotonic: A solution that has a lower concentration of solute outside the cell than inside. This will create a rush of liquid into the cell causing it to burst (lysis).
3. Hypertonic: A solution that has a higher concentration of solute outside the cell than inside. This will cause the cell to lose liquid and shrink (crenation).
4. Isotonic (normal) saline: Used as a diluent or solution for hematological assays. A common isotonic solution similar to the osmotic pressure of plasma is isotonic saline, 0.85 g/dL NaCl solution.

I. Blood collection: See Venipuncture, earlier this chapter.

IX. HEMATOPOIESIS: BLOOD CELL PRODUCTION

A. General
1. Fetal: The liver and spleen are the most active sites of blood cell production. At about 4 months gestation, the bone marrow begins functioning as a blood cell producer.
2. Newborn: Shortly after birth, the marrow is the only tissue that continues to produce RBCs, WBCs, and plts.
3. Childhood: Between 5 and 7 years, the long bones become inactive and fat cells appear to replace the active marrow.
4. Adulthood: Red marrow is gradually displaced by fat cells, thereby transforming the red marrow to yellow marrow. After age 18 to 20 years, red marrow remains only in the vertebrae, ribs, sternum, skull, and partially in the femur and humerus.
5. The marrow is able to become active again when necessary, as in sudden blood loss.
6. Normally, the production and destruction of the formed elements of the blood are balanced so that a constant supply is available.

B. Leukopoiesis: WBC production
1. The bone marrow produces the granulocytes, monocytes, and platelets.
2. Lymphocytes are produced primarily by the lymphoid tissue (lymph nodes, thymus, and spleen).
3. Developmental changes
   a. As WBCs mature they become smaller.
   b. Nucleoli disappear.
   c. Nuclear chromatin becomes coarser.
   d. Cytoplasm changes from blue to pinkish-red or light blue.

C. Erythropoiesis
1. Developmental changes
   a. The RBC begins as a nucleated cell within the bone marrow. As the cell matures in the bone marrow, its diameter decreases and the nucleus becomes denser, smaller, and is finally released from the cell (extruded).
   b. Hemoglobin concentration increases and the cytoplasm changes from blue to pinkish in appearance.
   c. Complete maturation takes three to five days.
2. Maturation stages
   Rubriblast → Prorubricyte → Rubricyte → Metarubricyte → Reticulocyte → Erythrocyte (discocyte).
3. RBCs have a total life span of about 120 days, and the body releases new red cells into the circulatory system every day.
4. Hemoglobin synthesis
   a. Complex process, starting in the bone marrow with the production of the erythrocytes.
   b. The heme (iron-containing) portion of the molecule combines with globin (the protein portion) and forms an activated form of hemoglobin that is ready to transport oxygen.
   c. Hemoglobin A: Comprises 90% of adult hemoglobin.
   d. Hemoglobin F: Comprises 5% or less. It is the major form found during gestation and at birth.
   e. Hemoglobin S: Abnormal hemoglobin that occurs almost exclusively in the black population and is responsible for sickle cell anemia.
   f. Hemoglobin C, D, E: Clinically important abnormal hemoglobins that are hereditary.
5. When red cells are worn out, the body recycles the protein (globin) and iron components and eliminates the nonreusable components.
6. The heme portion of the hemoglobin molecule is a waste product that is converted to bilirubin, concentrated in the bile, and eliminated in the feces, and to some extent in the urine as urobilin and urobilinogen.

X. ERYTHROCYTES

A. Mature RBCs are biconcave disks having a doughnut shape, with a depressed area rather than a hole in the center. They do not contain a nucleus and are about 6 to 8 micrometers in diameter.

B. RBC morphology (see Figure 20-11)
1. Erythrocyte color or hemoglobin content
   a. Normochromia: RBCs that appear pinkish red with normal hemoglobin content.

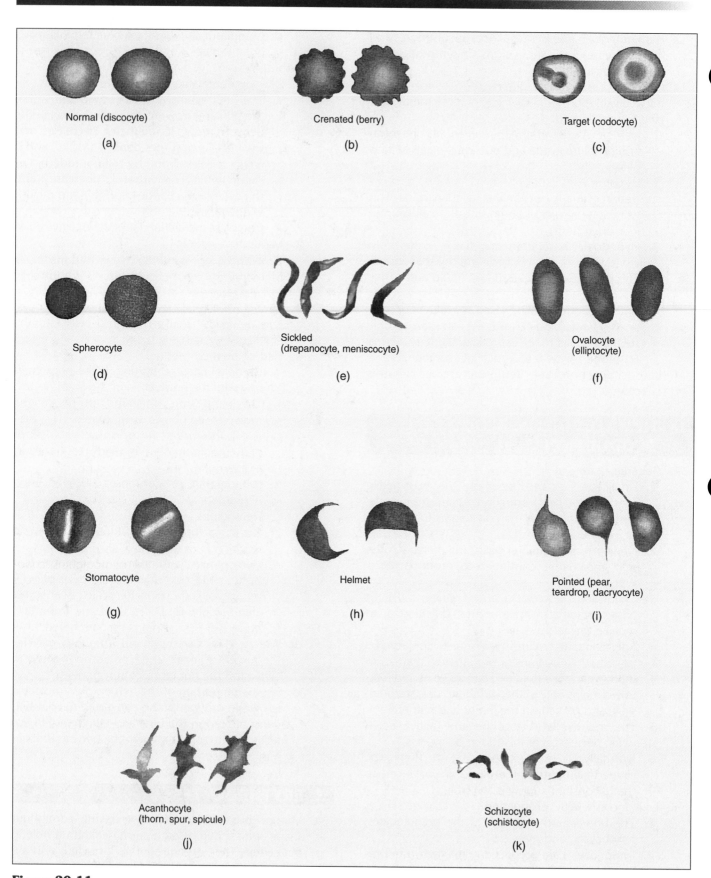

Figure 20-11

RBC morphology. Delmar/Cengage Learning.

b. Anisochromia: RBCs that have variable color, i.e., gray, pale to dark red.
  (1) Hypochromia: Pale RBCs with low hemoglobin content.
  (2) Hyperchromia: Dark RBCs with high hemoglobin content.
  (3) Polychromasia: Immature gray-light blue RBCs with low hemoglobin content.
2. Erythrocyte size: Anisocytosis describes general variation in RBC size.
  a. Macrocytosis: Large RBCs.
  b. Microcytosis: Small RBCs.
3. Erythrocyte shape: Poikilocytosis describes general variation in RBC shape.
  a. Discocytes: Normal shape.
  b. Ovalocytes: Oval shape.
  c. Elliptocytes: Thin oval shape.
  d. Drepanocytes: Sickle shape.
  e. Codocytes: Target shape.
  f. Spherocytes: Spherical shape with no central pallor.
  g. Stomatocytes: RBC with ellipsoid central pallor.
  h. Schistocytes: Fragmented RBCs.
  i. Dacryocytes: Teardrop shape.
  j. Echinocytes: Burrs along the RBC edge often resulting from improper drying (crenation).
  k. Acanthocytes: Sharp spikes along the RBC edge.
  l. Keratocytes: Half-moon or spindle shape (horn cells).

C. Anemias
1. Normochromic-normocytic
  a. RBCs are structurally normal.
  b. Results from a reduced number of circulating RBCs often because of acute blood loss.
  c. May result from an increase in plasma volume without a comparable increase in RBCs, such as pregnancy and overhydration.
2. Macrocytic: Megaloblastic anemias resulting from vitamin B_{12} or folic acid deficiency, or both.
  a. RBCs are slightly larger than normal RBCs, and may appear slightly paler than normally sized RBCs.
  b. Often results from either a nutritional deficiency or a malabsorption disorder.
  c. Causes the development of macrocytes having elevated MCV values (120 to 140).
3. Hypochromic-microcytic
  a. RBCs are smaller than normal RBCs, and may contain less hemoglobin concentration despite their size.
  b. The most common anemia resulting from iron deficiency.
4. Hemolytic: Anemias characterized by increased hemolysis of red cells.

  a. Often results from transfusion reactions, autoimmune disorders, or fetal blood that is incompatible with maternal blood.
  b. Increased production of red cells by the bone marrow causes nucleated RBCs and reticulocytes to appear on blood smears.

D. Polycythemia
1. Relative polycythemia
  a. Increase in RBC concentration due to decreased plasma volume.
  b. Slightly increased RBC count, hemoglobin, and hematocrit.
  c. Often caused by dehydration.
2. Absolute polycythemia
  a. A true increase in RBC concentration.
  b. Increased RBC count, hemoglobin, and hematocrit.
  c. Polycythemia vera: Cause unknown.
  d. Secondary polycythemia: Increased RBC production resulting from secondary factors involving oxygen deficiencies such as hypoxia, high altitudes, and pulmonary disease.

E. Hemoglobinopathies: Disorders of globin chain production that inhibit oxygen transport.
1. Alpha thalassemia
  a. Caused by a genetic defect in alpha chain production of the globin portion.
  b. Characterized by low hemoglobin, codocytes, microcytes, and hypochromasia.
2. Beta thalassemia
  a. Caused by a genetic defect in beta chain production of the globin portion.
  b. Characterized by low hemoglobin, codocytes, microcytes, hypochromasia, nucleated RBCs (NRBCs), increased retics, and basophilic stippling.
3. Sickle cell anemia
  a. Caused by a genetic structural defect of the beta globin chain that crystallizes the hemoglobin, making it insoluble under low oxygen conditions.
  b. Characterized by depranocytes, codocytes, ovalocytes, polychromasia, NRBCs, siderotic granules, and Howell-Jolly bodies.

F. Laboratory assays
1. Hemoglobin (hgb)
  a. Adult male: 15.7 (14.0 to 17.5) g/dL
  b. Adult female: 13.8 (12.3 to 15.3) g/dL
  c. Infant: 12.6 (11.1 to 14.1) g/dL
  d. Child: 13.4 (11.8 to 15.0) g/dL
2. Hematocrit (hct): Percent packed RBCs.
  a. Hematocrit is the relative volume of RBCs, expressed as a percent, as compared to the whole volume of blood.
  b. Hct = packed RBC height ÷ total blood height × 100.

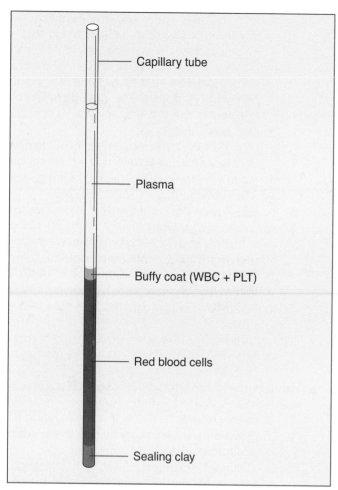

Figure 20-12A
Hematocrit tube. Delmar/Cengage Learning.

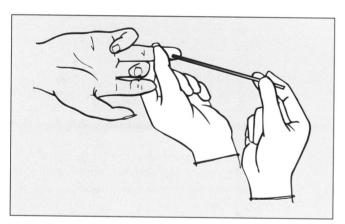

Figure 20-12B
Filling a capillary tube from a capillary puncture. Delmar/Cengage Learning.

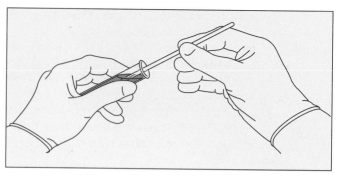

Figure 20-12C
Filling a capillary tube from a tube of blood. Delmar/Cengage Learning.

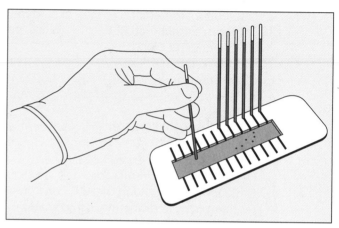

Figure 20-12D
Sealing the capillary tube with sealing clay. Delmar/Cengage Learning.

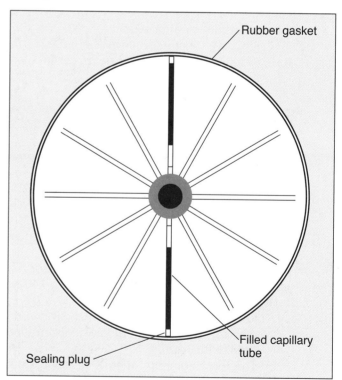

Figure 20-12E
Proper placement of sealed capillary tubes in microhematocrit centrifuge. Delmar/Cengage Learning.

c. The hematocrit measurement is more accurate than a manual RBC count because much less error is associated with it.
d. Hgb × 3 = Hct (+ or − 3 units).
e. Normal values
(1) Adult male: 46% (42% to 50%)
(2) Adult female: 40% (36% to 45%)

f. Procedure (see Figures 20-12A to E)
   (1) Fill two hematocrit (capillary) tubes at least three-fourths full with blood.
   (2) Wipe both tubes free of blood and plug the ends by inserting them into a clay preparation (Critoseal).
   (3) Place the tubes in a hematocrit centrifuge with stoppered ends facing toward the centrifuge rim; centrifuge 5 to 10 minutes.
   (4) Determine the hematocrit by using a reading device.
   (5) To be valid, both tubes should be within 2% of each other. If so, report the average. Otherwise, repeat the procedure.
3. RBC count: Number of RBCs in millions per cubic millimeter of blood.
   a. Normal value
      (1) Male: 4.5–6.0 × 10^6/mm³
      (2) Female: 4.0–5.0 × 10^6/mm³
4. RBC indices
   a. Mean corpuscular volume (MCV)
      (1) Measures the average volume of an RBC.
      (2) Normal MCV: 80 to 96.
      (3) The MCV indicates whether the RBCs will appear microcytic, normocytic, or macrocytic.

   (4) (Hct% × 10) ÷ RBC (in millions).
   b. Mean corpuscular hemoglobin
      (1) Measures the average weight of hemoglobin content in an RBC.
      (2) Normal MCH: 27 to 33.
      (3) (Hgb (g/dL) × 10) ÷ RBC (in millions).
   c. Mean corpuscular hemoglobin concentration (MCHC)
      (1) Measures the average hemoglobin concentration per unit volume of packed red cells.
      (2) Normal MCHC: 33 to 36 g/dL.
      (3) Values below 32 g/dL indicate hypochromia. Values greater than 37 are physiologically impossible and indicate an error.
      (4) Hgb (g/dL) ÷ hct (as a decimal).
   d. Example: RBC = 4.5 million, Hgb = 14 g/dL, Hct = 42%.
      (1) MCV = (42 × 10) ÷ 4.5 = 420 ÷ 4.5 = 93.3.
      (2) MCH = (14 × 10) ÷ 4.5 = 140 ÷ 4.5 = 31.1.
      (3) MCHC = 14 ÷ .42 = 33.3.
5. Erythrocyte sedimentation rate (ESR) (see Figures 20-13A and B)
   a. Measures the rate at which anticoagulated RBCs will fall when allowed to settle in a thin columnar tube.

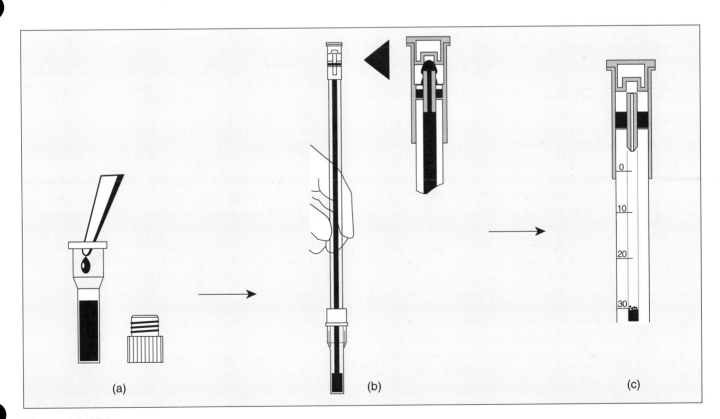

Figure 20-13A

Erythrocyte sedimentation rate (ESR), Westergren method. (a) Pipet blood into vial containing diluent; (b) Insert tube through vial stopper; tube will fill and autozero (inset); and (c) After 1 hour read sedimentation distance using calibrated markings (reported as mm/hr).
Delmar/Cengage Learning.

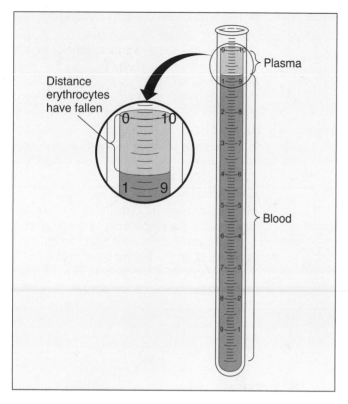

Figure 20-13B

Wintrobe tube showing sedimentation of cells. Example shown illustrates a sedimentation of 8 mm/hr. Delmar/Cengage Learning.

b. The ESR is a nonspecific screening test for inflammatory activity.
c. Methods: Westergren and Wintrobe method.
d. Normal values
   (1) Male: 0 to 15 mm/hr.
   (2) Female: 0 to 20 mm/hr.
e. Procedure
   (1) Fill the tube according to the manufacturer's instructions.
   (2) Place the tube in the sedimentation rack for 1 hour.
   (3) After 1 hour has expired, note the distance the cells have settled in millimeters and record.
6. Reticulocyte count
   a. Reticulocytes are immature RBCs that may be seen during anemia or after sudden blood loss.
   b. The reticulocyte count is used to follow therapeutic measures for anemias. A corresponding increase in the reticulocytes indicates a favorable response to therapy.
   c. The reticulocyte count is reported as the percentage of reticulocytes in the total red cells counted.
   d. Normal value: 0.9% to 2.1%.

XI. LEUKOCYTES

A. Normal leukocyte morphology (see Figure 20-14)
   1. Segmented neutrophils (segs)
      a. Most numerous granulocyte also known as polymorphonuclear neutrophils (PMNs).
      b. Distribution: Comprises 35% to 70% of normal peripheral WBCs.
      c. Size: 10 to 15 micrometers (2 or 3 RBCs).
      d. Nucleus: Lobular; being constricted in one to four places, it may have two to five lobes; stains deep reddish-purple.
      e. Cytoplasm: Abundant, having a light to dirty pink color containing many very small granules.
      f. Shift-to-the-right: Increased numbers of segs.
   2. Band neutrophils (bands)
      a. Immature form of the segmented neutrophil requiring a separate classification.
      b. Distribution: 1 to 5%
      c. Size: 10 to 15 micrometers (2 or 3 RBCs).
      d. Nucleus: Band, peanut, or rod-shaped with no constrictions or lobes.
      e. Cytoplasm: Same as a seg.
      f. When there is doubt, the cell should be classified as a seg.
      g. Shift-to-the-left: Increased numbers of bands.
      h. Neutrophilia: Increased neutrophils that may be found in acute infections; metabolic, chemical, and drug intoxications; acute hemorrhage; postoperative states; certain non-inflammatory conditions such as coronary thrombosis; malignant neoplasms; and after acute hemolytic episodes. It is usually accompanied by a shift to the left.
   3. Eosinophils (eos)
      a. Distribution: 1% to 5%.
      b. Size: 11 to 16 micrometers (2 or 3 RBCs).
      c. Nucleus: Not significant.
      d. Cytoplasm: Contains large, red-orange to dirty-pink granules.
      e. Eosinophilic granules contain histamine.
      f. Serve to ingest antigen-antibody complexes.
      g. Eosinophilia: Increased numbers of eosinophils seen in allergic reactions, inflammation, parasitic infections, and leukemia.
   4. Basophils (basos)
      a. Distribution: 0 to 1%.
      b. Size: 10 to 15 micrometers (2 or 3 RBCs).
      c. Nucleus: Indistinct.
      d. Cytoplasm: Large, dark purple to black granules.
      e. Basophilic granules contain histamine and heparin, and apparently play a role in allergic reactions.
      f. Basophilia: Increased numbers of basophils often associated with chronic myelocytic

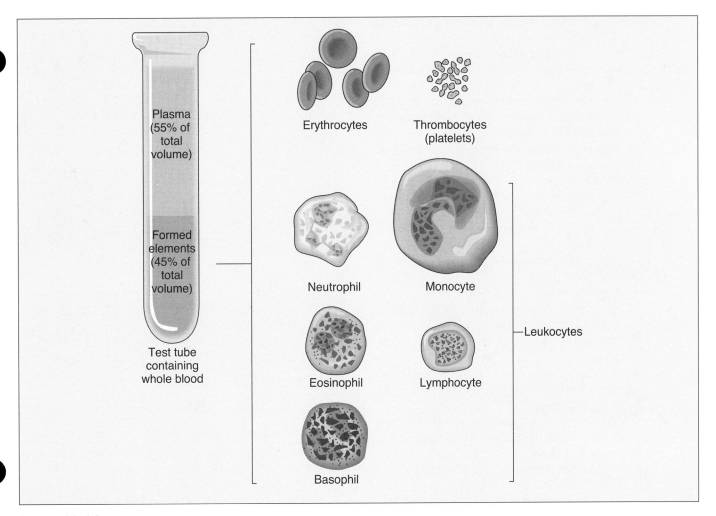

Figure 20-14

Major cellular components of blood. Delmar/Cengage Learning.

leukemia (CML), allergic reactions, radiation exposure, chronic hemolytic anemia, and after splenectomy.

5. Monocytes (monos)
   a. Largest normal WBC.
   b. Distribution: 3% to 5%.
   c. Size: 15 to 20 micrometers (3 to 5 RBCs).
   d. Nucleus: Large, foamy, rounded, elongated, horseshoe- or bean-shaped. Red-purple to medium-purple.
   e. Cytoplasm: Abundant, sky-blue to blue-gray, may contain azurophilic (reddish) granules and vacuoles.

6. Lymphocytes (lymphs)
   a. Smallest normal WBC.
   b. Distribution: 30% to 40%.
   c. Size: 6 to 10 micrometers (1 or 2 RBCs).
   d. Nucleus: Round, course, dark purple, filling most of the cytoplasm.
   e. Cytoplasm: Sky to medium-blue band encircling the nucleus.
   f. Infants and children normally have more lymphocytes and fewer neutrophils than adults.

   g. Lymphocytosis: Increased numbers of lymphocytes often seen in acute infections (e.g., mononucleosis, pertussis, mumps, and rubella) and chronic infections such as tuberculosis, brucellosis, and hepatitis.

B. Leukemias
   1. A neoplastic condition characterized by the proliferation of immature leukocytes in the peripheral blood.
   2. The proliferation of immature WBCs displaces normal WBCs.
   3. Leukemias are classified as acute or chronic on the basis of prognosis and the number of blasts present.
   4. Major symptoms: Fever, weight loss, night sweats, hepatomegaly, splenomegaly, enlarged lymph nodes, and bleeding tendencies.
   5. Acute leukemias
      a. Onset usually occurs suddenly accompanied by normocytic-normochromic anemia.
      b. Thrombocytopenia: Low platelet count is usually present.

c. Leukocytosis: WBC count of 50,000 to 100,000/mm³.

d. Blasts: Found in the peripheral blood; more than 60% blasts indicates an acute leukemic process.

e. Untreated acute leukemias can lead to death within 2 to 3 months. Death is often due to hemorrhage or infection.

f. Treatment: Chemotherapy and bone marrow transplantation.

g. Classifications
   (1) Acute myelocytic leukemia (AML):
   (2) Acute monocytic leukemia (AML):
   (3) Acute myelomonocytic leukemia (AMML):
   (4) Acute lymphocytic leukemia (ALL):

6. Chronic leukemias
   a. Asymptomatic, slow, insidious onset.
   b. Symptoms include fatigue, night sweats, weight loss, and fever.
   c. Anemia may develop as the disease progresses.
   d. Thrombocytosis: Occurs early in the disease.
   e. Thrombocytopenia: Occurs later as the disease progresses.
   f. Leukocytosis: Often in excess of 100,000/mm³.
   g. Blasts: Usually less than 10% seen in the peripheral blood.
   h. Average life expectancy: 3 to 4 years.
   i. Classifications
      (1) Chronic myelocytic leukemia (CML):
      (2) Chronic monocytic leukemia (CML):
      (3) Chronic myelomonocytic leukemia (CMML):
      (4) Chronic lymphocytic leukemia (CLL):

C. Laboratory assays

1. Leukocyte count: Normal value: 5000 to 10,000 WBCs/mm³.

2. Differential
   a. Microscopically observing a stained blood smear, the first 100 WBCs seen are classified.
   b. Normal value
      (1) Segmented neutrophils: 35% to 70%.
      (2) Band neutrophils: 1% to 5%.
      (3) Lymphocytes: 30% to 40%.
      (4) Monocytes: 3% to 5%.
      (5) Eosinophils: 1% to 5%.
      (6) Basophils: 0% to 1%.
   c. Procedure
      (1) Prepare a blood smear (see Figures 20-15 and 20-16)
         (a) Place a small drop of blood, using a safety device, about a half inch from the end of a glass slide.
         (b) Place the edge of a second (spreader) slide on the first near the blood drop at a 30- to 45-degree angle.

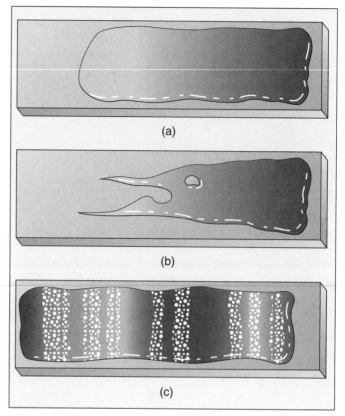

Figure 20-15

(a) Properly prepared blood smear. (b and c) Improperly prepared blood smears. Delmar/Cengage Learning.

         (c) Move the spreader slide back until it touches the blood drop. Just before the blood spreads completely across the spreader slide's edge, draw it smoothly and gently away from the blood drop. Allow to dry.
         (d) There should be a smooth feather edge; if not, repeat the procedure.
      (2) Stain (Wright's stain) the smear following the manufacturer's instructions.
      (3) Differential: The slide is observed under 100×, and the first 100 cells seen using a differential counter are recorded.
      (4) RBC morphology: 10 fields are observed, and any anisocytosis, poikilocytosis, and cytochromia is recorded.
      (5) Platelet estimate: 10 fields are observed at 100×; the number of platelets seen is counted and an average is calculated.
         (a) Average of 7 to 20 seen, report *adequate*.
         (b) Average of less than 7 seen, report *decreased*.
         (c) Average of greater than 20 seen, report *increased*.

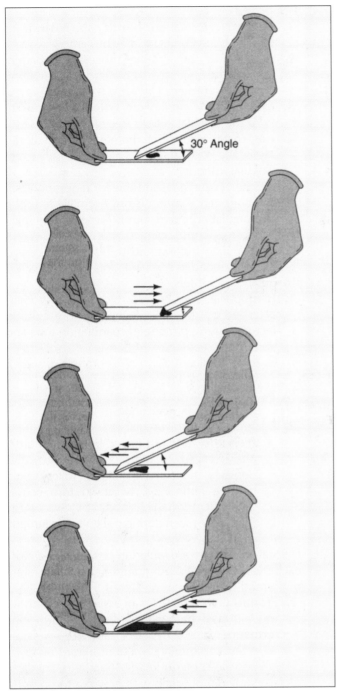

Figure 20-16

Preparing a smear. Delmar/Cengage Learning.

XII. THROMBOCYTES

A. Platelets are round or oval, small bodies 1 to 4 micrometers in diameter. Platelets have a colorless to pale blue background substance containing centrally located reddish to violet granules.

B. Platelets are produced in the bone marrow by cells called megakaryocytes, which are large and multinucleated.

C. Platelets do not have a nucleus and are not actually cells—they are portions of cytoplasm pinched off from megakaryocytes and released into the bloodstream.

D. Hemostasis: They serve an essential part of the coagulation process in that they maintain the integrity of the endothelial lining of the blood vessels. They act as plugs around the opening of a wound, and they release platelet factor 3 (PF3), a necessary component of coagulation.

E. Laboratory assays

1. Platelet count: Normal value: 150,000 to 400,000 plts/mm³.

2. Bleeding time: Measures platelet function by making a small incision in the patient's arm (Ivy method) or earlobe (Duke method) and noting the length of time it takes for the wound to stop bleeding. Anticoagulant therapy will not influence bleeding time.

   a. Normal value: Ivy: 1 to 7 minutes.

   b. Procedure (Ivy)

      (1) Observe standard precautions; wash hands.

      (2) Place a sphygmomanometer on the patient's upper arm and inflate to 40 mmHg; maintain this pressure for the entire procedure.

      (3) Locate an area on the patient's forearm free of observable superficial blood vessels and cleanse with 70 percent isopropyl alcohol.

      (4) Using an automatic lancet device, make an incision in the patient's forearm.

      (5) Activate a stopwatch when the first drop of blood appears.

      (6) Every 30 seconds blot away the blood using filter paper without touching the incision.

      (7) When the bleeding stops, the time is noted.

      (8) Apply a butterfly bandage to the wound; clean up.

XIII. HEMOSTASIS

A. Introduction

1. Hemostasis is the cessation of blood flow from an injured blood vessel.

2. Encompasses the entire process by which bleeding from an injured blood vessel is controlled and finally stopped.

3. It is a series of physical and biochemical changes normally initiated by an injury to the blood vessel and tissues, culminating in the transformation of fluid blood into a thrombus or clot; which effectively seals the injured vessel.

4. Extravascular effects

a. Physical effects: Muscle, skin, and elastic tissue tend to close and seal the tear in the injured vessel.
b. Biochemical effects: Substances released from the injured tissues that react with plasma and platelet factors to stimulate coagulation.

5. Vascular effects
   a. Vascular injury: Exposure of the underlying basement membrane layer of the vessel causes the vessel to constrict.
   b. Platelet plug: Thrombocytes make contact with the basement membrane, causing biochemical and structural changes resulting in the formation of platelet aggregates and a fibrin clot, thereby plugging the gaps in the endothelial lining.

B. Coagulation
   1. All the elements necessary for clot formation are normally present in the circulating blood.
   2. The process of coagulation is a series of biochemical reactions described as the coagulation cascade.
   3. Roman numerals (I to XIII) have been assigned to the various coagulation factors in the order of their discovery and have nothing to do with their activation sequence.
   4. Coagulation factors: Mainly proteins, except calcium and the phospholipid of platelets (PF3). Most of the factors become active enzymes after undergoing a physiochemical change.
   5. Stages of coagulation
      a. The mechanism of coagulation takes place in three major steps:
         (1) Thromboplastin formation.
         (2) Thrombin formation.
         (3) Fibrin formation.
      b. Intrinsic pathway: Activates the coagulation factors within the blood when endothelial lining of the vessel is damaged.
      c. Extrinsic pathway: Activation of the coagulation cascade when damaged tissue outside the circulatory system releases factor III into the circulatory system.
      d. Common pathway: By activating either the intrinsic or extrinsic pathway, or both, the coagulation cascade proceeds to final clot formation.
         (1) The intrinsic or extrinsic pathway activates factor X.
         (2) Factor V, PF3, and calcium all work with factor X to convert prothrombin (II) to thrombin.
         (3) Thrombin, in turn, converts fibrinogen (I) to fibrin.
         (4) Factor XIII stabilizes and strengthens the fibrin clot.

C. Fibrinolysis
   1. Besides clot formation, the body also has a means by which the fibrin clot may be removed.
   2. As soon as the clotting process has begun, fibrinolysis is initiated to break down the fibrin clot that is formed.
   3. Normally, the fibrinolytic system functions to keep the vascular system free of fibrin clots.
   4. Homeostasis: Through hemostasis and fibrinolysis, the body maintains a delicate balance of vascular integrity.
   5. Plasmin: Enzyme responsible for digesting fibrin or fibrinogen. Plasmin is not normally found in the circulating blood, but is present in an inactive form, plasminogen.
   6. Plasminogen is converted to plasmin by certain enzymes found in small amounts in most tissues.

D. Coagulation disorders
   1. Hemophilia: A hereditary blood disease characterized by the lack of one or more clotting factors causing prolonged coagulation time and abnormal bleeding.
      a. Hemophilia A (Von Willebrand's disease): Caused by a factor VIII deficiency.
      b. Hemophilia B (Christmas disease): Caused by a factor IX deficiency.
   2. Disseminated intravascular coagulation (DIC)
      a. A disorder, often triggered by tissue trauma, characterized by massive coagulation that depletes the clotting factors, followed by massive fibrinolysis, which in turn causes severe hemorrhage.
      b. Sometimes seen during difficult or traumatic childbirth.

E. Laboratory assays: Coagulation assays are almost exclusively performed using automation, and rarely performed manually.
   1. Prothrombin time (PT): an assay that monitors the extrinsic pathway leading to fibrin clot formation.
      a. A test commonly used to monitor therapeutic values of Coumadin (warfarin) medication for individuals with previous thrombotic episodes.
      b. Normal value for individual not on warfarin therapy: 10 to 13 seconds.
      c. Patients on warfarin therapy usually have a PT 2 to 3 times the normal range.
      d. INR usually complements PT to monitor warfarin therapy.
   2. International normalized ratio (INR): A standardized ratio that compares the therapeutic PT to a normal PT.
      a. Normal range: 0.9 to 1.3.
      b. Patients on routine anticoagulant therapy should have an INR of 2 to 3.

c. Patients with high risk of clot formation might have an INR of 2.5 to 3.5.

d. INR greater than 3.5 increases the risk of hemorrhage.

3. PTT: Partial thromboplastin time; an assay that monitors the intrinsic pathway leading to fibrin clot formation.

a. Used to monitor heparin therapy.

b. Normal value: 25 to 40 seconds.

4. FDP: Fibrin degradation products, an assay that measures the fragments of disintegrating fibrin during fibrinolysis.

a. The FDP is elevated following thrombotic events such as DIC and deep vein thrombosis (DVT).

b. Normal range: less than 10 mcg/mL.

5. D-dimer: Measures a specific FDP fragment.

a. Indicates an abnormally high level of FDPs resulting from significant coagulation and fibrinolysis, i.e., DIC, DVT, and pulmonary embolism.

b. Normal range: 0 to 300 ng/mL.

XIV. MICROBIOLOGY

A. Microbiological precautions

1. Always place culture plates facedown.

2. Do not pass open culture plates to colleagues.

3. Sterilize inoculating loops immediately after use.

B. Infectious process

1. Reservoir host: Organisms that harbor a pathogenic agent.

2. Mode of exit: The means by which the pathogen escapes the host environment usually through body orifices or wounds.

3. Mode of transmission: The means by which the pathogen is transported from the reservoir host to a new host.

a. Direct contact: Host to host contact.

b. Indirect contact: Host touching contaminated objects.

c. Vectors: Transmission from host to host via another organism such as insects.

4. Mode of entry: Means by which the pathogen enters the new host. Same as means of exit.

5. Susceptible host: A host that is capable of becoming infected by the pathogen.

C. Defensive mechanisms

1. Normal flora: Harmless microorganisms inhabiting the body that inhibit proliferation of pathogenic organisms.

2. Anatomical barriers: Skin, mucous membranes, and body fluids that create physical or chemical barriers to pathogens.

3. Inflammation: An immune response that attempts to remove pathogenic agents and their byproducts.

4. Phagocytosis: Cellular attack, ingestion, and destruction of pathogens.

5. Immune system: Coordinated body defense system that recognizes, attacks, and eliminates harmful foreign substances.

XV. CELLULAR ANATOMY

A. Eukaryotic cells: Review cellular anatomy in Chapter 5, Anatomy and Physiology.

B. Prokaryocytes: Cells found in less complex organisms such as bacteria and blue-green algae (cyanobacteria).

1. Capsule (slime layer): Outermost layer composed of a thick, sticky gelatinous layer.

a. Provides a protective covering.

b. Serves as a reservoir for stored nutrients.

c. Encapsulates most pathogenic bacteria and increases its virulence.

2. Cell wall: Lies between the outer capsule and the inner cytoplasmic membrane.

a. Rigid wall that provides shape and strength.

b. Cell wall properties allow it to be stained different colors to help identify specific genera.

3. Cytoplasmic membrane: Innermost membrane that envelopes the cytoplasm similar to the eukaryocytic cell membrane.

4. Mesosomes: Inward folding of the cytoplasmic membrane.

a. Increases cellular surface area.

b. Involved in cellular respiration.

c. Helps generate a new cell wall during cellular division.

5. Nucleoid: DNA material that is not enveloped by a nuclear membrane, but is bound by a protein layer.

6. Plasmids: Extrachromosomal DNA (outside the nucleoid).

a. Conjugation: Reproduction via DNA transfer between bacteria.

b. Resistance: Helps develop resistance to certain antibiotics.

7. Ribosomes: Similar to eukaryotic cells.

8. Flagella: Similar to eukaryotic cells.

9. Pili (fimbriae): Hairlike protrusions similar to cilia.

a. Found almost entirely in gram-negative bacteria.

b. Allows bacteria to stick to one another and to surfaces.

c. Aids the process of conjugation.

10. Endospore: During hostile conditions, some bacteria develop a protective covering.
  a. Composed of many layers of protein that can protect a bacteria for many thousands of years.
  b. When conditions are right, the bacteria will germinate.
  c. Some spores produce toxins.

C. Taxonomy: Classification of organisms.
  1. Hierarchy
    Kingdom: Common collection of phyla.
    Phylum: Common collection of classes.
    Class: Common collection of orders.
    Order: Common collection of families.
    Family: Common collection of genera.
    Genus: Common collection of species.
    Species: Same organism.
  2. Example: Human (*Homo sapien*)
    a. Kingdom: Animalia.
    b. Phylum: Chordata.
    c. Class: Mammalia.
    d. Order: Primatae.
    e. Family: Hominidae.
    f. Genus: *Homo*.
    g. Species: *sapien*.
  3. Binomial nomenclature: *Genus species*.
    a. Genus is capitalized.
    b. Species is in lowercase.
    c. Both are italicized or underlined.

XVI. BACTERIOLOGY

A. Bacteria: Microorganisms 0.5 to 1.0 microns in length.
B. Common morphological/differential characteristics (see Figure 20-17)
  1. Shape
    a. Cocci: Spherical in shape.
    b. Bacilli: Rod-shaped.
    c. Vibrio: Comma-shaped.
    d. Spirilla: Spiral-shaped.
    e. Spirochete: Corkscrew-shaped.
  2. Physical arrangement
    a. Diplo: Diplococci or diplobacilli are arranged in pairs.
    b. Strepto: Streptococci or streptobacilli are arranged in chains.
    c. Staphylo: Staphylococci are arranged in clusters.
  3. Staining properties
    a. Gram stain
      (1) Gram-positive: Gram-positive cocci (GPC) or gram-positive bacilli (rods) (GPR) stain dark purple to blue.
      (2) Gram-negative: Gram-negative cocci (GNC) or gram-negative bacilli (rods) (GNR) stain red or pink.

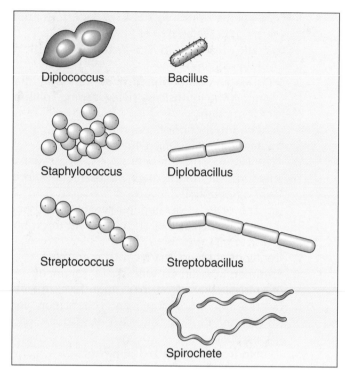

Figure 20-17

Bacterial morphology. Delmar/Cengage Learning.

    b. Acid-fast stain: Some bacteria are difficult to stain, but once stained resist decolorization with an alcohol-acid preparation and are thus "acid-fast"; e.g., the genera *Mycobacterium* that causes tuberculosis.
  4. Oxygen requirements
    a. Aerobic: Bacteria that require oxygen for survival.
    b. Microaerophilic: Bacteria that require reduced oxygen levels.
    c. Anaerobic: Bacteria that require an oxygen-free environment.
    d. Facultative: Bacteria that can survive in either an oxygen or oxygen-free environment.
  5. Pattern of colony growth on culture media
    a. Size, shape, elevation, texture, marginal appearance, and color.
    b. Patterns of hemolysis: Bacteria grown on blood agar.
      (1) Alpha: Incomplete zone of hemolysis, appearing yellow-green, surrounding the bacterial colony.
      (2) Beta: Clear, colorless zone of hemolysis surrounding the colonies.
      (3) Gamma: No hemolysis.
  6. Biochemical reactions: Bacteria respond differently to certain chemical reagents.
C. Gram stain procedure
  1. Apply the specimen to the slide by spreading it around in a circular fashion creating a thin layer. Let it dry.

2. Affix the bacterium to the slide by passing the underside of the slide over a flame two to four times, just until it is hot to the touch. The heat coagulates the cellular protein of the bacteria, causing it to stick to the slide.
3. Flood the slide with crystal violet stain and let sit for 20 to 60 seconds. This will stain the bacteria purple.
4. Gently rinse the stain off with water.
5. Rinse the slide with iodine solution, then flood it, letting it sit for 20 to 60 seconds. The iodine is a mordant, that is, it combines with the crystal violet, forming a dye-iodine complex that fixes the crystal violet to the bacteria by decreasing its ability to dissolve out of the bacterial cell wall.
6. Gently rinse the iodine off with water.
7. Apply the alcohol-acetone decolorizer drop by drop until the purple color no longer runs off the slide. Gram-positive bacteria will retain the purple stain, whereas gram-negative bacteria will lose it and appear colorless.
8. Gently rinse the slide with water.
9. Flood the slide with safranin stain and let sit for 20 to 60 seconds. The bacteria that lost the purple dye during decolorization will accept and retain the red safranin dye and appear reddish-pink or gram-negative.
10. Gently rinse with water.
11. Let stand until dry. View under the microscope using oil immersion, 100× objective.

D. Common pathogenic bacteria
1. Gram-positive cocci (GPC)
   a. *Staphylococcus:* GPC appearing in clusters.
      (1) *S. aureus:* Causes skin, wound, burn, and nosocomial infections, and impetigo.
      (2) *S. saprophyticus:* Implicated in urinary tract infections (UTI) among sexually active females.
      (3) *S. epidermis:* Normal flora of skin.
   b. *Streptococcus:* GPC appearing in chains.
      (1) *S. pyogenes:* Beta-hemolytic group A streptococci found in the respiratory tract. Implicated in pharyngitis, cellulitis, and rheumatic fever.
      (2) *S. pneumoniae* (Pneumococcus): Gamma-hemolytic streptococci found in the nasopharynx. Implicated in pneumonia, meningitis, sinusitis, and otitis media.
      (3) *S. viridans:* Alpha-hemolytic streptococci found in the mouth. Implicated in gum disease and subacute endocarditis (SBE).
2. Gram-negative cocci (GNC): *Neisseria:* Gram-negative diplococci.
   a. *N. meningitidis:* Found in the nasopharynx. Implicated in meningitis.
   b. *N. gonorrhoeae:* Causes gonorrhea, urethritis, vulvovaginitis, and ophthalmia neonatorium.
3. Gram-negative bacilli (GNR)
   a. *Escherichia coli:* Found in the colon. Commonly causes urinary tract infection (UTI) and nosocomial infections.
   b. *Salmonella:* Widely distributed in nature, commonly causes food poisoning.
      (1) *S. typhi:* Causes enteric fever and constipation.
      (2) *S. cholerae-suis:* Causes septicemia.
      (3) *S. enteritidis:* Causes gastroenteritis.
   c. *Shigella:* Causes bacillary dysentery acquired from contaminated food and water.
      (1) *S. sonnei:* Mild dysentery.
      (2) *S. flexneri:* Medium in severity.
      (3) *S. dysenteriae:* Severe dysentery.
   d. *Klebsiella pneumoniae:* Found in water and soil; normal flora of the bowel and upper respiratory tract. Causes UTI, bacteremia, peritonitis, wound infections, and severe pneumonia.
   e. *Proteus vulgaris:* Found in soil and intestinal tract. Causes UTI, wound infections, and bacteremia.
   f. *Yersinia:* Found in wild animals; creates fecal contamination.
      (1) *Y. enterocolitica:* Causes ileitis, lymphadenitis, and diarrhea.
      (2) *Y. pestis:* Causes plague.
   g. *Pseudomonas aeruginosa:* Found in soil and feces. Commonly causes UTI; also wound, burn, and respiratory infections, and septicemia.
   h. *Haemophilus influenzae:* Sometimes normal flora of the nasopharynx, it causes meningitis, and severe epiglottitis, as well as otitis media.
4. Gram-negative coccobacilli
   a. *Gardnerella vaginalis:* Causes nonspecific vaginitis.
   b. *Francisaella tularensis:* Causes tularemia (deer fly or rabbit fever), an infectious plaguelike disease transmitted by infected insects or animals.
   c. *Bordetella pertussis:* Causes whooping cough.
5. Gram-negative spirilla, spirochetes, and vibrio
   a. *Campylobacter jejuni:* Gram-negative spirilla. Common cause of febrile gastroenteritis.
   b. *Treponema pallidum:* Gram-negative spirochetes that cause syphilis.
   c. *Borrelia burgdorferi:* Gram-negative spirochete that causes Lyme disease.
   d. *Vibrio:* Comma-shaped bacillus.
      (1) *V. cholerae:* Causes cholera from contaminated water.

(2) *V. parahaemolyticus:* Causes gastroenteritis from contaminated seafood.

6. Gram-positive bacilli (GPR)
   a. *Bacillus cereus:* Causes food poisoning.
   b. *Corynebacterium diphtheriae:* GPR that is curved and club-shaped causes diphtheria.
   c. *Mycobacterium:* Acid-fast GPR.
      (1) *M. tuberculosis:* Causes tuberculosis.
      (2) *M. leprae:* Causes leprosy.
7. Anaerobic bacteria
   a. Gram-positive cocci: Generally found in a variety of infections. Normal flora of the bowel, female genital tract, and oral cavity.
      (1) *Streptococcus intermedius.*
      (2) *Peptococcus niger:* Rarely seen clinically but implicated in some septicemias.
      (3) *Peptostreptococcus anaerobius.*
   b. Gram-negative bacilli: Normal flora of the mouth, intestines, urethra, and female genital tract.
      (1) *Bacteroides fragilis:* Opportunistic, causing infection in these areas.
      (2) *Fusobacterium nucleatum:* Similar to *Bacteroides.*
   c. Gram-positive bacilli
      (1) *Lactobacillus acidophilus:* Normal flora of the vagina, it maintains its acid pH, but causes infection elsewhere.
      (2) *Propionibacterium acnes:* Normal flora of the skin. Implicated in endocarditis.
      (3) *Clostridium:* Spore-forming GPR.
         (a) *C. perfringens:* Causes gangrene.
         (b) *C. tetani:* Causes tetanus.
         (c) *C. botulinum:* Causes botulism and muscle paralysis.
         (d) *C. difficile:* Causes pseudomembranous colitis.

E. Rickettsias, chlamydias, and mycoplasmas
   1. *Rickettsia:* Very small, gram-negative, nonmotile, pleomorphic bacteria.
      a. Obligate intracellular parasites: Require living cells to live.
      b. Transmitted by the bite of fleas, lice, ticks, and mites.
      c. *R. rickettsii:* Causes Rocky Mountain spotted fever.
      d. *R. prowazekii:* Causes louseborn typhus.
      e. *R. typhi:* Causes fleaborn typhus.
   2. *Chlamydia:* Intracellular, gram-negative cocci.
      a. Depend on host cells for their energy source.
      b. *C. psittaci:* Causes psittacosis or ornithosis (parrot fever), an infectious disease transmitted by birds.
      c. *C. trachomatis:* Causes conjunctivitis.
   3. *Mycoplasma:* Simplest of bacteria comprising only a cell membrane, prokaryotic nucleus, and ribosomes.
      a. Normal flora of the genitalia and respiratory system.
      b. Commonly causes inflammation of these tissues as well as arthritis.
      c. *M. pneumoniae:* Causes upper respiratory infections as well as walking pneumonia.
      d. *M. hominis:* Causes urethritis.

F. Bacteriological cultures
   1. General
      a. Culture media contains a measured quantity of substances for optimal bacterial growth and diagnostic properties.
      b. Contains some or all of the following: Amino acids, sugars, vitamins, minerals, and diagnostic dyes.
      c. Media forms
         (1) Liquid: Media broths are generally used as a general growth media or to study the production of gas or changes in pH, especially among anaerobes.
         (2) Solid/semisolid: Agar, a seaweed extract, is a stiff, gelatinous material that is used as a general growth media or diagnostic media where bacterial colony size, shape, and color can be identified.
      d. Media must support bacterial growth requirements.
         (1) Nutrients: Different species require different nutrients such as peptone, salt, blood, carbohydrates, vitamins, and other minerals.
         (2) Temperature: Most bacteria thrive between 15° and 43°C; however, most human pathogens prefer normal body temperature (37°C).
         (3) Oxygen: Depending on the species, bacteria require differing levels of oxygen.
         (4) pH: Most bacteria thrive between a pH of 3 to 9; however, most human pathogens prefer a neutral pH (7). Substances such as blood, milk, and seawater that are neutral and resist significant changes in pH are often good media constituents.
         (5) Sterile: The media must be sterile and not contaminated.
         (6) Moisture: Most bacteria require some level of moisture.
      e. Media classifications
         (1) Supportive: Media that allow most bacteria to grow at a normal rate without any one species having an advantage.

(2) Selective: Media that inhibit the growth of some species but not others; are especially useful for specimens that have a variety of normal flora, such as fecal or throat specimens.

(3) Enrichment: Media that permit one organism to grow and inhibit all others.

(4) Differential: Media that contain substances such as a dye that gives organisms a distinctive, easily recognizable characteristic.

2. Common culture media

a. Tryptocase soy broth (TSB): General, all-purpose broth allowing most bacteria to grow well including anaerobes. Contains dextrose, peptone, salt, water, and a little agar.

b. Thioglycolate broth (Thio): Broth designed to grow anaerobes.

c. Blood agar (BAP): Supportive media used for primary plating. Good media for suspected *Staphylococcus* and *Streptococcus* because it demonstrates hemolysis. Contains sheep's blood.

d. Eosin-methylene blue (EMB): Selective medium that promotes gram-negative organisms while inhibiting gram-positive organisms. Some bacteria have a characteristic morphology on EMB.

e. MacConkey (Mac): Selective medium that inhibits gram-positive and most nonpathogenic gram-negative bacteria; especially used to culture urine to diagnose UTI. As a differential medium it gives rise to specific morphological characteristics depending on the species. Often used interchangeably with EMB.

f. Phenylethyl alcohol agar (PEA): Selective medium that promotes gram-positive bacteria while inhibiting gram-negative bacteria except *P. aeruginosa*. Contains sheep's blood with phenylethyl alcohol.

g. Chocolate agar (Choc): Rich medium of denatured blood and increased moisture used for fastidious organisms such as *Neisseria* and *Haemophilus influenzae*.

h. Thayer-Martin agar (TM): Enrichment medium that is selective for *N. gonorrhoeae* and *N. meningitidis*.

i. *Salmonella-Shigella* agar (SS): Selective for *Salmonella* and *Shigella* species.

j. Mueller-Hinton agar (MH): Selective for *Neisseria*, it is often used for sensitivity testing.

3. Procedure for streaking culture plates: Method of culturing bacterial specimens to isolate individual colonies for differential identification (see Figure 20-18A).

a. Collect the specimen or load a sterile inoculating loop with the specimen or isolate.

b. Primary streak: Rub the collected specimen using a swab or inoculating loop over one-fourth of the plate, starting at the edge and using a scribbling motion. Be careful not to apply too much pressure, to prevent gouging the agar.

c. Secondary streak: Flame or sterilize the inoculating loop and let it cool for a few seconds. Turn the plate in your hand counterclockwise (if right-handed) about 45 degrees; using the same scribbling motion, touch the primary streak with the inoculating loop three times as you draw out the streak to cover about one-quarter of the plate.

d. Tertiary streak: Flame and cool the inoculating loop as before. Turn the plate another 45 degrees and prepare a third streak just as you did the secondary streak.

e. Quaternary streak: Complete the fourth streak as you did the secondary and tertiary streaks. After touching the tertiary streak for the third time, streak the remaining

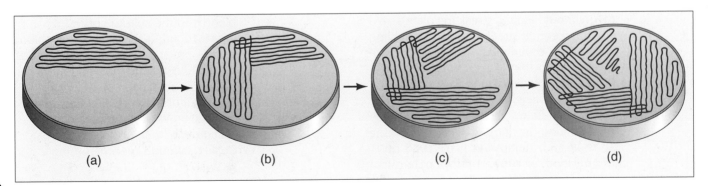

(a)   (b)   (c)   (d)

Figure 20-18A

Streaking an agar plate for isolation. Delmar/Cengage Learning.

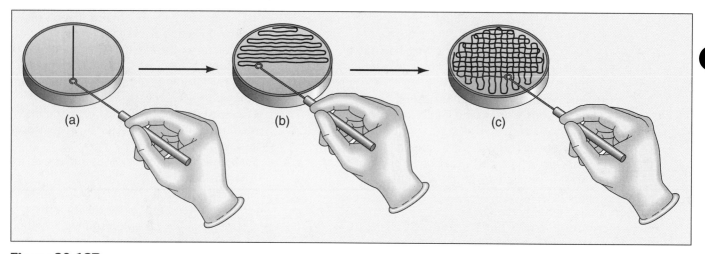

Figure 20-18B

Streaking a urine culture plate for colony count. Delmar/Cengage Learning.

unstreaked portion of the plate, being cautious not to touch any of the other streaks.

f. Flame the loop and properly incubate the culture plate.

4. Collection and cultivation of bacteriological specimens.

a. Throat culture
   (1) A sterile dacron or polyester swab is used to swab the posterior pharyngeal and tonsillar area.
   (2) If transport to the lab will be delayed, use a transport media.
   (3) Culture by streaking a blood agar plate (BAP).

b. Urine culture (see Figure 20-18B)
   (1) Collect a clean-catch, midstream urine in a sterile specimen container.
   (2) Dip a sterile calibrated loop (.01 or .001 mL) into the urine after it has been well mixed.
   (3) Touch the loop at the top center of the plate and draw the loop down the center to the bottom of the plate.
   (4) Without flaming, streak the plate across the central streak using a scribbling motion covering the entire plate from top to bottom.
   (5) Streak both a BAP and EMB or Mac.
   (6) Incubate at 37°C for 24 to 48 hours.
   (7) A quantitative result is determined by counting the number of colonies on the BAP and multiplying it by 1000 (.001 mL loop) or 100 (.01 mL loop) to calculate the number of colony-forming units (CFU) per milliliter of urine.
   (8) A 100,000 CFU/mL of urine is clinically significant for UTI in asymptomatic patients;

whereas a 1000 CFU/mL is clinically significant for symptomatic patients.

c. Genitourinary culture (see Figure 20-18C)
   (1) Collect a cervical or urethral specimen using a swab.
   (2) Roll the swab over the plate in a Z or W pattern.
   (3) Streak across the Z or W pattern using a sterile inoculating loop.
   (4) Incubate anaerobically at 37°C for 24 to 48 hours.
   (5) Streak both a Choc and TM.

d. Blood culture
   (1) Cleanse the tops of the culture bottles with iodine solution.
   (2) Select the phlebotomy site and vigorously cleanse with 75% alcohol in a circle 5 mm in diameter.
   (3) Apply 2% iodine solution in a concentric fashion over the phlebotomy site and let dry for 1 minute.
   (4) Insert the needle into the vein and withdraw approximately 20 mL of blood.
   (5) Change the needle before injecting the blood into the culture bottles.
   (6) Inject 10 mL into each of two blood culture broth preparation bottles. One is used to culture aerobic and the other, anaerobic bacteria.
   (7) Blood cultures are usually repeated two or three times over a timed interval.

e. Wound culture
   (1) Collect a wound specimen using a sterile swab.
   (2) Streak both a BAP and Mac.
   (3) Deep wounds are probably infected by anaerobic bacteria and require special handling.

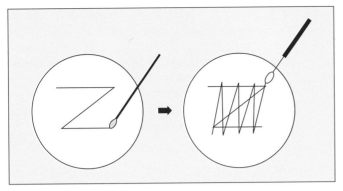

Figure 20-18C

Cross-streaking the Thayer-Martin genitourinary plate culture.
Delmar/Cengage Learning.

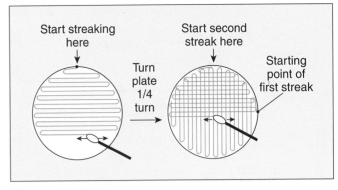

Figure 20-18D

Streaking the Mueller-Hinton plate for disc diffusion susceptibility testing. Delmar/Cengage Learning.

f. Fecal culture
  (1) Collect a fecal sample in a clean container.
  (2) Streak a BAP, Mac, one other selective media, and a broth.
g. Disc diffusion susceptibility testing (sensitivity culture) (see Figure 20-18D).
  (1) Once an infective agent has been identified, a suspension of the agent is prepared.
  (2) An agar plate, usually Mueller-Hinton, is inoculated with the pure suspension of the microorganism.
  (3) Following inoculation of the plate, paper discs containing specified quantities of antimicrobial agents are applied to the agar surface.
  (4) The agents diffuse into the agar; when an agent is effective, inhibition of bacterial growth occurs.
  (5) Following a specified period of incubation, the zone(s) of inhibition is measured and reported in reference to effectiveness of the antibiotics tested (see Figure 20-19). Areas where growth in prevented (zone of inhibition) by the antibiotic demonstrate that the microorganism is susceptible to that antibiotic; growth occurring up to the disc (no zone of inhibition) shows that the microorganism displays a resistance to that antibiotic, thus being ineffective against the infection.
h. Minimum inhibitory concentration (MIC)
  (1) Alternative approach to disc diffusion susceptibility testing; expensive, automated, and can be time-consuming.
  (2) Defined as the lowest concentration of an antimicrobial agent that will prevent visible growth of a microorganism.

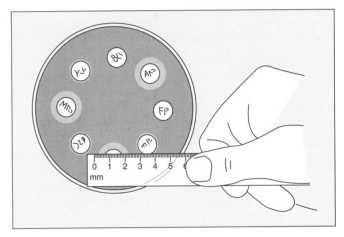

Figure 20-19

Susceptibility culture, measuring zones of inhibition to the antibiotic discs. Delmar/Cengage Learning.

  (3) Organism is exposed to various dilutions of said agents and incubated; following incubation, culture medium is inspected for identification of lowest dose of an agent for which no growth is visible.
  (4) Method that may help in cost-effectiveness for prescription antibiotics in ambulatory and in-patient health care settings.
G. Bacterial control
  1. Bactericides: Agents that destroy bacteria.
  2. Bacteriostats: Agents that inhibit bacterial growth.
  3. Sterilization: Destruction of all microorganisms.
  4. Physical agents of destruction
    a. Cold: Generally has a bacteriostatic effect.
    b. Drying: Some bacteria can resist prolonged drying and are only bacteriostatic.
    c. Lyophilization: Freeze-drying; often useful for food and biologicals.
    d. Ultraviolet radiation: Bacteriocidal effect on airborne and surface microbes.

e. High energy radiation: Beta, gamma, and X-rays are bacteriocidal.
f. Heat: Most effective bacteriocidal.
  (1) Flame.
  (2) Incineration.
  (3) Dry oven: Sterilizes glassware.
  (4) Boiling water.
  (5) Autoclave: Stream under pressure.
g. Filtration: Using microscopically porous material to collect bacteria.
h. Ultrasound: Using sound waves to destroy bacteria.

5. Chemical agents of destruction
a. Disinfectants: Surface bacteriocide.
b. Germicides: Skin bacteriocide.
c. Bactericide: Antibiotics taken internally.

XVII. MYCOLOGY

A. General
  1. Mycology is the study of fungi: Microscopic plantlike organisms having a eukaryotic cellular structure and no chlorophyll.
  2. All fungi reproduce asexually, but some can reproduce sexually.
  3. Fungi are gram-positive and resistant to bacterial antibiotics.
  4. Fungi can be either saprophytic (thrive on decaying or dead matter) or parasitic (thrive on living matter).
  5. Medical mycology includes two fungal forms, molds and yeast.
    a. Yeast: Unicellular microorganisms that multiply by budding. On culture media, yeast produce moist, creamy, opaque, or pasty colonies.
    b. Mold (filamentous fungi): Multicellular microorganisms that are composed of hyphae. On culture media, molds produce fluffy, cottony, wooly, or powdery colonies.
  6. Classification of clinically significant fungi
    a. Cutaneous mycoses: Superficial fungal infections of the hair, skin, or nails, typically the dermatophytes.
    b. Subcutaneous mycoses: Fungal infections confined to the subcutaneous layers.
    c. Systemic mycoses: Widespread infections especially involving the lungs and internal organs.
    d. Opportunistic mycoses: Fungal infections resulting from immune disorders.
B. Basic fungal anatomy
  1. Hyphae: Long, tubelike filamentous structures appearing similar to tree branches.
  2. Septa: Divisions along the hyphae that appear similar to tree-branch joints.
  3. Mycelium: Mass of hyphae.
    a. Rhizoids (vegetative mycelium): Root-like hyphae masses buried in the culture medium.
    b. Aerial mycelium: Hyphae masses suspended above the medium.
  4. Conidia: Asexual spores produced by fungi.
    a. Arthroconidia: Spores produced by septation from the tips of aerial hyphae of molds.
    b. Blastoconidia: Spores produced by budding of yeast.
C. Common pathogenic fungi
  1. Dermatophytes: Collection of genera, especially the three noted, that typically cause cutaneous fungal infections.
    a. *Trichophyton:* Causes various forms of tinea (ringworm and athlete's foot). The most common types in the United States are:
      (1) *T. rubrum.*
      (2) *T. mentagrophytes.*
    b. *Microsporum:* Transmitted by humans and animals, causing ringworm.
      (1) *M. audovinii:* Transmitted by humans.
      (2) *M. canis:* Transmitted by dogs and cats.
      (3) *M. gypseum:* Transmitted by humans and animals.
    c. *Epidermophyton floccosum.*
  2. Yeast
    a. *Candida albicans:* Normal flora of the bowel and skin, it is a dimorphic yeast that causes opportunistic or systemic infections; most commonly causing thrush, vulvovaginitis, endocarditis, and meningitis.
    b. *Cryptococcus neoformans:* A yeast that has been isolated from soil and pigeon droppings that is usually implicated in systemic infections such as meningitis and encephalitis.
  3. Opportunistic fungi: Fungi that are generally non-pathogenic, but among debilitated or immuno-suppressed patients may become pathogenic.
    a. *Aspergillus fumigatus:* Commonly affects the ears, skin, and respiratory tract.
    b. *Penicillium notatum:* Commonly used to make penicillin; can cause pulmonary infections, ear infections, and UTI.
    c. *Phycomycetes mucor:* Commonly causes opportunistic infections among poorly controlled diabetics.
D. Mycological identification methods
  1. Common media
    a. Sabouraud agar with chloramphenicol (SAB): Selective media that promotes fungal growth while inhibiting bacteria. Always incubate at room temperature.
    b. Sabhi medium: Contains equal parts of Sabouraud and brain infusion agar to culture clinically significant fungi and bacteria.

2. KOH preparation: Identification of fungal elements in tissues and fluids.
    a. Place specimen on a glass slide.
    b. Flood the slide with 10% potassium hydroxide (KOH) and coverslip.
    c. Allow specimen to sit for 20 minutes to clear viscosity. Warming may dissipate viscosity.
    d. Observe microscopically under low power.
3. India ink preparation: Identification of capsular material of *C. neoformans* in body fluid.
    a. A drop of body fluid is mixed with a drop of India ink on a slide and coverslip and observed microscopically under low and high power for cells having a clear halo surrounded by a dark background created by the ink.

XVIII. VIROLOGY

A. General
    1. Viruses are microscopic intracellular parasites that require host cells to carry out their metabolic functions and reproductive activities.
    2. Comprising only nucleic acid (RNA or DNA) and a protective protein layer, viruses do not have a cellular structure.
    3. The protein layer determines what sort of cell the virus will parasitize.
    4. Replication process
        a. Attachment: The virus attaches itself to a cell wall such as a lymphocyte or monocyte.
        b. Penetration: The virus produces a lysozyme that dissolves part of the cell wall, allowing the virus to penetrate it.
        c. Uncoating: The virus injects its nucleic acid into the cell, leaving the protective protein layer behind.
        d. Replication: The viral DNA takes control of the cell's biochemical processes to synthesize only viral DNA and protein coats.
        e. Maturation: Viral replication occurs rapidly.
        f. Release: Near the end of viral maturation, lysozymes burst open the cell to release new viruses in search of other cells to repeat the process.
B. Common viruses
    1. Picornavirus: Small viruses containing RNA.
        a. Poliomyelitis: Causes polio.
        b. Coxsackie virus: Causes herpangina, a childhood disease characterized by sore throat, vomiting, and abdominal pain.
        c. Echovirus: Enteric cytopathogenic human orphan virus that causes meningitis and encephalitis.
        d. Rhinovirus: Causes common cold.
        e. Hepatitis A virus (HAV): Causes infectious hepatitis.

2. Arbovirus: Arthropodborne viruses transmitted by insects, ticks, or mites. Causes yellow fever and encephalitis.
3. Myxovirus: Causes influenza.
4. Paramyxovirus: Causes parainfluenza, mumps, and measles (rubeola).
5. Rhabdovirus: Causes rabies.
6. Adenovirus: Causes conjunctivitis and pneumonia.
7. Papovirus: Causes verruca (warts).
8. Herpes virus: Causes herpes simplex, varicella (chicken pox), varicella-zoster (shingles), cytomegalovirus, and Epstein-Barr virus.
C. AIDS virus
    1. General
        a. Caused by the human immunodeficiency virus (HIV).
        b. Causes acquired immune deficiency syndrome, a disease that severely suppresses the immune system, allowing normally nonpathogenic agents to cause opportunistic infections and diseases.
        c. Retrovirus: Caused by a retrovirus or RNA-containing tumor virus that produces DNA from RNA.
        d. Thought to have originated from the bite of an African monkey, then transported to Haiti and then the United States.
        e. HIV can be transmitted by blood, genital secretions (semen, vaginal fluids), breast milk, and umbilical cord from mother to fetus.
        f. High-risk factors: Homosexuality, promiscuity, unprotected sex, and IV drug use.
    2. Signs and symptoms
        a. Prolonged fatigue of unknown etiology.
        b. Persistent fevers and night sweats.
        c. Persistent, unexplained cough.
        d. A thick, opaque coating of the pharynx and tongue.
        e. Easily bruised.
        f. Persistent, purplish lesions of the mucous membranes.
        g. Chronic diarrhea.
        h. Shortness of breath.
        i. Persistent, swollen glands.
        j. Unexplained weight loss.
D. Viral cultures: Generally performed using tissue cultures; beyond the scope of medical assisting practice.

XIX. PARASITOLOGY

A. General
    1. Host/Parasite relationships
        a. Symbiosis: General term describing a dependent relationship between two dissimilar organisms.

b. Parasitism: A symbiotic relationship in which one organism benefits at the expense of the other.

c. Commensalism: A symbiotic relationship in which neither organism is harmed; however, one may benefit.

d. Mutualism: A symbiotic relationship in which both organisms benefit.

e. Neutralism: A symbiotic relationship in which both organisms are neither harmed nor benefited.

f. Antibiosism: Two organisms cannot coexist and one will produce an antibiotic to kill the other.

2. Infection: The invasion of unicellular, microscopic parasites causing disease.

3. Infestation: The internal or external harboring of animal parasites (macroscopic organisms).

4. Basic classification of medical parasites.

a. Protozoans: Unicellular, eukaryotic microorganisms.

   (1) Amoebae: Microorganisms that move by means of pseudopodia.

   (2) Flagellates: Microorganisms that move by means of flagella.

   (3) Ciliates: Microorganisms that move by means of cilia.

   (4) Sporozoans: Microorganisms that have no obvious means of locomotion, but have both sexual and asexual reproductive cycles.

b. Helminths: Wormlike organisms.

   (1) Nematodes: Roundworms.

   (2) Cestodes: Tapeworms.

   (3) Trematodes: Flukes (flat, leaf-shaped organisms).

c. Arthropods: Organisms with an exoskeleton and jointed appendages.

   (1) Crustacea: Crabs, shrimp, and crayfish.

   (2) Insects: Flies, fleas, mosquitoes, lice.

   (3) Arachnids: Ticks and mites.

B. Protozoans (see Figures 20-20A to C)

1. Forms: Protozoans have two forms.

a. Trophozoite: Motile, reproductive, feeding stage.

b. Cyst: Nonmotile, nonfeeding stage.

2. Transmission

a. Usually occurs by ingestion of the infective cysts in fecally contaminated food or water.

b. Once ingested they excyst, becoming trophozoites and multiply in the lower intestine.

3. Amoeba: *Entamoeba hystolytica*: Causes amebic dysentery.

4. Intestinal flagellates

a. *Giardia lamblia:* Causes traveler's diarrhea.

b. *Dientamoeba fragilis.*

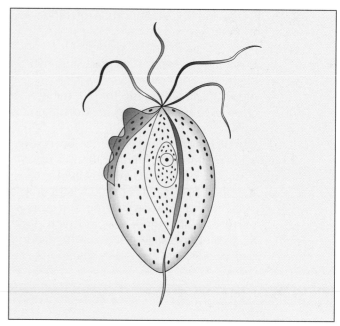

Figure 20-20A

Trichomonas vaginalis. Delmar/Cengage Learning.

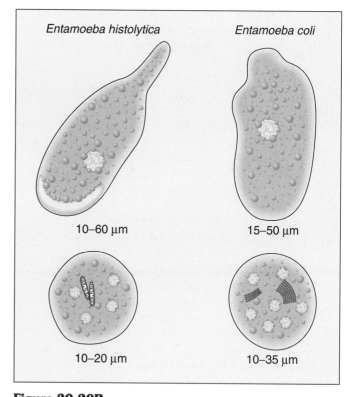

Figure 20-20B

Intestinal amoebae. Delmar/Cengage Learning.

5. Vaginal flagellate: *Trichomonas vaginalis* causes parasitic vaginitis.

6. Hemoflagellates

a. *Trypanosoma*

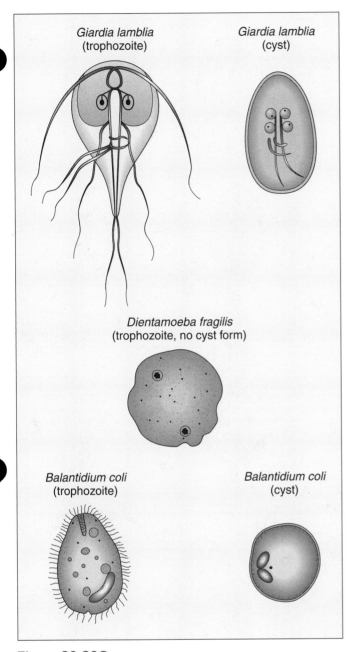

Figure 20-20C

Intestinal ciliates and flagellates. Delmar/Cengage Learning.

(1) *T. rhodesiense:* Causes East African sleeping sickness.
(2) *T. gambiense:* Causes West African sleeping sickness.
(3) *T. cruzi:* Causes Chagas' disease.
  b. *Leishmania*
(1) *L. tropica:* Causes oriental sore.
(2) *L. mexicana:* Causes New World cutaneous leishmaniasis.
(3) *L. braziliensis:* Causes New World leishmaniasis.

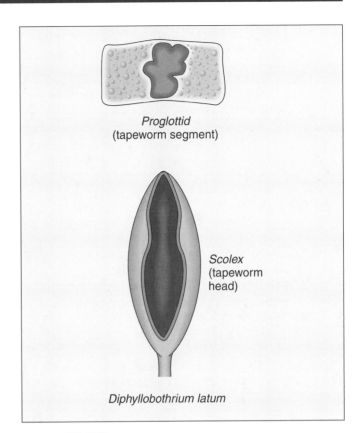

Figure 20-20D

Morphology of D. latum. Delmar/Cengage Learning.

(4) *L. donovani:* Causes Kala azar or deumdum fever.
  7. Ciliate: *Balantidium coli:* Largest protozoan and only pathogenic ciliate; causes balantidial dysentery.
  8. Sporozoans
    a. *Plasmodium:* Causes malaria.
(1) *P. vivax:* Causes benign tertian malaria.
(2) *P. falciparum:* Causes malignant tertian malaria.
(3) *P. malariae:* Causes quarten malaria.
(4) *P. ovale:* Causes ovale malaria.
    b. *Toxoplasma gondii:* Causes toxoplasmosis.
    c. *Pneumocystis carinii:* Causes parasitic pneumonia, especially among AIDS patients.
  C. Helminths: Parasitic wormlike organisms (see Figures 20-20D and E).
    1. Nematodes: Roundworms.
      a. *Enterobius vermicularis:* Causes pinworm infections.
      b. *Trichuris trichiura:* Causes whipworm infections.
      c. *Ascaris lumbricoides:* Large intestinal roundworm.
      d. *Trichinella spiralis:* Trichina worm infection.
      e. *Necator americanus:* New World hookworm disease.

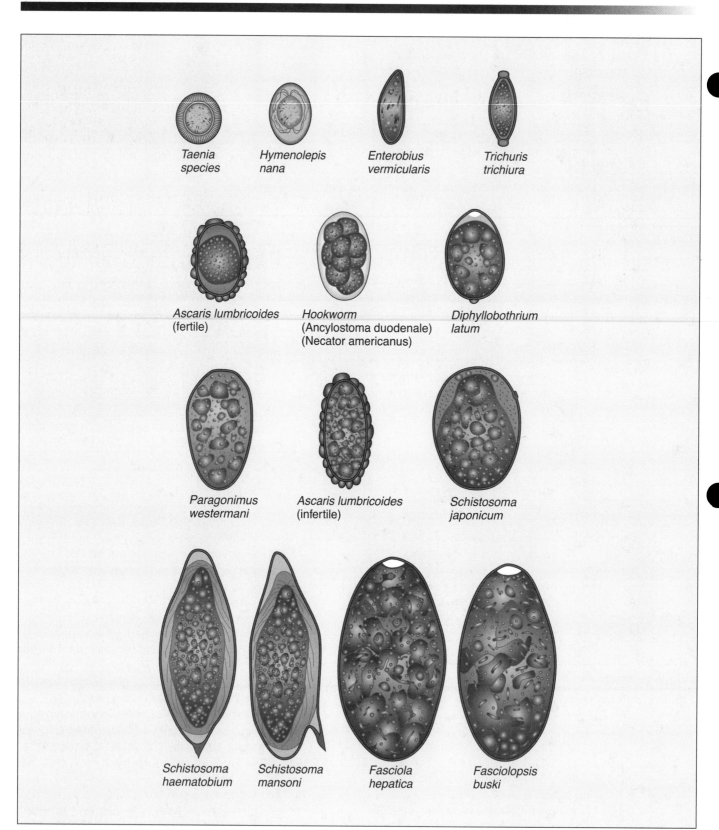

Figure 20-20E

Helminth eggs. Delmar/Cengage Learning.

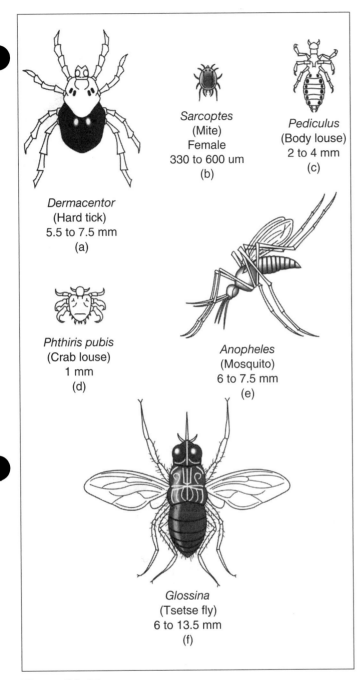

Figure 20-21

Significant arthropods. Delmar/Cengage Learning.

Within the figure:

Dermacentor
(Hard tick)
5.5 to 7.5 mm
(a)

Sarcoptes
(Mite)
Female
330 to 600 um
(b)

Pediculus
(Body louse)
2 to 4 mm
(c)

Phthiris pubis
(Crab louse)
1 mm
(d)

Anopheles
(Mosquito)
6 to 7.5 mm
(e)

Glossina
(Tsetse fly)
6 to 13.5 mm
(f)

  f. *Ancylostoma duodenale:* Old World hookworm disease.
  g. *Strongyloides stercoralis:* Threadworm disease.
  h. *Dracunculus medinensis:* Guinea worm disease.
 2. Cestodes: Tapeworms.
  a. *Hymenolepis nana:* Dwarf tapeworm disease.
  b. *Taenia saginata:* Beef tapeworm disease.
  c. *Taenia solium:* Pork tapeworm disease.
  d. *Diphyllobothrium latum:* Broad tapeworm disease.

  e. *Echinococcus granulosus:* Dog tapeworm disease.
 3. Trematodes: Flukes.
  a. Intestinal flukes
   (1) *Fasciolopsis buski:* Large intestinal fluke.
   (2) *Fasciola hepatica:* Sheep liver fluke.
   (3) *Clonorchis sinensis:* Chinese liver fluke.
   (4) *Paragonimus westermani:* Oriental lung fluke.
  b. Blood flukes
   (1) *Schistosoma mansoni:* Manson's blood fluke.
   (2) *Schistosoma japonicum:* Blood fluke.
   (3) *Schistosoma haematobium:* Bladder fluke.
D. Arthropods: Organisms that serve as a vector for parasitic diseases or as an intermediate host (see Figure 20-21).
 1. Crustaceans: Marine arthropods.
  a. *Cyclops spp:* Tiny crustacean that is an intermediate host for *D. latum* and *D. medinensis.*
  b. Crabs/crayfish: Intermediate host for *P. westermani.*
 2. Insects
  a. Lice: *Pediculus spp.* causes head and body lice. *Phthirus pubis* causes pubic (crab) lice.
  b. Fleas: *Xenopsylla cheopis* transmits plague (*Y. pestis*).
  c. Flies/gnats:
   (1) *Glossina spp.* (Tsetse fly) transmits trypanosomiasis.
   (2) *Phlebotomus spp.* transmits leishmaniasis.
  d. Mosquitoes: *Anopheles spp.* transmits malaria.
 3. Arachnids
  a. Mites: *Liponyssoides spp.* transmits rickettsia. *Sarcoptes scabiei* (itch mite) causes scabies.
  b. Ticks: *Dermacentor spp.* transmits rickettsia.
E. Diagnostic procedures
 1. Scotch-tape preparation: For diagnosing pinworm (*Enterobius vermicularis*).
  a. As the adult female lays her eggs on the area surrounding the anus during resting hours, the best time to collect the specimen is early in the morning before the patient bathes or sometime during the night.
  b. Use either a commercially prepared specimen collector or affix a piece of cellophane tape onto the end of a slide and drape it over the slide so that the adhesive side faces outward.
  c. Gently touch the anus and surrounding area with the adhesive side of the tape.
  d. Undrape the tape and adhere it onto the slide; label the slide; wash hands.
  e. Transport the slide to the clinic or laboratory for examination.

f. The technician will view the slide under 10x and 40×, observing for the distinctively shaped ova.

2. Ova and parasite (O&P): Fecal examination for parasites and/or their ova.

   a. Instruct the patient to collect a fecal sample in the clean dry container provided. Do not allow the feces to touch any liquid such as water or urine.

   b. Using a spatula, scoop out the appropriate amount of fecal material and place it in the commercially prepared specimen containers as directed; label the specimens; wash hands.

   c. Transport the specimens to the laboratory for analysis.

   d. Explain to the patient that a total of three specimens over a 3-day period will probably have to be collected for proper analysis.

CHAPTER 21

Nutrition and Diet Therapy

I. INTRODUCTION

A. General
1. Nutrition is considered an integral part of patient care, along with the physical, social, psychiatric, and economic aspects.
2. Although health may be restored without medicine, it cannot be maintained without proper nutrition.
3. Nutrients: Food elements that supply energy and material needed for normal cellular activity.
4. Recommended dietary allowances (RDA): RDAs are the levels of intake of essential nutrients that are judged by the Food and Nutrition Board to be adequate to meet the known nutrient needs of practically all healthy persons.

B. Dietary guidelines for Americans (2005).
1. Consume adequate nutrients within calorie needs: Adopt a balanced eating pattern that includes nutrient-dense foods among the basic food groups; limit selected fats, cholesterol, sugars, salt, and alcohol.
2. Weight management: Maintain body weight in a healthy range.
3. Physical activity: Engage in regular physical activity and reduce sedentary activities.
4. Food groups to encourage: Consume sufficient amounts of fruits, vegetables, whole-grain products, and low-fat milk products.
5. Fats: Limit intake of fats and oils high in saturated and trans fatty acids.
6. Carbohydrates: Consume fiber-rich fruits, vegetables, and whole grains; restrict added sugars and caloric sweeteners.
7. Sodium and potassium: Consume foods with little sodium (less than 1 tsp—2300 mg); consume potassium-rich foods.
8. Alcoholic beverages: Those who consume alcohol safely should restrict daily consumption to 1 or 2 drinks.
9. Food safety: Cleanliness of hands and food processing surfaces; cook to a safe temperature; chill and defrost foods properly; avoid raw and unpasteurized foods.

C. Food pyramid (MyPyramid): (see Figure 21-1)
D. Vegetarian diets
1. Lacto-ovo vegetarian: Plant foods are supplemented with dairy products and eggs. Most common type of vegetarian diet.
2. Lacto-vegetarian: Dairy products are included, but eggs are not.
3. Total vegetarian (vegan): Animal food sources (including both eggs and dairy products) are completely excluded. For this reason, this diet is low or inadequate in iodine, vitamin B_{12}, iron, calcium, zinc, riboflavin, and vitamin D.

E. Metabolism: A general term covering all physical and chemical changes that food nutrients undergo after their absorption from the gastrointestinal tract.
1. Anabolism: Constructive process of building up new substances.
2. Catabolism: Destructive process of breaking down substances resulting in the release of energy.
3. Basal metabolism: The amount of energy required to sustain normal processes. On the average, basal metabolism requires 1200 to 1400 kilocalories daily for women, and 1600 to 1800 kilocalories daily for men.
4. Regulated primarily through the thyroid gland.

F. Calorie: Unit of heat.
1. calorie (small c): Describes the amount of energy required to heat 1 g of water 1 degree Celsius.
2. Calorie (capital C or kilocalorie): The amount of energy required to heat 1 kg (1000 g) of water 1 degree Celsius.

G. Enrichment: Replacing nutritional elements lost during the processing of food.

H. Fortification: Process of adding nutrients in higher amounts than naturally provided or others generally not present.

I. Nutritional elements:
1. Carbohydrates
2. Proteins
3. Fats
4. Vitamins
5. Minerals
6. Water

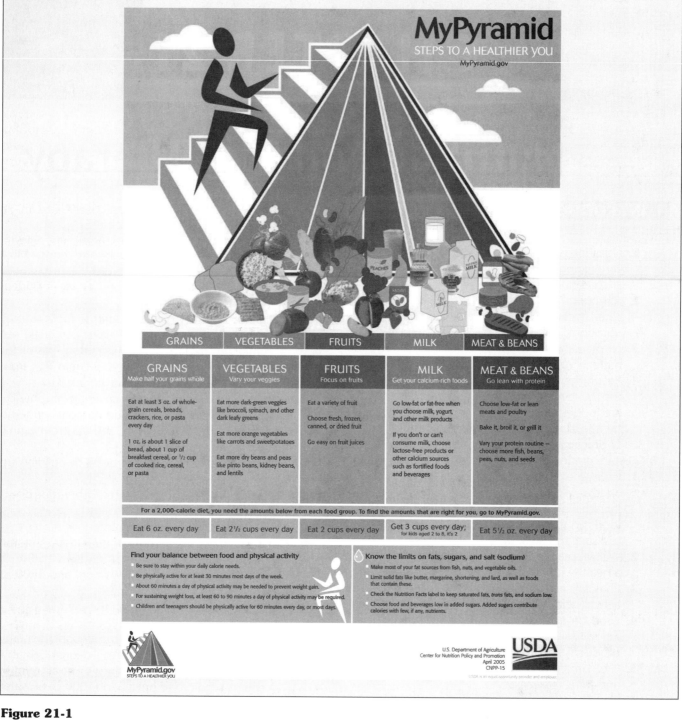

Figure 21-1

The U.S. Department of Agriculture's food pyramid, MyPyramid. Courtesy of the Department of Agriculture.

II. CARBOHYDRATES

A. Mostly plant products in origin; composed of the elements carbon, hydrogen, and oxygen.

B. Grains and grain products, fruits, vegetables, legumes, sugars, and syrups are the chief sources of carbohydrates in the average diet.

C. One gram yields 4 kilocalories of energy.

D. Function: Primarily to meet the body's specific needs for energy.

1. Spare the burning of protein for energy (protein has more important functions).

2. Aid in the more efficient and complete oxidation (burning) of fats for energy.

3. As dietary fiber (insoluble and indigestible), it aids in the normal functioning of the intestines. Soluble forms are believed to lower serum cholesterol levels and control blood glucose levels. Insoluble forms provide bulk for water absorption and regularity.

III. PROTEINS

A. Composed of amino acid links that are made up of carbon, hydrogen, oxygen, and nitrogen.
B. Can also be broken down and stripped of its nitrogen to be used as an energy source.
C. Essential amino acids: Twenty-two amino acids are known to be necessary. Most of them can be synthesized by the human body; however, there are nine amino acids that cannot be synthesized and must be obtained from the diet: Histidine, isoleucine, leucine, valine, lysine, methionine, phenylalanine, threonine, and tryptophan.
D. Functions
1. Repairs and replaces worn-out tissue.
2. Essential for growth, supplying material for tissue building.
3. Supplies some energy (4 kilocalories/g), but is not as efficient as carbohydrates and fats.
4. Essential to the construction and function of important body compounds such as enzymes, hormones, hemoglobin, antibodies, other blood proteins, and glandular secretions.
E. Humans must get their protein preformed from plants and animals.
1. Animal sources: Milk, cheese, eggs, meat, fish, and poultry. The protein found in these foods provides all of the essential amino acids; however, these sources tend to be high in fat and cholesterol.
2. Plant sources: Beans, lentils and other legumes, breads and cereals, and nuts and seeds. Protein from these sources must be complemented either with another plant protein or with an animal protein.
F. Biological value: Describes the degree to which a particular protein contains all amino acids needed by the body. A complete protein contains all of the essential amino acids, whereas an incomplete protein lacks some.
1. Animal sources of protein have high biological value.
2. Plants must be consumed in combinations to achieve complete proteins. For example, corn and beans together provide a complete protein because beans provide the lusine that corn lacks, and corn provides the methionine that beans lack. Lentils complement rice and peanut butter complements bread.

IV. FATS

A. Lipids: Fats, oils, and fatlike substances that are insoluble in water.
a. Oils: Lipids that are of a liquid consistency at room temperature.
b. Fats: Lipids that are solid at room temperature.

B. Composed of carbon, hydrogen, and oxygen.
C. One gram yields 9 kilocalories of energy.
D. Classified according to hydrogen concentration.
1. Saturated: Fatty acids with the most hydrogen atoms; mostly from animal sources.
2. Polyunsaturated: Fatty acids with the least hydrogen atoms; mostly from plant sources.
E. Essential fatty acids: Necessary for the nutritional well-being of all animals. The principal ones for humans are linoleic and arachidonic acid. Essential fatty acids are not synthesized in the body and must be supplied by food.
F. Common sources
1. Animal sources: Milk, butter, cheese, lard, meat, and eggs.
2. Plant sources: Vegetable oils, margarine, chocolate, nuts, olives, and avocados.
G. Functions
1. Energy: The primary function of fat is to serve as a concentrated source of heat and energy.
2. Furnish essential fatty acids.
3. Spare burning of protein for energy.
4. Add flavor and palatability to the diet.
5. Give satiety value to the diet (fat slows the digestive process and retards the development of hunger).
6. Promotes absorption of fat-soluble vitamins A, D, E, K.
7. Insulates and protects organs and nerves.
8. Lubricates the intestinal tract.
9. Cholesterol has an essential role in the structure of sex and adrenal hormones and is converted to vitamin D by the action of ultraviolet light on the skin.
H. Good fat: Polyunsaturated and monounsaturated fats, and high-density lipoproteins (HDL).
I. Bad fat: Cholesterol, saturated fat, low-density lipoprotein (LDL) and very low-density lipoprotein (VLDL); however, neither should be consumed freely, because the total fat intake should be less than 30% of the total kilocalories consumed.

V. VITAMINS

A. Natural forms of vitamins in food are far superior to vitamin pill technology.
B. Only individuals with conditions that increase vitamin and mineral needs or impair the absorption and utilization of these essential nutrients need worry about supplements.
C. Vitamins are needed by the body in only minute amounts for proper growth and development. Some may be synthesized in the body, but most must be supplied in the daily diet.
D. Vitamins, although organic in nature, do not provide energy, but act as catalysts for efficient metabolism.

E. Vitamins serve a regulatory function.
1. They regulate the synthesis of many body compounds such as bones, skin, glands, nerves, brain, and blood.
2. They participate in the metabolism of protein, carbohydrates, and fats.

F. Fat-soluble vitamins
1. Vitamins A, D, E, and K. The absorption of fat-soluble vitamins is enhanced with dietary fat.
2. Vitamin A (retinoic acid)
   a. Source: Deep orange and dark green, leafy vegetables, fruits, milk fat, and egg yolks.
   b. Deficiency: Nyctalopia, keratinosis.
   c. Toxicity: Anorexia, hair loss, arthralgia, organomegaly.
3. Vitamin D (cholecalciferol)
   a. Source: Fortified in milk because it enhances the absorption of calcium. Sunlight exposure stimulates vitamin D production.
   b. Deficiency: Rickets, osteomalacia.
   c. Toxicity: Soft-tissue calcification, nephrolithiasis.
4. Vitamin E (tocopherol): Identified as a potent antioxidant that helps to rid the body of free radicals. Free radicals are natural by-products of the body's metabolism that can ultimately damage healthy cells if not kept under control. Although there are no known toxic effects of Vitamin E, there is also no medical justification for the use of large doses, particularly because it is widely distributed in common foods.
5. Vitamin K (menadione): Essential for blood coagulation.
   a. Source: Green, leafy vegetables, soybean, cauliflower; also synthesized by bacteria in the intestine.
   b. Deficiency: Hemorrhage.
   c. Toxicity: Hemolytic anemia, hepatopathies.

G. Water-soluble vitamins
1. Vitamin B complex and vitamin C (ascorbic acid). A regular daily supply is needed as these vitamins are not stored to any great degree, and excess intake is often eliminated in the urine.
2. Twelve factors in the vitamin B complex are recognized today. The RDA has been established for six: thiamine (vitamin B_1), riboflavin (vitamin B_2), niacin (vitamin B_3), vitamins B_6 and B_{12}, and folacin.
   a. Source: Well distributed among plant and animal products.
   b. Deficiency: Anemia, beriberi, pallegra, muscle disorders, glossitis, etc.
   c. Toxicity: Nausea, vomiting, anaphylactic shock, anorexia, ataxia, hypotension, and nervous system disorders.
3. Vitamin C (ascorbic acid): Aids in iron absorption and the formation and maintenance of the intracellular cement substance of body tissue, and is important for tooth dentin, bones, cartilage, connective tissue, and blood vessels.
   a. Source: Citrus fruits and vegetables.
   b. Deficiency: Scurvy, bruising, loose teeth.
   c. Toxicity: Nephrolithiasis.

VI. MINERALS

A. Minerals are elemental inorganic substances that help build the following tissues:
1. Bony tissue: Calcium and phosphorus in bones and teeth, and fluoride in teeth.
2. Soft body tissue (muscles, nerves, glands): All salts, especially phosphorus, potassium, sulfur, and chloride.
3. Hair, nails, skin: Sulfur.
4. Blood: All salts, iron for hemoglobin and copper for RBCs.
5. Glandular secretions: Chlorine in gastric juice, sodium in intestinal juice, iodine in thyroxine, manganese in endocrine secretions, and zinc in enzymes.

B. Regulatory role
1. Fluid pressure: All salts, especially sodium and potassium.
2. Muscle contraction and relaxation: Calcium, potassium, sodium, phosphorus, chlorine.
3. Nerve responses: All salts, with a balance between calcium and sodium.
4. Blood clotting: Calcium.
5. Oxidation in tissue and blood: Iron, iodine.

C. Major minerals: Macrominerals that are present in amounts greater than 5g in the human body.
1. Calcium: Ninety-nine percent of calcium is found in bones and teeth, providing their rigid structure.
   a. Source: Milk products, dark, green leafy vegetables.
   b. Deficiency: Poor bone growth and tooth development, stunted growth, rickets, osteomalacia, osteoporosis in adults, thin and fragile bones, and poor blood clotting.
   c. Toxicity: Nephrolithiasis.
2. Phosphorus: The largest amount of phosphorus is with calcium in the bones and teeth. Phosphorus helps in oxidation of carbohydrates and fats, helps enzymes act in energy metabolism, and aids in maintaining the body's acid-base balance.
   a. Source: Milk, meat, eggs, cheese, dry beans, nuts, and whole-grain cereals.
   b. Deficiency: Anorexia, weakness, stiff joints.
   c. Toxicity: Muscle spasms.
3. Sodium: As an electrolyte it is a key element in the maintenance of fluid and acid-base balance. It transmits nerve impulses, helps control muscle

contractions, and regulates cell permeability. The recommended range for healthy individuals is between 2000 and 4000 mg daily.
   a. Source: Salt, milk, vegetables.
   b. Deficiency: Hyponatremia.
   c. Toxicity: Hypertension, heart and kidney disease.
4. Potassium: Serves a role similar to sodium.
   a. Source: Citrus fruits, bananas, tomatoes, potatoes, meat, and milk.
   b. Deficiency: Arrhythmia, hypertension, renal hypertrophy, muscle cramps.
   c. Toxicity: Cardiac disturbances.
5. Chloride: As an electrolyte, it is involved in the maintenance of fluid and acid-base balance. It provides an acidic medium for activation of gastric enzymes and aids in maintaining osmotic pressure.
   a. Source: Salt, chlorinated water.
   b. Deficiency/toxicity: Acid-base imbalance.
6. Magnesium: Is a component of bones and teeth. It plays a role in metabolic processes and muscle contractions.
   a. Source: Nuts, whole grains, seafoods, coffee, tea, cocoa, and in hard (versus soft) water.
   b. Deficiency: Neuromuscular disturbances.
   c. Toxicity: Paralysis, depressed nervous function.
7. Sulfur: Is a component of skin, hair, nails, cartilage, and some organ tissue. It is a component of all body proteins, along with thiamine and biotin. Unknown deficiency or toxicity.
D. Trace minerals: Microminerals that are found in the human body in amounts less than 5g.
   1. Iron: More than one-half of the 4 to 5g of iron in the body is hemoglobin. About one-third of the body's iron is in the liver, spleen, and bone marrow, and small amounts are found in muscles and in oxidative enzymes in cells.
      a. Source: Organ meats, especially liver.
      b. Deficiency: Anemia.
      c. Toxicity: Cirrhosis, cardiomyopathies.
   2. Iodine: A constituent of the thyroid hormones thyroxine and thyroglobulin. It helps regulate energy metabolism.
      a. Source: Iodized salt, ocean or salt-water fish.
      b. Deficiency: Goiter. Rare toxicity.
   3. Zinc: Is a component of more than 50 enzymes and is essential for normal growth, wound healing, immune function, and cellular differentiation. It also influences taste sensitivity.
      a. Source: High-protein foods, especially oysters and liver, and whole grains.
      b. Deficiency: Depressed immunity, dwarfism.
      c. Toxicity: Anemia, nausea, vomiting.
   4. Copper: Aids in the absorption of iron from the intestinal tract, the production and survival of red blood cells, and is essential to many enzymes.
      a. Source: Dark chocolate, legumes, liver, kidney, nuts, seeds, whole grains, and raisins.
      b. Deficiency: Anemia, nervous system disorders.
      c. Toxicity: Wilson's disease, Huntington's chorea.
   5. Fluoride: This mineral helps in the formation of solid bones and teeth.
      a. Source: Fluoridated water, fish.
      b. Deficiency: Dental caries.
      c. Toxicity: Dental mottling.
E. Miscellaneous trace minerals: The minerals chromium, cobalt, manganese, molybdenum, selenium, nickel, tin, vanadium, and silicone have an important role in enzyme activity, metabolism, and proper organ function.

VII. WATER

A. Principal body constituent: Water aids digestion, absorption, circulation, and excretion. Functions as a solvent for body constituents and as a medium for all chemical changes in the body.
B. Thermal regulation: Participates in the regulation of body temperature.
C. Lubrication: Lubricates the moving parts of the body.
D. Anabolism: Necessary for building and repair processes.
E. Foods contain from 10% to 98% water. It is also formed in the body's metabolic processes and is an end-product of oxidation.
F. Adult requirement: 1 mL/kcalorie, and for infants it is 1.5 ml/kcalorie. Fluid requirements are closely related to salt requirements.

VIII. MATERNAL & INFANT NUTRITION

A. Proper nutrition is critical during the first trimester, when major fetal development occurs.
B. The best pregnancy outcomes occur when women of normal weight gain about 27 lb, women who are underweight gain at least 30 lb, and women who are grossly overweight gain about 15 lb.
C. Clinical problems during pregnancy
   1. Nausea: Eating high-carbohydrate foods, such as dry toast or crackers, before arising may alleviate the problem. Fried foods and other high-fat foods are a common cause of nausea and should be avoided.
   2. Hyperemesis: It can cause serious dehydration and weight loss. Some women respond to vitamin B_6 therapy, but this form of management should be performed under an obstetrician's care.

3. Anemia: Anemia from iron deficiency may occur during pregnancy when iron intake and stores do not meet the demand. Supplements are usually prescribed.

4. Overweight: For obese women, a weight reduction regimen should not be initiated at any time during pregnancy.

5. Pica: Is an abnormal craving for nonfood substances. Laundry starch, clay, and chalk are the most common nonfood cravings during pregnancy.

6. Constipation: Often related to iron supplementation as well as to decreased intestinal motility. Adequate fiber, fluid, and appropriate exercise can help control constipation.

7. Heartburn: Usually due to the pressure of the growing fetus on the stomach, resulting in hydrochloric acid being forced up into the esophagus. It may help to eat more frequent, smaller meals, and to avoid a reclining position after meals.

8. Diabetes: Control of maternal glycemia is important to good fetal outcomes, because fetal death may occur during periods of early-morning hypoglycemia.

D. Lactation: Adequate diet becomes more critical.

1. Kilocalorie intake can affect the quantity of milk produced, and thus is important for a breast-feeding woman to lose any excess weight slowly.

2. Breast milk is an important source of vitamins for the infant.

3. An additional health benefit to the infant from breast milk is increased immunological resistance.

4. Generally about every 2 hours is a good feeding schedule.

E. Solid food: Introducing some solid foods into the infant's diet serves to replenish the depleting stores of iron between 4 and 6 months of age. Solid food should not be given until 4 to 6 months of age.

F. Food restrictions

1. Honey: Honey should not be given because of the potential for botulism, because honey contains botulism spores.

2. Processed food: The high sodium content of some processed foods can be detrimental to the infant's immature kidneys.

3. Hard texture: Hard food or food in large pieces should also be avoided to prevent choking until the infant is old enough to chew adequately.

IX. CHILD TO ADOLESCENT NUTRITION

A. Preschool nutrition

1. As children grow, their eating habits change. These changes are reflective of their stage of development.

a. When compared with the infant, there is a slowing in the rate of growth and development in the preschool child. A decrease in the consumption of food parallels this decrease in metabolic rate.

b. A pattern of strong food preferences and aversions with a general disinterest in food.

c. Erratic desires for food (food jags): Settling on a few foods only to discard them for another pattern of food choices shortly thereafter.

2. The preschool child seems to prefer foods that are simply prepared.

a. Mixed foods are generally unpopular with this age group.

b. Finger foods are well accepted.

c. Different food textures interest children. Each meal might include something soft and easy to chew, something crispy, and something chewy to promote the use of newly learned chewing skills.

3. The child should be offered only small amounts of food at a time. Even giving one bite of each food served, with second or third helping allowed, can stimulate a child's interest in eating, in part because of feelings of accomplishment and control.

4. A child should never be forced to eat.

B. School-age nutrition

1. Meeting the nutritional requirements of the 6- to 12-year-old child requires larger amounts of the same foods needed by the preschool child.

2. Meal patterns are likely to change once school starts. Breakfast may have to be eaten earlier to allow sufficient time to get to school. Children who skip breakfast are less well fed, because it is difficult to make up missed nutrients at other meals.

3. Lunch should supply approximately one-third of the RDA for all nutrients.

C. Adolescent nutrition

1. The need for self-worth and a sense of identity can take priority over good nutritional practices.

2. Barriers to good nutrition

a. Society's emphasis on slimness.

b. Access to jobs and spending money.

c. More time spent away from home.

3. Adolescence is a period of rapid growth and development. Girls tend to grow more rapidly between 12 and 14 years of age, and boys experience this rapid growth between 14 and 16 years of age.

4. Caloric and nutrient needs are higher to provide for increases in bone density, muscle mass, blood volume, and endocrine system development.

5. There is an increased need for calories, calcium, iron, and iodine. Nutrient needs can be met easily by increasing the serving size of foods from the four basic food groups.

X. NUTRITION OF THE ELDERLY

A. The older adult experiences social, physiological, and economic changes that affect nutrition.

B. Decreased BMR: The aging process slows the basal metabolic rate (BMR) and reduces the amount of lean body mass (muscle tissue).

C. Loss of sense acuity
1. Taste: A decrease in the number of taste buds diminishes taste acuity. Older adults may compensate by excessive use of salt and sugar. Seasonings such as herbs, spices, and lemon juice can be recommended as an alternative.
2. Smell, sight, hearing: A reduced ability to hear, see, and detect odors may reduce the enjoyment of the social aspects of eating.
3. Thirst: Sense of thirst diminishes with age. It is important to be aware of the need for fluids to promote the removal of wastes through the gastrointestinal tract and kidneys.

D. Edentulous: Loss of teeth may lead to altered food choices that may decrease the nutritive value of the diet. If refined foodstuffs are eaten instead of raw fruits and vegetables, constipation may become a problem. The fiber content of the diet can be increased by the use of whole-grain breads and cereals, and raw bran may be added to cereals for additional fiber.

E. Calcium deficiency: A woman may lose 20% to 30% of her total skeleton during a 20-year period encompassing menopause. As much as 1500 mg of calcium daily may be needed to maintain calcium balance because of a reduced ability of the body to absorb this nutrient and because vitamin D synthesis in the skin is decreased in elderly individuals.

F. Six small meals a day are often more appropriate than three full-sized meals.

XI. WEIGHT MANAGEMENT

A. Overweight: Excess body weight; if a person's weight is 10% greater than the standard, the person is considered to be overweight.

B. Obesity: Excess body fat. Weight is 20% (or more) greater than the standard weight for height. A more accurate means of determining obesity is by first estimating the percentage of body fat in relation to total weight. Individuals with a body fat content of more than 24% of total body weight for men and 33% for women are considered obese.
1. Generally, obesity occurs as a result of long-term positive energy balance: weight gain occurs when kilocalorie intake exceeds kilocalorie expenditure.
2. A gain of 1 lb of body fat is the result of approximately 3500 kilocalories that have been ingested, but not used. A deficit of 3500 kilocalories must, therefore, be achieved in order to lose 1lb of body fat.
3. Fat cell theory: When the body stores energy in the form of fat, existing fat cells grow larger (hypertrophy), and sometimes new fat cells are created (hyperplasia). Once a fat cell is created it exists for life. Therefore, when an obese person loses weight, fat cells do not disappear, they only shrink. Shrinkage then triggers a strong desire for food; as a result, the individual eats and regains the weight.
4. Set point theory: Each individual has a "natural" weight, which is predetermined by a number of biological factors. Attempts to change weight above the set point are thwarted by various mechanisms in the body. The body defends its set point, even though it may be a weight 10 or 20 lb greater than what is considered ideal.
5. For safe and permanent weight loss, an individual should lose no more than 1 to 2 lb per week. More rapid weight loss will compel the body to use protein for energy instead of fat. This is highly undesirable because it decreases muscle mass and promotes rapid fuel loss.
6. To lose weight at the optimal 1 to 2 lb per week, most women need to consume about 1200 kilocalories per day; men should consume 1500 to 1800 kilocalories per day.
7. Vitamin and mineral supplementation should be ordered when energy intake is less than 1200 kilocalories per day.

C. Food exchange system: A tool often used in reducing caloric intake. It breaks all foods into six separate groups. Foods in the same group have similar proportions of carbohydrate, fat, and protein and about the same number of kilocalories. By allowing a given number of exchanges in each group, a daily diet pattern can be developed that offers the dieter a choice of a variety of foods within the given pattern.

D. Physical activity: Uses the body's energy stores. Activity is also important because it causes more kilocalories to be expended even after the exercise is finished. Physical activity can increase the metabolic rate as much as 10% for as long as 48 hours after the activity ceases. Also, physical activity decreases appetite.

E. Aerobic exercise: Activity that uses large muscle groups in a rhythmic movement over a period of 5 minutes or more. This type of activity tends to use the highest percentage of body fat for fuel, thus promoting the most beneficial weight loss. Brisk walking, bicycle riding, and cross-country skiing are excellent activities.

F. A duration of at least 30 minutes, 3 days per week is needed to promote weight loss. A higher frequency would be even more beneficial.

G. Behavior modification: Principles used to assist obese individuals in identifying the personal eating behaviors that have been promoting weight gain and maintaining obesity.
   1. Food diary: Is kept by the individual to find out what specific factors are triggering unhealthy eating behaviors.
   2. Eat slowly: Take not less than 20 minutes to eat your food to allow time for nerve receptors in the digestive tract to send satiety signals to the brain. Do not take more than 30 minutes to mitigate the temptation to eat more.
      a. Put down your fork between each bite.
      b. Chew and swallow food completely before taking another bite.
   3. Drink water: Drink a glass of water before, during, and after a meal.
   4. Do not clean your plate: Especially when dining out, leave some food on your plate when you finish.
H. Surgical techniques: These techniques have been developed for the morbidly obese person as a last treatment resort. Treatments include gastric bypass, gastric stapling, intestinal bypass, and jaw wiring, which prevents the ingestion of solid foods.
I. Underweight treatment: A high-kilocalorie diet is used to restore and maintain normal weight. Kilocalories in excess of expenditure will result in storage of fatty tissue.

XII. PSYCHOLOGICAL EATING DISORDERS

A. Estimates indicate that 10% to 15% of adolescent girls and young women are affected by anorexia nervosa, and approximately 19% of college women are known to have bulimia.
B. Obsessive dieting, refusal to eat, binging and gorging, purging, fasting, and laxative and diuretic abuse can all lead to malnutrition, electrolyte imbalance, and cardiac arrhythmia, which can result in death.
C. Anorexia nervosa
   1. The person with anorexia nervosa has an intense fear of becoming obese that does not lessen as weight loss progresses.
   2. There is a disturbance of body image, such as claiming to feel fat even when emaciated.
   3. This condition is characterized by a lack of desire to eat resulting from anxiety, irritation, anger, and fear. There is no real loss of appetite, but the person refuses to eat. The syndrome occurs mainly in girls after puberty.
   4. There is a weight loss of at least 25% of original body weight with subsequent amenorrhea.
   5. There is no known physical illness that would account for the weight loss.

6. Dietary treatment:
   a. Plan a diet with the patient that includes a variety of foods from each of the four food groups.
   b. Kilocalories should be increased slowly so that the patient can adjust psychologically to weight gain. Once the goal for weight gain is reached, weight maintenance requires an educational approach with emphasis on moderation, variety, and regularity in eating.
D. Bulimia
   1. This condition is characterized by binge eating followed by purging through self-induced vomiting and abusive use of laxatives. The person is afraid of becoming overweight and is aware that the eating pattern is abnormal.
   2. High-kilocalorie, easily ingested foods are chosen during binge episodes. Fasting then follows, often resulting in a weight fluctuation of as much as 10 lb.
   3. Dietary treatment: Food intake should be restricted to mealtimes, with close supervision after eating to control vomiting. The patient must be counseled on the importance of the need to stop using laxatives and to accept a higher body weight.

XIII. NUTRITION THERAPY

A. The role of food and nutrition in the treatment of various diseases and disorders.
B. Purpose
   1. To maintain or improve nutritional status or deficiencies.
   2. To maintain, decrease, or increase body weight.
   3. To rest certain organs or the whole body.
   4. To eliminate allergic foods.
C. Therapeutic diets may modify the following:
   1. Consistency: Soft, liquid, or parenteral diets for edentulous patients or patients with afflictions that prevent normal chewing, swallowing, or digestion of food.
   2. The energy value (kilocalories) may be increased or decreased.
   3. Fiber (bulk, roughage) may be increased, or decreased.
   4. Specific nutrients may be increased or decreased.
   5. Specific foods or types of foods may be increased or decreased.
D. Diet prescription: Written in terms of energy requirements and the nutritional elements needed to treat the condition. This prescription is translated into foods and meals by the dietitian who, in turn, instructs the patient regarding the diet.

E. Nutritional status assessment
1. Dietary history
    a. Types and frequency of foods the individual eats over a 24-hour period or for an average of 3 to 7 days.
    b. Appetite and weight changes. It is important to note if the patient has lost more than 10 lb within the last 6 months.
    c. Medications and illnesses, especially those involving the gastrointestinal tract, are noted.
    d. Elimination practices.
    e. Cultural and religious food habits.
2. Anthropometry: Body measurements such as size, weight, and proportions.
    a. Triceps skin fold: Index of the body's fat or energy stores. A low skin-fold thickness measurement may indicate malnutrition. The most common site for measuring skin-fold thickness is on the posterior side of the upper arm at the midpoint.
    b. Mid-arm circumference: Measures the level of the body's protein stores, which are found mainly in the muscles. The nondominant arm is flexed at a 90-degree angle and the circumference is measured with a non-stretchable measuring tape at the midpoint of the upper arm.
    c. Elbow breadth: Measures frame size. It is a reliable measurement that changes little with age and is not affected by body fat stores. Calipers are applied to either side of the two prominent bones of the elbow while the forearm is bent upward at a 90-degree angle. The fingers are straight, and the inside of the wrist is turned toward the body.
    d. Body weight.
3. Biochemical and clinical data: Several laboratory tests of the blood, urine, and skin are frequently used in assessing nutritional status.

XIV. METABOLIC DISORDERS

A. Diabetes mellitus
1. Diabetes mellitus is a disorder related to carbohydrate metabolism. Diabetes mellitus primarily is due to a lack of insulin.
2. Complex carbohydrates and fiber are advocated for the control of diabetes and its complications.
3. Etiological classifications
    a. Insulin-dependent diabetes mellitus (IDDM, type 1): Accounts for approximately 10% to 15% of diabetic cases. Onset is usually sudden and severe. Control is usually accomplished through diet and insulin regulation.
        1. Type 1A: Develops during childhood and the young adult years.
        2. Type 1B: Develops in older individuals.
    b. Non–insulin-dependent diabetes melitus (NIDDM, type 2): Comprises the majority of diabetic individuals, most of whom are overweight.
        1. Insulin may be produced in too short a supply for body needs, or it may be produced in normal amounts but meet insulin resistance at receptor sites.
        2. The onset is slow and gradual. It is more stable and can usually be controlled with diet alone or diet plus oral hypoglycemics.
        3. Gestational diabetes: Temporary form of NIDDM that occurs during pregnancy. Diet control focuses on slow but steady weight gain, avoidance of concentrated sugar sources, and frequent small balanced meals.
4. Signs and symptoms
    a. Diabetes mellitis
        1. Hyperglycemia: Elevated blood glucose level occurs because there is not enough insulin to allow glucose to be taken up by the tissue cells for energy.
        2. Glycosuria: Glucose is excreted in the urine when the kidneys exceed their capacity for reabsorption (renal threshold).
        3. Ketonuria: Without insulin, carbohydrates are unavailable for energy utilization. Instead, the body metabolizes fat as an energy source. Ketones are the by-product of fat metabolism that is excreted in the urine.
        4. Dehydration: Excretion of excess glucose and ketones by the kidneys requires more water.
        5. Polydipsia, polyphagia, and polyuria: Increased thirst, hunger, and frequent urination.
        6. Weight loss.
    b. Insulin shock (insulin reaction): Occurs when there is too much insulin from an injection.
        1. It can be the result of omitting foods from the diet, increased activity and exercise, or an error in insulin injection.
        2. Hypoglycemia: Decreased blood glucose level.
        3. Diaphoresis: Profuse perspiration and nervousness.
        4. Shock: Pale, cold, clammy skin.
        5. Disorientation: Mental confusion. If untreated will result in unconsciousness and ultimately death.
    c. Diabetic coma (acidosis, ketoacidosis): Occurs when the body breaks down too much fat for energy needs. This is caused

by insufficient transfer of blood glucose to the cell tissues because of inadequate amounts of insulin.

   1. It can result from an overconsumption of food, an illness, or an error in insulin injection.
   2. Hyperglycemia.
   3. Ketonuria.
   4. Ketoacidosis: Ketones lower blood pH. Causes a fruity breath odor.
   5. Drowsiness, lethargy.
   6. Hot, dry skin.
   7. Deep, labored breathing. Coma and death will occur without insulin and fluids.
5. Nutritional management
   a. Balanced/RDA diet.
   b. Fiber: Lowers blood glucose levels postprandially. A fresh orange, for example, is more beneficial than orange juice. Whole wheat bread would be better than eating white bread.

B. Food allergies: Hypersensitivity to certain food substances called allergens.
   1. Food allergens are usually proteins that cause symptoms involving the skin, nasal passages, and respiratory or gastrointestinal tract.
   2. Common food allergens: Milk, fish, shellfish, nuts, eggs, chocolate, corn, wheat, pork, and legumes (green peas, lima beans, and peanuts) and some fresh fruits, especially peaches and strawberries.

C. Inborn errors of metabolism: Group of diseases generally characterized by an enzyme deficiency requiring the diet to be modified to prevent toxicity from the excessive accumulation of poisonous by-products.
   1. Phenylketonuria (PKU): A lack of the enzyme necessary to metabolize phenylalanine, one of the essential amino acids.
      a. High levels accumulate and cause the excretion of phenylketones in the urine.
      b. When untreated, infants are hyperactive and irritable with an unpleasant personality and a *musty* or gamy odor.
      c. Severe retardation results if treatment is delayed. Requires restriction of milk, meats, bread, etc.
   2. Others include galactosemia, homocystinuria, tyrosinosis, histidinemia, and maple syrup urine disease.

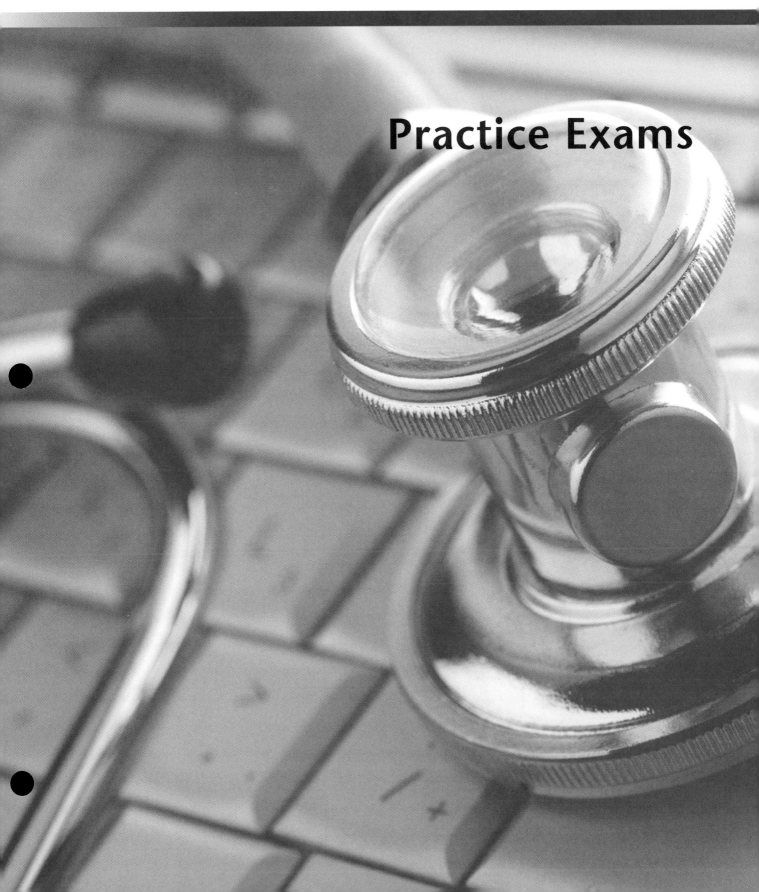

SECTION VI

Practice Exams

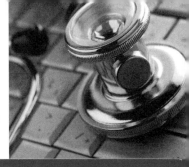

CMA SIMULATION TEST

Post-Test

198-question, 2-hour, 40 minutes timed practice exam

PART 1: GENERAL

1. Which of the following word parts is a suffix?
   a. ante
   b. post
   c. organ/o
   d. itis
   e. stoma

2. In the structural hierarchy of organisms, which of the following immediately precedes the organ level?
   a. organism
   b. systems
   c. tissues
   d. cells
   e. atoms

3. Which of the following is true regarding the principles of growth and development?
   a. They are continuous, orderly, sequential processes.
   b. Humans generally follow the same pattern of growth and develoment
   c. The sequence of each stage is predictable.
   d. Time of onset, length, and effects of each stage are individual.
   e. All of the above

4. A facilitative communication technique that repeats what the patient has said to demonstrate understanding is
   a. accepting
   b. mirroring
   c. clarification
   d. focusing
   e. exploring

5. All of the following are reasons for revocation or suspension of a health care provider's license **EXCEPT**
   a. conviction of a crime
   b. unprofessional conduct
   c. administering atypical treatments
   d. physical incapacity
   e. mental incapacity

6. A standard or principle that guides our behavior regarding what is right and what is wrong is a(n)
   a. norm
   b. moral
   c. morale
   d. ethic
   e. duty

7. Which of the following word parts is a prefix?
   a. pre
   b. cleid/o
   c. osis
   d. rrhea
   e. cephal/o

8. Which of the following tissues consists of neurons?
   a. epithelial
   b. nervous
   c. connective
   d. muscle
   e. glandular

9. Behavioral responses resulting from the conflicts of inner impulses and the anxiety they create best defines:
   a. Defense (adaptive) mechanisms
   b. Personality
   c. Libigo
   d. Ego
   e. Superego

10. All of the following are facilitative communication techniques **EXCEPT**
    a. exploring
    b. clarifying
    c. focusing
    d. advising
    e. accepting

11. Behavior or an action that can be reasonably presumed to be consensual is
    a. express consent
    b. self-determination
    c. informed consent
    d. improper consent
    e. implied consent

12. Telling the truth best defines
    a. beneficence
    b. nonmaleficence
    c. justice
    d. veracity
    e. fidelity

13. Which of the following is an ENT specialist?
    a. otologist
    b. rhinologist
    c. audiologist
    d. ophthalmologist
    e. otorhinolaryngologist

14. Which of the following is considered an appendage of the skin?
    a. dermis
    b. epidermis
    c. subcutaneous
    d. sudoriferous glands
    e. hypodermis

15. The source of energy for satisfying the sexual urges that influence the three levels of personality.
    a. Personality
    b. Libido
    c. Id
    d. Ego
    e. Superego

16. An unconscious defense mechanism characterized by behaving in the opposite way to one's actual feelings is
    a. introjection
    b. projection
    c. reaction formation
    d. sublimation
    e. denial

17. Which of the following may require notification of the appropriate health agencies?
    a. auto accident
    b. roseola
    c. staph infection
    d. strep throat
    e. phenylketonuria

18. Positive character traits are
    a. duties
    b. virtues
    c. justice
    d. ethics
    e. rights

19. Which of the following terms relates to a respiratory disorder?
    a. MI
    b. HBP
    c. COPD
    d. RIH
    e. HIV

20. Which if the following best describes a bony projection?
    a. spine
    b. fissure
    c. process
    d. fossa
    e. foramen

21. According to Sigmund Freud, this is the development stage focusing on physical and intellectual activity where sexual impulses are repressed, e.g. 6 to 12 years old.
    a. Oral
    b. Anal
    c. Phallic
    d. Latency
    e. Genital

22. Mimicking the behavior of another to cope with feelings of inadequacy is called
    a. dissociation
    b. rationalization
    c. substitution
    d. identification
    e. suppression

23. Confidentiality is legally supported by the
    a. Self-Determination Act
    b. Health Care Quality Improvement Act
    c. Americans with Disabilities Act
    d. Standards of Care Act
    e. Privacy Act

24. Disclosing unpleasant information to a patient is best supported by the ethical concept of
    a. duty
    b. right
    c. nonmaleficence
    d. justice
    e. veracity

25. Which of the following terms relates to a gynecological disorder?
    a. epididymitis
    b. salpingitis
    c. stomatitis
    d. rhinitis
    e. vasitis

26. Turning a body part inward, especially the sole of the foot is
    a. flexion
    b. abduction
    c. circumduction
    d. eversion
    e. inversion

27. Psychosexual stage that focuses on attaining a mature sexual relationship.
    a. Oral
    b. Anal
    c. Phallic
    d. Latency
    e. Genital

28. The reasons a patient may desire to continue the sick role is
    a. fear of reestablishing responsibility
    b. financial gain such as Workers' Compensation
    c. to generate sympathy and attention
    d. (A) and (B) only
    e. (A), (B), and (C)

29. Confidentiality is ethically supported by the concept of
    a. beneficence
    b. nonmaleficence
    c. fidelity
    d. all of the above
    e. none of the above

30. Informed consent is most related to the concept of
    a. justice
    b. autonomy
    c. role fidelity
    d. code of ethics
    e. benevolent deception

31. Which of the following terms is spelled incorrectly?
    a. sinusitis
    b. hysterectomy
    c. arteriosclerosis
    d. lymphadenopathy
    e. rabdomyoma

32. The right atrioventricular valve is known as the
    a. bicuspid
    b. mitral
    c. semilunar
    d. tricuspid
    e. aortic

33. The psychosexual stage where the Oedipus or Electra complex will most likely occur.
    a. Oral
    b. Anal
    c. Phallic
    d. Latency
    e. Genital

34. All of the following may be considered losses associated with adopting the sick role **EXCEPT**
    a. autonomy
    b. privacy
    c. mobility or function
    d. normal appearance
    e. none of the above

35. A civil wrong committed against other persons or their property is
    a. a tort
    b. a breach of contract
    c. negligence
    d. malpractice
    e. assault and battery

36. An argument supporting not disclosing unpleasant information to a patient for his own good is
    a. veracity
    b. duty
    c. deception
    d. benevolent deception
    e. justice

37. Unclear vision caused by hardening of the crystal-line lens common among the elderly is known as
    a. diplopia
    b. presbyopia
    c. amblyopia
    d. myopia
    e. hyperopia

38. The structure known as the voice box is the
    a. pharynx
    b. larynx
    c. epiglottis
    d. oropharynx
    e. nasopharynx

39. The psychosexual stage where fixation may create mistrust along with nail-biting, drug abuse, smoking, and overeating.
    a. Oral
    b. Anal
    c. Phallic
    d. Latency
    e. Genital

40. Methods of discovering what is important to a patient include
    a. asking the patient
    b. observing patient behavior
    c. asking family and friends
    d. reviewing the medical chart
    e. all of the above

41. A health-care provider who guarantees the outcome of a course of treatment may be in jeopardy of committing
    a. a tort
    b. a breach of contract
    c. negligence
    d. malpractice
    e. assault and battery

42. A malingerer or hypochondriac may be inappropriately labeled a
    a. crock
    b. gork
    c. GOMER
    d. vegetable
    e. gimp

43. Inflammation of the gallbladder is known as
    a. cholelithiasis
    b. colitis
    c. cholecystitis
    d. cystitis
    e. cholelithectomy

44. A fingerlike projection of the soft palate is a(n)
    a. uvula
    b. frenulum
    c. epiglottis
    d. villi
    e. cilia

45. The psychosexual stage where toilet training provides pleasure and control.
    a. Oral
    b. Anal
    c. Phallic
    d. Latency
    e. Genital

46. Adopting the view of other persons relative to their situation and experience is known as
    a. empathy
    b. sympathy
    c. reinforcement
    d. projection
    e. introjection

47. Negligence of a professional person is known as
    a. nonfeasance
    b. misfeasance
    c. malfeasance
    d. criminal negligence
    e. malpractice

48. Suicide is often viewed as
    a. an act against God
    b. socially irresponsible
    c. a sign of insanity
    d. a way of "copping out"
    e. any of the above

49. Radiographic study involving the urinary system is called
    a. intravenous pyelogram
    b. intravenous infusion
    c. intravenous cardiogram
    d. intravenous injection
    e. intravenous feeding

50. The structure that houses the glomerulus is the
    a. loop of Henle
    b. proximal convoluted tubule
    c. Bowman's capsule
    d. distal convoluted tubule
    e. collecting duct

51. Erik Erikson's Theory of Psychosocial Development consists of how many stages?
    a. Four
    b. Five
    c. Six
    d. Seven
    e. Eight

52. Which of the following will most likely promote the perception of professional competence?
    a. shaking when performing a procedure
    b. behaving in a nonchalant manner
    c. poor enunciation
    d. lack of eye contact
    e. appearing confident

53. The least serious degree of negligence is
    a. minor
    b. ordinary
    c. inconsequential
    d. gross
    e. misdemeanor

54. A document serving to appoint an individual, chosen by the patient, to represent the patient's interests is a(n)
    a. advance directive
    b. living will
    c. durable power of attorney
    d. subpoena duces tecum
    e. guardian ad litem

55. The medical abbreviation meaning *by mouth* is
    a. ad lib
    b. p.o.
    c. n.p.o.
    d. b.i.d.
    e. t.i.d.

56. The innermost layer of the uterus is the
    a. epimetrium
    b. fimbria
    c. myometrium
    d. oviduct
    e. endometrium

57. Jean Piaget's Theory of Cognitive Development consists of how many stages?
    a. Four
    b. Five
    c. Six
    d. Seven
    e. Eight

58. Interacting with a health professional as one would interact with a parental figure is known as
    a. inference
    b. dependence
    c. transference
    d. countertransference
    e. overidentification

59. The principle that the provider has a professional obligation to care for a patient is known as
    a. duty
    b. dereliction of duty
    c. direct causation
    d. damage
    e. due care

60. An argument supporting euthanasia is
    a. fidelity
    b. self-determination
    c. justice
    d. duty
    e. right

61. The medical abbreviation meaning *as desired* is
    a. stat
    b. p.r.n.
    c. ad lib
    d. q.o.d.
    e. cc

62. Neuronal structures that receive and conduct impulses toward the cell body are
    a. axons
    b. dendrites
    c. synapses
    d. neurilemmas
    e. nodes of Ranvier

63. James Fowler's Theory of Spirtitual Development consists of how many stages?
    a. Four
    b. Five
    c. Six
    d. Seven
    e. Eight

64. The process of converting meaning into understandable symbols is known as
    a. communication
    b. deciphering
    c. decoding
    d. encoding
    e. feedback

65. In most states, there is no legal duty to rescue victims **EXCEPT**
   a. family members
   b. innocent bystanders
   c. if you witness the accident
   d. close friends
   e. helpless young children

66. Manipulating the genes of offspring through either breeding or alteration is known as
   a. euthanasia
   b. eupnea
   c. eugenics
   d. euphoria
   e. eupraxia

PART 2: ADMINISTRATIVE

DIRECTIONS

Each of the questions or incomplete statements below is followed by five suggested answers or completions. Select the *one* answer or completion that is *best* in each case and fill in the circle containing the corresponding letter on the answer sheet.

1. The smallest piece of information processed by a computer is the
   a. data
   b. bit
   c. byte
   d. ASCII
   e. output

2. When a pharmaceutical representative arrives unannounced, it is best to
   a. request a business card and see if the health care provider is available for a visit
   b. immediately escort her to the provider's office
   c. ask the representative to wait until the provider is free
   d. refer the representative to the next available medical assistant
   e. indicate that visitors are not seen without an appointment

3. A signature card must be completed to
   a. file medical practice income taxes
   b. authorize reconciliation of bank statements
   c. pay medical practice professional dues
   d. open a checking account
   e. deposit funds in a bank

4. A direction to consider additional codes is
   a. See condition
   b. NEC
   c. See category
   d. NOS
   e. See also

5. The person most likely to handle equipment purchases is the
   a. receptionist
   b. medical assistant
   c. office manager
   d. nurse
   e. health-care provider

6. Integrating the various resources to meet organizational objectives is known as
   a. planning
   b. organizing
   c. coordinating
   d. directing
   e. controlling

7. Which of the following would be indexed first?
   a. Allison B. Wilson
   b. Alice A. Wilson
   c. Mrs. Anthony (Alma) Wilson
   d. Alice B. Wilson
   e. Alicia A. Wilsonn

8. Ideally, the phone should be answered by the
   a. first ring
   b. second ring
   c. third ring
   d. fourth ring
   e. fifth ring

9. Special characters that simplify the sorting and routing of financial documents are
   a. FONT
   b. PITCH
   c. MICR
   d. OCR
   e. MICRO

10. An organizational arrangement that provides medical services for a fixed, prepaid fee best describes
   a. PPO
   b. SEC
   c. HMO
   d. HRM
   e. IPA

11. Which of the following statutes requires public facilities to be made accessible?
   a. ADA
   b. ADEA
   c. FLSA
   d. FMLA
   e. OSHA

12. An employee's ability to perform a task is a function of all of the following **EXCEPT**
    a. knowledge
    b. skill
    c. experience
    d. commitment
    e. past performance

13. The process of activating the input of the operating system into main memory is known as
    a. start-up
    b. shutdown
    c. booting
    d. program installation
    e. disk formatting

14. When a second line rings, it is best to
    a. answer with "please hold"
    b. ask the first caller if she can hold
    c. indicate to the first caller, "My other line is ringing, I will place you on hold for a moment"
    d. ignore it until you have finished with the first caller
    e. indicate to the first caller, "please hold"

15. Which of the following most characterizes an ABA number?
    a. 1012-231678-55
    b. 17-7000/2910
    c. 504.10
    d. 1052
    e. 27

16. The underlined portion of: Hypertension (<u>orthostatic, benign, simple</u>) identifies a(n)
    a. main term
    b. subterm modifier
    c. essential modifier
    d. nonessential modifier
    e. fourth-digit modifier

17. According to ADA regulations, private businesses are required to make their facilities accessible to the public except when
    a. it is time consuming.
    b. it financially harms the business.
    c. it is inconvenient.
    d. it concerns an already existing structure.
    e. it is expensive.

18. An employee's willingness to perform a task is a function of all of the following **EXCEPT**
    a. confidence
    b. performance
    c. commitment
    d. desire
    e. motivation

19. Which of the following would be indexed last?
    a. John P. St. John
    b. John Q. St. George
    c. Paul M. St. Paul
    d. Alfred O. San Luis
    e. Arthur R. San Jose

20. All of the following are typically recorded on a telephone message **EXCEPT**
    a. date and time of call
    b. person called
    c. message
    d. person taking message
    e. caller's demographic data

21. A check that a bank refuses to pay is
    a. postdated
    b. debited
    c. honored
    d. credited
    e. dishonored

22. An insurance policy designed to pay fees not covered by conventional plans is a
    a. commercial plan
    b. government plan
    c. private plan
    d. medigap plan
    e. companion plan

23. A business that serves the public must remove physical "barriers." Which of the following statements governing this provision is true?
    a. It is an absolute requirement.
    b. It is based on the size and resources of the business.
    c. It is based on the relative profitability of the business.
    d. It is based on existing economic conditions.
    e. It is based on the type of business.

24. Close supervision of an employee is most required when the employee is
    a. unable and unwilling
    b. unable but willing
    c. able but unwilling
    d. able and willing
    e. none of the above

25. The process of organizing a blank disk into sectors so that it can store data is known as
    a. booting
    b. configuration
    c. WYSIWYG
    d. formatting
    e. icon

26. The MA's telephone voice should convey all of the following **EXCEPT**
   a. confidence
   b. warmth
   c. disinterest
   d. concern
   e. courteousness

27. A personal record of relevant information regarding a check and checking account balance is a
   a. deposit ticket
   b. debit memo
   c. check register
   d. credit memo
   e. bank statement

28. A term after the brace (}) indicates
   a. completion of the main statement before the brace
   b. a required modifier of the statement before the brace
   c. that a fifth-digit modifier is required
   d. that the conditions listed do not qualify
   e. the clarification of a code description

29. The highest priority for barrier removal to improve accessibility to a facility refers to which of the following?
   a. Sidewalks
   b. Toilet rooms
   c. Telephones
   d. Drinking fountains
   e. Service areas

30. Delegating the authority and responsibility for completing a task is most effective when the employee is
   a. unable and unwilling
   b. unable but willing
   c. able but unwilling
   d. able and willing
   e. all of the above

31. Which of the following would be indexed first?
   a. Karen A. Lane
   b. Karin B. Lone
   c. Karen Lane
   d. Kristen F. Line
   e. Kristy G. Lin

32. When dialing direct, the caller dials
   a. 0 + area code + seven-digit number
   b. 1 + area code + seven-digit number
   c. 1 + 800 + seven-digit number
   d. caller ID number + seven-digit number
   e. caller ID number + area code + seven-digit number

33. Carbonless copies of checks use a special paper known as
   a. NCR paper
   b. OCR paper
   c. MICR paper
   d. DOD paper
   e. DOE paper

34. AOB means
   a. actual observable behavior
   b. assignment of benefits
   c. average objective benefits
   d. archives of business records
   e. achievable objectives

35. Which of the following are true regarding accessible parking?
   a. There must be an access aisle on either side of the parking space.
   b. A sign with the international symbol of accessibility must be located in front of the parking space.
   c. An accessible route must be provided between the access aisle and the accessible entrance.
   d. Should be the spaces closest to the accessible entrance.
   e. All of the above.

36. Goals developed and documented by employees themselves are
   a. strategic plans
   b. MBOs
   c. day planners
   d. to do lists
   e. work plans

37. A key that moves the cursor to the left, right, top, or bottom margins when pressed is the
   a. Backspace key
   b. Tab key
   c. Delete key
   d. Escape key
   e. Home key

38. The long-distance directory assistance number is
   a. 0 + area code + 411
   b. 1 + area code + 411
   c. 0 + area code + 555-1212
   d. 1 + area code + 555-1212 or 411
   e. 1 + 800 + 555-1212

39. A check that has been honored and appropriately stamped to prevent it from being reissued is a(n)
   a. NSF check
   b. postdated check
   c. dishonored check
   d. unpaid check
   e. cancelled check

40. Brackets ([]) in ICD-9-CM are used to enclose
    a. synonyms, alternative words, or explanatory phrases
    b. essential modifiers
    c. ill-defined or ambiguous terms
    d. directions to seek an alternative code
    e. instructions on fourth- and fifth-digit modifiers

41. A van accessible parking space must have an access aisle that is at least how wide?
    a. Four feet
    b. Five feet
    c. Six feet
    d. Seven feet
    e. Eight feet

42. All of the following are devices used to manage one's time EXCEPT a
    a. day planner
    b. to do list
    c. directory
    d. pocket calendar
    e. white-, chalk-, or corkboard

43. Annual reports are best filed using a(n)
    a. alphabetical system
    b. subject system
    c. geographic system
    d. numerical system
    e. terminal digit system

44. The time zone difference between California and New Jersey is
    a. 1 hour
    b. 2 hours
    c. 3 hours
    d. 4 hours
    e. 5 hours

45. The bank statement shows a balance of $4250, deposits in transit total $1200, and outstanding checks that equal $300. The check register balance should be
    a. $2750
    b. $3350
    c. $4550
    d. $5150
    e. $5750

46. A fixed, prepaid fee per person enrolled in a managed care program describes
    a. copayment
    b. premium
    c. balance billing
    d. capitation
    e. exclusion

47. Accessible parking spaces for cars must have an access aisle that is at least how wide?
    a. Four feet
    b. Five feet
    c. Six feet
    d. Seven feet
    e. Eight feet

48. When interviewing job applicants, all of the following should be considered EXCEPT
    a. social affiliations
    b. education and training
    c. experience
    d. personality and temperament
    e. references

49. A blinking dash or small rectangle that identifies where on the computer screen data will be entered is the
    a. pause/break
    b. icon
    c. cursor
    d. page-up
    e. end

50. WATS stands for
    a. Washington Tax Service
    b. Western Area Transit System
    c. World Arena Telephone Systems
    d. Whirlpool and Therapeutic Sauna
    e. Wide Area Telephone Service

51. Upon receiving checks in the mail, the MA should first
    a. deposit them immediately
    b. place them in the safe until deposited
    c. restrictively endorse them
    d. endorse them with the MA's signature
    e. temporarily store them in the cash drawer

52. After locating a code in ICD-9-CM Volume II, the MA should
    a. record the code
    b. include the term *Rule Out* as indicated
    c. locate the appropriate E-code
    d. verify the code in Volume I
    e. cross-check the code in Volume III

53. The slope of an access ramp to a facility must be no more than:
    a. 1:10
    b. 1:12
    c. 1:14
    d. 1:16
    e. 1:18

54. Which of the following interview questions is illegal?
    a. "Where did you receive your training?"
    b. "Do you have any hobbies?"
    c. "May I contact your references?"
    d. "Are you aware of anything that may interfere with your ability to perform the/job?"
    e. "Do you have any children?"

55. The best method of controlling charts removed from the office is with a(n)
    a. out guide
    b. subpoena duces tecum
    c. borrowed charts log
    d. archival record
    e. chart retention plan

56. An effective answering service is necessary to avoid
    a. liability
    b. malpractice
    c. negligence
    d. abandonment charges
    e. carelessness

57. An organization's ability to pay its debts is known as
    a. solvency
    b. profitability
    c. effectiveness
    d. efficiency
    e. liability

58. The person or party designated by the policyholder to receive the value of a policy is the
    a. carrier
    b. beneficiary
    c. provider
    d. insured
    e. insurer

59. Doors must be wide enough to be accessible, usually at least:
    a. 30 inches
    b. 32 inches
    c. 34 inches
    d. 36 inches
    e. 38 inches

60. Orientation of new employees serves to
    a. impart the philosophy and mission of the organization
    b. identify performance expectations
    c. provide a protected period of time to learn a new job
    d. assess the employee's skills and learning needs
    e. all of the above

61. The number of characters contained within an inch is the
    a. macro
    b. font
    c. widow
    d. default
    e. pitch

62. The appointment scheduling system should reflect the needs of
    a. the health-care provider
    b. the staff
    c. patients
    d. (A) and (C) only
    e. (B) and (C) only

63. The property of value owned or controlled by an organization is known as
    a. capital
    b. liability
    c. asset
    d. revenue
    e. expense

64. According to ICD-9-CM coding conventions, malignant hypertension is
    a. mild and in control
    b. a systole greater than 140 mmHg
    c. a diastole greater than 90 mmHg
    d. a severe form with vascular damage
    e. coded the same as simple hypertension

65. Generally there should be at least ___ cubic feet of outside air per minute/per person for an office environment.
    a. 10
    b. 20
    c. 30
    d. 40
    e. 50

66. Which of the following purposes is most in line with assigning a new employee a preceptor?
    a. to report positive and negative employee characteristics
    b. to make recommendations regarding the employee's "fit" with the job
    c. to help the new employee navigate through the system
    d. to carry out a background check to protect the organization
    e. to make recommendations regarding the employee's likelihood of remaining with the organization

PART 3: CLINICAL

DIRECTIONS

Each of the questions or incomplete statements below is followed by five suggested answers or completions. Select the *one* answer or completion that is *best* in each case and fill in the circle containing the corresponding letter on the answer sheet.

1. Details regarding the health status of the patient's parents and siblings are known as the
   a. chief complaint
   b. social history
   c. past medical history
   d. occupational history
   e. family history

2. All of the following are methods of disinfection **EXCEPT**
   a. alcohol
   b. boiling
   c. antiseptics
   d. acids
   e. dessication

3. All of the following may be consulted for drug information **EXCEPT**
   a. PDR
   b. medical dictionary
   c. product insert
   d. USP/NF
   e. desk reference for nonprescription drugs

4. All of the following are common causes of breathing emergencies **EXCEPT**
   a. choking
   b. obstruction
   c. strains
   d. asthma
   e. allergic reactions

5. Which of the following illustrates an engineering control?
   a. sharps container
   b. handwashing
   c. lab coat
   d. treating all body fluids as potentially infectious
   e. all of the above

6. The best source of vitamin D is
   a. beef
   b. green vegetables
   c. cheese
   d. fruits
   e. cereals

7. An examination method that requires the use of a stethoscope is
   a. palpation
   b. manipulation
   c. mensuration
   d. auscultation
   e. percussion

8. A grooved instrument used to guide the direction and depth of a surgical incision is a(n)
   a. scalpel
   b. obturator
   c. applicator
   d. trocar
   e. director

9. An example of a Schedule IV drug is
   a. acetaminophen
   b. codeine
   c. heroin
   d. valium
   e. morphine

10. Shock caused by sudden blood or body fluid loss is
    a. anaphylactic
    b. psychogenic
    c. neurogenic
    d. cardiogenic
    e. hypovolemic

11. The normal transparency of freshly voided urine is
    a. opaque
    b. turbid
    c. cloudy
    d. hazy
    e. clear

12. Replacing nutritional elements lost during the processing of food is known as
    a. enhancement
    b. homogenization
    c. fortification
    d. pasteurization
    e. enrichment

13. A bipolar limb lead is
    a. V_2
    b. I
    c. aVR
    d. aVL
    e. V_6

14. All of the following are endoscopes **EXCEPT** the
    a. stethoscope
    b. sigmoidoscope
    c. bronchoscope
    d. proctoscope
    e. laparoscope

15. A medication given to a patient for a fee is
    a. prescribed
    b. injected
    c. dispensed
    d. subscribed
    e. administered

16. All of the following are common signs or symptoms of shock **EXCEPT**
    a. nausea
    b. polyphagia
    c. tachycardia
    d. cool, moist skin
    e. unconsciousness

17. The term hemopoiesis is best associated with
    a. hematology
    b. bacteriology
    c. microbiology
    d. serology
    e. parasitology

18. Nutritional elements that help replace and repair worn out tissue are
    a. carbohydrates
    b. proteins
    c. vitamins
    d. fats
    e. minerals

19. The following identifies the action to be taken to solve a medical problem such as treatment, medication, surgery, referral, etc.
    a. subjective
    b. objective
    c. assessment
    d. plan
    e. POMR

20. All of the following are steps for proper instrument care **EXCEPT**
    a. Do not stack instruments to avoid entangling them.
    b. Keep instruments with differing finishes separate.
    c. Use the instrument only for the purpose for which it is designed.
    d. Keep ratcheted instruments in a closed position.
    e. Keep sharp and delicate instruments separate from the rest to avoid dulling or damaging them.

21. Schedule II inventories must be made every
    a. year
    b. 2 years
    c. 3 years
    d. 4 years
    e. 5 years

22. The first aid priority for an injured victim is to
    a. create a patent airway
    b. initiate breathing
    c. stop bleeding
    d. immoblize injuries
    e. treat for shock

23. *Neisseria gonorrhoeae* is morphologically described as
    a. GPC
    b. GNC
    c. GNR
    d. GPR
    e. none of the above

24. Nutritional elements that are concentrated sources of energy that add satiety value to foods are
    a. carbohydrates
    b. minerals
    c. fats
    d. vitamins
    e. proteins

25. All of the following instruments are commonly used during a routine physical examination **EXCEPT**
    a. stethoscope
    b. otoscope
    c. percussion hammer
    d. ophthalmoscope
    e. thumb forceps

27. Drug inventory records must include the following information **EXCEPT**
    a. health care provider's name
    b. DEA registration number
    c. date of inventory
    d. signature of person who has taken the inventory
    e. signature of patients who accepted drugs

28. Common signs and symptoms of myocardial infarction include
    a. diaphoresis
    b. angina pectoris
    c. dyspnea
    d. nausea
    e. all of the above

29. All of the following are included in the chemical examination of urine **EXCEPT**
    a. ketones
    b. urobilinogen
    c. specific gravity
    d. glucose
    e. nitrite

30. Nutritional elements that serve as catalysts for efficient metabolism are
    a. carbohydrates
    b. minerals
    c. fats
    d. vitamins
    e. proteins

31. Placement at the fourth intercostal space to the left of the sternum is known as
    a. V_1
    b. V_2
    c. V_3
    d. V_4
    e. V_6

32. All of the following are proper aseptic techniques **EXCEPT**
    a. Transfer forceps are held facing down.
    b. Bottles containing sterile solution should not touch the sterile receptacle when poured.
    c. Lids are placed down on the table.
    d. Do not reach over a sterile field.
    e. Cover a sterile tray with a sterile towel if not used immediately.

33. The form completed when damaged or contaminated controlled substances are destroyed is
    a. DEA-41
    b. DEA-106
    c. DEA-222
    d. DEA-335
    e. DEA-457

34. The most common cause of convulsions is
    a. fever
    b. dehydration
    c. diarrhea
    d. epilepsy
    e. hyperemesis

35. The abnormal hemoglobin molecule responsible for sickle cell anemia is
    a. hemoglobin A
    b. hemoglobin C
    c. hemoglobin F
    d. hemoglobin S
    e. hemoglobin D

36. All of the following are fat-soluble vitamins **EXCEPT**
    a. A
    b. D
    c. E
    d. K
    e. B

37. The patient's name, date of birth, marital status, education, occupation, etc., is known as the
    a. social history
    b. demographics
    c. family history
    d. past illnesses
    e. personal history

38. A surgical wound that becomes infected and must be reopened is a
    a. first intention wound
    b. second intention wound
    c. third intention wound
    d. fourth intention wound
    e. fifth intention wound

39. The Rx symbol is classified as the
    a. prescription
    b. subscription
    c. signature
    d. inscription
    e. superscription

40. According to the Rule of Nines, the amount of body surface represented by the head and neck is
    a. 1 %
    b. 4.5 %
    c. 9 %
    d. 18 %
    e. 36 %

41. The species of bacteria that commonly causes food poisoning is
    a. *Escherichia coli*
    b. *Streptococcus pyogenes*
    c. *Salmonella typhi*
    d. *Staphylococcus aureus*
    e. *Klebsiella pneumoniae*

42. The societal factor having the most negative impact on adolescent nutrition is
    a. peer pressure
    b. emphasis on slimness
    c. teen pregnancy
    d. drug abuse
    e. commercialism

43. Initial examination of the breasts is usually performed when the patient is in which of the following positions?
    a. lithotomy
    b. Trendelenberg
    c. sitting
    d. dorsal recumbent
    e. prone

44. The sterile cover placed over a wound to prevent contamination is the
   a. dressing
   b. wrap
   c. Band-Aid
   d. cast
   e. bandage

45. The acronym p.c. means
   a. after meals
   b. as needed
   c. with meals
   d. as desired
   e. before meals

46. Dry, hot, red skin is characteristic of
   a. hyperthermia
   b. heat exhaustion
   c. heat cramps
   d. heat stroke
   e. hypothermia

47. The specific gravity testing method requiring the least amount of urine is by
   a. reagent strip
   b. microscopy
   c. refractometer
   d. litmus paper
   e. urinometer

48. The metabolic disorder characterized by the lack of the enzyme needed to metabolize phenylalanine is known as
   a. galactosemia
   b. homocystinuria
   c. tyrosinosis
   d. PKU
   e. histidinemia

49. Each large block of five small squares represent how many seconds on ECG paper?
   a. .04 seconds
   b. .05 seconds
   c. .1 seconds
   d. .2 seconds
   e. .3 seconds

50. All of the following would be needed for a laceration repair **EXCEPT**
   a. surgical scissors
   b. hemostatic forcep
   c. needle holder
   d. tissue forceps
   e. Penrose drain

51. The generic name for Lopressor is
   a. nitroglycerin
   b. metoprolol
   c. nifedipine
   d. alprazolam
   e. Prozac

52. When in doubt about whether a conscious victim is suffering from diabetic coma or insulin shock, first
   a. administer sugar
   b. administer fluids
   c. treat for shock
   d. lay the victim down
   e. perform a primary survey

53. All of the following are examples of anisochromia in RBCs **EXCEPT**
   a. normochromia
   b. hypochromia
   c. polychromia
   d. hyperchromia
   e. none of the above

54. A common sign of diabetes mellitus is
   a. polycythemia
   b. hypoglycemia
   c. polyuria
   d. hypoxia
   e. polycrotism

55. Questions regarding each of the major body systems and parts are known as
   a. CC
   b. PMH
   c. FH
   d. ROS
   e. PI

56. Which of the following is considered a dissecting instrument?
   a. thumb forceps
   b. hemostat
   c. surgical scissor
   d. probe
   e. sound

57. A drug that is used to prevent disease is
   a. therapeutic
   b. prophylactic
   c. diagnostic
   d. cathartic
   e. analgesic

58. Which of the following is not appropriate for the treatment of shock?
    a. Elevate the legs 12 inches.
    b. Keep the victim warm.
    c. Activate EMS.
    d. Give the victim water.
    e. Monitor ABCs.

59. A common liquid culture media is
    a. BAP
    b. MAC
    c. PEA
    d. TSB
    e. TM

60. A diet of plant foods supplemented with dairy products and eggs is called
    a. lacto-ovo vegetarian
    b. vegan
    c. lacto-vegetarian
    d. vegetarian
    e. regular

61. The Ishihara test is associated with which of the following examinations?
    a. otological
    b. ophthalmological
    c. gynecological
    d. orthopedic
    e. dermatological

62. An instrument used to grasp or clamp down objects is a(n)
    a. scalpel
    b. bandage scissor
    c. obturator
    d. forceps
    e. retractor

63. A drug's generic name is best illustrated by which one of the following?
    a. Tylenol
    b. Aspirin
    c. Achromycin
    d. Salicylic acid
    e. Ibuprofn

64. The treatment for poison ivy includes:
    a. applying a paste of baking soda and water
    b. applying vinegar
    c. applying water that is as hot as can be tolerated
    d. applying ice
    e. applying ammonia

65. A glass tube used to measure small quantities of liquid is a
    a. beaker
    b. cuvette
    c. bottle
    d. flask
    e. pipette

66. The constructive process of building up new substances is called
    a. metabolism
    b. anabolism
    c. catabolism
    d. cannibalism
    e. basal metabolism

CMA POST-TEST SCORE SHEET

DIRECTIONS:

1. Comparing your answer sheet with the correct answers listed below for each section, circle the incorrect responses below.
2. Tally the number of incorrect responses in each column and record the total in the space provided.
3. Score each of the three sections as described in Chapter 1. Identify the section (general, administrative, or clinical) having the lowest score.
4. In the section having the lowest overall score, identify the column having the most incorrect responses and turn to the chapter indicated for further study.
5. Concentrate your study on the section with the lowest score by studying the next weakest area and the next, and so on.
6. After completing your study of the weakest content section, turn to the section having the next lowest score, concentrating your study on the column with the lowest score, and so on.

ADMINISTRATIVE: Percent correct: _____%

1 = B	2 = A	3 = D	4 = E	5 = C	6 = C
7 = B	8 = C	9 = C	10 = C	11 = A	12 = D
13 = C	14 = B	15 = B	16 = D	17 = B	18 = B
19 = D	20 = E	21 = E	22 = E	23 = B	24 = A
25 = D	26 = C	27 = C	28 = B	29 = A	30 = D
31 = C	32 = B	33 = A	34 = B	35 = E	36 = B
37 = E	38 = D	39 = E	40 = A	41 = E	42 = C
43 = B	44 = C	45 = D	46 = D	47 = B	48 = A
49 = C	50 = E	51 = C	52 = D	53 = B	54 = E
55 = A	56 = D	57 = A	58 = B	59 = D	60 = E
61 = E	62 = D	63 = C	64 = D	65 = B	66 = C
_____	_____	_____	_____	_____	_____
Ch. 10	Ch. 11	Ch. 12	Ch. 13	Ch. 14	Ch. 15

GENERAL: Percent correct: _____%

1 = D	2 = C	3 = E	4 = B	5 = C	6 = B
7 = A	8 = B	9 = A	10 = D	11 = E	12 = D
13 = E	14 = D	15 = B	16 = C	17 = E	18 = B
19 = C	20 = C	21 = D	22 = D	23 = E	24 = E
25 = B	26 = E	27 = E	28 = E	29 = D	30 = B
31 = E	32 = D	33 = C	34 = E	35 = A	36 = D
37 = B	38 = B	39 = A	40 = E	41 = B	42 = A
43 = C	44 = A	45 = B	46 = A	47 = E	48 = E
49 = A	50 = C	51 = E	52 = E	53 = B	54 = C
55 = B	56 = E	57 = A	58 = C	59 = A	60 = B
61 = C	62 = B	63 = D	64 = D	65 = A	66 = C
_____	_____	_____	_____	_____	_____
Ch. 4	Ch. 5	Ch. 6	Ch. 7	Ch. 8	Ch. 9

CLINICAL: Percent correct: _____%

1 = E	2 = C	3 = B	4 = C	5 = A	6 = C
7 = D	8 = E	9 = D	10 = E	11 = E	12 = E
13 = B	14 = A	15 = C	16 = B	17 = A	18 = B
19 = D	20 = D	21 = B	22 = A	23 = B	24 = C
25 = E	26 = D	27 = E	28 = E	29 = C	30 = D
31 = B	32 = C	33 = A	34 = D	35 = D	36 = E
37 = B	38 = C	39 = E	40 = C	41 = C	42 = B
43 = C	44 = A	45 = A	46 = D	47 = A	48 = D
49= D	50 = E	51 = B	52 = A	53 = A	54 = C
55 = D	56 = C	57 = B	58 = D	59 = D	60 = A
61 = B	62 = D	63 = D	64 = A	65 = E	66 = B
_____	_____	_____	_____	_____	_____
Ch. 16	Ch. 17	Ch. 18	Ch. 19	Ch. 20	Ch. 21

General:

If you answered 6 or more questions incorrectly in any of the columns, turn to the appropriate chapter for further study.

Administrative:

If you answered 6 or more questions incorrectly in any of the columns, turn to the appropriate chapter for further study.

Clinical:

If you answered 6 or more questions incorrectly in any of the columns, turn to the appropriate chapter for further study.

Total percent correct (_____ /198 × 100): _____%

CMA standard score = (Raw score × 10) − 200 (Standard score ≥ 445 is passing)

CMA POST-TEST ANSWERS AND RATIONALES

General:

1. D. -itis is a suffix meaning inflammation. Ante- and post- are prefixes; organ/o is a combining form; stoma is a word standing alone.

2. C. Structurally this order from bottom to top is: atoms, cells, tissues, organs, systems, and organism.

3. E. They all represent true statements regarding human growth and development.

4. B. By mirroring the patient's conversation, any discrepancy in what the medical assistant heard and what the patient actually said will be immediately identified.

5. C. With informed consent, providers may administer atypical treatments to attempt curing and/or treating their patients.

6. B. Option A is a custom; C is a positive spirit; D is a study of moral thought; E is an obligation.

7. A. B and E are combining forms; C and D are suffixes.

8. B. Neurons are the cells composing the nervous system.

9. A. B is the outward expression of the inner self; C and D are Freud's three levels of personality.

10. D. Unsolicited advice may cause a roadblock in the communication process rather than facilitating it.

11. E. Implied consent may be an action such as a patient agreeing to take an injection or allowing the medical assistant to take blood.

12. D. Option A means to do good; B means to do no harm; C means fairness; E means loyalty.

13. E. ENT is a common abbreviation for "ear, nose, and throat." The medical term for this specialist is otorhinolaryngologist (-logist = one who specializes; ot/o = ear; rhin/o = nose; laryng/o=throat).

14. D. The sudoriferous glands are the sweat glands, which are accessory skin structures; A, B, C, and E are layers of the skin.

15. B. A is the outward expression of the inner self; C and D are Freud's three levels of personality.

16. C. By acting opposite to one's actual feelings, such as laughing when you want to cry, an individual forms a reaction to a situation. The other terms listed are defense mechanisms that operate in different ways, such as adopting another's values for your own, blaming others for feelings of inadequacy, channeling or suggesting other more socially acceptable behaviors, or refusing to accept a situation.

17. E. Phenylketonuria (PKU) is mandated to be reported because when left untreated in infants, it will cause mental retardation.

18. B. Option A means obligations; C means fairness; D means the study of moral principles; E means legal claims.

19. C. COPD is the common abbreviation for "chronic obstructive pulmonary (lung) disease." The others do not apply to the respiratory system.

20. C. The spine is a series of bones; a fissure is a break in a bone; a fossa is a depression; a foramen is an opening.

21. D. The others represent different psychosexual stages.

22. D. Through identification, an insecure person will imitate another's behavior and act just as the other person would. Dissociation, rationalization, substitution, and suppression are other defense mechanisms for dealing with feelings of inadequacy.

23. E. The Privacy Act protects the rights of patients, their medical information, and confidential issues regarding their care.

24. E. Being truthful to the patient regardless of the unpleasantness involved is our duty and the patient's right.

25. B. Salpingitis is an inflammation of the fallopian tubes. The other terms listed do not relate to the female reproductive system.

26. E.   In- relates to inward in the term inversion. Flexion is the act of flexing; abduction means moving away from the midline; circumduction would be moving in a circle; eversion would be turning outward.

27. E.   The others represent different psychosexual stages.

28. E.   Many individuals crave sympathy and attention and so will continue to act sick. In other cases, individuals are afraid to accept responsibility, and some are comfortable to remain off the job while getting paid.

29. D.   A, B, and C are terms related to a beneficial nature or outcome and so relate to the concept of confidentiality.

30. B.   Making informed decisions is consistent with the notion of autonomy or self-determination.

31. E.   The correct spelling is *rhabdomyoma.*

32. D.   The valve between the right atrium and right ventricle is composed of three flaps—the tricuspid valve.

33. C.   The others do not typically include these complexes.

34. E.   When assuming a sick role, a patient can lose the ability to function on his or her own, a degree of privacy, mobility/function, and/or a normal appearance depending on the circumstance.

35. A.   Whereas the other answers refer to wrongs committed against others, the common legal term to encompass any civil wrong against persons and/or their property is tort.

36. D.   To deceive patients for their own good. Option A means truthfulness; B means obligation; C means to deceive; E means fairness.

37. B.   Presby- is the prefix meaning aging or elderly.

38. B.   The larynx is the structure holding the vocal chords, which allow us to speak. The other structures do not relate to the ability for speech.

39. A.   Fixation during the other stages creates other developmental issues.

40. E.   All of the methods are essential clues in determining what a patient feels is important.

41. B.   Promising a patient that she or he will be cured and not being able to provide that outcome would constitute a breach of contract. Negligence is a disregard for human life; malpractice is not performing in a manner in which another equally qualified person would perform; assault and battery is physically touching someone without their permission, such as striking them; a tort is any civil wrongdoing against a person or their property.

42. A.   A crock is a derogatory term for a malingerer or hypochondriac.

43. C.   -itis = inflammation, cholecyst/o = gallbladder. Option A refers to the presence of gallstones; B is the inflammation of the colon; D is inflammation of the bladder; E is the surgical removal of a gallstone.

44. A.   The uvula is the structure projecting from the top of the soft palate that closes off the nasal cavity when swallowing to prevent food or liquid to pass up the nasal passageway.

45. B.   The others represent different psychosexual stages.

46. A.   Putting one in another's position to understand their views or positions based on an experience or circumstance is empathy.

47. E.   Malpractice is the failure of a professional person to use reasonable care or judgment in treatment of a case.

48. E.   Suicide may be viewed as all those listed.

49. A.   Pyelogram is a term meaning a record of the renal pelvis (pyel/o). The other terms are not related to the urinary system.

50. C.   The functional unit of the kidney, the nephron, consists of two primary components. The renal corpuscle consists of the glomerulus enclosed within the Bowman's capsule. The tubules are structures outside of the corpuscle where urine is filtered, secreted, and substances reabsorbed.

51. E.   Eight stages.

52. E.   Confidence displayed by speaking clearly, making eye contact, caring behavior, and performing procedures with ease are all signs of professional competence.

53. B.   Negligence is classified as ordinary or gross. Ordinary negligence is the failure of a professional person to use the same level of care or judgment that another professional person would under the same or similar circumstances.

54. C.   Durable power of attorney allows another to represent the patient's interests.

55. B. p.o. is the abbreviation for *per os,* or by mouth.

56. E. The uterus is composed of the epimetrium (outer membranous layer), the myometrium (muscular layer), and the endometrium (innermost membranous layer). The fimbria and oviduct are not uterine structures.

57. A. Four stages.

58. C. When a patient views another as a parental figure, their feelings, fear, and/or emotions are transferred to that professional as a mother or father figure.

59. A. Failure to use due care in the line of duty or dereliction of duty can result in direct causation of a patient's illness or damage to a patient's health.

60. B. Self-rule is a common argument to justify allowing one's self to die.

61. C. Ad lib is the abbreviation for the Latin term *ad libitum,* meaning to take as desired. Stat refers to immediately; p.r.n. is as needed (not to be confused with as desired); q.o.d. is every other day; cc is the abbreviation for cubic centimeter.

62. B. Axons conduct impulses away from the neuron, synapses are the "gaps" between the neurons; neurilemmas are the coatings of the neurons; the nodes of Ranvier are areas along the axon not encased in myelin.

63. D. Seven stages.

64. D. The communication process includes a sender, receiver, and a message. In order to send a message, the sender must first *encode* the message; subsequently, the receiver will decode and/ or decipher the message for feedback to the sender.

65. A. States expect present family members to respond to emergencies regarding victims of the family out of family obligation. Other rescues by unqualified persons could result in litigation.

66. C. Eugenics refers to gene manipulation.

Administrative:

1. B. A bit is the smallest piece of data processed by a computer.

2. A. The remaining options may require a long wait or are inappropriate.

3. D. A signature card is required to open a checking account.

4. E. See also directs one to consider additional codes.

5. C. Equipment being a capital expense is generally handled by the office manager.

6. C. Option A refers to developing objectives; B is assembling organizational resources; D is overseeing the use of the resources; E is comparing planned results with actual results.

7. B. In order they would be B, D, A, C, and E.

8. C. The phone should not be allowed to ring more than three times.

9. C. Magnetic ink character recognition.

10. C. HMO is a plan that provides medical services for a fixed, prepaid fee.

11. A. B refers to prohibiting age discrimination, C refers to wage and work hours, D refers to medical leave, and E refers to safe working conditions.

12. D. A person's commitment is not a function of ability.

13. C. Booting activates the operating system of a computer.

14. B. This is the most courteous response.

15. B. ABA numbers are presented as a fraction.

16. D. The underlined portion may or may not be considered when assigning a code.

17. B. The other conditions are not relevant to meet the ADA requirements.

18. B. Performance is not a function of one's willingness to perform a task.

19. D. In order: B, A, C, E, and D.

20. E. Demographic data is of little use for most phone messages.

21. E. Dishonored checks are ones the bank refuses to pay.

22. E. A companion plan covers fees not covered by a conventional plan.

23. B. The other conditions are not relevant.

24. A. An employee who is unwilling and unable to perform a task must be closely supervised.

25. D. Formatting organizes a disk into sectors.

26. C. The MA should convey interest not disinterest.

27. C. The check register records the pertinent information regarding a check and the account balance.

28. B. Terms after a brace are required modifiers.

29. A. Making sidewalks accessible to businesses has the highest priority.

30. D. When an employee is both willing and able to perform a task, that task should be delegated.

31. C. In order: C, A, E, D, and B

32. B. 1 + area code + seven-digit number is direct dialing.

33. A. No carbon required.

34. B. Assignment of benefits.

35. E. All are true.

36. B. Management by objectives.

37. E. The Home key moves the cursor to the margins.

38. D. Depending on the location, 411 or 1 + area code + 555-1212 is long-distance directory assistance.

39. E. Checks that have been stamped to prevent their reuse are cancelled.

40. A. Brackets enclose synonyms, alternative words, or explanatory phrases.

41. E. 8 feet.

42. C. A directory is not used to manage one's time.

43. B. First filed by subject then chronologically (numerically).

44. C. There is a 3-hour difference between California and New Jersey.

45. D. 4250 + 1200 − 300 = 5150.

46. D. Capitation is a fixed, prepaid fee per person.

47. B. 5 feet.

48. A. Social affiliations are the least important and may be considered illegal.

49. C. The cursor is the blinking dash that identifies where data will be entered on the screen.

50. E. Wide Area Telephone Sevice.

51. C. The MA should restrictively endorse all checks received by the clinic.

52. D. Before assigning an ICD code, it should always be verified in Volume I.

53. B. 1:12. A is too steep. C through E have a lesser slope and are permissible.

54. E. Asking about children is illegal.

55. A. Using out guides is an effective method of controlling removed charts.

56. D. If a provider or her alternate cannot be contacted, a patient may be able to sue for abandonment.

57. A. Option B refers to the positive difference between revenue and expense; C refers to achieving goals; D refers to using the least amount of resources; E is a debt obligation.

58. B. The beneficiary is the person entitled to the value of a policy.

59. D. A through C are too narrow; E exceeds the minimum standard.

60. E. All of the options serve as reasons for orientation.

61. E. Pitch represents the number of characters contained within an inch.

62. D. The best choice is D.

63. C. Option A is assets less liabilities; B is a debt obligation; D is business income; E is business cost.

64. D. Malignant hypertension is a severe form with vascular damage.

65. B. A is below the standard. C through E exceed the standard.

66. C. The remaining options should have been determined before the person was hired.

Clinical:

1. E. Family history is a detailed account of the illnesses and health status of family members. The chief complaint is the primary reason the patient sought medical care; the social history involves topics such as smoking, alcohol and/or drug use, and sexual behavior. The past medical history includes events that have occurred through the patient's lifetime that are significant; the occupational history directly applies to work-related events that could adversely affect health.

2. C. An antiseptic is a substance that will prevent or reduce the risk of infection rather than just disinfecting.

3. B. Medical dictionaries do not have drug information printed in the text as do the *Physicians' Desk Reference* and *US Pharmacopeia/National Formulary,* the product insert, or a desk reference for nonprescription medications.

4. C. Although strains are painful, they will not cause a breathing emergency.

5. A. An engineering control is a device designed to be used with work practices. Options B and D are work practice controls while C is an example of personal protective equipment (PPE).

6. C. Vitamin D is found in milk and milk products such as cheese. The other foods listed do not have vitamin D or have negligible amounts.

7. D. Except for mensuration and auscultation, the other examination methods do not require use of an instrument.

8. E. A scalpel is used for cutting into tissue, whereas an obturator is used to close an opening and may be placed within a director. An applicator is used for placing substances onto a surface or taking samples from a surface; a trocar is an instrument usually used for extracting fluid from body cavities.

9. D. Acetaminophen is not a controlled drug; codeine and morphine are Schedule II drugs; heroin is a Schedule I drug (illegal).

10. E. Hypovolemic means pertaining to a decreased volume, which could be either blood loss or loss of body fluid. Anaphylactic shock is the result of a severe allergic reaction; psychogenic shock is mind induced; neurogenic is from the nervous system; cardiogenic relates to the heart.

11. E. When freshly voided urine specimens are not clear in appearance, it may indicate a disease process such as infection.

12. E. This process provides a richer base of nutrients for patients who have not been able to assimilate nutrients for various health reasons.

13. B. V_2 and V_6 are precordial (chest leads); aVR and aVL are augmented, unipolar leads.

14. A. An endoscope is a lighted instrument for viewing inside the body. A stethoscope is neither lighted nor used inside the body.

15. C. An example of dispensing a medication is a patient who takes a prescription to a pharmacy, has it filled, pays a fee for the service, and takes the medication home for future use.

16. B. Polyphagia is not a common sign of shock because in states of shock, salivary production is decreased, usually resulting in less swallowing rather than more.

17. A. Hemopoiesis is the formation of new blood cells; therefore, it would be associated with hematology, the study of the blood and blood-forming organs.

18. B. Carbohydrates and fats are nutrients that provide energy, but not the basic building blocks for repairing/replacing tissue. Vitamins and minerals are important to maintain tissue.

19. D. Subjective is data reported by the patient; objective is data found on examination; assessment is adding the subjective and objective data together. Once the assessment is completed, a plan is formulated. POMR is the abbreviation for problem-oriented medical records.

20. D. If ratcheted instruments are not open during the sterilization process, surfaces not exposed to the sterilant will remain contaminated.

21. B. The Drug Enforcement Agency mandates that Schedule II drugs be inventoried every 2 years and records retained for an additional 2 years.

22. A. A viable airway is essential before a rescuer can even initiate breathing in victims with respiratory arrest. When the brain is deprived of oxygen, brain damage and/or death can occur quickly.

23. B. Neisseria gonorrheae is typically described as gram-negative [diplo] cocci. The bacteria, when observed microscopically, appear in pairs of round-shaped microorganisms and are red to pink when stained.

24. C. Fats provide more flavor and thus more satisfaction when used in food preparation. Fats also have a caloric value of 9 calories/gram and so are more concentrated than proteins or carbohydrates.

25. E. A routine physical examination would not necessitate the use of thumb forceps, which could be used to extract a foreign body. The other instruments are used to assess heart and lung sounds, ears, reflexes, and the eyes.

26. D. Temperatures less than 250° to 270° F may result in not sterilizing the contents within the autoclave. The autoclave design is steam under pressure, and temperatures exceeding 270° F may damage the instrument and/or the contents.

27. E. The responsibility of the drug inventory is the health-care provider's, not the patients who have accepted the drugs. The first four items are essential information relating to the provider's responsibility of the inventory.

28. E. Patients having a heart attack often have complaints of increased sweating, intense chest pain, shortness of breath, and/or sick stomach.

29. C. Specific gravity is one of the parameters performed in the physical examination of the urinalysis.

30. D. Carbohydrates, fats, and proteins are nutrients; although minerals play a role in regulating many body functions, they do not act as catalysts for metabolism.

31. B. V_1 is placed to the right of the sternum at the 4th intercostal space; V_4 is placed in the 5th intercostal space at the junction of the left midclavicular line; V_3 is placed midway between V_2 and V_4; V_5 and V_6 follow in the same line with placement at the axillary line and midaxillary line, respectively.

32. C. When lids are placed down, the inner surface of the cap could become contaminated.

33. A. DEA-106 is the form to be completed when a controlled substance is lost, and DEA-222 is the form for narcotics shipments. The DEA does not have a form 335 or 457.

34. D. Epilepsy is characterized by uncontrolled seizures or convulsions. The other conditions do not commonly cause convulsions.

35. D. Hemoglobin A is normal hemoglobin; hemoglobin C is an abnormal hemoglobin that substitutes lysine for glutamic acid; hemoglobin F is the hemoglobin found in fetal cells; hemoglobin D does not exist.

36. E. All of the B vitamins are water soluble.

37. B. The demographic area is not part of the actual medical history of the patient but yields important information for future reference and in case of emergency.

38. C. A first intention wound is part of the healing process in which there is no contamination and no complications. Second intention wound healing demonstrates a postoperative complication such as an infection. A third intention wound demonstrates where the healing process has been interrupted by gross infection and requires surgical intervention. There are no fourth or fifth intention wounds.

39. E. *Signetur* means "write on label." The prescription is the complete form with all of the individual components. The subscription is the section including the amount of drug to be dispensed and special directions to the pharmacist when preparing the drug. The inscription is the area including the patient's name, address, and date of prescription.

40. C. According to the Rule of Nines, the head and neck area represents 9% of the total body surface: each arm is 9%; the trunk is 36%; each leg is 18%; the genitalia account for 1%.

41. C. *Salmonella* bacteria cause a form of gastroenteritis when foods contaminated with them are consumed. Adequate cooking, good refrigeration, and handwashing help to control outbreaks.

42. B. Adolescents have constant exposure to various media that continually emphasize and entice them into the illusion they need to be as thin as models to be desirable and attractive.

43. C. After the initial inspection/examination of the breasts in the sitting position, a patient is usually placed in the supine position for palpation of the breasts.

44. A. The dressing is immediately applied over wounds; following this application, the dressing may be covered by a wrap, bandage, or cast to hold it in place. Only the small pad area of a Band-Aid is sterile and would be applied to a wound.

45. A. p.c. is the abbreviation for the Latin phrase *post cibum,* post meaning after. PRN would be the abbreviation for as needed; ad lib represents as desired; a.c. is the abbreviated form of *ante cibum,* ante meaning before.

46. D. In cases of heat stroke, the body conserves water for the internal organs, resulting in dry, hot, and red skin.

47. A. The reagent strip requires less than a drop of urine for testing specific gravity or other components on the strip. Specific gravity cannot be assessed through microscopy or litmus paper. The urinometer, though no longer used in current practices, uses the largest amount of urine for testing since the quantity must be sufficient to float a calibrated stem.

48. D. PKU is the recognized abbreviation for *phenylketonuria.* Galactosemia is the presence of galactose in the blood; and homocystinuria is the rare presence of homocystine in the urine; tyrosinosis is an abnormal condition of tyrosine (crystals); histidinemia is the presence of histidine in the blood. All are inherited metabolic disorders.

49. D. The distance across each small square is 0.04 second. The distance across one large square block is 0.2 second (five times greater because one large block contains five small squares). The distance across five large squares is equal to 1 second.

50. E. A Penrose drain is a thin rubber tube used as a surgical drain device. Its use would not be indicated in a laceration repair.

51. B. Nitroglycerin is the generic name for Nitrostat or Nitroquick. Nifedipine is the generic name for Procardia, while alprazolam is generic for Xanax. Prozac is the brand name, not a generic.

52. A. Because insulin shock is more life-threatening than a diabetic coma, since the brain and other vital organs cannot function without adequate energy, it is best to administer sugar. Once evaluation of the patient has been performed, if the blood sugar is high, insulin can be administered.

53. A. Anisochromia of RBCs relates to varying concentrations of color within the RBCs. Hypochromia, polychromia, and hyperchromia are all abnormal concentrations of hemoglobin (color) within the cells; normochromia refers to a normal concentration of color or hemoglobin.

54. C. One of the most common signs of diabetes mellitus is excessive urination.

55. D. ROS is the abbreviation for "review of systems," which includes questions directed at each of the major body systems. The other abbreviations represent the following: CC—chief complaint; PMH—past medical history; FH—family history; and PI—present illness.

56. C. The other instruments are not used to cut tissue.

57. B. A is used for treatment, C is used to identify a disease, D is used to promote defecation, and E is used to relieve pain.

58. D. Water should not be given to someone suffering from shock.

59. D. BAP (blood agar plates), MAC (MacConkey plates), PEA (phenylethyl alcohol plates), and TM (Thayer-Martin plates) are all examples of agar that are semisolid. TSB (trypticase soy broth) is the only liquid medium listed and is contained in a tube rather than on a plate.

60. A. Lacto, meaning milk and ovo, meaning egg is the correct response.

61. B. The Ishihara test is a specialized test to assess color blindness and could only be associated with an ophthalmological examination.

62. D. The other instruments are not used to grasp or clamp tissue.

63. D. The others are trade names.

64. A. The other applications will either have no effect or exacerbate the condition.

65. E. Beakers, cuvettes, bottles, and flasks are designed to hold and measure larger quantities of liquids than pipettes.

66. B. A is the process of converting nutrients into energy, C is the destruction of substances to release energy, D is a nonsense distracter, and E is the energy required to maintain normal processes.

RMA SIMULATION TEST

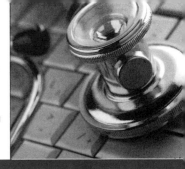

Post-Test

200-question, 3-hour, timed practice exam

PART 1: GENERAL

DIRECTIONS

Each of the questions or incomplete statements below is followed by four suggested answers or completions. Select the *one* answer or completion that is *best* in each case and fill in the circle containing the corresponding letter on the answer sheet. Perforated answer sheets are located at the back of the book.

1. A basic word element that identifies the central meaning of a word is a
   a. root
   b. prefix
   c. suffix
   d. combining form

2. The opposite of distal is
   a. anterior
   b. lateral
   c. medial
   d. proximal

3. Law developed and enforced by government agencies best describes
   a. common law
   b. statutory law
   c. administrative law
   d. constitutional law

4. Communication is best defined as the
   a. process of orally speaking to each other
   b. process of nonverbally speaking to each other
   c. process of sharing meaning
   d. process of talking

5. Which of the following prefixes refers to a color?
   a. uni-
   b. hemi-
   c. circum-
   d. melan/o-

6. The control center of a cell best describes the
   a. nucleus
   b. cytoplasm
   c. cell membrane
   d. organelles

7. Which of the following is considered a mandatory credential?
   a. registration
   b. certification
   c. licensure
   d. accreditation

8. The means by which meaning is conveyed best describes
   a. source
   b. message
   c. receiver
   d. channel

9. All of the following are adjectival suffixes **EXCEPT**
   a. -al
   b. -oma
   c. -ic
   d. -ical

10. All of the following are functions of the integumentary system **EXCEPT**
    a. protection
    b. sensation
    c. thermoregulation
    d. calcium storage

11. In order for consent to be informed, which of the following elements should be present?
    a. nature of the patient's condition
    b. nature and purpose of the proposed treatment
    c. risks and benefits of the proposed treatment
    d. all of the above

12. Anything that interferes with the communication process best describes
    a. source
    b. receiver
    c. noise
    d. message

13. Which of the following is a proper plural?
    a. bursa
    b. irises
    c. ovum
    d. irides

14. The shaft of a bone best describes the
    a. epiphysis
    b. diaphysis
    c. endosteum
    d. periosteum

15. The health care provider is required to report the following to the appropriate local agencies **EXCEPT**
    a. AIDS
    b. cholera
    c. tuberculosis
    d. strep throat

16. The objective of therapeutic communication includes
    a. communicating technical information in a form the patient can understand
    b. providing comfort
    c. indicating that patients are important
    d. all of the above

17. All of the following terms are spelled correctly **EXCEPT**
    a. sphygmomanometer
    b. arteriosclerosis
    c. synovialectomy
    d. angioplasty

18. Muscles that can be controlled consciously best describes
    a. smooth muscle
    b. involuntary muscle
    c. striated muscle
    d. cardiac muscle

19. Which of the following charting situations may create liability?
    a. failing to properly document care
    b. scribbling out errors
    c. altering a medical document
    d. all of the above

20. All of the following are considered facilitative communication techniques **EXCEPT**
    a. advising
    b. accepting
    c. encouraging
    d. clarifying

21. Myring/o- means which of the following?
    a. eyelid
    b. eye
    c. eardrum
    d. earflap

22. The chamber of the heart that receives deoxygenated blood returning from the body is the
    a. right ventricle
    b. left ventricle
    c. right atrium
    d. left atrium

23. Which of the following best describes the omission of care when one had the duty to provide such care?
    a. misfeasance
    b. malfeasance
    c. nonfeasance
    d. malpractice

24. Which of the following may create communication barriers?
    a. shame
    b. embarrassment
    c. misunderstanding
    d. all of the above

25. The underlined part of the word salpingopathy represents which of the following word parts?
    a. root
    b. prefix
    c. suffix
    d. combining form

26. Which of the following best describes a function of the respiratory system?
    a. hormone production
    b. movement
    c. oxidation
    d. air exchange

27. Which of the following is considered an intentional tort?
    a. negligence
    b. malpractice
    c. misfeasance
    d. defamation

28. Among Maslow's Hierarchy of Needs, the need for shelter and freedom from anxiety best describes
    a. physiological need
    b. safety need
    c. social need
    d. self-esteem need

29. Which of the following describes bacteria arranged in clusters?
    a. Staphylococci
    b. Streptococci
    c. Diplococci
    d. Micrococci

30. Which of the following organs is best described as an accessory organ of the digestive system?
    a. esophagus
    b. stomach
    c. intestines
    d. liver

31. The AMA Code of Ethics subscribes to which of the following general principles?
    a. respect for persons
    b. confidentiality
    c. work within one's scope of practice
    d. all of the above

32. Assuming the patient role may interfere with which of the following needs?
    a. social
    b. safety
    c. self-esteem
    d. all of the above

33. A provider who specializes in diagnosing and treating conditions of the eye is an
    a. ophthalmologist
    b. ophthalmology
    c. ophthalmological
    d. ophthalmopathy

34. Which of the following structures connects the kidney and the urinary bladder?
    a. ureter
    b. urethra
    c. Bowman's capsule
    d. glomerulus

35. Uncooperative patients are frustrating to work with because
    a. they obviously do not understand their condition
    b. the health professional is denied experiencing the satisfaction associated with helping the patient
    c. they do not care about themselves
    d. they are immature and stubborn

36. Setting aside unpleasant th___ ___nd feelings best describes which of the ___ ___ uncon-scious defense mechanisms?
    a. repression
    b. regression
    c. aggression
    d. rationalization

37. An increased number of white blood cells be___ describes
    a. leukocyte
    b. leukemia
    c. leukocytosis
    d. leukopenia

38. All of the following structures are part of the female reproductive system **EXCEPT** the
    a. uterus
    b. fallopian tubes
    c. epididymis
    d. vulva

39. Arguments supporting abortion include
    a. killing another is wrong
    b. all living things have a right to life
    c. a woman's right to self-determination
    d. the unborn fetus is helpless and therefore deserves protection

40. Which of the following represents a duty when adopting the sick role?
    a. exemption from responsibility
    b. make every effort to get well
    c. exemption from social obligations
    d. both (A) and (B)

41. An increased rate of breathing best describes
    a. bradypnea
    b. hyperpnea
    c. apnea
    d. tachypnea

42. All of the following are part of the peripheral nervous system **EXCEPT** the
    a. brain
    b. spinal nerves
    c. afferent nerves
    d. autonomic nervous system

43. In distributing scarce resources, the following criteria may be considered ethical **EXCEPT**
    a. to each an equal share
    b. to each according to need
    c. to each according to probability of benefit
    d. to each according to social class

...with adopting the sick role may

44. Losses a̶s̶tractiveness
include̶l̶y̶
   a. n̶e̶
   b̶.̶f the above

̶n̶e who specializes in the study of tissue is a(n)
   a. histology
   b. histologist
   c. cytology
   d. cytologist

46. Olfaction relates to which of the following senses?
   a. taste
   b. sight
   c. smell
   d. touch

47. "To do no harm" best describes
   a. nonmaleficence
   b. beneficence
   c. fidelity
   d. veracity

48. The stages of dying as described by Dr. Elisabeth Kübler-Ross include all of the following **EXCEPT**
   a. denial
   b. anger
   c. bargaining
   d. humiliation

49. Which of the following words best describes a muscular disorder?
   a. tendonitis
   b. metrorrhagia
   c. emphysema
   d. amyotrophic lateral sclerosis

50. All of the following hormones are produced by the anterior pituitary **EXCEPT**
   a. somatotropic hormone
   b. prolactin
   c. thyroid-stimulating hormone
   d. oxytocin

51. A defense against malpractice may include acts of independent agents that stand in the way of the causal connection between the negligent act and the damage suffered. This is called
   a. tolling of the statute of limitations
   b. intervening cause
   c. contributory negligence
   d. comparative negligence

52. If a patient is in obvious pain, the medical assistant should
   a. ignore the signs of pain
   b. interact with the patient in the usual manner
   c. indicate to the patient that he appears uncomfortable and offer assistance
   d. consult the healthcare provider immediately

53. The destruction of blood cells is called
   a. hematology
   b. hematoma
   c. hemolysis
   d. cytolysis

54. The body region representing the neck region is the
   a. axilla
   b. patellar
   c. cervical
   d. buccal

55. A standard or principle that guides our behavior regarding what is right and what is wrong is a
   a. norm
   b. moral
   c. morale
   d. duty

56. If an upset patient expresses frustration concerning a long wait, the medical assistant should say
   a. "Yeah, I know, it's a busy day."
   b. "We are very sorry; the doctor is way behind."
   c. "I am sorry; excuse me while I check to see when you may expect to be seen."
   d. "This is a very busy clinic; please be patient."

57. A herniation of a joint capsule is called
   a. arthrocele
   b. arthrosis
   c. arthritis
   d. orchidocele

58. The organelle responsible for energy production is the
   a. nucleus
   b. ribosome
   c. Golgi body
   d. mitochondria

59. An obligation to act in certain ways is a(n)
   a. norm
   b. moral
   c. duty
   d. ethic

60. A patient enters the clinic and collapses on the floor. The medical assistant should
    a. call 911
    b. yell for help
    c. calmly page the provider and immediately check the patient's airway
    d. send a waiting patient to the back office to summon help

61. A decrease in size of an organ or tissue is known as
    a. dystrophy
    b. myopathy
    c. atrophy
    d. organopenia

62. The middle layer of the skin (true skin) is the
    a. epidermis
    b. hypodermis
    c. dermis
    d. subcutaneous

63. Telling the truth best defines
    a. beneficence
    b. nonmaleficence
    c. fidelity
    d. veracity

64. Reasons patients may be reluctant to ask that instructions be repeated include
    a. fear
    b. embarrassment
    c. bewilderment
    d. all of the above

65. The medical abbreviation meaning *every other day* is
    a. q.i.d.
    b. q.o.d.
    c. q.h.s.
    d. q.o.n.

66. The bone that forms the inferior, posterior aspect of the skull is the
    a. parietal
    b. temporal
    c. mandible
    d. occipital

PART 2: ADMINISTRATIVE

DIRECTIONS

Each of the questions or incomplete statements below is followed by four suggested answers or completions. Select the *one* answer or completion that is *best* in each case and fill in the circle containing the corresponding letter on the answer sheet.

1. A medium-size computer that can handle multiple users is a
   a. supercomputer
   b. mainframe
   c. minicomputer
   d. microcomputer

2. The purpose of records management includes which of the following?
   a. classifying
   b. arranging
   c. storage
   d. all of the above

3. Which of the following are important attributes of an effective receptionist?
   a. positive attitude
   b. professional appearance
   c. proper etiquette
   d. all of the above

4. A restrictive endorsement is when
   a. the payee signs the back of the check
   b. the drawer signs the back of the check
   c. the payee directs how the check is to be made payable
   d. the drawee signs the back of the check

5. The purpose of medical coding includes
   a. tracking diseases
   b. classifying diseases
   c. providing comparable data for research
   d. all of the above

6. An insurance policy clause that restricts the overpayment of benefits when an insured has more than one policy is called
   a. coordination of benefits
   b. assignment of benefits
   c. copayment
   d. exclusions

7. Which of the following factors should be considered when scheduling a meeting?
   a. meeting objectives
   b. time, place, and duration
   c. expected attendance
   d. all of the above

8. Which of the following is considered a peripheral?
   a. central processing unit
   b. read only memory
   c. read access memory
   d. monitor

9. Checking for and repairing damaged documents is part of what step in the filing process?
   a. conditioning
   b. inspecting
   c. indexing
   d. sorting

10. Which of the following visitors should be immediately announced and escorted to the provider's office?
    a. pharmaceutical representatives
    b. healthcare providers
    c. vendors
    d. former patients

11. Which of the following documents is prepared when money is placed in an account?
    a. check
    b. deposit ticket
    c. bank statement
    d. debit memo

12. All of the following coding systems are associated with medical procedures **EXCEPT**
    a. CPT
    b. HCPCS
    c. RBRVS
    d. ICD-9-CM

13. An insurance company that sells or administers an insurance contract is also known as the
    a. provider
    b. carrier
    c. beneficiary
    d. policy

14. A typed list of the items to be discussed during a meeting is called the
    a. minutes
    b. motion
    c. agenda
    d. facilitation

15. All of the following are input devices **EXCEPT** the
    a. mouse
    b. joystick
    c. printer
    d. light pen

16. All of the following indexing rules are true **EXCEPT**
    a. The surname is indexed as unit 1.
    b. Initials come after complete names.
    c. Apostrophes in a name are disregarded.
    d. Numbers are indexed as if written out.

17. Which of the following represents improper telephone technique?
    a. answering a call with "please hold"
    b. asking the caller if (s)he can hold and waiting for a reply
    c. thanking the caller for holding
    d. checking periodically with callers who are on hold

18. MICR stands for
    a. mathematical index of cash and receipts
    b. magnetic ink character recognition
    c. monetary input of cash and receivables
    d. magnetically inked cash receipts

19. The ICD of ICD-9-CM stands for
    a. International Classification of Diseases
    b. Internal Coding of Disorders
    c. International College of Diagnosticians
    d. Index of Codes Directory

20. Contractual clauses that identify additional coverage beyond what is standard are called
    a. premiums
    b. copayments
    c. riders
    d. policies

21. The minutes of a meeting typically do *not* include which of the following?
    a. name of the organization
    b. place, date, and time of meeting
    c. those in attendance and absent
    d. salutation

22. All of the following are considered secondary storage devices **EXCEPT**
    a. hard disk
    b. floppy disk
    c. magnetic tape reel
    d. modem

23. A filing system that organizes items chronologically for action when the date arrives is called a(n)
   a. alphabetical file
   b. alphanumeric file
   c. numerical file
   d. tickler file

24. Which of the following information is typically *not* included in a telephone message?
   a. date and time of call
   b. name of person called
   c. reason for the call
   d. the location of the person who was called

25. A check may be dishonored for which of the following reasons?
   a. NSF
   b. postdated check
   c. overdraft
   d. all of the above

26. Which of the following ICD-9-CM codes might require an External cause code (E-code)?
   a. 011
   b. 210
   c. 420.1
   d. 890

27. All of the following are government sponsored programs **EXCEPT**
   a. Medicare
   b. Medicaid
   c. Workers' Compensation
   d. Blue Cross/Blue Shield

28. A method of generating ideas without judgment or criticism is
   a. brainstorming
   b. facilitating
   c. chairing
   d. monitoring

29. Which of the following is considered software?
   a. monitor
   b. Microsoft® Word
   c. disk drive
   d. printer

30. A mail classification that includes books and manuscripts is
   a. first class
   b. second class
   c. third class
   d. special fourth class

31. Which of the following calls should be transferred to the provider?
   a. calls requesting billing information
   b. unidentified callers
   c. patients expressing problems associated with treatment or medication
   d. calls from office suppliers

32. When completing the check register, all of the following information is recorded **EXCEPT**
   a. the date the check is written
   b. the check number
   c. the payee
   d. the date the check is expected to clear

33. Which of the following ICD-9-CM codes refer to factors that influence health status?
   a. V-codes
   b. Volume I codes
   c. E-codes
   d. Volume II codes

34. Which of the following is funded by both federal and state revenues?
   a. Medicare
   b. Medicaid
   c. Workers' Compensation
   d. Tri care

35. All of the following are part of the management process **EXCEPT**
   a. planning
   b. organizing
   c. directing
   d. reporting

36. Which of the following is not considered a part of the data processing cycle?
   a. input
   b. processing
   c. output
   d. informing

37. All of the following are considered the closing part of the letter **EXCEPT** the
   a. complimentary close
   b. salutation
   c. signature line
   d. reference notation

38. Which of the following actions would *not* be taken when speaking to an angry caller?
   a. Remain calm
   b. Determine and record the reason for the anger
   c. Resolve the problem if within your power
   d. Project a disrespectful tone

39. Which of the following information is typically *not* shown on the bank statement?
   a. balance on deposit at the beginning of the period
   b. amount of deposits credited during the period
   c. amount of checks honored during the period
   d. names of payees paid during the period

40. Which of the following diagnoses would be coded as indicated?
   a. rule out appendicitis
   b. suspected skull fracture
   c. questionable ETOH abuse
   d. definitive poliomyelitis

41. Which of the following programs is available to active duty military dependents?
   a. Medicare
   b. Medicaid
   c. Workers' Compensation
   d. Tricare

42. Leadership is best described as
   a. the process of developing, implementing, and achieving organizational objectives
   b. the process of achieving goals in a timely fashion
   c. the process of achieving goals using the least amount of resources
   d. the process of working with and through people to achieve organizational objectives willingly

43. The process of activating the input of the operating system into main memory best describes
   a. booting
   b. installing
   c. formatting
   d. copying

44. When a letter requires a second page, the following information is typed in which order near the top of the second page?
   a. recipient's name, page number, date
   b. recipient's name, date, page number
   c. page number, recipient's name, date
   d. page number, date, recipient's name

45. Which of the following conditions has the highest emergency priority?
   a. loss of consciousness
   b. cessation of breathing
   c. shock
   d. bleeding

46. All of the following items are subtracted from the bank statement during reconciliation **EXCEPT**
   a. outstanding checks
   b. outstanding withdrawals
   c. outstanding deposits
   d. bank errors that incorrectly increased your account balance

47. CPT stands for
   a. common procedural terminology
   b. current procedural terminology
   c. common provider treatments
   d. current provider treatments

48. Which of the following commonly serves as a fiscal intermediary for the Medicare program?
   a. Blue Cross/Blue Shield
   b. Medicaid
   c. Tricare
   d. Workers' Compensation

49. An employee's ability to properly perform a task is a function of
   a. knowledge
   b. experience
   c. performance
   d. all of the above

50. The process of loading the software instructions onto the hard disk is called
   a. booting
   b. installing
   c. formatting
   d. copying

51. Mail inadvertently opened should be
   a. stapled shut
   b. left as is
   c. resealed with tape with the notation "opened in error"
   d. immediately hand delivered

52. The long-distance directory assistance number is
   a. 0 + area code + 411
   b. 1 + area code + 411
   c. 411 or 1+ area code + 555-1212
   d. none of the above

53. The bank statement shows a balance of $4250, deposits in transit total $1200, and outstanding checks equal $300. The check register balance should be
   a. $2750
   b. $3350
   c. $4550
   d. $5150

54. Which CPT modifier indicates that multiple modifiers have been assigned?
    a. -22
    b. -47
    c. -66
    d. -99

55. Who of the following is most likely eligible for Medicaid?
    a. persons age 65 and older
    b. dependents of retired military personnel
    c. workers afflicted with end-stage renal disease
    d. persons receiving Supplemental Security Income (SSI) for the aged and disabled

56. When interviewing job applicants, all of the following should be considered **EXCEPT**
    a. social affiliations
    b. education and training
    c. experience
    d. references

57. A predefined computer setting that is automatically loaded with each new document unless changed by the user is the
    a. default
    b. directory
    c. menu
    d. macro

58. Upon receiving checks in the mail, the MA should first
    a. deposit them immediately
    b. place them in the safe until deposited
    c. restrictively endorse them
    d. temporarily store them in the cash drawer

59. The time zone difference between California and New Jersey is
    a. 1 hour
    b. 2 hours
    c. 3 hours
    d. 4 hours

60. An organization's ability to pay its debts is known as
    a. solvency
    b. profitability
    c. effectiveness
    d. efficiency

61. According to CPT coding conventions, terms after a semicolon (;)
    a. indicate synonyms
    b. are part of, or clarify, a main term
    c. identify ill-defined or ambiguous terms
    d. provide directions to seek an alternative code

62. Which of the following is the universal claim form?
    a. DD-214
    b. COBRA-1990
    c. CMS-1500
    d. Form 1904

63. Which of the following interview questions is illegal?
    a. "Where did you receive your training?"
    b. "Do you have any children?"
    c. "Do you have any hobbies?"
    d. "May I contact your references?"

64. An index of files on a disk is known as the
    a. macro
    b. directory
    c. menu
    d. window

65. Documents that have the important information highlighted have been
    a. annotated
    b. dictated
    c. circulated
    d. restricted

66. WATS stands for
    a. Washington Tax Service
    b. Western Area Transit System
    c. Wide Area Telephone Service
    d. Whirlpool and Therapeutic Sauna

67. The property of value owned or controlled by an organization is known as
    a. capital
    b. liability
    c. asset
    d. expense

PART 3: CLINICAL

DIRECTIONS

Each of the questions or incomplete statements below is followed by four suggested answers or completions. Select the *one* answer or completion that is *best* in each case and fill in the circle containing the corresponding letter on the answer sheet.

1. Which of the following is typically *not* found in the medical chart?
    a. chief complaint
    b. past medical history
    c. physical examination
    d. patient ledger card

2. Measuring a body part is called
   a. inspection
   b. palpation
   c. percussion
   d. mensuration

3. According to the food pyramid, which of the following nutrients should be consumed least?
   a. grains
   b. vegetables
   c. oils
   d. fruits

4. Cardiac cells in a resting, negatively charged state are known as
   a. polarization
   b. depolarization
   c. repolarization
   d. any of the above

5. Which of the following is considered a dissecting instrument?
   a. thumb forceps
   b. hemostat
   c. surgical scissor
   d. probe

6. A drug that is used to prevent disease is
   a. therapeutic
   b. prophylactic
   c. diagnostic
   d. cathartic

7. Which of the following should be assessed first when rendering first aid?
   a. pulse
   b. pupillary reaction
   c. pain or injury to limbs
   d. emotional state

8. Which of the following is a subdivision of the microbiology department?
   a. serology
   b. chemistry
   c. parasitology
   d. hematology

9. All of the following are signs of decomposing urine **EXCEPT**
   a. bacterial growth
   b. pH becomes acidic
   c. cellular structures disintegrate
   d. acetone evaporates

10. The study of blood and blood-forming tissues is known as
    a. hematology
    b. microbiology
    c. bacteriology
    d. clinical chemistry

11. Which of the following is the smallest pathogen?
    a. *Escherichia coli*
    b. *Enterobius vermicularis*
    c. *Rickettsia rickettsii*
    d. Epstein-Barr virus

12. Which of the following documents is usually found only in the problem oriented medical record?
    a. medical history
    b. progress notes
    c. diagnostic reports
    d. problem list

13. An instrument used to test hearing is a(n)
    a. stethoscope
    b. tuning fork
    c. ophthalmoscope
    d. otoscope

14. A diet of plant foods supplemented with dairy products and eggs is called
    a. lacto-ovo vegetarian
    b. vegan
    c. lacto-vegetarian
    d. regular

15. All of the following are included in the cardiac electrical conduction system **EXCEPT**
    a. sinoatrial node
    b. atrioventricular node
    c. bundle of His
    d. sinoatrial septum

16. An instrument used to grasp or clamp down objects is a(n)
    a. scalpel
    b. bandage scissor
    c. obturator
    d. forceps

17. A drug's generic name is best illustrated by which one of the following?
    a. Tylenol
    b. Aspirin
    c. Achromycin
    d. Salicylic acid

18. When rendering first aid to a choking infant, all of the following may be performed **EXCEPT**
    a. back blows
    b. chest thrust
    c. open mouth
    d. finger sweep

19. Which of the following health personnel are trained to perform the majority of laboratory procedures?
    a. pathologist
    b. histocytologist
    c. medical technologist
    d. medical laboratory technician

20. The physical examination of urine includes
    a. color
    b. transparency
    c. odor
    d. all of the above

21. Equal concentration of solute inside and outside a cell is known as
    a. isotonic
    b. hypotonic
    c. ionic pressure
    d. hypertonic

22. All of the following are included in a Gram stain **EXCEPT**
    a. crystal violet
    b. new methylene blue
    c. safranin
    d. iodine

23. Which of the following materials *does not* require the use of universal precautions?
    a. blood
    b. semen
    c. feces
    d. vaginal secretions

24. Examination of the back may be performed when the patient is in all of the following positions **EXCEPT**
    a. sitting
    b. Trendelenburg
    c. prone
    d. standing

25. The constructive process of building up new substances is called
    a. metabolism
    b. anabolism
    c. catabolism
    d. basal metabolism

26. Atrial depolarization is represented by the
    a. P wave
    b. PR interval
    c. QRS complex
    d. ST segment

27. Which of the following suture sizes is the largest?
    a. 00
    b. 000
    c. 0000
    d. 00000

28. All of the following are liquid preparations **EXCEPT**
    a. syrup
    b. suspension
    c. troche
    d. elixir

29. When performing CPR on an adult, chest compressions should be
    a. one-half to 1 inch
    b. 1 to 1 and one-half inches
    c. 1 and one-half to 2 inches
    d. 2 to 2 and one-half inches

30. The most common bloodborne pathogen is
    a. HIV
    b. HBV
    c. *Salmonella*
    d. *Streptococcus*

31. The unit of measure for urine specific gravity is
    a. mg/dL
    b. mg
    c. mL
    d. none of the above

32. The first step when performing a capillary puncture is to
    a. cleanse the site with alcohol
    b. select the site
    c. don gloves
    d. identify the patient

33. All of the following are Gram-positive cocci **EXCEPT**
    a. *Streptococcus pyogenes*
    b. *Staphylococcus aureus*
    c. *Neisseria meningitidis*
    d. *Micrococcus tetragenus*

34. Which of the following may affect body temperature?
    a. age
    b. environment
    c. activity
    d. all of the above

35. All of the following materials are associated with an ophthalmological exam **EXCEPT**
    a. otoscope
    b. Snellen chart
    c. tonometer
    d. Ishihara plates

36. A unit of heat energy is
    a. RDA
    b. metabolism
    c. calorie
    d. enrichment

37. Ventricular depolarization is represented by the
    a. P wave
    b. PR interval
    c. QRS complex
    d. ST segment

38. Which of the following surgical procedures is used to remove abscesses?
    a. incision and drainage
    b. laceration repair
    c. cyst removal
    d. toenail resection

39. Common signs and symptoms of drug abuse include
    a. changes in appearance
    b. changes in attitude and mood
    c. increased friendliness
    d. (A) and (B) only

40. The compression to ventilation ratio for adult, one-rescuer CPR is
    a. 15:1
    b. 15:2
    c. 30:1
    d. 30:2

41. Treating all body fluids as if they are infectious regardless of their true pathogenicity is called
    a. employee-right-to-know
    b. MSDS
    c. OSHA
    d. universal precautions

42. Microscopic structures found in the urine that are composed of precipitated protein are called
    a. blood cells
    b. casts
    c. crystals
    d. bacteria

43. RBCs that are pale in color indicate
    a. hypochromia
    b. hyperchromia
    c. anisochromia
    d. polychromasia

44. A bacillus that stains red with Gram stain is
    a. GPC
    b. GNC
    c. GPR
    d. GNR

45. All of the following are characteristics of the pulse **EXCEPT**
    a. rate
    b. rhythm
    c. volume
    d. depth

46. Diagnostic imaging is best associated with which of the following specialties?
    a. pediatrics
    b. gynecology
    c. internal medicine
    d. orthopedics

47. Nutritional elements containing the most calories per gram are
    a. carbohydrates
    b. proteins
    c. fats
    d. vitamins

48. Process of cleaning or freeing materials from dirt is called
    a. sterilization
    b. disinfection
    c. asepsis
    d. sanitization

49. Most drugs are metabolized by the
    a. lungs
    b. pancreas
    c. intestines
    d. liver

50. Burns that require immediate activation of local EMS include
    a. first-degree burns on the arms
    b. second-degree burns on the shoulders
    c. third-degree burn over a small area
    d. burns that cause breathing difficulties

51. Common signs and symptoms of myocardial infarction include
    a. diaphoresis
    b. angina pectoris
    c. dyspnea
    d. all of the above

52. An instrument that uses a spinning force to separate solids of differing mass is a(n)
    a. spectrophotometer
    b. centrifuge
    c. autoclave
    d. seralyzer

53. When centrifuging urine for microscopic analysis, the MA should use
    a. 4 to 6 mL
    b. 6 to 8 mL
    c. 8 to 10 mL
    d. 10 to 12 mL

54. The normal adult hemoglobin is approximately
    a. 10 to 12 g/dL
    b. 12 to 14 g/dL
    c. 14 to16 g/dL
    d. 16 to 18 g/dL

55. *Enterobius vermicularis* is commonly known as
    a. tapeworm
    b. pinworm
    c. roundworm
    d. flatworm

56. A common acronym meaning the left ear is
    a. AD
    b. OD
    c. AS
    d. OS

57. The process of measuring range of motion of a joint is
    a. arthrometry
    b. goniometry
    c. cystometry
    d. electromyography

58. All of the following are fat-soluble vitamins **EXCEPT**
    a. A
    b. D
    c. E
    d. B

59. Which of the following body parts requires use of the Potter-Bucky diaphragm for X-ray?
    a. hand
    b. ankle
    c. foot
    d. thigh

60. All of the following are proper aseptic techniques **EXCEPT**
    a. Transfer forceps are held facing down.
    b. Bottles containing sterile solution should not touch the sterile receptacle when poured.
    c. Lids are placed down on the table.
    d. Do not reach over a sterile field.

61. The form completed when damaged or contaminated controlled substances are destroyed is
    a. DEA-41
    b. DEA-106
    c. DEA-222
    d. DEA-335

62. The most common cause of convulsions is
    a. fever
    b. dehydration
    c. diarrhea
    d. epilepsy

63. A condition commonly caused by hyperbilirubinemia is
    a. lipemia
    b. hemolysis
    c. icterus
    d. melanosis

64. Which of the following is the by product of incomplete fat metabolism?
    a. casts
    b. urobilinogen
    c. ketones
    d. glucose

65. Another name for percent packed RBCs is
    a. CBC
    b. hematocrit
    c. hemoglobin
    d. MCV

66. The study of fungus is
    a. microbiology
    b. mycology
    c. parasitology
    d. virology

67. Which of the following acronyms refers to physical examination of the eye?
    a. CCE
    b. PERRLA
    c. HCM
    d. T&A

RMA POST-TEST SCORE SHEET

DIRECTIONS

1. Comparing your answer sheet with the correct answers listed below for each section, circle the incorrect responses below.
2. Tally the number of incorrect responses in each column and record the total in the space provided.
3. Score each of the three sections as described in Chapter 1. Identify the section (general, administrative, or clinical) having the lowest score.
4. In the section having the lowest overall score, identify the column having the most incorrect responses and turn to the chapter indicated for further study.
5. Concentrate your study on the section with the lowest score by studying the next weakest area and the next, and so on.
6. After completing your study of the weakest content section, turn to the section having the next lowest score, concentrating your study on the column with the lowest score, and so on.

GENERAL: Percent correct: _____%

1=A	2=D	3=C	4=C
5=D	6=A	7=C	8=D
9=B	10=D	11=D	12=C
13=D	14=B	15=D	16=D
17=C	18=C	19=D	20=A
21=C	22=C	23=C	24=D
25=D	26=D	27=D	28=B
29=A	30=D	31=D	32=D
33=A	34=A	35=B	36=A
37=C	38=C	39=C	40=B
41=D	42=A	43=D	44=D
45=B	46=C	47=A	48=D
49=D	50=D	51=B	52=C
53=C	54=C	55=B	56=C
57=A	58=D	59=C	60=C
61=C	62=C	63=D	64=D
65=B	66=D		
_____	_____	_____	_____
Ch.4	Ch.5	Chs.8-9	Chs.6-7

ADMINISTRATIVE: Percent correct: _____%

1=C	2=D	3=D	4=C	5=D	6=A	7=D
8=D	9=A	10=B	11=B	12=D	13=B	14=C
15=C	16=B	17=A	18=B	19=A	20=C	21=D
22=D	23=D	24=D	25=D	26=D	27=D	28=A
29=C	30=D	31=C	32=D	33=A	34=B	35=D
36=D	37=B	38=D	39=D	40=D	41=D	42=D
43=A	44=A	45=B	46=C	47=B	48=A	49=D
50=B	51=C	52=C	53=D	54=D	55=D	56=A
57=A	58=C	59=C	60=A	61=B	62=C	63=B
64=B	65=A	66=C	67=C			
_____	_____	_____	_____	_____	_____	_____
Ch.10	Ch.10	Ch.11	Ch.12	Ch.13	Ch.13	Chs.14-15

1=D	2=D	3=C	4=B	5=C	6=B	7=A	8=C	9=B	10=A	11=D
12=D	13=B	14=A	15=D	16=D	17=D	18=D	19=C	20=D	21=A	22=B
23=C	24=B	25=B	26=A	27=A	28=C	29=C	30=B	31=D	32=D	33=C
34=D	35=A	36=C	37=C	38=A	39=D	40=C	41=D	42=B	43=A	44=D
45=D	46=D	47=C	48=D	49=D	50=D	51=D	52=B	53=D	54=C	55=B
56=C	57=B	58=D	59=D	60=C	61=A	62=D	63=C	64=C	65=B	66=B
67=B										

_____	_____	_____	_____	_____	_____	_____	_____	_____	_____	_____
Ch.16	Ch.16	Ch.21	Ch.16	Ch.17	Ch.18	Ch.19	Ch.20	Ch.20	Ch.20	Ch.20

General:

If you answered nine or more questions incorrectly in any of the columns, turn to the appropriate chapter for further study.

Administrative:

If you answered six or more questions incorrectly in any of the columns, turn to the appropriate chapter for further study.

Clinical:

If you answered three or more questions incorrectly in any of the columns, turn to the appropriate chapter for further study.

Total percent correct (_____ /200 × 100): _____%

RMA scaled score = (Raw score × 0.6) + 40
(Scaled score ≥ 70 is passing)

RMA POST-TEST ANSWERS AND RATIONALES

General:

1. A. The word root is altered by suffixes and/or prefixes; the combining form occurs by placing a vowel immediately following the root to make the word easier to pronounce.

2. D. The opposite of anterior is posterior; the opposite of lateral is medial.

3. C. Common law comes from previous similar decisions in cases; statutory laws are enacted by statutes; constitutional law is based on tenets in the U.S. Constitution.

4. C. Although the other answers do pertain to methods of communication, the idea behind communication is having the ability to share the meaning with others and have them understand you as well.

5. D. Uni- is a prefix for one; hemi- is a prefix for half; circum- is a prefix for around.

6. A. The nucleus of a cell is the "brain" of the cell; the other structures are found within the cell's cytoplasm.

7. C. Registration and certification are voluntary; accreditation is a process for institutions to gain recognition.

8. D. The *source* delivers a *message* through a channel to a *receiver* and gets *feedback*.

9. B. -oma is a suffix meaning tumor; the other suffixes are adjectives added to word roots.

10. D. The skin and its associated structures has no capability to store calcium. The other processes are essential functions of the integumentary system.

11. D. A patient needs to fully understand his or her condition, the nature and purpose of the treatments, and the risks and/or benefits of the proposed treatment to be considered informed in order to consent.

12. C. Noise is the only element listed that is not an integral part of the communication process.

13. D. To be in proper plural form, bursa would be *bursae;* irises is not a medical term; ovum would become *ova.*

14. B. The epiphysis refers to the end of the bone; endosteum is the membrane lining the inside

of the bone cavity; periosteum is the membrane lining the outside of the bone's surface.

15. D. Although strep throat is certainly a contagious disease, the other diseases listed are considered by the Centers for Disease Control and Prevention and other agencies to be communicable and a threat to the public health.

16. D. In communicating with patients, if all of the three elements listed are not conveyed to the patient, there is no therapeutic value in the process.

17. C. The correct spelling for this word is synovectomy.

18. C. Striated muscle is skeletal muscle, which is under the mind's voluntary control; the other muscle types listed are involuntary and thus, not under conscious control.

19. D. Because the medical record is considered a legal document, if any of the events listed occur each or all of them would contribute to provider liability because of inappropriate or inadequate documentation.

20. A. Facilitative means to help; while we may in good faith consider advising helpful, offering unsolicited advice may hinder the communication process, whereas the other techniques will foster it.

21. C. Blephar/o is a combining form referring to eyelid; ophthalm/o is the combining form for the eye. Another way of referring to the earflap is either the auricle or pinna.

22. C. The right ventricle receives blood from the right atrium; the left ventricle receives blood from the left atrium; the right atrium receives blood from the vena cavae; the vena cavae routes deoxygenated blood from the circulatory system back through the heart.

23. C. The prefix *non-* found in the word *nonfeasance* refers to the omission.

24. D. Each of the listed topics would not be conducive to effective communication and as a result create a barrier between the sender and receiver.

25. D. The presence of the "o" following the word root of *salping* demonstrates the combining form, making the word easier to pronounce.

26. D. Option A is an endocrine function; B is musculoskeletal function; C is muscular function.

27. D. Options A–C represent broad categories of negligence (unintentional torts).

28. B. Option A represents the need for water and food; C represents the need for love and belonging; D represents the need for respect and prestige.

29. A. Option B relates to bacteria arranged in chains; C is double cocci; D is small cocci.

30. D. An accessory organ is one that complements the main organs of a system. In this case, the liver is considered an accessory organ of the digestive system.

31. D. All are general principles of the code of ethics.

32. D. All needs may be affected by adopting the sick role.

33. A. Option B means the study of the eyes; C means pertaining to the study of the eyes; D means disease of the eyes.

34. A. Option B is the tube that connects the urinary bladder to the outside of the body; C and D are structures of the nephron.

35. B. Health professionals are motivated to help patients. When patients are uncooperative, they mitigate the satisfaction one experiences by serving in a helping role.

36. A. Option B means to turn to more immature forms of behavior to cope with anxiety; C means to become confrontational; D means to justify one's thoughts, feelings, and behavior.

37. C. Option A means white blood cell; B means a neoplastic blood condition; D means a decreased number of white blood cells.

38. C. The epididymis is part of the male reproductive system.

39. C. The remaining options are all arguments against abortion.

40. B. Options A and C are rights not duties.

41. D. Option A means slow breathing; B means increased depth of breathing; C means lack of breathing.

42. A. The brain is part of the central nervous system.

43. D. Of the options given, this is the least justifiable as social class is of little importance when deciding who should and should not receive limited resources.

44. D. All are potential losses associated with being sick.

45. B. Option A means the study of tissue; C means the study of cells; D means one who studies cells.

46. C. Olfaction refers to the sense of smell.

47. A. Option B means to do good; C means to be loyal; D means to be truthful.

48. D. Humiliation is not a stage of dying.

49. D. Option A means inflammation of a tendon; B means uterine discharge; C is a respiratory disorder.

50. D. Oxytocin is produced by the hypothalamus and stored in the posterior pituitary.

51. B. Option A is the time limit in which a lawsuit can be filed; C and D are defenses when the plaintiff is jointly responsible for the injuries.

52. C. Option A is never done; B fails to acknowledge the pain the patient is suffering; D is usually unnecessary.

53. C. Option A is the study of blood; B is a bruise; D is the destructions of cells.

54. C. Option A is the armpit; B is the kneecap; D is the cheek.

55. B. Option A is a custom; C is positive spirit of an individual or group; D is an obligation.

56. C. The other options indicate to the patient that nothing will be done to expedite the visit.

57. A. Option B is an abnormal joint condition; C is inflammation of a joint; D is a herniation of a testicle.

58. D. Option A is the control center of a cell; B is the site of protein synthesis; C modifies and packages proteins.

59. C. Option A refers to a custom; B and D represent rules that govern right and wrong.

60. C. Of the options given, this is the best response.

61. C. Option A is abnormal development; B is muscle disease; D is a nonsense word.

62. C. Option A is the outer skin layer; B and D represent the inner skin layer.

63. D. Option A means to do good; B means to do no harm; C means loyalty.

64. D. All are reasons patients may be reluctant to ask that instructions be repeated.

65. B. Option A is four times a day; C is at every bedtime; D is a nonsense distracter.

66. D. Option A is the upper side bones; B is the lower side bones; C is the lower jaw bone.

Administrative:

1. C. A medium-size computer is a minicomputer.

2. D. Records management includes all of these tasks.

3. D. All are attributes of an effective receptionist.

4. C. The payee directs how the check is to be paid, such as "for deposit only."

5. D. All are purposes of medical coding.

6. A. Coordination of benefits is a policy clause that prevents the overpayment of benefits when more than one policy is in force.

7. D. All of these factors should be considered when scheduling a meeting.

8. D. The monitor is a peripheral. A–C are part of the main computer.

9. A. Conditioning is the process of checking for and repairing damaged documents.

10. B. Of those listed, visiting health care providers should be announced and escorted to the provider's office.

11. B. A deposit ticket is prepared when money will be placed into an account.

12. D. CPT, HCPCS, and RBRVS are used to code medical procedures; whereas ICD is used to code medical diagnoses.

13. B. An insurance company is also called the carrier.

14. C. The agenda is a typed list of the topics to be discussed in a meeting.

15. C. The printer is an output device.

16. B. Initials come before complete names, not after.

17. A. The MA should never answer an incoming call with "please hold."

18. B. Magnetic ink character recognition.

19. A. International Classification of Diseases.

20. C. Riders are clauses that identify additional coverage.

21. D. Salutation is not included in meetings minutes.

22. D. All are secondary storage devices except the modem.

23. D. A tickler file is organized by date.

24. D. Of the options listed, the location of the person called is least likely to be included in a phone message.

25. D. All are reasons for the bank to dishonor a check.

26. D. 800 and 900 codes cover accidents and injuries. These may require an additional code identifying the cause of the accident or injury.

27. D. All are government sponsored programs except Blue Cross/Blue Shield.

28. A. Brainstorming is a method for generating ideas without criticism.

29. B. Microsoft Word is a word processing software program. The others are all hardware.

30. D. Special fourth class includes books and manuscripts.

31. C. Patients with treatment problems should always be transferred to the provider. The other calls listed can be handled by someone other than the provider, e.g., MA or office manager.

32. D. The date the check is expected to clear is variable and never recorded.

33. A. V-codes refer to factors that influence health status.

34. B. Medicaid is funded by both federal and state revenue.

35. D. Reporting is not one of the elements of the management process.

36. D. Informing is not a part of the data processing cycle.

37. B. All are considered part of the closing except the salutation, which is the opening.

38. D. It is never wise to be disrespectful to anyone, including an angry caller.

39. D. The names of payees are not recorded on the bank statement.

40. D. All but D are speculative diagnoses and never coded.

41. D. Tricare is an insurance program that is available to active duty military personnel and their dependents.

42. D. A defines management; B and C define efficiency.

43. A. Booting is the process of activating the operating system.

44. A. Name, page number, and date is the correct order.

45. B. If the patient is not getting any oxygen, death is likely to occur within 4 minutes.

46. C. Outstanding deposits add funds to that stated on the bank statement and should be added not subtracted.

47. B. Current procedural terminology.

48. A. Blue Cross/Blue Shield may serve as the fiscal intermediary for the Medicare program.

49. D. An employee's ability to perform a task is a function of knowledge, experience, and performance.

50. B. Software instructions are installed onto the hard drive.

51. C. Mail that has been opened by mistake should be resealed with tape along with a note stating it was opened in error.

52. C. Depending on the area, 411 or 1 + area code + 555-1212 can be called for long distance directory assistance.

53. D. $4250 + 1200 - 300 = 5150$

54. D. The modifier -99 indicates that multiple modifiers are in effect.

55. D. A and C are eligible for Medicare; B is eligible for Tricare.

56. A. Of those listed, social affiliations is the least important.

57. A. The default setting is automatically loaded with each new document unless changed by the user.

58. C. It is prudent that each check be restrictively endorsed with "for deposit only."

59. C. There is a 3-hour difference between California and New Jersey.

60. A. Solvency is the ability to pay one's debts in a timely fashion.

61. B. Terms after a semicolon are part of, or clarify, a main term.

62. C. CMS-1500 is the universal claim form.

63. B. It is illegal to ask job applicants if they have children.

64. B. An index of files on a disk is known as a directory.

65. A. Important information that has been highlighted on a document has been annotated.

66. C. Wide Area Telephone Service.

67. C. Assets are property of value owned or controlled by a business.

Clinical:

1. D. The patient's ledger card is part of the financial record, not the medical record or chart.

2. D. Inspection is a visualization; palpation is examination through feel; percussion is resonance of sounds within the body.

3. C. Because oils are high in fats, and fats are recommended to be restricted within most diets, these should compose the smallest part of a healthy diet.

4. A. Depolarization is the energy-expending phase of the cycle, which is immediately followed by repolarization. The next step in the cycle is polarization.

5. C. Surgical scissors are used for cutting tissue; none of the other instruments have the capability to take tissue apart.

6. B. Prophylactic means "before" disease; therapeutic drugs are used after a disease has been diagnosed and are used for treatment. Diagnostic drugs help to define a medical problem. Cathartic is a medication used for the lower intestinal tract.

7. A. It is most important to assess the pulse and airway before assessing any of the other listed topics.

8. C. All of the other listings are commonly departments themselves. Microbiology is devoted to the study of microorganisms such as bacteria, fungi, viruses, and parasites.

9. B. Part of the decomposition process of a urine specimen for a prolonged period of time is that the normally acidic urine will become more alkaline due to the breakdown of elements in the urine.

10. A. Microbiology is the study of microorganisms; bacteriology is the study of bacteria; clinical chemistry analyzes the serum or plasma.

11. D. The other listed microorganisms are either bacteria or fungi; viruses are considered the smallest living microorganisms.

12. D. Because problem oriented medical records are based on the complaint or illness bringing the patient into the office, the problem list would only be found in this type of record. The others listed would be found in source oriented medical records typically.

13. B. An otoscope is used to examine the ear, not test it; a stethoscope is used for auscultation of body parts; an ophthalmoscope is used to examine the eye.

14. A. The descriptive terms *lacto* (milk) and *ovo* (eggs) in addition to vegetarian define the diet of plant foods supplemented with dairy products and eggs.

15. D. No electrical impulse is conducted in the sinoatrial septum.

16. D. Scalpels are blades used for cutting; bandage scissors are designed for cutting away dressings; an obturator is a device fitted inside a scope or cannula.

17. D. Salicylic acid is the chemical name for aspirin; the others are brand names assigned by the manufacturers.

18. D. The finger sweep should be performed only on adults.

19. C. Medical technologists hold a 4-year bachelor's degree in laboratory technology and therefore are qualified to perform tests in the waived, moderate-complexity, and high-complexity areas. Pathologists oversee medical laboratories but usually do not perform laboratory tests. A histocytologist is specialized in processing tissues for examination as well as slides. Medical laboratory technicians are not qualified under CLIA '88 to perform high-complexity testing.

20. D. Although odor is usually not documented, all of these should be observed during the physical examination of the urine.

21. A. The prefix *iso-* denotes the "same" or equal concentration. Hypotonic refers to a lesser concentration where hypertonic means a greater concentration. Ionic pressure does not apply to the definition.

22. B. Crystal violet is the primary stain; safranin is the counterstain; iodine is the mordant. New methylene blue is not one of the reagents found in Gram stain.

23. C. Feces are one of the few materials that do not require the use of universal precautions.

24. B. The Trendelenburg position places a patient on the back with the head slightly lowered for treatment of shock; therefore, examination of the back could not be performed in this position.

25. B. Metabolism is the sum of anabolism (building) minus catabolism (breaking down). Basal metabolism is the minimum amount of energy required to maintain the body without expending energy.

26. A. The P wave always represents the beginning of the cardiac cycle when the atria contract;

the QRS complex represents ventricular contraction. The PR interval and ST segments are measurements.

27. A. The fewer the number of "0"s, the larger the suture size.

28. C. A troche is a lozenge, which is a solid preparation of a medication.

29. C. Compressions of less than 1 1/2 to 2 inches will not be sufficient to stimulate the heart and compressions greater than this can cause physical damage.

30. B. *Salmonella* and *Streptococcus* are not blood-borne pathogens. Although HIV is a bloodborne pathogen, it is less common than HBV.

31. D. Specific gravity is always recorded with 1.xxx on a report and does not have units assigned to the measurement.

32. D. Identification of the patient is always the first step of any procedure to ascertain the medical assistant is testing the correct patient.

33. C. *Neisseria* species always stain gram-negative.

34. D. Any of the factors listed can either elevate or lower the body temperature, depending on individual circumstances.

35. A. An otoscope is only used to examine the ear.

36. C. The definition of a calorie is the amount of heat or energy required to raise the temperature of 1 kilogram of water 1 degree Celsius.

37. C. The QRS complex represents ventricular contraction; the P wave always represents the beginning of the cardiac cycle when the atria contract. The PR interval and ST segments are measurements.

38. A. The surgical procedure to remove an abscess includes cutting into the abscess (incision) and removing the infectious material (draining).

39. D. Persons abusing drugs will withdraw from society rather than become more friendly.

40. D. The compression to ventilation ratio is 30:2; this ratio is the same for adults and children, per AHA guidelines.

41. D. All of the other listed components are essential in complying with OSHA requirements, but universal precautions is the part of the bloodborne pathogen standard that mandates treating all body fluids as if infectious.

42. B. Tamm-Horsfall protein is the primary constituent of casts found in urines; when renal function

is impaired, this protein may precipitate within the tubules and be seen microscopically.

43. A. *-ia* is a suffix referring to a condition; *hypo-* is the prefix meaning below normal (pale); *chrom/o-* is the combining form for color. Therefore, *hypochromia* is the most appropriate term.

44. D. The common word for *bacillus* is rod, and organisms that stain red or pink are gram positive. GNR is an abbreviation denoting gram-negative rod.

45. D. The depth of the pulse cannot be measured.

46. D. Because of the nature of most orthopedic visits, such as broken bones, diagnostic imaging (radiology) would be most often associated with this specialty.

47. C. Fats have 9 calories, whereas carbohydrates and proteins have 4 calories. Vitamins have no calories.

48. D. Sanitization can be the first step in the process of preparing instruments for sterilization and includes cleaning grossly visible materials from the surface.

49. D. The liver is the organ responsible for metabolizing and detoxifying drugs. None of the others listed have a part in this metabolism although the kidneys usually excrete the waste products after hepatic metabolism.

50. D. Any breathing difficulty requires emergency services immediately.

51. D. Myocardial infarction or heart attack may include all of the symptoms listed. Diaphoresis is sweating; angina pectoris is chest pain; dyspnea is difficulty breathing.

52. B. Option A is an instrument that passes light through a liquid to measure the concentration of selected substances; C is an instrument that uses steam under pressure to sterilize selected options; D is an instrument that analyzes serum for various substances.

53. D. Ten to twelve milliliters of urine is centrifuged for microscopic analysis.

54. C. The normal adult hemoglobin is generally 14–16 g/dL.

55. B. Pinworm is the common name for *E. vermicularis*.

56. C. AS (auris sinister) is the Latin abbreviation for left ear. Option A, auris dexter, means right ear. Option B, oculus dexter, means right eye. Option D, oculus sinister, means left eye.

57. B. Option A means the process of measuring a joint; C means the process of measuring the bladder; D means the process of recording the electrical activity of a muscle.

58. D. Vitamin B is a water soluble vitamin. The fat soluble vitamins include A, D, E, and K.

59. D. The Potter-Bucky diaphragm is used to enhance the x-rays of thicker body parts like the thigh.

60. C. Lids are placed face up on the table.

61. A. Form DEA -41 is completed when controlled substances are destroyed.

62. D. The most common cause of convulsions is epilepsy.

63. C. Icterus is a yellow discoloration caused by hyperbilirubinemia. Option A means lipids in the blood; B means destruction of blood cells; D means abnormal darkening, especially the skin.

64. C. Ketones are the byproduct of incomplete fat metabolism.

65. B. Hematocrit is also known as percent packed red blood cells. Option A means complete blood count; C is an oxygen carrying blood protein, and D means corpuscular volume.

66. B. Mycology is the study of fungus. Option A is the study of microorganisms; C is the study of parasites; D is the study of viruses.

67. B. Pupils equal, round, and reactive to light and accommodation. Option A means cyanosis, clubbing, and edema; C means health care maintenance; D means tonsillectomy and adenoidectomy.

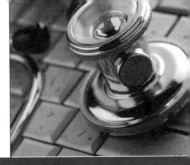

Post-Test

200-question, 3-hour, timed diagnostic practice exam

Each of the questions or incomplete statements below is followed by four suggested answers or completions. Select the *one* answer or completion that is *best* in each case and fill in the circle containing the corresponding letter on the answer sheet. Perforated answer sheets are located at the back of the book.

1. Which of the following combining forms means "eyelid"?
   a. cost/o
   b. or/o
   c. ocul/o
   d. blephar/o

2. The most common connecting vowel found in combining forms is
   a. a
   b. i
   c. o
   d. u

3. The term tachycardia is synonymous with
   a. fast heart rate
   b. slow heart rate
   c. normal heart rate
   d. irregular heart rate

4. Balanitis refers to which body system?
   a. nervous system
   b. reproductive system
   c. digestive system
   d. circulatory system

5. Hematopoiesis means
   a. blood condition
   b. hemorrhage
   c. blood formation
   d. bloody discharge

6. Which of the following word parts is a suffix?
   a. ante
   b. post
   c. organ/o
   d. itis

7. Which of the following word parts is a prefix?
   a. pre
   b. cleid/o
   c. osis
   d. rrhea

8. Who of the following is an ENT specialist?
   a. otologist
   b. rhinologist
   c. otorhinolaryngologist
   d. ophthalmologist

9. Which of the following terms relates to a respiratory disorder?
   a. MI
   b. HBP
   c. COPD
   d. RIH

10. Which of the following terms relates to a gynecological disorder?
    a. epididymitis
    b. salpingitis
    c. stomatitis
    d. rhinitis

11. Which of the following terms is spelled incorrectly?
    a. rabdomyoma
    b. sinusitis
    c. hysterectomy
    d. arteriosclerosis

12. Unclear vision resulting from hardening of the crystalline lens, common among the elderly, is known as
    a. diplopia
    b. presbyopia
    c. ambliopia
    d. myopia

13. Inflammation of the gallbladder is known as
    a. cholelithiasis
    b. colitis
    c. cholecystitis
    d. cystitis

14. The medical abbreviation meaning *by mouth* is
    a. ad lib
    b. p.o.
    c. n.p.o.
    d. b.i.d.

15. The medical abbreviation meaning *as desired* is
    a. stat
    b. p.r.n.
    c. ad lib
    d. cc

16. The medical term meaning *disease of the blood vessel(s)* is
    a. angiopathy
    b. cardiopathy
    c. angioplasty
    d. angiectomy

17. Surgical removal of the iris is called an
    a. irisectomy
    b. irisostomy
    c. iridotomy
    d. iridectomy

18. Lou Gehrig's disease is also known as
    a. lymphadenoma
    b. amyotrophic lateral sclerosis
    c. idiopathic thrombocytopenia
    d. polycythemia purpura

19. Excision of a small piece of tissue is a(n)
    a. autopsy
    b. necropsy
    c. biopsy
    d. endoscopy

20. Swelling of the eyelids is known as
    a. blepharoptosis
    b. blepharitis
    c. blepharedema
    d. blepharoma

21. The twelfth cranial nerve is
    a. acoustic
    b. trigeminal
    c. olfactory
    d. hypoglossal

22. The structure that prevents material from entering the windpipe is
    a. trachea
    b. epiglottis
    c. bronchus
    d. alveolus

23. The wristbones are collectively known as
    a. metatarsals
    b. tarsals
    c. metacarpals
    d. carpals

24. The tube extending from the kidney to the bladder is the
    a. ureter
    b. urethra
    c. epididymis
    d. seminal vesicle

25. The aqueous humor is situated _____ to the lens.
    a. lateral
    b. distal
    c. medial
    d. anterior

26. In the structural hierarchy of organisms, which of the following immediately precedes the organ level?
    a. organism
    b. systems
    c. tissues
    d. cells

27. Which of the following tissues consists of neurons?
    a. epithelial
    b. nervous
    c. connective
    d. muscle

28. Which of the following is considered an appendage of the skin?
    a. dermis
    b. epidermis
    c. sudoriferous glands
    d. hypodermis

29. Which of the following best describes a bony projection?
    a. spine
    b. fissure
    c. foramen
    d. process

30. Turning a body part inward, especially the sole of the foot is
    a. flexion
    b. abduction
    c. inversion
    d. eversion

31. The right atrioventricular valve is known as the
    a. bicuspid
    b. mitral
    c. tricuspid
    d. semilunar

32. The structure known as the voice box is the
    a. pharynx
    b. larynx
    c. epiglottis
    d. nasopharynx

33. A fingerlike projection of the soft palate is the
    a. uvula
    b. frenulum
    c. epiglottis
    d. villi

34. The structure that houses the glomerulus is the
    a. loop of Henle
    b. proximal convoluted tubule
    c. Bowman's capsule
    d. distal convoluted tubule

35. The innermost layer of the uterus is the
    a. epimetrium
    b. fimbria
    c. myometrium
    d. endometrium

36. Neuronal structures that receive and conduct impulses toward the cell body are
    a. axons
    b. dendrites
    c. synapses
    d. nodes of Ranvier

37. Sensory receptors responsible for the sense of taste are
    a. olfactory
    b. auditory
    c. visual
    d. gustatory

38. The small gland located in the posterior hypothalamus is the
    a. pituitary
    b. adrenal
    c. pineal
    d. parathyroid

39. The ability of a muscle to be stimulated by nervous impulses is
    a. irritability
    b. flexibility
    c. contractility
    d. elasticity

40. The double membranous sac that envelopes the heart is called the
    a. epicardium
    b. pericardium
    c. endocardium
    d. mesocardium

41. A consent form is not required if the patient is
    a. a minor
    b. elderly
    c. incompetent
    d. unconscious and critically injured

42. Failing to act when one has the duty to act describes which tort?
    a. nonfeasance
    b. misfeasance
    c. malfeasance
    d. negligence

43. Defamation of character employing the written word describes
    a. invasion of privacy
    b. libel
    c. slander
    d. fraud

44. Negligence requires the following elements **EXCEPT**
    a. inconvenience
    b. duty
    c. causation
    d. damage

45. Defenses against negligence include which of the following?
    a. tolling of the statute of limitations
    b. contributory negligence
    c. assumption of the risk
    d. all of the above

46. All of the following are reasons for revocation or suspension of a healthcare provider's license **EXCEPT**
    a. conviction of a crime
    b. unprofessional conduct
    c. mental incapacity
    d. administering atypical treatments

47. Behavior or an action that can be reasonably presumed to be consensual is
    a. express consent
    b. implied consent
    c. informed consent
    d. rescinded consent

48. Which of the following may require notification of the appropriate health agencies?
    a. auto accident
    b. roseola
    c. phenylketonuria
    d. strep throat

49. Confidentiality is legally supported by the
    a. Self-Determination Act
    b. Health Care Quality Improvement Act
    c. Americans with Disabilities Act
    d. Privacy Act

50. Confidentiality is ethically supported by the concept of
    a. beneficence
    b. nonmaleficence
    c. fidelity
    d. all of the above

51. A civil wrong committed against other persons or their property is
    a. a tort
    b. a breach of contract
    c. negligence
    d. malpractice

52. A healthcare provider who guarantees the outcome of a course of treatment may be in jeopardy of committing
    a. a tort
    b. a breach of contract
    c. negligence
    d. malpractice

53. Negligence of a professional person is known as
    a. nonfeasance
    b. misfeasance
    c. malfeasance
    d. malpractice

54. The least serious degree of negligence is
    a. minor
    b. ordinary
    c. inconsequential
    d. gross

55. The principle that the provider has a professional obligation to care for a patient is known as
    a. duty
    b. dereliction of duty
    c. direct causation
    d. damage

56. In most states, there is no legal duty to rescue victims **EXCEPT**
    a. family members
    b. innocent bystanders
    c. if you witness the accident
    d. helpless young children

57. In most states, rescuers can abandon an accident victim if
    a. the victim is a family member
    b. the victim is not placed in further peril
    c. the victim regains consciousness
    d. the victim cannot be saved

58. Positive character traits are
    a. duties
    b. virtues
    c. justice
    d. rights

59. Disclosing unpleasant information to a patient is best supported by the ethical concept of
    a. duty
    b. right
    c. justice
    d. veracity

60. Informed consent is most related to the concept of
    a. justice
    b. autonomy
    c. role fidelity
    d. code of ethics

61. In Abraham Maslow's Hierarchy of Needs, the need to be respected describes the
    a. physiological need
    b. safety need
    c. social need
    d. self-esteem need

62. Exhibiting immature behavior as a result of stress or anxiety describes
    a. regression
    b. denial
    c. sublimation
    d. repression

63. An unconscious defense mechanism characterized by behavior that is the opposite of one's true feelings describes
    a. introjection
    b. dissociation
    c. rationalization
    d. reaction formation

64. Elisabeth Kübler-Ross is credited with establishing the
    a. elements of the communication process
    b. steps in dealing with the emotionally distressed client
    c. five stages of dying
    d. development of the unconscious defense mechanisms

65. A patient expresses fear about dying; the medical assistant should
    a. ask the patient to discuss something more cheerful
    b. indicate that fearing death is futile
    c. describe in detail the stages of dying
    d. attempt to be attentive and understanding

66. A facilitative communication technique that repeats what the patient has said to demonstrate understanding is
    a. accepting
    b. mirroring
    c. clarification
    d. exploring

67. All of the following are facilitative communication techniques **EXCEPT**
    a. exploring
    b. focusing
    c. advising
    d. accepting

68. An unconscious defense mechanism characterized by diverting unacceptable thoughts, feelings, and impulses into acceptable behaviors.
    a. introjection
    b. projection
    c. reaction formation
    d. sublimation

69. Mimicking the behavior of another to cope with feelings of inadequacy is called
    a. dissociation
    b. rationalization
    c. substitution
    d. identification

70. The reasons a patient may desire to continue the sick role is
    a. fear of reestablishing responsibility
    b. financial gain
    c. to generate sympathy and attention
    d. all of the above

71. All of the following may be considered losses associated with adopting the sick role **EXCEPT**
    a. autonomy
    b. privacy
    c. mobility or function
    d. none of the above

72. Methods of discovering what is important to a patient include
    a. asking the patient
    b. observing patient behavior
    c. reviewing the medical chart
    d. all of the above

73. Adopting the view of other persons relative to their situation and experience is known as
    a. empathy
    b. sympathy
    c. reinforcement
    d. projection

74. Which of the following will most likely promote the perception of professional competence?
    a. trembling
    b. poor enunciation
    c. appearing confident
    d. lack of eye contact

75. Interacting with a health professional as one would interact with a parental figure is known as
    a. inference
    b. transference
    c. countertransference
    d. dependence

76. The process of converting meaning into understandable symbols is known as
    a. communication
    b. deciphering
    c. decoding
    d. encoding

77. Mrs. Jonathan (Wilma) Wilson would be most properly addressed as
    a. Wilma
    b. Mrs. Wilson
    c. Ms. Wilma
    d. Mrs. "W"

78. Encouraging a patient to stay on a topic is known as
    a. mirroring
    b. focusing
    c. reflecting
    d. exploring

79. A common stereotype associated with persons having communication disabilities is
    a. disinterest
    b. indigence
    c. lack of intelligence
    d. indifference

80. A malingerer or hypochondriac may be inappropriately labeled a
    a. crock
    b. gork
    c. GOMER
    d. gimp

81. When using a typewriter to complete a preprinted form, pica pitch consists of what number of characters per inch?
    a. 8
    b. 10
    c. 12
    d. 14

82. The tab key allows one to
    a. set the margins
    b. move the cursor a predetermined number of spaces to the right
    c. center the cursor
    d. return the cursor to the left margin

83. What number of lines of text represent 1 inch?
    a. 6
    b. 8
    c. 10
    d. 12

84. The keyboard keys most commonly used with function keys (F1–F12) are
    a. alt
    b. space bar
    c. ctrl
    d. (A) and (C)

85. In word processing, to remove a portion of text and transport it to another section of the document describes
    a. cut and paste
    b. concatenate
    c. copy and paste
    d. purging

86. The smallest piece of information processed by a computer is the
    a. data
    b. bit
    c. byte
    d. ASCII

87. The process of activating the input of the operating system into main memory is known as
    a. start-up
    b. shutdown
    c. booting
    d. installing

88. The process of organizing a blank disk into sectors so that it can store data is known as
    a. booting
    b. configuring
    c. WYSIWYG
    d. formatting

89. A key that moves the cursor to the left, right, top, or bottom margins when pressed is the
    a. Backspace key
    b. Tab key
    c. Delete key
    d. Home key

90. A blinking dash or small rectangle that identifies where on the computer screen data will be entered is the
    a. pause/break
    b. icon
    c. cursor
    d. ctrl

91. The number of characters contained within an inch is the
    a. font
    b. pitch
    c. macro
    d. widow

92. Which of the following permits the printing of identical information at the top of each page?
    a. header
    b. footer
    c. orphan
    d. widow

93. The last paragraph line appearing alone at the top of a page is a(n)
    a. widow
    b. orphan
    c. header
    d. footer

94. The computer command that organizes data alphabetically or numerically in ascending or descending order is
    a. sort
    b. presort
    c. macro
    d. function

95. A computer application that allows multiple applications to operate simultaneously is
    a. spreadsheet
    b. Windows
    c. DOS
    d. CD-ROM

96. The software program that permits rapid calculations to be applied to a table of numerical data is
    a. word processing
    b. spreadsheet
    c. desktop publishing
    d. Windows

97. The data entered into a spreadsheet comprising alphanumeric characters primarily used as column and row headings is known as the
    a. value
    b. label
    c. formula
    d. cell

98. Cell A3 is located at
    a. column A, row 3
    b. row A, column 3
    c. columns 1 to 3, and row A
    d. rows 1 to 3, and column A

99. An optical disk that can store, erase, and restore data best describes a
    a. DVD
    b. CD-ROM
    c. CD-R
    d. CD-RW

100. A USB or flash drive is an example of what type of storage medium?
    a. floppy disk
    b. DVD
    c. CD-R
    d. solid state

101. The number of lines separating the inside address and the salutation is
    a. 2
    b. 4
    c. 10
    d. 15

102. Open punctuation refers to
    a. placing a comma after the complimentary close
    b. placing a semicolon after the complimentary close
    c. placing a colon after the salutation
    d. placing no punctuation after the salutation

103. The acronym "bc" indicates
    a. a letter is the typed copy of the original
    b. a letter is a carbon copy of the original
    c. a letter has not been copied from the original
    d. a copy has been sent to a third party without the original party's knowledge

104. Semiblock describes a letter format in which
    a. all lines begin at the left margin
    b. all lines begin at the left margin except the date line and complimentary close, which begin at the center
    c. the first line of each paragraph is indented five spaces
    d. the salutation and complimentary close are omitted

105. Which of the following comprises the opening of a letter?
    a. inside address
    b. complimentary close
    c. copy notation
    d. signature line

106. Which of the following would be indexed first?
    a. Allison B. Wilson
    b. Alice A. Wilson
    c. Mrs. Anthony (Alma) Wilson
    d. Alice B. Wilson

107. Which of the following would be indexed last?
    a. John P. St. John
    b. John Q. St. George
    c. Paul M. St. Paul
    d. Alfred O. San Luis

108. Which of the following would be indexed first?
    a. Karen A. Lane
    b. Karen B. Lone
    c. Karen Lane
    d. Kristen F. Line

109. Annual reports are best filed using a(n)
    a. alphabetical system
    b. subject system
    c. geographic system
    d. numerical system

110. The most common color coding filing system color codes the
    a. patient's surname
    b. patient's given name
    c. patient's Social Security number
    d. patient's identification card number

111. A simple method to check the accuracy of a postal scale is to see if 1 ounce is displayed when weighing
    a. 6 pennies
    b. 7 pennies
    c. 8 pennies
    d. 9 pennies

112. The class of mail delivery of books and manuscripts of at least 24 pages is
    a. second class
    b. third class
    c. fourth class
    d. special fourth class

113. First-class mail that is insured is
    a. priority mail
    b. certified mail
    c. registered mail
    d. express mail

114. "Dear Mrs. Smith:" is an example of
    a. inside address
    b. salutation
    c. complimentary close
    d. signature line

115. "Dear Mrs. Smith:" demonstrates
    a. open punctuation
    b. mixed punctuation
    c. closed punctuation
    d. semiblock punctuation

116. Reference notation comes right after the
    a. copy notation
    b. enclosure notation
    c. postscript notation
    d. signature line

117. A provider's resumé is often in the form of a
    a. bibliography
    b. curriculum vitae
    c. biography
    d. portfolio

118. The number of lines separating the complimentary close and the signature line typically is
    a. 2
    b. 3
    c. 4
    d. 5

119. Long letters will typically have what size margins?
    a. 1/2 inch
    b. 1 inch
    c. 1 1/2 inch
    d. 2 inch

120. A summary of a manuscript in 100 to 200 words is a(n)
    a. abstract
    b. acknowledgement
    c. footnote
    d. bibliography

121. Scheduling the number of patients that can be seen in 1 hour based on the average appointment describes the
    a. time specified
    b. wave system
    c. modified wave system
    d. double booking system

122. All of the following should be considered when scheduling appointments **EXCEPT**
    a. patient need
    b. day of the week
    c. provider preference
    d. available facilities

123. Scheduling patients with similar diagnoses, treatments, or needs within a specified time frame describes
    a. double booking
    b. grouping (clustering)
    c. time specified
    d. wave

124. To mitigate potential legal difficulties, appointments should be recorded in
    a. indelible ink
    b. erasable ink
    c. pencil
    d. any of the above

125. When it is 2 p.m. in Minnesota, it is _____ in Georgia.
    a. 1 p.m.
    b. 2 p.m.
    c. 3 p.m.
    d. 4 p.m.

126. The person most likely to handle equipment purchases is the
    a. receptionist
    b. medical assistant
    c. office manager
    d. nurse

127. When a pharmaceutical representative arrives unannounced, it is best to
    a. request a business card and see if the healthcare provider is available for a visit
    b. immediately escort her to the provider's office
    c. ask the representative to wait until the provider is free
    d. refer the representative to the next available medical assistant

128. When the second line rings, it is best to
    a. answer with "please hold"
    b. ask the caller if she can hold
    c. ignore it until you are finished with the first caller
    d. indicate to the first caller, "please hold"

129. All of the following are typically recorded on a telephone message **EXCEPT**
    a. date and time of call
    b. person called
    c. message
    d. caller's demographic data

130. The MA's telephone voice should convey all of the following **EXCEPT**
    a. confidence
    b. warmth
    c. disinterest
    d. concern

131. When dialing direct, the caller dials
    a. 0 + area code + seven-digit number
    b. 1 + area code + seven-digit number
    c. 1 + 800 + seven-digit number
    d. 0 + 800 + seven-digit number

132. An effective answering service is necessary to avoid
    a. liability
    b. malpractice
    c. negligence
    d. abandonment charges

133. The appointment scheduling system should reflect the needs of the
    a. provider
    b. staff
    c. patients
    d. all of the above

134. When scheduling appointments, all of the following should be considered **EXCEPT**
    a. needs of the patient
    b. location of clinic
    c. amount of time needed
    d. available facilities

135. A different color ink is commonly used when recording appointments to denote
    a. new patients
    b. patients with a disability
    c. cardiac patients
    d. patients who are typically late

136. When making international calls, the international access code is
    a. 009
    b. 010
    c. 011
    d. 012

137. Time slots used as "catch-up" periods are known as
    a. buffers
    b. waves
    c. clustering
    d. modified waves

138. Patients arriving with an emergency condition should be
    a. seen right away
    b. advised to call 911
    c. scheduled for the next available appointment
    d. refused an appointment

139. The ideal waiting time for a clinic visit is
    a. 20 minutes
    b. 30 minutes
    c. 40 minutes
    d. 50 minutes

140. The most effective means of conveying a cheerful tone while speaking on the phone is to
    a. speak slowly
    b. smile
    c. frown
    d. chew gum

141. The bank is also known as the
    a. drawee
    b. drawer
    c. payee
    d. payer

142. The bank statement shows a balance of $4,050.00. Outstanding deposits total $1,025.00, and outstanding checks total $700.00. The checkbook balance should be
   a. $2,325.00
   b. $3,725.00
   c. $4,375.00
   d. $5,775.00

143. Categorizing accounts according to the number of days the accounts are past-due describes
   a. aging accounts receivable
   b. accounts receivable turnover
   c. accounts receivable analysis
   d. none of the above

144. A medical assistant who is compensated every other Friday is being paid
   a. semimonthly
   b. biweekly
   c. bimonthly
   d. semiannually

145. A property or right owned by a business defines
   a. capital
   b. liability
   c. asset
   d. revenue

146. A signature card must be completed to
   a. file income taxes
   b. reconcile a bank statement
   c. pay practice expenses
   d. open a checking account

147. Special characters that simplify the sorting and routing of financial documents are
   a. FONT
   b. MICR
   c. OCR
   d. MICRO

148. Which of the following most characterizes an ABA number?
   a. 27
   b. 1052
   c. 504.10
   d. 17-700/2910

149. A check that the bank refuses to pay is
   a. postdated
   b. debited
   c. dishonored
   d. credited

150. A personal record of relevant information concerning a check and the checking account balance is a
   a. deposit ticket
   b. debit memo
   c. check register
   d. bank statement

151. Carbonless copies of checks use a special paper known as
   a. NCR paper
   b. OCR paper
   c. MICR paper
   d. OSS paper

152. A check that has been honored and stamped to prevent its reuse is a(n)
   a. NSF check
   b. postdated check
   c. cancelled check
   d. outstanding check

153. All of the following are common users of a clinic's accounting information **EXCEPT**
   a. owners
   b. patients
   c. managers
   d. creditors

154. Funds legally removed from a practice for personal use are often classified as
   a. revenue
   b. expense
   c. income
   d. drawing

155. An accounting document that serves to record all daily transactions is a
   a. pegboard
   b. journal
   c. ledger
   d. superbill

156. A financial statement that summarizes revenue and expense for a specified period is the
   a. trial balance
   b. balance sheet
   c. income statement
   d. statement of retained earnings

157. An amount maintained to cover minor expenses is
   a. accounts receivable
   b. accounts payable
   c. petty cash
   d. capital

158. A fee a provider most frequently charges for a service is
    a. usual
    b. customary
    c. reasonable
    d. scheduled

159. Lower fees typically paid by third-party payers refer to
    a. uncollectible accounts allowance
    b. charity allowance
    c. contractual allowance
    d. courtesy allowance

160. Billing segments of the patient population describes
    a. time of service billing
    b. cycle billing
    c. credit card billing
    d. computerized billing

161. Which of the following would require an ICD-9 (or 10)-CM code?
    a. hysterosalpingo-oophorectomy
    b. cystopexy
    c. cleidorrhexis
    d. glossitis

162. All of the following would require a CPT code **EXCEPT**
    a. myringotomy
    b. atherosclerosis
    c. herniorrhaphy
    d. rhinoplasty

163. A healthcare entitlement program for the indigent that is funded by both state and federal revenues but is administered by the state is
    a. Medicare
    b. Medicaid
    c. Blue Cross
    d. Tricare

164. An amount that is paid on an insurance contract prior to the payment of benefits is called
    a. deductible
    b. coinsurance
    c. assignment
    d. exclusion

165. A prepaid health plan that emphasizes health prevention and promotion is a(n)
    a. HMO
    b. PPO
    c. IPA
    d. PID

166. A purchase agreement provision that covers the cost of repair due to faulty design or manufacturing is a
    a. service agreement
    b. garnishee
    c. guarantee
    d. warranty

167. The meeting chairperson is responsible for which of the following?
    a. developing the meeting agenda
    b. determining who should be present
    c. deciding on the meeting time, place, and duration
    d. all of the above

168. Protocol regarding who reports to whom within an organization's hierarchy is the
    a. chain of custody
    b. organizational chart
    c. chain of authority
    d. chain of infection

169. A gratuitous payment for professional services for which custom or propriety forbids a price to be set is a(n)
    a. professional fee
    b. honorarium
    c. gratuity
    d. tip

170. The amount of supplies used as a buffer while awaiting receipt of additional supplies is
    a. safety stock
    b. stock-out
    c. replenishment
    d. inventory

171. A direction to consider additional codes is
    a. See condition
    b. NEC
    c. See category
    d. See also

172. The underlined portion of Hypertension (<u>orthostatic, benign, simple</u>) identifies a(n)
    a. main term
    b. subterm modifier
    c. essential modifer
    d. nonessential modifier

173. An organizational arrangement that provides medical services for a fixed, prepaid fee best describes a(n)
    a. PPO
    b. SEC
    c. HMO
    d. HRM

174. Integrating the various resources to meet organizational objectives is known as
a. planning
b. organizing
c. coordinating
d. controlling

175. A term after the brace (}) indicates
a. completion of a main statement before the brace
b. a required modifier of the statement before the brace
c. that a fifth-digit modifier is required
d. the clarification of a code description

176. AOB means
a. actual observable behavior
b. assignment of benefits
c. archives of business records
d. achievable objectives

177. A fixed, prepaid fee per person enrolled in a managed care program is a(n)
a. copayment
b. premium
c. capitation
d. exclusion

178. The person or party designated by the policyholder to receive the value of a policy is the
a. carrier
b. beneficiary
c. insured
d. insurer

179. According to ICD-9 (or 10)-CM coding conventions, malignant hypertension is
a. mild and in control
b. a systole greater than 140 mmHg
c. a severe form with vascular damage
d. coded the same as simple hypertension

180. Title 18 of the Social Security Act best describes
a. Medicare
b. Tricare
c. Medicaid
d. CHAMPVA

181. The acronym PERRLA is typically recorded in what part of the Review of Systems?
a. head and neck
b. cardiovascular
c. respiratory
d. urinary

182. The "S" of SOAP notes comprises
a. data acquired through examination and testing
b. data provided by the patient describing signs, symptoms, and feelings
c. the provider's diagnosis
d. the course of treatment

183. Which of the following represents hypotension?
a. 130/84
b. 120/80
c. 142/90
d. 90/58

184. The typical pulse range for adults is
a. 50–70
b. 60–80
c. 70–90
d. 60–100

185. Which of the following factors affects body temperature?
a. age
b. environment
c. activity
d. all of the above

186. The position of choice for orthopnea is
a. lithotomy
b. dorsal recumbent
c. Fowler's
d. supine

187. Attempting to assess a patient's condition by ruling out certain possibilities describes
a. suspected diagnosis
b. differential diagnosis
c. definitive diagnosis
d. tentative diagnosis

188. All of the following describe examination methods **EXCEPT**
a. inspection
b. palpation
c. percussion
d. recitation

189. All of the following may be used in a routine physical exam **EXCEPT**
a. stethoscope
b. otoscope
c. reflex hammer
d. sigmoidoscope

190. A percussion hammer is more commonly used for which of the following medical specialties?
a. family practice
b. ophthalmology
c. internal medicine
d. (A) and (C)

191. Details regarding the health status of the patient's parents and siblings are known as the
    a. chief complaint
    b. social history
    c. past medical history
    d. family history

192. An examination method that requires the use of a stethoscope is
    a. palpation
    b. auscultation
    c. mensuration
    d. percussion

193. The following identifies the action to be taken to solve a medical problem such as treatment, medication, surgery, referral, etc.
    a. subjective
    b. objective
    c. assessment
    d. plan

194. The patient's name, date of birth, marital status, education, occupation, etc., is known as the
    a. social history
    b. family history
    c. past illnesses
    d. demographics

195. Initial examination of the breasts is usually performed when the patient is in which of the following positions?
    a. sitting
    b. dorsal recumbent
    c. prone
    d. supine

196. The Romberg test is associated with which of the following examinations?
    a. gastroenterological
    b. ophthalmological
    c. oncological
    d. otorhinolaryngological

197. Questions regarding each of the major body systems and parts are known as
    a. CC
    b. ROS
    c. PMH
    d. FH

198. A common abbreviation for biopsy is
    a. (B)
    b. Bx
    c. bpsy
    d. bsy

199. An agent that mechanically removes contaminants from objects is a(n)
    a. detergent
    b. disinfectant
    c. alcohol
    d. chemical

200. A normal adult respiratory rate is
    a. 8 to 10/min
    b. 14 to 16/min
    c. 20 to 24/min
    d. 26 to 28/min

CMAS POST-TEST SCORE SHEET

DIRECTIONS:

1. Comparing your answer sheet with the correct answers listed below for each section, circle the incorrect responses below.
2. Tally the number of incorrect responses in each column and record the total in the space provided.
3. Identify the column having the lowest score and turn to the chapters indicated for further study.
4. Focus your attention on the columns having the lowest scores.
5. After completing your study of the weakest content area, turn to the column having the next lowest score, concentrating on that area, and so on.

CMAS: Percent correct: _____ %

1=D	21=D	41=D	61=D	81=B	101=A	121=B	141=A	161=D	181=A
2=C	22=B	42=A	62=A	82=B	102=D	122=B	142=C	162=B	182=B
3=A	23=D	43=B	63=D	83=A	103=D	123=B	143=A	163=B	183=D
4=B	24=A	44=A	64=C	84=D	104=C	124=A	144=B	164=A	184=D
5=C	25=D	45=D	65=D	85=A	105=A	125=C	145=C	165=A	185=D
6=D	26=C	46=D	66=B	86=B	106=B	126=C	146=D	166=D	186=C
7=A	27=B	47=B	67=C	87=C	107=D	127=A	147=B	167=D	187=B
8=C	28=C	48=C	68=D	88=D	108=C	128=B	148=D	168=C	188=D
9=C	29=D	49=D	69=D	89=D	109=B	129=D	149=C	169=B	189=D
10=B	30=C	50=D	70=D	90=C	110=A	130=C	150=C	170=A	190=D
11=A	31=C	51=A	71=D	91=B	111=D	131=B	151=A	171=D	191=D
12=B	32=B	52=B	72=D	92=A	112=D	132=D	152=C	172=D	192=B
13=C	33=A	53=D	73=A	93=A	113=C	133=D	153=B	173=C	193=D
14=B	34=C	54=B	74=C	94=A	114=B	134=B	154=D	174=C	194=D
15=C	35=D	55=A	75=B	95=B	115=B	135=A	155=B	175=B	195=A
16=A	36=B	56=A	76=D	96=B	116=D	136=C	156=C	176=B	196=D
17=D	37=D	57=B	77=B	97=B	117=B	137=A	157=C	177=C	197=B
18=B	38=C	58=B	78=B	98=A	118=C	138=A	158=A	178=B	198=B
19=C	39=A	59=D	79=C	99=D	119=B	139=A	159=C	179=C	199=A
20=C	40=B	60=B	80=A	100=D	120=A	140=B	160=B	180=A	200=B
___	___	___	___	___	___	___	___	___	___
Ch.4	Ch.5	Chs.8-9	Chs.6-7	Ch.10	Ch.10	Ch.11	Ch.12	Chs.13-15	Ch.16

If you answered eleven or more questions incorrectly in any of the columns, turn to the appropriate chapter for further study.

Total percent correct (____ /200 × 100): ____%

CMAS scaled score = (Raw score × 0.6) + 40
(Scaled score ≥ 70 is passing)

CMAS POST-TEST ANSWERS AND RATIONALES

1. D. Option A means rib; B means mouth; C means eye.

2. C. O is the most common connecting vowel found in combining forms.

3. A. Tachycardia is a fast heart rate.

4. B. Balanitis means inflammation of the glans penis—a reproductive system organ.

5. C. Hematopoiesis means blood formation.

6. D. Option A is a prefix meaning before; B is a prefix meaning after; C is a combining form meaning organ.

7. A. Option B is a combining form for clavicle (collar bone); C is a suffix for abnormal condition; D is a suffix for discharge or flow.

8. C. Option A is one who studies the ear; B is one who studies the nose; D is one who studies the eyes.

9. C. Chronic obstructive pulmonary disease—a respiratory disorder. Option A is myocardial infarction, a cardiovascular disorder; B is high blood pressure, a vascular disorder; D is right inguinal hernia, a digestive disorder.

10. B. Salpingitis means inflammation of the fallopian tubes, a gynecological disorder. Option A means inflammation of the epididymis, a male reproductive disorder; C is inflammation of the mouth, an oral disorder; D is inflammation of the nose, a respiratory disorder.

11. A. It should be spelled rhabdomyoma.

12. B. Option A means double vision; C means dulled vision; D means nearsightedness.

13. C. Option A means gallstones; B means inflammation of the colon; D means inflammation of the urinary bladder.

14. B. L. *per os.* Option A means *as desired;* C means *nothing by mouth;* D means *twice a day.*

15. C. Option A means *immediately;* B means *as needed;* D means *cubic centimeter.*

16. A. Option B means disease of the heart; C means plastic surgery of the blood vessel; D means surgical removal of a blood vessel.

17. D. Options A and B are spelled incorrectly; C means an opening into the iris.

18. B. Lou Gehrig's disease is an eponym for amyotrophic lateral sclerosis (ALS).

19. C. Options and A and B are synonymous and mean to examine a dead body. Option D means the process of visualizing the internal body.

20. C. Option A means a drooping eyelid; B means inflammation of the eyelid; D means a tumor of the eyelid.

21. D. Option A is the 8th cranial nerve; B is the 5th cranial nerve; C is the 1st cranial nerve.

22. B. Option A is the windpipe; C is the branches of the windpipe that enter each lung; D is the air sacs of the lungs.

23. D. Option A is the foot bones; B is the ankle bones; C is the hand bones.

24. A. Option B is the tube that connects the bladder to the outside of the body; C is the tube that transports sperm from the testicles; D is a bilateral pouch behind the bladder that secretes seminal fluid.

25. D. The aqueous humor is situated anterior (in front of) the lens.

26. C. A collection of similar cells comprise tissue; a collection of similar tissues comprise an organ; a collection of organs having a similar function comprise a system; a collection of systems necessary to sustain life comprise an organism. Tissues, therefore, precede the organ level.

27. B. Nervous tissue consists of neurons.

28. C. An appendage is a structure that complements the primary function of an organ or system. In this case, the sudoriferous glands serve this role.

29. D. Option A is a sharp boney projection; B is a groove in a bone; C is an opening in a bone.

30. C. Option A is a body part bending in on itself; B is a body part that is moved away from the midline; D is turning a body part outward.

31. C. Options A and B are synonymous for the left atrioventricular valve; D is a half-moon–shaped valve located in the great vessels.

32. B. The structure known as the voice box is the larynx.

33. A. Option B is the web of tissue under the tongue; C is the flap of tissue that closes the trachea during swallowing; D is the fingerlike projections of the small intestine.

34. C. The structure that houses the glomerulus is the Bowman's capsule.

35. D. Option A is the outermost layer of the uterus; B is part of the fallopian tubes; C is the muscular layer of the uterus.

36. B. Option A conducts impulses away from the cell body; C is the junction between dendrites and synapses; D is the gaps in the myelin sheath.

37. D. Option A relates to smell; B relates to hearing; C relates to seeing.

38. C. The small gland located in the posterior hypothalamus is the pineal.

39. A. The ability of a muscle to be stimulated by nervous impulses is irritability.

40. B. Option A is the outermost layer of the heart; C is the innermost layer of the heart; D is the middle layer of the heart.

41. D. A consent form is generally required for many medical procedures; however, if one cannot be acquired because the patient is unconscious and a relative is unavailable to provide it, it is assumed that the patient would wish to receive care.

42. A. Option B means performing an improper act; C means performing a bad act; D is performing a careless act.

43. B. Option A means illegally prying into personal matters; C means defamation of character in the spoken form; D means to illegally deceive someone.

44. A. Duty, dereliction of duty, direct causation, and damage are the required elements of negligence, not inconvenience.

45. D. All are defenses against negligence.

46. D. Healthcare providers are free to offer treatments to patients that may not be considered mainstream as long as doing so does not constitute malpractice.

47. B. A is consent communicated orally or in writing; C is consent that is documented before risky procedures; D is taking back one's consent.

48. C. Most state public health agencies require that cases of phenylketonuria (PKU) be reported.

49. D. Confidentiality is legally supported by the Privacy Act.

50. D. Confidentiality is ethically supported by all of the concepts listed.

51. A. B is failing to carry out the terms of an agreement; C is the tort of carelessness; D is negligence of a professional person.

52. B. A provider who guarantees the outcome of a course of treatment and that outcome does not materialize could be sued for breach of contract.

53. D. Negligence of a professional person such as a provider, nurse, or allied health practitioner constitutes malpractice.

54. B. Options A and C are not legal terms used to describe negligence. Option D is a more serious form than ordinary negligence.

55. A. Option B means to breach one's duty; C means the carelessness was the direct cause of the patient's injuries; D means the injuries suffered by the patient.

56. A. In most states there is no general duty to rescue anyone who is in peril except family members and those you have imperiled.

57. B. In most states, if you begin to assist someone in peril, you are free to abandon the rescue as long as you do not put the victim in any additional peril.

58. B. Option A relates to obligations; C relates to fairness; D relates to legal claims.

59. D. Veracity means to be truthful. Even though information communicated to the patient may be unpleasant, providers have an obligation to be truthful about such information.

60. B. Informed consent means that patients have been given sufficient information to make an informed decision about their care. Failing to disclose such information violates the patient's right to self-determination, i.e., autonomy.

61. D. Option A relates to what is needed to physically stay alive, e.g., food and water; B relates to the need to be free from harm and anxiety; C relates to the need to be loved and to belong.

62. A. Option B means to not acknowledge reality; C means to divert unacceptable thoughts and feelings into acceptable behaviors; D means to put unpleasant thoughts or feelings out of one's mind.

63. D. Option A means to adopt the feelings of others; B means to disconnect emotional significance from specific ideas or events; C means to justify one's thoughts, feelings, or behavior.

64. C. Elisabeth Kübler-Ross is credited with establishing the five stages of dying.

65. D. Options A–C are ineffective means of helping patients cope with their fears.

66. B. Repeating what the patient has said in one's own words to communicate understanding is mirroring.

67. C. Advising is communicating to a patient what one feels the patient should do or not do. It is better to communicate the facts and let the patient make the decision independently.

68. D. Option A means to adopt the feelings of others; B means to ascribe to others one's own feelings; C means behavior that is the opposite of one's true feelings.

69. D. Option A means to disconnect emotional significance from specific ideas or events; B means to justify one's thoughts, feelings, or behavior; C means to make up for an area of deficiency by concentrating on a more easily attainable goal.

70. D. The patient may wish to continue the sick role for all of the listed reasons.

71. D. All are considered losses associated with adopting the sick role, therefore, this is the best response.

72. D. All are methods that may be used to determine what is important to a patient.

73. A. Option B means to feel sorry for someone; C means to strengthen a behavior; D means to ascribe to another one's own thoughts and feelings.

74. C. The remaining options will likely have the opposite effect.

75. B. Option A means to draw a conclusion based on incomplete information; C means the provider interacts with a patient as one would a sibling or son or daughter; D means to need a provider's interaction to the detriment of care.

76. D. Option A means to share meaning; B and C mean to interpret the meaning of a communication.

77. B. The other options are too familiar, at least initially.

78. B. Encouraging a patient to stay on topic is focusing.

79. C. Lack of intelligence is a common stereotype ascribed to those who have communication difficulties.

80. A. Option B refers to someone in a vegetative state; C refers to one who habitually visits the emergency room; D refers to someone who has a physical disability.

81. B. Pica pitch is 10 characters per inch.

82. B. The tab key allows one to move the cursor a predetermined number of spaces to the right.

83. A. Six lines of text represent 1 inch.

84. D. The alt and ctrl keys triple the tasks the function keys can perform.

85. A. Option B means to combine the contents of a document; C means to reproduce text and place it in another section of the document; D means to eliminate records or their contents.

86. B. The smallest piece of information processed by a computer is a bit.

87. C. The process of activating the input of the operating system into main memory is booting.

88. D. The process of organizing a blank disk into sectors so that it can store data is known as formatting.

89. D. A key that moves the cursor to the margins when pressed is the Home key.

90. C. A blinking dash that identifies where on the computer screen data will be entered is the cursor.

91. B. The number of characters contained within an inch is the pitch.

92. A. Option B permits the printing of identical information at the bottom of each page; C is the first line of a paragraph appearing alone at the bottom of a page; D is the last line of a paragraph appearing alone at the top of a page.

93. A. Option B is the first line of a paragraph appearing alone at the bottom of a page; C permits the printing of identical information at the top of each page; D permits the printing of identical information at the bottom of each page.

94. A. The computer command that organizes data alphabetically or numerically is sort.

95. B. Windows is a computer application that allows multiple applications to operate simultaneously.

96. B. A spreadsheet permits rapid calculations to be applied to a table of numerical data.

97. B. Alphanumeric characters primarily used as headings are known as labels.

98. A. Column A, row 3 is located at cell A3.

99. D. CD-RW (read/write) is an optical disk storage medium that allows one to store, erase, and restore data.

100. D. Solid state because it involves no moving parts.

101. A. Two lines separate the inside address and the salutation.

102. D. Open punctuation refers to placing no punctuation after the salutation.

103. D. The acronym bc means blind copy—a copy has been sent to a third party without the orginal party's knowledge.

104. C. A refers to full block; B refers to modified block; D refers to simplified.

105. A. The remaining options are part of the closing.

106. B. In order, they would be indexed as B, D, A, and C.

107. D. In order, they would be indexed as B, A, C, and D.

108. C. In order, they would be indexed as C, A, D, and B.

109. B. First filed by subject and then chronologically (numerically) by date.

110. A. Systems that color code patient charts do so using the patient's surname.

111. D. Approximately 9 pennies equal 1 ounce.

112. D. Special fourth class is used to deliver books and manuscripts.

113. C. First-class mail that is insured is registered mail.

114. B. "Dear Mrs. Smith:" is an example of a salutation.

115. B. "Dear Mrs. Smith:" demonstrates mixed punctuation.

116. D. The reference notation comes after the signature line.

117. B. A provider's resumé is often in the form of a curriculum vitae.

118. C. Four lines typically separate the complimentary close and the signature line.

119. B. Long letters typically have 1 inch margins.

120. A. A summary of a manuscript in 100 to 200 words is an abstract.

121. B. Option A refers to scheduling patients for a specified time; C is a staggered wave system; D refers to scheduling more than one patient for the same time slot.

122. B. All may be considered; however, option B is the least important of those given.

123. B. Scheduling patients with similar needs within a specified time frame describes grouping (clustering).

124. A. The appointment book is a legal record and should ideally be recorded in ink that cannot be erased.

125. C. When it is 2 p.m. in Minnesota, it is 3 p.m. in Georgia.

126. C. Equipment being a capital item is typically purchased by the office manager.

127. A. Options B and C may cause the representative to unduly wait. With option D, medical assistants do not select drugs.

128. B. Never begin with "please hold" and never ignore a ringing line.

129. D. Demographic data such as age, education, income, and the like are rarely recorded on a message slip.

130. C. Conveying disinterest is discourteous.

131. B. When dialing direct, the caller dials 1 + area code + seven-digit number.

132. D. If a provider or an alternate cannot be reached, a patient could file a lawsuit based on abandonment.

133. D. The appointment scheduling system should reflect the needs of the provider, staff, and patients.

134. B. The location of the clinic is the least important consideration given.

135. A. Red ink is often used to identify new patients.

136. C. The international access code is 011.

137. A. Time slots used as "catch-up" periods are known as buffer periods.

138. A. Patients arriving with an emergency condition should be seen right away.

139. A. Twenty minutes or less is ideal.

140. B. The most effective means of conveying a cheerful tone while speaking on the phone is to smile.

141. A. Option B is the depositor; C is the party to receive the money (check); D is the person making out the check.

142. C. $4050 + 1025 - 700 = 4375$.

143. A. Categorizing accounts according to the number of days the accounts are past-due describes aging accounts receivable.

144. B. Option A is twice a month; C is every 2 months; D is twice a year.

145. C. Option A is the difference between assets and liabilities; B is a debt obligation; D is business income.

146. D. A signature card must be completed to open a checking account.

147. B. MICR—magnetic ink character recognition.

148. D. ABA numbers are expressed as a fraction.

149. C. A check the bank refused to pay has been dishonored.

150. C. A personal record of the checks written and the account balance is a check register.

151. A. NCR—no carbon required.

152. C. A check that has been stamped to prevent its reuse is cancelled.

153. B. All may be called upon to review a clinic's accounting records except patients.

154. D. Options A and C refer to business income; B is business costs.

155. B. A journal serves to record all daily transactions.

156. C. Option A is a list of all account balances to determine whether the debits equal the credits; B is a statement that summarizes assets, liabilities, and capital balances; D is a statement used in corporations to identify that amount of income retained in the business.

157. C. An amount maintained for minor expenses is petty cash.

158. A. The usual fee is the one a provider most frequently charges for a service.

159. C. Option A refers to bad debts; B refers to allowances given to the indigent; D refers to allowances given to other providers, and the like.

160. B. Billing segments of the patient population describes cycle billing.

161. D. Glossitis is a diagnosis and is assigned an ICD code. Options A–C are procedures and are typically assigned a CPT code.

162. B. Atherosclerosis is a diagnosis and would require an ICD code.

163. B. Option A is available for the elderly and disabled; C is conventional insurance; D is available for military personnel and their dependents.

164. A. Option B is a policy that complements another policy; C is when the carrier pays the provider directly; D is a peril not covered by the policy.

165. A. A prepaid health plan that emphasizes health prevention and promotion is an HMO.

166. D. A provision that covers the cost of repair resulting from defects is a warranty.

167. D. The chairperson of a meeting is typically responsible for all of the tasks listed.

168. C. Option A is a legal document that identifies how evidence was handled; B is a chart that identifies the positions within an organization; D refers to the elements of the infectious process.

169. B. An honorarium is a gratuitous payment for professional services.

170. A. Option B is the depletion of stock; C is the replacement of stock; D is amount of stock on hand.

171. D. A direction to consider additional codes is "see also."

172. D. Nonessential modifier. The underlined portion can be included or excluded as part of the main term when assigning a code.

173. C. HMO is an organizational arrangement that provides medical services for a fixed, prepaid fee.

174. C. Option A is formulating objectives; B is assembling business resources; D is comparing actual results with planned results.

175. B. A term after the brace (}) indicates that it is a required modifier of the term before the brace.

176. B. AOB means assignment of benefits.

177. C. Option A refers to making a small payment at the time of visit; B is the monthly payment required to keep a policy in force; D is a peril that is not covered by the policy.

178. B. Options A and D refer to the insurance company; C is the policyholder.

179. C. Malignant hypertension is a severe form with vascular damage.

180. A. Medicare is Title 18 of the SSA.

181. A. Pupils equal, round, and reactive to light and accommodation is part of the head and neck of the ROS.

182. B. Option A refers to objective data (O); C is the assessment (A); D is the plan (P).

183. D. Hypotension is a systolic pressure less than 90 and/or a diastolic pressure less than 60.

184. D. Although any one of these ranges may be normal for selected adults, the best option is 60–100.

185. D. All of the options listed affect body temperature.

186. C. The position of choice for orthopnea is the Fowler's position.

187. B. Attempting to assess a patient's condition by ruling out certain possibilities describes differential diagnosis.

188. D. Recitation is not an examination method.

189. D. A sigmoidoscope is typically not used in a routine physical examination.

190. D. Ophthalmologists typically do not use a percussion hammer when diagnosing and treating disorders of the eye.

191. D. Details regarding the health status of the patient's parents and siblings are known as the family history.

192. B. Auscultation is the process of listening to body sounds using a stethoscope.

193. D. A is the patient report of the medical problem; B is the observations, measurements, and tests performed on the patient; C is the diagnosis.

194. D. Demographics includes the patient's DOB, marital status, education, occupation, and the like.

195. A. The sitting position is generally the initial position in which the breasts are examined. The breasts will also later be examined in the supine position as well.

196. D. The Romberg test is performed during an otorhinolaryngological examination.

197. B. Review of systems.

198. B. Option A is both; options C and D are nonsense distracters.

199. A. The other options are chemicals.

200. B. The best option is B.

CMA Simulation Test: Pre-Test

Name _____ **Date** _____

Last   First   Middle

DIRECTIONS:

1. Fill in only one circle using pencil representing your answer for each question.
2. Keeping your marks inside the circle, blacken the circle completely.
3. Completely erase any answer you wish to change, and make no stray marks.

Correct: Wrong:

GENERAL

1. Ⓐ Ⓑ Ⓒ Ⓓ Ⓔ
2. Ⓐ Ⓑ Ⓒ Ⓓ Ⓔ
3. Ⓐ Ⓑ Ⓒ Ⓓ Ⓔ
4. Ⓐ Ⓑ Ⓒ Ⓓ Ⓔ
5. Ⓐ Ⓑ Ⓒ Ⓓ Ⓔ
6. Ⓐ Ⓑ Ⓒ Ⓓ Ⓔ
7. Ⓐ Ⓑ Ⓒ Ⓓ Ⓔ
8. Ⓐ Ⓑ Ⓒ Ⓓ Ⓔ
9. Ⓐ Ⓑ Ⓒ Ⓓ Ⓔ
10. Ⓐ Ⓑ Ⓒ Ⓓ Ⓔ
11. Ⓐ Ⓑ Ⓒ Ⓓ Ⓔ
12. Ⓐ Ⓑ Ⓒ Ⓓ Ⓔ
13. Ⓐ Ⓑ Ⓒ Ⓓ Ⓔ
14. Ⓐ Ⓑ Ⓒ Ⓓ Ⓔ
15. Ⓐ Ⓑ Ⓒ Ⓓ Ⓔ
16. Ⓐ Ⓑ Ⓒ Ⓓ Ⓔ
17. Ⓐ Ⓑ Ⓒ Ⓓ Ⓔ
18. Ⓐ Ⓑ Ⓒ Ⓓ Ⓔ
19. Ⓐ Ⓑ Ⓒ Ⓓ Ⓔ
20. Ⓐ Ⓑ Ⓒ Ⓓ Ⓔ
21. Ⓐ Ⓑ Ⓒ Ⓓ Ⓔ
22. Ⓐ Ⓑ Ⓒ Ⓓ Ⓔ
23. Ⓐ Ⓑ Ⓒ Ⓓ Ⓔ
24. Ⓐ Ⓑ Ⓒ Ⓓ Ⓔ
25. Ⓐ Ⓑ Ⓒ Ⓓ Ⓔ
26. Ⓐ Ⓑ Ⓒ Ⓓ Ⓔ
27. Ⓐ Ⓑ Ⓒ Ⓓ Ⓔ
28. Ⓐ Ⓑ Ⓒ Ⓓ Ⓔ
29. Ⓐ Ⓑ Ⓒ Ⓓ Ⓔ
30. Ⓐ Ⓑ Ⓒ Ⓓ Ⓔ

ADMINISTRATIVE

1. Ⓐ Ⓑ Ⓒ Ⓓ Ⓔ
2. Ⓐ Ⓑ Ⓒ Ⓓ Ⓔ
3. Ⓐ Ⓑ Ⓒ Ⓓ Ⓔ
4. Ⓐ Ⓑ Ⓒ Ⓓ Ⓔ
5. Ⓐ Ⓑ Ⓒ Ⓓ Ⓔ
6. Ⓐ Ⓑ Ⓒ Ⓓ Ⓔ
7. Ⓐ Ⓑ Ⓒ Ⓓ Ⓔ
8. Ⓐ Ⓑ Ⓒ Ⓓ Ⓔ
9. Ⓐ Ⓑ Ⓒ Ⓓ Ⓔ
10. Ⓐ Ⓑ Ⓒ Ⓓ Ⓔ
11. Ⓐ Ⓑ Ⓒ Ⓓ Ⓔ
12. Ⓐ Ⓑ Ⓒ Ⓓ Ⓔ
13. Ⓐ Ⓑ Ⓒ Ⓓ Ⓔ
14. Ⓐ Ⓑ Ⓒ Ⓓ Ⓔ
15. Ⓐ Ⓑ Ⓒ Ⓓ Ⓔ
16. Ⓐ Ⓑ Ⓒ Ⓓ Ⓔ
17. Ⓐ Ⓑ Ⓒ Ⓓ Ⓔ
18. Ⓐ Ⓑ Ⓒ Ⓓ Ⓔ
19. Ⓐ Ⓑ Ⓒ Ⓓ Ⓔ
20. Ⓐ Ⓑ Ⓒ Ⓓ Ⓔ
21. Ⓐ Ⓑ Ⓒ Ⓓ Ⓔ
22. Ⓐ Ⓑ Ⓒ Ⓓ Ⓔ
23. Ⓐ Ⓑ Ⓒ Ⓓ Ⓔ
24. Ⓐ Ⓑ Ⓒ Ⓓ Ⓔ
25. Ⓐ Ⓑ Ⓒ Ⓓ Ⓔ
26. Ⓐ Ⓑ Ⓒ Ⓓ Ⓔ
27. Ⓐ Ⓑ Ⓒ Ⓓ Ⓔ
28. Ⓐ Ⓑ Ⓒ Ⓓ Ⓔ
29. Ⓐ Ⓑ Ⓒ Ⓓ Ⓔ
30. Ⓐ Ⓑ Ⓒ Ⓓ Ⓔ

CLINICAL

1. Ⓐ Ⓑ Ⓒ Ⓓ Ⓔ
2. Ⓐ Ⓑ Ⓒ Ⓓ Ⓔ
3. Ⓐ Ⓑ Ⓒ Ⓓ Ⓔ
4. Ⓐ Ⓑ Ⓒ Ⓓ Ⓔ
5. Ⓐ Ⓑ Ⓒ Ⓓ Ⓔ
6. Ⓐ Ⓑ Ⓒ Ⓓ Ⓔ
7. Ⓐ Ⓑ Ⓒ Ⓓ Ⓔ
8. Ⓐ Ⓑ Ⓒ Ⓓ Ⓔ
9. Ⓐ Ⓑ Ⓒ Ⓓ Ⓔ
10. Ⓐ Ⓑ Ⓒ Ⓓ Ⓔ
11. Ⓐ Ⓑ Ⓒ Ⓓ Ⓔ
12. Ⓐ Ⓑ Ⓒ Ⓓ Ⓔ
13. Ⓐ Ⓑ Ⓒ Ⓓ Ⓔ
14. Ⓐ Ⓑ Ⓒ Ⓓ Ⓔ
15. Ⓐ Ⓑ Ⓒ Ⓓ Ⓔ
16. Ⓐ Ⓑ Ⓒ Ⓓ Ⓔ
17. Ⓐ Ⓑ Ⓒ Ⓓ Ⓔ
18. Ⓐ Ⓑ Ⓒ Ⓓ Ⓔ
19. Ⓐ Ⓑ Ⓒ Ⓓ Ⓔ
20. Ⓐ Ⓑ Ⓒ Ⓓ Ⓔ
21. Ⓐ Ⓑ Ⓒ Ⓓ Ⓔ
22. Ⓐ Ⓑ Ⓒ Ⓓ Ⓔ
23. Ⓐ Ⓑ Ⓒ Ⓓ Ⓔ
24. Ⓐ Ⓑ Ⓒ Ⓓ Ⓔ
25. Ⓐ Ⓑ Ⓒ Ⓓ Ⓔ
26. Ⓐ Ⓑ Ⓒ Ⓓ Ⓔ
27. Ⓐ Ⓑ Ⓒ Ⓓ Ⓔ
28. Ⓐ Ⓑ Ⓒ Ⓓ Ⓔ
29. Ⓐ Ⓑ Ⓒ Ⓓ Ⓔ
30. Ⓐ Ⓑ Ⓒ Ⓓ Ⓔ

RMA Simulation Test: Pre-Test

Name _____   **Date** _____

Last   First   Middle

DIRECTIONS:

1. Fill in only one circle using pencil representing your answer for each question.
2. Keeping your marks inside the circle, blacken the circle completely.
3. Completely erase any answer you wish to change, and make no stray marks.

Correct: Ⓐ ● Ⓒ Ⓓ Ⓔ   Wrong: Ⓧ ◓ ◯ Ⓓ̸ Ⓔ̸

GENERAL

1. Ⓐ Ⓑ Ⓒ Ⓓ Ⓔ
2. Ⓐ Ⓑ Ⓒ Ⓓ Ⓔ
3. Ⓐ Ⓑ Ⓒ Ⓓ Ⓔ
4. Ⓐ Ⓑ Ⓒ Ⓓ Ⓔ
5. Ⓐ Ⓑ Ⓒ Ⓓ Ⓔ
6. Ⓐ Ⓑ Ⓒ Ⓓ Ⓔ
7. Ⓐ Ⓑ Ⓒ Ⓓ Ⓔ
8. Ⓐ Ⓑ Ⓒ Ⓓ Ⓔ
9. Ⓐ Ⓑ Ⓒ Ⓓ Ⓔ
10. Ⓐ Ⓑ Ⓒ Ⓓ Ⓔ
11. Ⓐ Ⓑ Ⓒ Ⓓ Ⓔ
12. Ⓐ Ⓑ Ⓒ Ⓓ Ⓔ
13. Ⓐ Ⓑ Ⓒ Ⓓ Ⓔ
14. Ⓐ Ⓑ Ⓒ Ⓓ Ⓔ
15. Ⓐ Ⓑ Ⓒ Ⓓ Ⓔ
16. Ⓐ Ⓑ Ⓒ Ⓓ Ⓔ
17. Ⓐ Ⓑ Ⓒ Ⓓ Ⓔ
18. Ⓐ Ⓑ Ⓒ Ⓓ Ⓔ
19. Ⓐ Ⓑ Ⓒ Ⓓ Ⓔ
20. Ⓐ Ⓑ Ⓒ Ⓓ Ⓔ
21. Ⓐ Ⓑ Ⓒ Ⓓ Ⓔ
22. Ⓐ Ⓑ Ⓒ Ⓓ Ⓔ
23. Ⓐ Ⓑ Ⓒ Ⓓ Ⓔ
24. Ⓐ Ⓑ Ⓒ Ⓓ Ⓔ
25. Ⓐ Ⓑ Ⓒ Ⓓ Ⓔ
26. Ⓐ Ⓑ Ⓒ Ⓓ Ⓔ
27. Ⓐ Ⓑ Ⓒ Ⓓ Ⓔ
28. Ⓐ Ⓑ Ⓒ Ⓓ Ⓔ
29. Ⓐ Ⓑ Ⓒ Ⓓ Ⓔ
30. Ⓐ Ⓑ Ⓒ Ⓓ Ⓔ

ADMINISTRATIVE

1. Ⓐ Ⓑ Ⓒ Ⓓ Ⓔ
2. Ⓐ Ⓑ Ⓒ Ⓓ Ⓔ
3. Ⓐ Ⓑ Ⓒ Ⓓ Ⓔ
4. Ⓐ Ⓑ Ⓒ Ⓓ Ⓔ
5. Ⓐ Ⓑ Ⓒ Ⓓ Ⓔ
6. Ⓐ Ⓑ Ⓒ Ⓓ Ⓔ
7. Ⓐ Ⓑ Ⓒ Ⓓ Ⓔ
8. Ⓐ Ⓑ Ⓒ Ⓓ Ⓔ
9. Ⓐ Ⓑ Ⓒ Ⓓ Ⓔ
10. Ⓐ Ⓑ Ⓒ Ⓓ Ⓔ
11. Ⓐ Ⓑ Ⓒ Ⓓ Ⓔ
12. Ⓐ Ⓑ Ⓒ Ⓓ Ⓔ
13. Ⓐ Ⓑ Ⓒ Ⓓ Ⓔ
14. Ⓐ Ⓑ Ⓒ Ⓓ Ⓔ
15. Ⓐ Ⓑ Ⓒ Ⓓ Ⓔ
16. Ⓐ Ⓑ Ⓒ Ⓓ Ⓔ
17. Ⓐ Ⓑ Ⓒ Ⓓ Ⓔ
18. Ⓐ Ⓑ Ⓒ Ⓓ Ⓔ
19. Ⓐ Ⓑ Ⓒ Ⓓ Ⓔ
20. Ⓐ Ⓑ Ⓒ Ⓓ Ⓔ
21. Ⓐ Ⓑ Ⓒ Ⓓ Ⓔ
22. Ⓐ Ⓑ Ⓒ Ⓓ Ⓔ
23. Ⓐ Ⓑ Ⓒ Ⓓ Ⓔ
24. Ⓐ Ⓑ Ⓒ Ⓓ Ⓔ
25. Ⓐ Ⓑ Ⓒ Ⓓ Ⓔ
26. Ⓐ Ⓑ Ⓒ Ⓓ Ⓔ
27. Ⓐ Ⓑ Ⓒ Ⓓ Ⓔ
28. Ⓐ Ⓑ Ⓒ Ⓓ Ⓔ
29. Ⓐ Ⓑ Ⓒ Ⓓ Ⓔ
30. Ⓐ Ⓑ Ⓒ Ⓓ Ⓔ

CLINICAL

1. Ⓐ Ⓑ Ⓒ Ⓓ Ⓔ
2. Ⓐ Ⓑ Ⓒ Ⓓ Ⓔ
3. Ⓐ Ⓑ Ⓒ Ⓓ Ⓔ
4. Ⓐ Ⓑ Ⓒ Ⓓ Ⓔ
5. Ⓐ Ⓑ Ⓒ Ⓓ Ⓔ
6. Ⓐ Ⓑ Ⓒ Ⓓ Ⓔ
7. Ⓐ Ⓑ Ⓒ Ⓓ Ⓔ
8. Ⓐ Ⓑ Ⓒ Ⓓ Ⓔ
9. Ⓐ Ⓑ Ⓒ Ⓓ Ⓔ
10. Ⓐ Ⓑ Ⓒ Ⓓ Ⓔ
11. Ⓐ Ⓑ Ⓒ Ⓓ Ⓔ
12. Ⓐ Ⓑ Ⓒ Ⓓ Ⓔ
13. Ⓐ Ⓑ Ⓒ Ⓓ Ⓔ
14. Ⓐ Ⓑ Ⓒ Ⓓ Ⓔ
15. Ⓐ Ⓑ Ⓒ Ⓓ Ⓔ
16. Ⓐ Ⓑ Ⓒ Ⓓ Ⓔ
17. Ⓐ Ⓑ Ⓒ Ⓓ Ⓔ
18. Ⓐ Ⓑ Ⓒ Ⓓ Ⓔ
19. Ⓐ Ⓑ Ⓒ Ⓓ Ⓔ
20. Ⓐ Ⓑ Ⓒ Ⓓ Ⓔ
21. Ⓐ Ⓑ Ⓒ Ⓓ Ⓔ
22. Ⓐ Ⓑ Ⓒ Ⓓ Ⓔ
23. Ⓐ Ⓑ Ⓒ Ⓓ Ⓔ
24. Ⓐ Ⓑ Ⓒ Ⓓ Ⓔ
25. Ⓐ Ⓑ Ⓒ Ⓓ Ⓔ
26. Ⓐ Ⓑ Ⓒ Ⓓ Ⓔ
27. Ⓐ Ⓑ Ⓒ Ⓓ Ⓔ
28. Ⓐ Ⓑ Ⓒ Ⓓ Ⓔ
29. Ⓐ Ⓑ Ⓒ Ⓓ Ⓔ
30. Ⓐ Ⓑ Ⓒ Ⓓ Ⓔ

CMAS Simulation Test: Pre-Test

Name _____ **Date** _____

Last   First   Middle

DIRECTIONS:

1. Fill in only one circle using pencil representing your answer for each question.
2. Keeping your marks inside the circle, blacken the circle completely.
3. Completely erase any answer you wish to change, and make no stray marks.

Correct: Ⓐ ● Ⓒ Ⓓ Ⓔ   Wrong: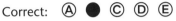

1. Ⓐ Ⓑ Ⓒ Ⓓ Ⓔ
2. Ⓐ Ⓑ Ⓒ Ⓓ Ⓔ
3. Ⓐ Ⓑ Ⓒ Ⓓ Ⓔ
4. Ⓐ Ⓑ Ⓒ Ⓓ Ⓔ
5. Ⓐ Ⓑ Ⓒ Ⓓ Ⓔ
6. Ⓐ Ⓑ Ⓒ Ⓓ Ⓔ
7. Ⓐ Ⓑ Ⓒ Ⓓ Ⓔ
8. Ⓐ Ⓑ Ⓒ Ⓓ Ⓔ
9. Ⓐ Ⓑ Ⓒ Ⓓ Ⓔ
10. Ⓐ Ⓑ Ⓒ Ⓓ Ⓔ
11. Ⓐ Ⓑ Ⓒ Ⓓ Ⓔ
12. Ⓐ Ⓑ Ⓒ Ⓓ Ⓔ
13. Ⓐ Ⓑ Ⓒ Ⓓ Ⓔ
14. Ⓐ Ⓑ Ⓒ Ⓓ Ⓔ
15. Ⓐ Ⓑ Ⓒ Ⓓ Ⓔ
16. Ⓐ Ⓑ Ⓒ Ⓓ Ⓔ
17. Ⓐ Ⓑ Ⓒ Ⓓ Ⓔ
18. Ⓐ Ⓑ Ⓒ Ⓓ Ⓔ
19. Ⓐ Ⓑ Ⓒ Ⓓ Ⓔ
20. Ⓐ Ⓑ Ⓒ Ⓓ Ⓔ
21. Ⓐ Ⓑ Ⓒ Ⓓ Ⓔ
22. Ⓐ Ⓑ Ⓒ Ⓓ Ⓔ
23. Ⓐ Ⓑ Ⓒ Ⓓ Ⓔ
24. Ⓐ Ⓑ Ⓒ Ⓓ Ⓔ
25. Ⓐ Ⓑ Ⓒ Ⓓ Ⓔ

26. Ⓐ Ⓑ Ⓒ Ⓓ Ⓔ
27. Ⓐ Ⓑ Ⓒ Ⓓ Ⓔ
28. Ⓐ Ⓑ Ⓒ Ⓓ Ⓔ
29. Ⓐ Ⓑ Ⓒ Ⓓ Ⓔ
30. Ⓐ Ⓑ Ⓒ Ⓓ Ⓔ
31. Ⓐ Ⓑ Ⓒ Ⓓ Ⓔ
32. Ⓐ Ⓑ Ⓒ Ⓓ Ⓔ
33. Ⓐ Ⓑ Ⓒ Ⓓ Ⓔ
34. Ⓐ Ⓑ Ⓒ Ⓓ Ⓔ
35. Ⓐ Ⓑ Ⓒ Ⓓ Ⓔ
36. Ⓐ Ⓑ Ⓒ Ⓓ Ⓔ
37. Ⓐ Ⓑ Ⓒ Ⓓ Ⓔ
38. Ⓐ Ⓑ Ⓒ Ⓓ Ⓔ
39. Ⓐ Ⓑ Ⓒ Ⓓ Ⓔ
40. Ⓐ Ⓑ Ⓒ Ⓓ Ⓔ
41. Ⓐ Ⓑ Ⓒ Ⓓ Ⓔ
42. Ⓐ Ⓑ Ⓒ Ⓓ Ⓔ
43. Ⓐ Ⓑ Ⓒ Ⓓ Ⓔ
44. Ⓐ Ⓑ Ⓒ Ⓓ Ⓔ
45. Ⓐ Ⓑ Ⓒ Ⓓ Ⓔ
46. Ⓐ Ⓑ Ⓒ Ⓓ Ⓔ
47. Ⓐ Ⓑ Ⓒ Ⓓ Ⓔ
48. Ⓐ Ⓑ Ⓒ Ⓓ Ⓔ
49. Ⓐ Ⓑ Ⓒ Ⓓ Ⓔ
50. Ⓐ Ⓑ Ⓒ Ⓓ Ⓔ

51. Ⓐ Ⓑ Ⓒ Ⓓ Ⓔ
52. Ⓐ Ⓑ Ⓒ Ⓓ Ⓔ
53. Ⓐ Ⓑ Ⓒ Ⓓ Ⓔ
54. Ⓐ Ⓑ Ⓒ Ⓓ Ⓔ
55. Ⓐ Ⓑ Ⓒ Ⓓ Ⓔ
56. Ⓐ Ⓑ Ⓒ Ⓓ Ⓔ
57. Ⓐ Ⓑ Ⓒ Ⓓ Ⓔ
58. Ⓐ Ⓑ Ⓒ Ⓓ Ⓔ
59. Ⓐ Ⓑ Ⓒ Ⓓ Ⓔ
60. Ⓐ Ⓑ Ⓒ Ⓓ Ⓔ
61. Ⓐ Ⓑ Ⓒ Ⓓ Ⓔ
62. Ⓐ Ⓑ Ⓒ Ⓓ Ⓔ
63. Ⓐ Ⓑ Ⓒ Ⓓ Ⓔ
64. Ⓐ Ⓑ Ⓒ Ⓓ Ⓔ
65. Ⓐ Ⓑ Ⓒ Ⓓ Ⓔ
66. Ⓐ Ⓑ Ⓒ Ⓓ Ⓔ
67. Ⓐ Ⓑ Ⓒ Ⓓ Ⓔ
68. Ⓐ Ⓑ Ⓒ Ⓓ Ⓔ
69. Ⓐ Ⓑ Ⓒ Ⓓ Ⓔ
70. Ⓐ Ⓑ Ⓒ Ⓓ Ⓔ
71. Ⓐ Ⓑ Ⓒ Ⓓ Ⓔ
72. Ⓐ Ⓑ Ⓒ Ⓓ Ⓔ
73. Ⓐ Ⓑ Ⓒ Ⓓ Ⓔ
74. Ⓐ Ⓑ Ⓒ Ⓓ Ⓔ
75. Ⓐ Ⓑ Ⓒ Ⓓ Ⓔ

76. Ⓐ Ⓑ Ⓒ Ⓓ Ⓔ
77. Ⓐ Ⓑ Ⓒ Ⓓ Ⓔ
78. Ⓐ Ⓑ Ⓒ Ⓓ Ⓔ
79. Ⓐ Ⓑ Ⓒ Ⓓ Ⓔ
80. Ⓐ Ⓑ Ⓒ Ⓓ Ⓔ
81. Ⓐ Ⓑ Ⓒ Ⓓ Ⓔ
82. Ⓐ Ⓑ Ⓒ Ⓓ Ⓔ
83. Ⓐ Ⓑ Ⓒ Ⓓ Ⓔ
84. Ⓐ Ⓑ Ⓒ Ⓓ Ⓔ
85. Ⓐ Ⓑ Ⓒ Ⓓ Ⓔ
86. Ⓐ Ⓑ Ⓒ Ⓓ Ⓔ
87. Ⓐ Ⓑ Ⓒ Ⓓ Ⓔ
88. Ⓐ Ⓑ Ⓒ Ⓓ Ⓔ
89. Ⓐ Ⓑ Ⓒ Ⓓ Ⓔ
90. Ⓐ Ⓑ Ⓒ Ⓓ Ⓔ
91. Ⓐ Ⓑ Ⓒ Ⓓ Ⓔ
92. Ⓐ Ⓑ Ⓒ Ⓓ Ⓔ
93. Ⓐ Ⓑ Ⓒ Ⓓ Ⓔ
94. Ⓐ Ⓑ Ⓒ Ⓓ Ⓔ
95. Ⓐ Ⓑ Ⓒ Ⓓ Ⓔ
96. Ⓐ Ⓑ Ⓒ Ⓓ Ⓔ
97. Ⓐ Ⓑ Ⓒ Ⓓ Ⓔ
98. Ⓐ Ⓑ Ⓒ Ⓓ Ⓔ
99. Ⓐ Ⓑ Ⓒ Ⓓ Ⓔ
100. Ⓐ Ⓑ Ⓒ Ⓓ Ⓔ

CMA Simulation Test: Post-Test

Name _____ **Date** _____

Last   First   Middle

DIRECTIONS:

1. Fill in only one circle using pencil representing your answer for each question.
2. Keeping your marks inside the circle, blacken the circle completely.
3. Completely erase any answer you wish to change, and make no stray marks.

Correct: Ⓐ ● Ⓒ Ⓓ Ⓔ   Wrong: Ⓧ ◓ ○ Ⓓ Ⓔ

GENERAL

1. Ⓐ Ⓑ Ⓒ Ⓓ Ⓔ
2. Ⓐ Ⓑ Ⓒ Ⓓ Ⓔ
3. Ⓐ Ⓑ Ⓒ Ⓓ Ⓔ
4. Ⓐ Ⓑ Ⓒ Ⓓ Ⓔ
5. Ⓐ Ⓑ Ⓒ Ⓓ Ⓔ
6. Ⓐ Ⓑ Ⓒ Ⓓ Ⓔ
7. Ⓐ Ⓑ Ⓒ Ⓓ Ⓔ
8. Ⓐ Ⓑ Ⓒ Ⓓ Ⓔ
9. Ⓐ Ⓑ Ⓒ Ⓓ Ⓔ
10. Ⓐ Ⓑ Ⓒ Ⓓ Ⓔ
11. Ⓐ Ⓑ Ⓒ Ⓓ Ⓔ
12. Ⓐ Ⓑ Ⓒ Ⓓ Ⓔ
13. Ⓐ Ⓑ Ⓒ Ⓓ Ⓔ
14. Ⓐ Ⓑ Ⓒ Ⓓ Ⓔ
15. Ⓐ Ⓑ Ⓒ Ⓓ Ⓔ
16. Ⓐ Ⓑ Ⓒ Ⓓ Ⓔ
17. Ⓐ Ⓑ Ⓒ Ⓓ Ⓔ
18. Ⓐ Ⓑ Ⓒ Ⓓ Ⓔ
19. Ⓐ Ⓑ Ⓒ Ⓓ Ⓔ
20. Ⓐ Ⓑ Ⓒ Ⓓ Ⓔ
21. Ⓐ Ⓑ Ⓒ Ⓓ Ⓔ
22. Ⓐ Ⓑ Ⓒ Ⓓ Ⓔ
23. Ⓐ Ⓑ Ⓒ Ⓓ Ⓔ
24. Ⓐ Ⓑ Ⓒ Ⓓ Ⓔ
25. Ⓐ Ⓑ Ⓒ Ⓓ Ⓔ
26. Ⓐ Ⓑ Ⓒ Ⓓ Ⓔ
27. Ⓐ Ⓑ Ⓒ Ⓓ Ⓔ
28. Ⓐ Ⓑ Ⓒ Ⓓ Ⓔ
29. Ⓐ Ⓑ Ⓒ Ⓓ Ⓔ
30. Ⓐ Ⓑ Ⓒ Ⓓ Ⓔ
31. Ⓐ Ⓑ Ⓒ Ⓓ Ⓔ
32. Ⓐ Ⓑ Ⓒ Ⓓ Ⓔ
33. Ⓐ Ⓑ Ⓒ Ⓓ Ⓔ
34. Ⓐ Ⓑ Ⓒ Ⓓ Ⓔ
35. Ⓐ Ⓑ Ⓒ Ⓓ Ⓔ
36. Ⓐ Ⓑ Ⓒ Ⓓ Ⓔ
37. Ⓐ Ⓑ Ⓒ Ⓓ Ⓔ
38. Ⓐ Ⓑ Ⓒ Ⓓ Ⓔ
39. Ⓐ Ⓑ Ⓒ Ⓓ Ⓔ
40. Ⓐ Ⓑ Ⓒ Ⓓ Ⓔ
41. Ⓐ Ⓑ Ⓒ Ⓓ Ⓔ
42. Ⓐ Ⓑ Ⓒ Ⓓ Ⓔ
43. Ⓐ Ⓑ Ⓒ Ⓓ Ⓔ
44. Ⓐ Ⓑ Ⓒ Ⓓ Ⓔ
45. Ⓐ Ⓑ Ⓒ Ⓓ Ⓔ
46. Ⓐ Ⓑ Ⓒ Ⓓ Ⓔ
47. Ⓐ Ⓑ Ⓒ Ⓓ Ⓔ
48. Ⓐ Ⓑ Ⓒ Ⓓ Ⓔ
49. Ⓐ Ⓑ Ⓒ Ⓓ Ⓔ
50. Ⓐ Ⓑ Ⓒ Ⓓ Ⓔ
51. Ⓐ Ⓑ Ⓒ Ⓓ Ⓔ
52. Ⓐ Ⓑ Ⓒ Ⓓ Ⓔ
53. Ⓐ Ⓑ Ⓒ Ⓓ Ⓔ
54. Ⓐ Ⓑ Ⓒ Ⓓ Ⓔ
55. Ⓐ Ⓑ Ⓒ Ⓓ Ⓔ
56. Ⓐ Ⓑ Ⓒ Ⓓ Ⓔ
57. Ⓐ Ⓑ Ⓒ Ⓓ Ⓔ
58. Ⓐ Ⓑ Ⓒ Ⓓ Ⓔ
59. Ⓐ Ⓑ Ⓒ Ⓓ Ⓔ
60. Ⓐ Ⓑ Ⓒ Ⓓ Ⓔ
61. Ⓐ Ⓑ Ⓒ Ⓓ Ⓔ
62. Ⓐ Ⓑ Ⓒ Ⓓ Ⓔ
63. Ⓐ Ⓑ Ⓒ Ⓓ Ⓔ
64. Ⓐ Ⓑ Ⓒ Ⓓ Ⓔ
65. Ⓐ Ⓑ Ⓒ Ⓓ Ⓔ
66. Ⓐ Ⓑ Ⓒ Ⓓ Ⓔ

ADMINISTRATIVE

1. Ⓐ Ⓑ Ⓒ Ⓓ Ⓔ
2. Ⓐ Ⓑ Ⓒ Ⓓ Ⓔ
3. Ⓐ Ⓑ Ⓒ Ⓓ Ⓔ
4. Ⓐ Ⓑ Ⓒ Ⓓ Ⓔ
5. Ⓐ Ⓑ Ⓒ Ⓓ Ⓔ
6. Ⓐ Ⓑ Ⓒ Ⓓ Ⓔ
7. Ⓐ Ⓑ Ⓒ Ⓓ Ⓔ
8. Ⓐ Ⓑ Ⓒ Ⓓ Ⓔ
9. Ⓐ Ⓑ Ⓒ Ⓓ Ⓔ
10. Ⓐ Ⓑ Ⓒ Ⓓ Ⓔ
11. Ⓐ Ⓑ Ⓒ Ⓓ Ⓔ
12. Ⓐ Ⓑ Ⓒ Ⓓ Ⓔ
13. Ⓐ Ⓑ Ⓒ Ⓓ Ⓔ
14. Ⓐ Ⓑ Ⓒ Ⓓ Ⓔ
15. Ⓐ Ⓑ Ⓒ Ⓓ Ⓔ
16. Ⓐ Ⓑ Ⓒ Ⓓ Ⓔ
17. Ⓐ Ⓑ Ⓒ Ⓓ Ⓔ
18. Ⓐ Ⓑ Ⓒ Ⓓ Ⓔ
19. Ⓐ Ⓑ Ⓒ Ⓓ Ⓔ
20. Ⓐ Ⓑ Ⓒ Ⓓ Ⓔ
21. Ⓐ Ⓑ Ⓒ Ⓓ Ⓔ
22. Ⓐ Ⓑ Ⓒ Ⓓ Ⓔ
23. Ⓐ Ⓑ Ⓒ Ⓓ Ⓔ
24. Ⓐ Ⓑ Ⓒ Ⓓ Ⓔ
25. Ⓐ Ⓑ Ⓒ Ⓓ Ⓔ
26. Ⓐ Ⓑ Ⓒ Ⓓ Ⓔ
27. Ⓐ Ⓑ Ⓒ Ⓓ Ⓔ
28. Ⓐ Ⓑ Ⓒ Ⓓ Ⓔ
29. Ⓐ Ⓑ Ⓒ Ⓓ Ⓔ
30. Ⓐ Ⓑ Ⓒ Ⓓ Ⓔ
31. Ⓐ Ⓑ Ⓒ Ⓓ Ⓔ
32. Ⓐ Ⓑ Ⓒ Ⓓ Ⓔ
33. Ⓐ Ⓑ Ⓒ Ⓓ Ⓔ
34. Ⓐ Ⓑ Ⓒ Ⓓ Ⓔ
35. Ⓐ Ⓑ Ⓒ Ⓓ Ⓔ
36. Ⓐ Ⓑ Ⓒ Ⓓ Ⓔ
37. Ⓐ Ⓑ Ⓒ Ⓓ Ⓔ
38. Ⓐ Ⓑ Ⓒ Ⓓ Ⓔ
39. Ⓐ Ⓑ Ⓒ Ⓓ Ⓔ
40. Ⓐ Ⓑ Ⓒ Ⓓ Ⓔ
41. Ⓐ Ⓑ Ⓒ Ⓓ Ⓔ
42. Ⓐ Ⓑ Ⓒ Ⓓ Ⓔ
43. Ⓐ Ⓑ Ⓒ Ⓓ Ⓔ
44. Ⓐ Ⓑ Ⓒ Ⓓ Ⓔ
45. Ⓐ Ⓑ Ⓒ Ⓓ Ⓔ
46. Ⓐ Ⓑ Ⓒ Ⓓ Ⓔ
47. Ⓐ Ⓑ Ⓒ Ⓓ Ⓔ
48. Ⓐ Ⓑ Ⓒ Ⓓ Ⓔ
49. Ⓐ Ⓑ Ⓒ Ⓓ Ⓔ
50. Ⓐ Ⓑ Ⓒ Ⓓ Ⓔ
51. Ⓐ Ⓑ Ⓒ Ⓓ Ⓔ
52. Ⓐ Ⓑ Ⓒ Ⓓ Ⓔ
53. Ⓐ Ⓑ Ⓒ Ⓓ Ⓔ
54. Ⓐ Ⓑ Ⓒ Ⓓ Ⓔ
55. Ⓐ Ⓑ Ⓒ Ⓓ Ⓔ
56. Ⓐ Ⓑ Ⓒ Ⓓ Ⓔ
57. Ⓐ Ⓑ Ⓒ Ⓓ Ⓔ
58. Ⓐ Ⓑ Ⓒ Ⓓ Ⓔ
59. Ⓐ Ⓑ Ⓒ Ⓓ Ⓔ
60. Ⓐ Ⓑ Ⓒ Ⓓ Ⓔ
61. Ⓐ Ⓑ Ⓒ Ⓓ Ⓔ
62. Ⓐ Ⓑ Ⓒ Ⓓ Ⓔ
63. Ⓐ Ⓑ Ⓒ Ⓓ Ⓔ
64. Ⓐ Ⓑ Ⓒ Ⓓ Ⓔ
65. Ⓐ Ⓑ Ⓒ Ⓓ Ⓔ
66. Ⓐ Ⓑ Ⓒ Ⓓ Ⓔ

CLINICAL

1. Ⓐ Ⓑ Ⓒ Ⓓ Ⓔ
2. Ⓐ Ⓑ Ⓒ Ⓓ Ⓔ
3. Ⓐ Ⓑ Ⓒ Ⓓ Ⓔ
4. Ⓐ Ⓑ Ⓒ Ⓓ Ⓔ
5. Ⓐ Ⓑ Ⓒ Ⓓ Ⓔ
6. Ⓐ Ⓑ Ⓒ Ⓓ Ⓔ
7. Ⓐ Ⓑ Ⓒ Ⓓ Ⓔ
8. Ⓐ Ⓑ Ⓒ Ⓓ Ⓔ
9. Ⓐ Ⓑ Ⓒ Ⓓ Ⓔ
10. Ⓐ Ⓑ Ⓒ Ⓓ Ⓔ
11. Ⓐ Ⓑ Ⓒ Ⓓ Ⓔ
12. Ⓐ Ⓑ Ⓒ Ⓓ Ⓔ
13. Ⓐ Ⓑ Ⓒ Ⓓ Ⓔ
14. Ⓐ Ⓑ Ⓒ Ⓓ Ⓔ
15. Ⓐ Ⓑ Ⓒ Ⓓ Ⓔ
16. Ⓐ Ⓑ Ⓒ Ⓓ Ⓔ
17. Ⓐ Ⓑ Ⓒ Ⓓ Ⓔ
18. Ⓐ Ⓑ Ⓒ Ⓓ Ⓔ
19. Ⓐ Ⓑ Ⓒ Ⓓ Ⓔ
20. Ⓐ Ⓑ Ⓒ Ⓓ Ⓔ
21. Ⓐ Ⓑ Ⓒ Ⓓ Ⓔ
22. Ⓐ Ⓑ Ⓒ Ⓓ Ⓔ

(continued)

23. Ⓐ Ⓑ Ⓒ Ⓓ Ⓔ
24. Ⓐ Ⓑ Ⓒ Ⓓ Ⓔ
25. Ⓐ Ⓑ Ⓒ Ⓓ Ⓔ
26. Ⓐ Ⓑ Ⓒ Ⓓ Ⓔ
27. Ⓐ Ⓑ Ⓒ Ⓓ Ⓔ
28. Ⓐ Ⓑ Ⓒ Ⓓ Ⓔ
29. Ⓐ Ⓑ Ⓒ Ⓓ Ⓔ
30. Ⓐ Ⓑ Ⓒ Ⓓ Ⓔ
31. Ⓐ Ⓑ Ⓒ Ⓓ Ⓔ
32. Ⓐ Ⓑ Ⓒ Ⓓ Ⓔ
33. Ⓐ Ⓑ Ⓒ Ⓓ Ⓔ

34. Ⓐ Ⓑ Ⓒ Ⓓ Ⓔ
35. Ⓐ Ⓑ Ⓒ Ⓓ Ⓔ
36. Ⓐ Ⓑ Ⓒ Ⓓ Ⓔ
37. Ⓐ Ⓑ Ⓒ Ⓓ Ⓔ
38. Ⓐ Ⓑ Ⓒ Ⓓ Ⓔ
39. Ⓐ Ⓑ Ⓒ Ⓓ Ⓔ
40. Ⓐ Ⓑ Ⓒ Ⓓ Ⓔ
41. Ⓐ Ⓑ Ⓒ Ⓓ Ⓔ
42. Ⓐ Ⓑ Ⓒ Ⓓ Ⓔ
43. Ⓐ Ⓑ Ⓒ Ⓓ Ⓔ
44. Ⓐ Ⓑ Ⓒ Ⓓ Ⓔ

45. Ⓐ Ⓑ Ⓒ Ⓓ Ⓔ
46. Ⓐ Ⓑ Ⓒ Ⓓ Ⓔ
47. Ⓐ Ⓑ Ⓒ Ⓓ Ⓔ
48. Ⓐ Ⓑ Ⓒ Ⓓ Ⓔ
49. Ⓐ Ⓑ Ⓒ Ⓓ Ⓔ
50. Ⓐ Ⓑ Ⓒ Ⓓ Ⓔ
51. Ⓐ Ⓑ Ⓒ Ⓓ Ⓔ
52. Ⓐ Ⓑ Ⓒ Ⓓ Ⓔ
53. Ⓐ Ⓑ Ⓒ Ⓓ Ⓔ
54. Ⓐ Ⓑ Ⓒ Ⓓ Ⓔ
55. Ⓐ Ⓑ Ⓒ Ⓓ Ⓔ

56. Ⓐ Ⓑ Ⓒ Ⓓ Ⓔ
57. Ⓐ Ⓑ Ⓒ Ⓓ Ⓔ
58. Ⓐ Ⓑ Ⓒ Ⓓ Ⓔ
59. Ⓐ Ⓑ Ⓒ Ⓓ Ⓔ
60. Ⓐ Ⓑ Ⓒ Ⓓ Ⓔ
61. Ⓐ Ⓑ Ⓒ Ⓓ Ⓔ
62. Ⓐ Ⓑ Ⓒ Ⓓ Ⓔ
63. Ⓐ Ⓑ Ⓒ Ⓓ Ⓔ
64. Ⓐ Ⓑ Ⓒ Ⓓ Ⓔ
65. Ⓐ Ⓑ Ⓒ Ⓓ Ⓔ
66. Ⓐ Ⓑ Ⓒ Ⓓ Ⓔ

RMA Simulation Test: Post-Test

Name _____   **Date** _____

Last   First   Middle

DIRECTIONS:

1. Fill in only one circle using pencil representing your answer for each question.
2. Keeping your marks inside the circle, blacken the circle completely.
3. Completely erase any answer you wish to change, and make no stray marks.

Correct: Ⓐ ● Ⓒ Ⓓ Ⓔ   Wrong: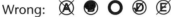

GENERAL

1. Ⓐ Ⓑ Ⓒ Ⓓ Ⓔ
2. Ⓐ Ⓑ Ⓒ Ⓓ Ⓔ
3. Ⓐ Ⓑ Ⓒ Ⓓ Ⓔ
4. Ⓐ Ⓑ Ⓒ Ⓓ Ⓔ
5. Ⓐ Ⓑ Ⓒ Ⓓ Ⓔ
6. Ⓐ Ⓑ Ⓒ Ⓓ Ⓔ
7. Ⓐ Ⓑ Ⓒ Ⓓ Ⓔ
8. Ⓐ Ⓑ Ⓒ Ⓓ Ⓔ
9. Ⓐ Ⓑ Ⓒ Ⓓ Ⓔ
10. Ⓐ Ⓑ Ⓒ Ⓓ Ⓔ
11. Ⓐ Ⓑ Ⓒ Ⓓ Ⓔ
12. Ⓐ Ⓑ Ⓒ Ⓓ Ⓔ
13. Ⓐ Ⓑ Ⓒ Ⓓ Ⓔ
14. Ⓐ Ⓑ Ⓒ Ⓓ Ⓔ
15. Ⓐ Ⓑ Ⓒ Ⓓ Ⓔ
16. Ⓐ Ⓑ Ⓒ Ⓓ Ⓔ
17. Ⓐ Ⓑ Ⓒ Ⓓ Ⓔ
18. Ⓐ Ⓑ Ⓒ Ⓓ Ⓔ
19. Ⓐ Ⓑ Ⓒ Ⓓ Ⓔ
20. Ⓐ Ⓑ Ⓒ Ⓓ Ⓔ
21. Ⓐ Ⓑ Ⓒ Ⓓ Ⓔ
22. Ⓐ Ⓑ Ⓒ Ⓓ Ⓔ
23. Ⓐ Ⓑ Ⓒ Ⓓ Ⓔ
24. Ⓐ Ⓑ Ⓒ Ⓓ Ⓔ
25. Ⓐ Ⓑ Ⓒ Ⓓ Ⓔ
26. Ⓐ Ⓑ Ⓒ Ⓓ Ⓔ
27. Ⓐ Ⓑ Ⓒ Ⓓ Ⓔ
28. Ⓐ Ⓑ Ⓒ Ⓓ Ⓔ
29. Ⓐ Ⓑ Ⓒ Ⓓ Ⓔ
30. Ⓐ Ⓑ Ⓒ Ⓓ Ⓔ
31. Ⓐ Ⓑ Ⓒ Ⓓ Ⓔ
32. Ⓐ Ⓑ Ⓒ Ⓓ Ⓔ
33. Ⓐ Ⓑ Ⓒ Ⓓ Ⓔ
34. Ⓐ Ⓑ Ⓒ Ⓓ Ⓔ
35. Ⓐ Ⓑ Ⓒ Ⓓ Ⓔ
36. Ⓐ Ⓑ Ⓒ Ⓓ Ⓔ
37. Ⓐ Ⓑ Ⓒ Ⓓ Ⓔ
38. Ⓐ Ⓑ Ⓒ Ⓓ Ⓔ
39. Ⓐ Ⓑ Ⓒ Ⓓ Ⓔ

40. Ⓐ Ⓑ Ⓒ Ⓓ Ⓔ
41. Ⓐ Ⓑ Ⓒ Ⓓ Ⓔ
42. Ⓐ Ⓑ Ⓒ Ⓓ Ⓔ
43. Ⓐ Ⓑ Ⓒ Ⓓ Ⓔ
44. Ⓐ Ⓑ Ⓒ Ⓓ Ⓔ
45. Ⓐ Ⓑ Ⓒ Ⓓ Ⓔ
46. Ⓐ Ⓑ Ⓒ Ⓓ Ⓔ
47. Ⓐ Ⓑ Ⓒ Ⓓ Ⓔ
48. Ⓐ Ⓑ Ⓒ Ⓓ Ⓔ
49. Ⓐ Ⓑ Ⓒ Ⓓ Ⓔ
50. Ⓐ Ⓑ Ⓒ Ⓓ Ⓔ
51. Ⓐ Ⓑ Ⓒ Ⓓ Ⓔ
52. Ⓐ Ⓑ Ⓒ Ⓓ Ⓔ
53. Ⓐ Ⓑ Ⓒ Ⓓ Ⓔ
54. Ⓐ Ⓑ Ⓒ Ⓓ Ⓔ
55. Ⓐ Ⓑ Ⓒ Ⓓ Ⓔ
56. Ⓐ Ⓑ Ⓒ Ⓓ Ⓔ
57. Ⓐ Ⓑ Ⓒ Ⓓ Ⓔ
58. Ⓐ Ⓑ Ⓒ Ⓓ Ⓔ
59. Ⓐ Ⓑ Ⓒ Ⓓ Ⓔ
60. Ⓐ Ⓑ Ⓒ Ⓓ Ⓔ
61. Ⓐ Ⓑ Ⓒ Ⓓ Ⓔ
62. Ⓐ Ⓑ Ⓒ Ⓓ Ⓔ
63. Ⓐ Ⓑ Ⓒ Ⓓ Ⓔ
64. Ⓐ Ⓑ Ⓒ Ⓓ Ⓔ
65. Ⓐ Ⓑ Ⓒ Ⓓ Ⓔ
66. Ⓐ Ⓑ Ⓒ Ⓓ Ⓔ

ADMINISTRATIVE

1. Ⓐ Ⓑ Ⓒ Ⓓ Ⓔ
2. Ⓐ Ⓑ Ⓒ Ⓓ Ⓔ
3. Ⓐ Ⓑ Ⓒ Ⓓ Ⓔ
4. Ⓐ Ⓑ Ⓒ Ⓓ Ⓔ
5. Ⓐ Ⓑ Ⓒ Ⓓ Ⓔ
6. Ⓐ Ⓑ Ⓒ Ⓓ Ⓔ
7. Ⓐ Ⓑ Ⓒ Ⓓ Ⓔ
8. Ⓐ Ⓑ Ⓒ Ⓓ Ⓔ
9. Ⓐ Ⓑ Ⓒ Ⓓ Ⓔ
10. Ⓐ Ⓑ Ⓒ Ⓓ Ⓔ
11. Ⓐ Ⓑ Ⓒ Ⓓ Ⓔ

12. Ⓐ Ⓑ Ⓒ Ⓓ Ⓔ
13. Ⓐ Ⓑ Ⓒ Ⓓ Ⓔ
14. Ⓐ Ⓑ Ⓒ Ⓓ Ⓔ
15. Ⓐ Ⓑ Ⓒ Ⓓ Ⓔ
16. Ⓐ Ⓑ Ⓒ Ⓓ Ⓔ
17. Ⓐ Ⓑ Ⓒ Ⓓ Ⓔ
18. Ⓐ Ⓑ Ⓒ Ⓓ Ⓔ
19. Ⓐ Ⓑ Ⓒ Ⓓ Ⓔ
20. Ⓐ Ⓑ Ⓒ Ⓓ Ⓔ
21. Ⓐ Ⓑ Ⓒ Ⓓ Ⓔ
22. Ⓐ Ⓑ Ⓒ Ⓓ Ⓔ
23. Ⓐ Ⓑ Ⓒ Ⓓ Ⓔ
24. Ⓐ Ⓑ Ⓒ Ⓓ Ⓔ
25. Ⓐ Ⓑ Ⓒ Ⓓ Ⓔ
26. Ⓐ Ⓑ Ⓒ Ⓓ Ⓔ
27. Ⓐ Ⓑ Ⓒ Ⓓ Ⓔ
28. Ⓐ Ⓑ Ⓒ Ⓓ Ⓔ
29. Ⓐ Ⓑ Ⓒ Ⓓ Ⓔ
30. Ⓐ Ⓑ Ⓒ Ⓓ Ⓔ
31. Ⓐ Ⓑ Ⓒ Ⓓ Ⓔ
32. Ⓐ Ⓑ Ⓒ Ⓓ Ⓔ
33. Ⓐ Ⓑ Ⓒ Ⓓ Ⓔ
34. Ⓐ Ⓑ Ⓒ Ⓓ Ⓔ
35. Ⓐ Ⓑ Ⓒ Ⓓ Ⓔ
36. Ⓐ Ⓑ Ⓒ Ⓓ Ⓔ
37. Ⓐ Ⓑ Ⓒ Ⓓ Ⓔ
38. Ⓐ Ⓑ Ⓒ Ⓓ Ⓔ
39. Ⓐ Ⓑ Ⓒ Ⓓ Ⓔ
40. Ⓐ Ⓑ Ⓒ Ⓓ Ⓔ
41. Ⓐ Ⓑ Ⓒ Ⓓ Ⓔ
42. Ⓐ Ⓑ Ⓒ Ⓓ Ⓔ
43. Ⓐ Ⓑ Ⓒ Ⓓ Ⓔ
44. Ⓐ Ⓑ Ⓒ Ⓓ Ⓔ
45. Ⓐ Ⓑ Ⓒ Ⓓ Ⓔ
46. Ⓐ Ⓑ Ⓒ Ⓓ Ⓔ
47. Ⓐ Ⓑ Ⓒ Ⓓ Ⓔ
48. Ⓐ Ⓑ Ⓒ Ⓓ Ⓔ
49. Ⓐ Ⓑ Ⓒ Ⓓ Ⓔ
50. Ⓐ Ⓑ Ⓒ Ⓓ Ⓔ
51. Ⓐ Ⓑ Ⓒ Ⓓ Ⓔ
52. Ⓐ Ⓑ Ⓒ Ⓓ Ⓔ

53. Ⓐ Ⓑ Ⓒ Ⓓ Ⓔ
54. Ⓐ Ⓑ Ⓒ Ⓓ Ⓔ
55. Ⓐ Ⓑ Ⓒ Ⓓ Ⓔ
56. Ⓐ Ⓑ Ⓒ Ⓓ Ⓔ
57. Ⓐ Ⓑ Ⓒ Ⓓ Ⓔ
58. Ⓐ Ⓑ Ⓒ Ⓓ Ⓔ
59. Ⓐ Ⓑ Ⓒ Ⓓ Ⓔ
60. Ⓐ Ⓑ Ⓒ Ⓓ Ⓔ
61. Ⓐ Ⓑ Ⓒ Ⓓ Ⓔ
62. Ⓐ Ⓑ Ⓒ Ⓓ Ⓔ
63. Ⓐ Ⓑ Ⓒ Ⓓ Ⓔ
64. Ⓐ Ⓑ Ⓒ Ⓓ Ⓔ
65. Ⓐ Ⓑ Ⓒ Ⓓ Ⓔ
66. Ⓐ Ⓑ Ⓒ Ⓓ Ⓔ
67. Ⓐ Ⓑ Ⓒ Ⓓ Ⓔ

CLINICAL

1. Ⓐ Ⓑ Ⓒ Ⓓ Ⓔ
2. Ⓐ Ⓑ Ⓒ Ⓓ Ⓔ
3. Ⓐ Ⓑ Ⓒ Ⓓ Ⓔ
4. Ⓐ Ⓑ Ⓒ Ⓓ Ⓔ
5. Ⓐ Ⓑ Ⓒ Ⓓ Ⓔ
6. Ⓐ Ⓑ Ⓒ Ⓓ Ⓔ
7. Ⓐ Ⓑ Ⓒ Ⓓ Ⓔ
8. Ⓐ Ⓑ Ⓒ Ⓓ Ⓔ
9. Ⓐ Ⓑ Ⓒ Ⓓ Ⓔ
10. Ⓐ Ⓑ Ⓒ Ⓓ Ⓔ
11. Ⓐ Ⓑ Ⓒ Ⓓ Ⓔ
12. Ⓐ Ⓑ Ⓒ Ⓓ Ⓔ
13. Ⓐ Ⓑ Ⓒ Ⓓ Ⓔ
14. Ⓐ Ⓑ Ⓒ Ⓓ Ⓔ
15. Ⓐ Ⓑ Ⓒ Ⓓ Ⓔ
16. Ⓐ Ⓑ Ⓒ Ⓓ Ⓔ
17. Ⓐ Ⓑ Ⓒ Ⓓ Ⓔ
18. Ⓐ Ⓑ Ⓒ Ⓓ Ⓔ
19. Ⓐ Ⓑ Ⓒ Ⓓ Ⓔ
20. Ⓐ Ⓑ Ⓒ Ⓓ Ⓔ
21. Ⓐ Ⓑ Ⓒ Ⓓ Ⓔ

(continued)

22. Ⓐ Ⓑ Ⓒ Ⓓ Ⓔ   34. Ⓐ Ⓑ Ⓒ Ⓓ Ⓔ   46. Ⓐ Ⓑ Ⓒ Ⓓ Ⓔ   58. Ⓐ Ⓑ Ⓒ Ⓓ Ⓔ
23. Ⓐ Ⓑ Ⓒ Ⓓ Ⓔ   35. Ⓐ Ⓑ Ⓒ Ⓓ Ⓔ   47. Ⓐ Ⓑ Ⓒ Ⓓ Ⓔ   59. Ⓐ Ⓑ Ⓒ Ⓓ Ⓔ
24. Ⓐ Ⓑ Ⓒ Ⓓ Ⓔ   36. Ⓐ Ⓑ Ⓒ Ⓓ Ⓔ   48. Ⓐ Ⓑ Ⓒ Ⓓ Ⓔ   60. Ⓐ Ⓑ Ⓒ Ⓓ Ⓔ
25. Ⓐ Ⓑ Ⓒ Ⓓ Ⓔ   37. Ⓐ Ⓑ Ⓒ Ⓓ Ⓔ   49. Ⓐ Ⓑ Ⓒ Ⓓ Ⓔ   61. Ⓐ Ⓑ Ⓒ Ⓓ Ⓔ
26. Ⓐ Ⓑ Ⓒ Ⓓ Ⓔ   38. Ⓐ Ⓑ Ⓒ Ⓓ Ⓔ   50. Ⓐ Ⓑ Ⓒ Ⓓ Ⓔ   62. Ⓐ Ⓑ Ⓒ Ⓓ Ⓔ
27. Ⓐ Ⓑ Ⓒ Ⓓ Ⓔ   39. Ⓐ Ⓑ Ⓒ Ⓓ Ⓔ   51. Ⓐ Ⓑ Ⓒ Ⓓ Ⓔ   63. Ⓐ Ⓑ Ⓒ Ⓓ Ⓔ
28. Ⓐ Ⓑ Ⓒ Ⓓ Ⓔ   40. Ⓐ Ⓑ Ⓒ Ⓓ Ⓔ   52. Ⓐ Ⓑ Ⓒ Ⓓ Ⓔ   64. Ⓐ Ⓑ Ⓒ Ⓓ Ⓔ
29. Ⓐ Ⓑ Ⓒ Ⓓ Ⓔ   41. Ⓐ Ⓑ Ⓒ Ⓓ Ⓔ   53. Ⓐ Ⓑ Ⓒ Ⓓ Ⓔ   65. Ⓐ Ⓑ Ⓒ Ⓓ Ⓔ
30. Ⓐ Ⓑ Ⓒ Ⓓ Ⓔ   42. Ⓐ Ⓑ Ⓒ Ⓓ Ⓔ   54. Ⓐ Ⓑ Ⓒ Ⓓ Ⓔ   66. Ⓐ Ⓑ Ⓒ Ⓓ Ⓔ
31. Ⓐ Ⓑ Ⓒ Ⓓ Ⓔ   43. Ⓐ Ⓑ Ⓒ Ⓓ Ⓔ   55. Ⓐ Ⓑ Ⓒ Ⓓ Ⓔ   67. Ⓐ Ⓑ Ⓒ Ⓓ Ⓔ
32. Ⓐ Ⓑ Ⓒ Ⓓ Ⓔ   44. Ⓐ Ⓑ Ⓒ Ⓓ Ⓔ   56. Ⓐ Ⓑ Ⓒ Ⓓ Ⓔ
33. Ⓐ Ⓑ Ⓒ Ⓓ Ⓔ   45. Ⓐ Ⓑ Ⓒ Ⓓ Ⓔ   57. Ⓐ Ⓑ Ⓒ Ⓓ Ⓔ

CMAS SIMULATION TEST: POST-TEST

Name _____   **Date** _____

Last   First   Middle

DIRECTIONS:

1. Fill in only one circle using pencil representing your answer for each question.
2. Keeping your marks inside the circle, blacken the circle completely.
3. Completely erase any answer you wish to change, and make no stray marks.

Correct: Ⓐ ● Ⓒ Ⓓ Ⓔ   Wrong: Ⓐ̶ ◍ ○ Ⓓ̶ Ⓔ̶

1. Ⓐ Ⓑ Ⓒ Ⓓ Ⓔ	42. Ⓐ Ⓑ Ⓒ Ⓓ Ⓔ	83. Ⓐ Ⓑ Ⓒ Ⓓ Ⓔ	124. Ⓐ Ⓑ Ⓒ Ⓓ Ⓔ
2. Ⓐ Ⓑ Ⓒ Ⓓ Ⓔ	43. Ⓐ Ⓑ Ⓒ Ⓓ Ⓔ	84. Ⓐ Ⓑ Ⓒ Ⓓ Ⓔ	125. Ⓐ Ⓑ Ⓒ Ⓓ Ⓔ
3. Ⓐ Ⓑ Ⓒ Ⓓ Ⓔ	44. Ⓐ Ⓑ Ⓒ Ⓓ Ⓔ	85. Ⓐ Ⓑ Ⓒ Ⓓ Ⓔ	126. Ⓐ Ⓑ Ⓒ Ⓓ Ⓔ
4. Ⓐ Ⓑ Ⓒ Ⓓ Ⓔ	45. Ⓐ Ⓑ Ⓒ Ⓓ Ⓔ	86. Ⓐ Ⓑ Ⓒ Ⓓ Ⓔ	127. Ⓐ Ⓑ Ⓒ Ⓓ Ⓔ
5. Ⓐ Ⓑ Ⓒ Ⓓ Ⓔ	46. Ⓐ Ⓑ Ⓒ Ⓓ Ⓔ	87. Ⓐ Ⓑ Ⓒ Ⓓ Ⓔ	128. Ⓐ Ⓑ Ⓒ Ⓓ Ⓔ
6. Ⓐ Ⓑ Ⓒ Ⓓ Ⓔ	47. Ⓐ Ⓑ Ⓒ Ⓓ Ⓔ	88. Ⓐ Ⓑ Ⓒ Ⓓ Ⓔ	129. Ⓐ Ⓑ Ⓒ Ⓓ Ⓔ
7. Ⓐ Ⓑ Ⓒ Ⓓ Ⓔ	48. Ⓐ Ⓑ Ⓒ Ⓓ Ⓔ	89. Ⓐ Ⓑ Ⓒ Ⓓ Ⓔ	130. Ⓐ Ⓑ Ⓒ Ⓓ Ⓔ
8. Ⓐ Ⓑ Ⓒ Ⓓ Ⓔ	49. Ⓐ Ⓑ Ⓒ Ⓓ Ⓔ	90. Ⓐ Ⓑ Ⓒ Ⓓ Ⓔ	131. Ⓐ Ⓑ Ⓒ Ⓓ Ⓔ
9. Ⓐ Ⓑ Ⓒ Ⓓ Ⓔ	50. Ⓐ Ⓑ Ⓒ Ⓓ Ⓔ	91. Ⓐ Ⓑ Ⓒ Ⓓ Ⓔ	132. Ⓐ Ⓑ Ⓒ Ⓓ Ⓔ
10. Ⓐ Ⓑ Ⓒ Ⓓ Ⓔ	51. Ⓐ Ⓑ Ⓒ Ⓓ Ⓔ	92. Ⓐ Ⓑ Ⓒ Ⓓ Ⓔ	133. Ⓐ Ⓑ Ⓒ Ⓓ Ⓔ
11. Ⓐ Ⓑ Ⓒ Ⓓ Ⓔ	52. Ⓐ Ⓑ Ⓒ Ⓓ Ⓔ	93. Ⓐ Ⓑ Ⓒ Ⓓ Ⓔ	134. Ⓐ Ⓑ Ⓒ Ⓓ Ⓔ
12. Ⓐ Ⓑ Ⓒ Ⓓ Ⓔ	53. Ⓐ Ⓑ Ⓒ Ⓓ Ⓔ	94. Ⓐ Ⓑ Ⓒ Ⓓ Ⓔ	135. Ⓐ Ⓑ Ⓒ Ⓓ Ⓔ
13. Ⓐ Ⓑ Ⓒ Ⓓ Ⓔ	54. Ⓐ Ⓑ Ⓒ Ⓓ Ⓔ	95. Ⓐ Ⓑ Ⓒ Ⓓ Ⓔ	136. Ⓐ Ⓑ Ⓒ Ⓓ Ⓔ
14. Ⓐ Ⓑ Ⓒ Ⓓ Ⓔ	55. Ⓐ Ⓑ Ⓒ Ⓓ Ⓔ	96. Ⓐ Ⓑ Ⓒ Ⓓ Ⓔ	137. Ⓐ Ⓑ Ⓒ Ⓓ Ⓔ
15. Ⓐ Ⓑ Ⓒ Ⓓ Ⓔ	56. Ⓐ Ⓑ Ⓒ Ⓓ Ⓔ	97. Ⓐ Ⓑ Ⓒ Ⓓ Ⓔ	138. Ⓐ Ⓑ Ⓒ Ⓓ Ⓔ
16. Ⓐ Ⓑ Ⓒ Ⓓ Ⓔ	57. Ⓐ Ⓑ Ⓒ Ⓓ Ⓔ	98. Ⓐ Ⓑ Ⓒ Ⓓ Ⓔ	139. Ⓐ Ⓑ Ⓒ Ⓓ Ⓔ
17. Ⓐ Ⓑ Ⓒ Ⓓ Ⓔ	58. Ⓐ Ⓑ Ⓒ Ⓓ Ⓔ	99. Ⓐ Ⓑ Ⓒ Ⓓ Ⓔ	140. Ⓐ Ⓑ Ⓒ Ⓓ Ⓔ
18. Ⓐ Ⓑ Ⓒ Ⓓ Ⓔ	59. Ⓐ Ⓑ Ⓒ Ⓓ Ⓔ	100. Ⓐ Ⓑ Ⓒ Ⓓ Ⓔ	141. Ⓐ Ⓑ Ⓒ Ⓓ Ⓔ
19. Ⓐ Ⓑ Ⓒ Ⓓ Ⓔ	60. Ⓐ Ⓑ Ⓒ Ⓓ Ⓔ	101. Ⓐ Ⓑ Ⓒ Ⓓ Ⓔ	142. Ⓐ Ⓑ Ⓒ Ⓓ Ⓔ
20. Ⓐ Ⓑ Ⓒ Ⓓ Ⓔ	61. Ⓐ Ⓑ Ⓒ Ⓓ Ⓔ	102. Ⓐ Ⓑ Ⓒ Ⓓ Ⓔ	143. Ⓐ Ⓑ Ⓒ Ⓓ Ⓔ
21. Ⓐ Ⓑ Ⓒ Ⓓ Ⓔ	62. Ⓐ Ⓑ Ⓒ Ⓓ Ⓔ	103. Ⓐ Ⓑ Ⓒ Ⓓ Ⓔ	144. Ⓐ Ⓑ Ⓒ Ⓓ Ⓔ
22. Ⓐ Ⓑ Ⓒ Ⓓ Ⓔ	63. Ⓐ Ⓑ Ⓒ Ⓓ Ⓔ	104. Ⓐ Ⓑ Ⓒ Ⓓ Ⓔ	145. Ⓐ Ⓑ Ⓒ Ⓓ Ⓔ
23. Ⓐ Ⓑ Ⓒ Ⓓ Ⓔ	64. Ⓐ Ⓑ Ⓒ Ⓓ Ⓔ	105. Ⓐ Ⓑ Ⓒ Ⓓ Ⓔ	146. Ⓐ Ⓑ Ⓒ Ⓓ Ⓔ
24. Ⓐ Ⓑ Ⓒ Ⓓ Ⓔ	65. Ⓐ Ⓑ Ⓒ Ⓓ Ⓔ	106. Ⓐ Ⓑ Ⓒ Ⓓ Ⓔ	147. Ⓐ Ⓑ Ⓒ Ⓓ Ⓔ
25. Ⓐ Ⓑ Ⓒ Ⓓ Ⓔ	66. Ⓐ Ⓑ Ⓒ Ⓓ Ⓔ	107. Ⓐ Ⓑ Ⓒ Ⓓ Ⓔ	148. Ⓐ Ⓑ Ⓒ Ⓓ Ⓔ
26. Ⓐ Ⓑ Ⓒ Ⓓ Ⓔ	67. Ⓐ Ⓑ Ⓒ Ⓓ Ⓔ	108. Ⓐ Ⓑ Ⓒ Ⓓ Ⓔ	149. Ⓐ Ⓑ Ⓒ Ⓓ Ⓔ
27. Ⓐ Ⓑ Ⓒ Ⓓ Ⓔ	68. Ⓐ Ⓑ Ⓒ Ⓓ Ⓔ	109. Ⓐ Ⓑ Ⓒ Ⓓ Ⓔ	150. Ⓐ Ⓑ Ⓒ Ⓓ Ⓔ
28. Ⓐ Ⓑ Ⓒ Ⓓ Ⓔ	69. Ⓐ Ⓑ Ⓒ Ⓓ Ⓔ	110. Ⓐ Ⓑ Ⓒ Ⓓ Ⓔ	151. Ⓐ Ⓑ Ⓒ Ⓓ Ⓔ
29. Ⓐ Ⓑ Ⓒ Ⓓ Ⓔ	70. Ⓐ Ⓑ Ⓒ Ⓓ Ⓔ	111. Ⓐ Ⓑ Ⓒ Ⓓ Ⓔ	152. Ⓐ Ⓑ Ⓒ Ⓓ Ⓔ
30. Ⓐ Ⓑ Ⓒ Ⓓ Ⓔ	71. Ⓐ Ⓑ Ⓒ Ⓓ Ⓔ	112. Ⓐ Ⓑ Ⓒ Ⓓ Ⓔ	153. Ⓐ Ⓑ Ⓒ Ⓓ Ⓔ
31. Ⓐ Ⓑ Ⓒ Ⓓ Ⓔ	72. Ⓐ Ⓑ Ⓒ Ⓓ Ⓔ	113. Ⓐ Ⓑ Ⓒ Ⓓ Ⓔ	154. Ⓐ Ⓑ Ⓒ Ⓓ Ⓔ
32. Ⓐ Ⓑ Ⓒ Ⓓ Ⓔ	73. Ⓐ Ⓑ Ⓒ Ⓓ Ⓔ	114. Ⓐ Ⓑ Ⓒ Ⓓ Ⓔ	155. Ⓐ Ⓑ Ⓒ Ⓓ Ⓔ
33. Ⓐ Ⓑ Ⓒ Ⓓ Ⓔ	74. Ⓐ Ⓑ Ⓒ Ⓓ Ⓔ	115. Ⓐ Ⓑ Ⓒ Ⓓ Ⓔ	156. Ⓐ Ⓑ Ⓒ Ⓓ Ⓔ
34. Ⓐ Ⓑ Ⓒ Ⓓ Ⓔ	75. Ⓐ Ⓑ Ⓒ Ⓓ Ⓔ	116. Ⓐ Ⓑ Ⓒ Ⓓ Ⓔ	157. Ⓐ Ⓑ Ⓒ Ⓓ Ⓔ
35. Ⓐ Ⓑ Ⓒ Ⓓ Ⓔ	76. Ⓐ Ⓑ Ⓒ Ⓓ Ⓔ	117. Ⓐ Ⓑ Ⓒ Ⓓ Ⓔ	158. Ⓐ Ⓑ Ⓒ Ⓓ Ⓔ
36. Ⓐ Ⓑ Ⓒ Ⓓ Ⓔ	77. Ⓐ Ⓑ Ⓒ Ⓓ Ⓔ	118. Ⓐ Ⓑ Ⓒ Ⓓ Ⓔ	159. Ⓐ Ⓑ Ⓒ Ⓓ Ⓔ
37. Ⓐ Ⓑ Ⓒ Ⓓ Ⓔ	78. Ⓐ Ⓑ Ⓒ Ⓓ Ⓔ	119. Ⓐ Ⓑ Ⓒ Ⓓ Ⓔ	160. Ⓐ Ⓑ Ⓒ Ⓓ Ⓔ
38. Ⓐ Ⓑ Ⓒ Ⓓ Ⓔ	79. Ⓐ Ⓑ Ⓒ Ⓓ Ⓔ	120. Ⓐ Ⓑ Ⓒ Ⓓ Ⓔ	161. Ⓐ Ⓑ Ⓒ Ⓓ Ⓔ
39. Ⓐ Ⓑ Ⓒ Ⓓ Ⓔ	80. Ⓐ Ⓑ Ⓒ Ⓓ Ⓔ	121. Ⓐ Ⓑ Ⓒ Ⓓ Ⓔ	162. Ⓐ Ⓑ Ⓒ Ⓓ Ⓔ
40. Ⓐ Ⓑ Ⓒ Ⓓ Ⓔ	81. Ⓐ Ⓑ Ⓒ Ⓓ Ⓔ	122. Ⓐ Ⓑ Ⓒ Ⓓ Ⓔ	
41. Ⓐ Ⓑ Ⓒ Ⓓ Ⓔ	82. Ⓐ Ⓑ Ⓒ Ⓓ Ⓔ	123. Ⓐ Ⓑ Ⓒ Ⓓ Ⓔ	*(continued)*

163. Ⓐ Ⓑ Ⓒ Ⓓ Ⓔ
164. Ⓐ Ⓑ Ⓒ Ⓓ Ⓔ
165. Ⓐ Ⓑ Ⓒ Ⓓ Ⓔ
166. Ⓐ Ⓑ Ⓒ Ⓓ Ⓔ
167. Ⓐ Ⓑ Ⓒ Ⓓ Ⓔ
168. Ⓐ Ⓑ Ⓒ Ⓓ Ⓔ
169. Ⓐ Ⓑ Ⓒ Ⓓ Ⓔ
170. Ⓐ Ⓑ Ⓒ Ⓓ Ⓔ
171. Ⓐ Ⓑ Ⓒ Ⓓ Ⓔ
172. Ⓐ Ⓑ Ⓒ Ⓓ Ⓔ

173. Ⓐ Ⓑ Ⓒ Ⓓ Ⓔ
174. Ⓐ Ⓑ Ⓒ Ⓓ Ⓔ
175. Ⓐ Ⓑ Ⓒ Ⓓ Ⓔ
176. Ⓐ Ⓑ Ⓒ Ⓓ Ⓔ
177. Ⓐ Ⓑ Ⓒ Ⓓ Ⓔ
178. Ⓐ Ⓑ Ⓒ Ⓓ Ⓔ
179. Ⓐ Ⓑ Ⓒ Ⓓ Ⓔ
180. Ⓐ Ⓑ Ⓒ Ⓓ Ⓔ
181. Ⓐ Ⓑ Ⓒ Ⓓ Ⓔ
182. Ⓐ Ⓑ Ⓒ Ⓓ Ⓔ

183. Ⓐ Ⓑ Ⓒ Ⓓ Ⓔ
184. Ⓐ Ⓑ Ⓒ Ⓓ Ⓔ
185. Ⓐ Ⓑ Ⓒ Ⓓ Ⓔ
186. Ⓐ Ⓑ Ⓒ Ⓓ Ⓔ
187. Ⓐ Ⓑ Ⓒ Ⓓ Ⓔ
188. Ⓐ Ⓑ Ⓒ Ⓓ Ⓔ
189. Ⓐ Ⓑ Ⓒ Ⓓ Ⓔ
190. Ⓐ Ⓑ Ⓒ Ⓓ Ⓔ
191. Ⓐ Ⓑ Ⓒ Ⓓ Ⓔ
192. Ⓐ Ⓑ Ⓒ Ⓓ Ⓔ

193. Ⓐ Ⓑ Ⓒ Ⓓ Ⓔ
194. Ⓐ Ⓑ Ⓒ Ⓓ Ⓔ
195. Ⓐ Ⓑ Ⓒ Ⓓ Ⓔ
196. Ⓐ Ⓑ Ⓒ Ⓓ Ⓔ
197. Ⓐ Ⓑ Ⓒ Ⓓ Ⓔ
198. Ⓐ Ⓑ Ⓒ Ⓓ Ⓔ
199. Ⓐ Ⓑ Ⓒ Ⓓ Ⓔ
200. Ⓐ Ⓑ Ⓒ Ⓓ Ⓔ

References

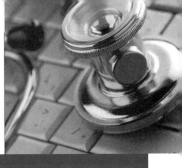

About Test Anxiety. (1987). A Scriptographic Booklet. South Deerfield, MA: Channing L. Bete Co.

Alton, T. (1986). *The First Aid Book*, 2nd ed. Upper Saddle River, NJ: Prentice-Hall.

Al-Ashkar, F., et al. (2003). "Interpreting Pulmonary Function Tests: Recognize the Pattern, and the Diagnosis Will Follow." *Cleveland Clinic Journal of Medicine*. 70:10. (pp. 866–881).

American Red Cross (2006). First Aid/CPR/AED for Schools and the Community, 3rd ed. The American National Red Cross.

Anderson, P. & Pendleton, A. *The Dental Assistant*, 7th ed. Clifton Park, NY: Delmar Cengage Learning.

Anderson, S. (1992). *Computer Literacy for Health Care Professionals*. Clifton Park, NY: Delmar Cengage Learning.

Andress, A. (1996). *Manual of Medical Office Management*. Philadelphia, PA: W. B. Saunders.

Annas, G., et al. (1990). *American Health Law*. Boston, MA: Little, Brown, & Company.

Asperheim, M. (2002). *Pharmacology: An Introductory Text*, 9th ed. Philadelphia, PA: W. B. Saunders.

Becklin, K. (2002). *Medical Office Procedures*, 5th ed. Chicago, IL: McGraw-Hill.

Birmingham, J. (2000). *Medical Terminology: A Self Learning Text*, 3rd ed. St. Louis, MO: Mosby.

Blanchard, K. & Peale, N. (1988). *The Power of Ethical Management*. New York, NY: Fawcett Crest.

Bonewit-West, K. (2004). *Clinical Procedures for Medical Assistants*, 6th ed. Philadelphia, PA: W. B. Saunders.

Brody, M. & Pachter, B. (1994). *Business Etiquette*. Chicago, IL: McGraw-Hill.

Burton, G. (2004). *Microbiology for the Health Sciences*, 7th ed. Philadelphia, PA: Lippincott Williams & Wilkins.

Carlton, R. & Adler, A. (2006). *Principles of Radiographic Imaging*, 4th ed. Clifton Park, NY: Delmar Cengage Learning.

Chabner, D. (2001). *The Language of Medicine*, 6th ed. Philadelphia, PA: W. B. Saunders.

Cody, J. (1991). "Measuring Your Study Skills." *The Professional Medical Assistant*, May/June, 24:3. (pp. 24–29).

Cody, J. (1992). "Preparing for the CDA Exam: Part 1." *The Dental Assistant Journal*, Winter, 61:1. (pp. 5–8).

Cody, J. (1992). "Preparing for the CDA Exam: Part 2." *The Dental Assistant Journal*, Spring, 61:2. (pp. 12–14).

Cohen, B. (1999). *Medical Terminology*, 3rd ed. Philadelphia, PA: J. B. Lippincott.

Collins & Davies. (1996). *Modern Medical Language*. Clifton Park, NY: Delmar Cengage Learning.

Corcoran, M. (1989). "Developing a Certification Study Group." *The Professional Medical Assistant*, S/O. (pp. 25f).

Davis, D. (1992). *How to Quickly and Accurately Master ECG Interpretation*. Philadelphia, PA: J. B. Lippincott.

DavisJones, B. (2008). *Comprehensive Medical Terminology*, 3rd ed. Clifton Park, NY: Delmar Cengage Learning.

Dean, T. & Whitlock, S. *The Clinical Lab Manual Series: Clinical Chemistry*. Clifton Park, NY: Delmar Cengage Learning.

Delmar's Anatomy and Physiology CD-ROM. (2002). Clifton Park, NY: Delmar Cengage Learning.

Dennerll, J. & Davis, P. (2010). *Medical Terminology: A Programmed Systems Approach*, 10th ed. Clifton Park, NY: Delmar Cengage Learning.

Edge, R. & Groves, J. (2006). *The Ethics of Health Care: A Guide for Clinical Practice*, 3rd ed. Clifton Park, NY: Delmar Cengage Learning.

Ehrlich, A. (2005). *Medical Terminology for Health Professions*, 5th ed. Clifton Park, NY: Delmar Cengage Learning.

Ehrlich, A. & Schroeder, C. (2009). *Introduction to Medical Terminology 2nd Ed*. Clifton Park, NY: Delmar Cengage Learning.

Ehrlich, A. & Schroeder, C. (2009). *Medical Terminology for Health Professions*, 6th ed. Clifton Park, NY: Delmar Cengage Learning.

Ellis, D. (2003). *Becoming a Master Student*, 10th ed. Rapid City, SD: College Survival, Inc.

Feinberg, J. (1982). "The Problem of Personhood." *Contemporary Issues in Bioethics*. Belmont, CA: Wadsworth.

Fischbach, F. (2004). *Laboratory and Diagnostic Tests*, 7th ed. Philadelphia, PA: J. B. Lippincott.

Fletcher, J. (1998). *Situation Ethics*. Louisville, KY: Westminster John Knox Press.

Flight, M. (2010). *Law, Liability, and Ethics*, 5th ed. Clifton Park, NY: Delmar Cengage Learning.

Flynn, J. & Whitlock, S. *The Clinical Lab Manual Series: Urinalysis*. Clifton Park, NY: Delmar Cengage Learning.

Fordney, M. (2004). *Insurance Handbook for the Medical Office*, 8th ed. Philadelphia, PA: W. B. Saunders.

Fordney, M., French, L. & Follis, J. (2008). *Administrative Medical Assisting*, 6th ed. Clifton Park, NY: Delmar Cengage Learning.

Frey, R. & Shearer-Cooper, L. (1996). *An Introduction to Nursing Assisting*: Building Language Skills. Clifton Park, NY: Delmar Cengage Learning.

Garner, B., editor in Chief. (2004). *Black's Law Dictionary*, 8th ed. St. Paul, MN: Thomson West.

Glylys, B. (1999). *Medical Terminology: Simplified*, 2nd ed. Philadelphia, PA: F. A. Davis.

Goldberger, et al. (1999). *Clinical Electrocardiography*, 6th ed. St. Louis, MO: Mosby.

Goodman, S. (1998). *Medical Cell Biology*, 2nd ed. Philadelphia, PA: Lippincott Williams & Wilkins.

Grad, F. (1990). *The Public Health Law Manual*, 2nd ed. Washington, DC: American Public Health Association, Washington.

Grover-Lakomia, L. & Fong, E. (1999). *Microbiology for Health Careers*, 6th ed. Clifton Park, NY: Delmar Cengage Learning.

Haddad, A. & Dougherty, C. (1991). "Whistle-Blowing in the O.R.: The Ethical Implications." *Today's O. R. Nurse*, March.

Hall, M. (2003). *Health Care Law and Ethics*, 6th ed. New York, NY: Aspen.

Hegner, B. & Caldwell, E. (2008). *Nursing Assistant*, 10th ed. Clifton Park, NY: Delmar Cengage Learning.

Heller, M. & Krebs, C. (2004). *Delmar Learning's Clinical Handbook for the Medical Office*, 2nd ed. Clifton Park, NY: Delmar Cengage Learning.

Hersey, P. & Blanchard, K. (2001). *Management of Organizational Behavior*, 8th ed. Englewood Cliffs, NJ: Prentice Hall.

Humphrey, D. (2004). *Medical Office Procedures*, 3rd ed., Clifton Park, NY: Delmar Cengage Learning.

Keir, L., et al. (2008). *Medical Assisting: Administrative and Clinical Competencies*, 6th ed. Clifton Park, NY: Delmar Cengage Learning.

Kelly, G. (1957). *Medico-moral Problems*. St. Louis, MO: St. Louis Catholic Hospital Association.

Kinn, S. et al. (2004). *The Medical Assistant: Administrative and Clinical*, 9th ed. Philadelphia, PA: W. B. Saunders.

Krager, D & Krager, C. (2005). *HIPAA for Medical Office Personnel*. Clifton Park, NY: Delmar Cengage Learning.

Lane, K. (1998). *Medications: A Guide for the Health Professions*, 2nd ed. Philadelphia, PA: F. A. Davis.

Leonard, P. (2003). *Quick and Easy Medical Terminology*, 4th ed. Philadelphia, PA: W. B. Saunders.

Leventhal, R. & Cheadle, F. (2002). *Medical Parasitology*, 5th ed. Philadelphia, PA: F. A. Davis.

Lewis, M. & Tamparo, C. (2002). *Medical Law, Ethics, and Bioethics in the Medical Office*, 5th ed. Philadelphia, PA: F. A. Davis.

Lindh, W., et al. (2010). *Delmar's Comprehensive Medical Assisting: Administrative and Clinical Competencies*, 3rd ed. Clifton Park, NY: Delmar Cengage Learning.

Linne, J. & Ringsrud, K. (2000). *Basic Techniques in Clinical Laboratory Science*, 4th ed. St. Louis, MO: Mosby.

Markell, E. et al. (2000). *Medical Parasitology*, 8th ed. Philadelphia, PA: W. B. Saunders.

McKeown, A. & Novak-Jandrey, M. (1991). *Human Resources Management in the Health Care Setting*. Dallas, TX: AHA.

Memmler, R., et al. (2000). *Structure and Function of the Human Body*, 7th ed. New York: Lippincott.

Miller, J. (2002). *Delmar's NCLEX-PN Review*. Clifton Park, NY: Delmar Cengage Learning.

Milliken, M. (2004). *Understanding Human Behavior*, 7th ed. Clifton Park, NY: Delmar Cengage Learning.

Miller-Keane. (2004). *Encyclopedia and Dictionary of Medicine, Nursing, and Allied Health*, 7th ed. PA: W. B. Saunders.

Monagle, J. & Thomasma, D. (2004). *Health Care Ethics*, 2nd ed. New York, NY: Aspen.

Office of Health and Safety (2000). *Office Safety*. Atlanta, GA: Centers for Disease Control and Prevention.

Passanisi, C. (2001). *Electrocardiography Essentials*. Clifton Park, NY: Delmar Cengage Learning.

Phyllis. (2000). *Administering Medication*, 4th ed. Chicago, IL: McGraw-Hill.

Pickar, G. (2008). *Dosage Calculations*, 8th ed. Clifton Park, NY: Delmar Cengage Learning.

Polman & Peckenpaugh. (2003). *Nutrition Essentials and Diet, Therapy*, 9th ed. Philadelphia, PA: W. B. Saunders.

Pozgar, G. (2005). *Legal Aspects of Health Care Administration*, 9th ed. Sudbury, MA: Jones & Bartlett Publishers.

Purtillo, R. (2005). *Ethical Dimensions in the Health Professions*, 4th ed. Philadelphia, PA: W. B. Saunders.

Reese, B. & Brandt, R. (2002). *Human Relations: Principles and Practice*, 5th ed. Boston, MA: Houghton-Mifflin.

Rescher, N. (1969). "The Allocation of Exotic Medical Life-saving Therapy." *Ethics*, 79:3.

Rice, J. (2004). *Medical Terminology with Human Anatomy*, 5th ed. Stamford, CT: Appleton & Lange.

Rice, J. (2006). *Pharmacology for Medical Assisting*, 4th ed. Clifton Park, NY: Delmar Cengage Learning.

Rizzo, D. (2010). *Delmar's Anatomy and Physiology*, 3rd ed. Clifton Park, NY: Delmar Cengage Learning.

Satinsky, M. (2007). *Medical Practice Management in the 21st Century*. Oxford, UK: Radcliffe Publishing.

Scott, A. & Fong, E. (2009). *Body Structures and Functions*, 11th ed. Clifton Park, NY: Delmar Cengage Learning.

Sherwood, L. (2005). *Fundamentals of Physiology: A Human Perspective*, 3rd ed. Florence, KY: Brooks-Cole.

Shimeld, L. (1999). *Essentials of Diagnostic Microbiology*. Clifton Park, NY: Delmar Cengage Learning.

Sloane, S. (1997). *Medical Abbreviations and Eponyms*, 2nd ed. Philadelphia, PA: W. B. Saunders.

Stanley, J. (2002). *Essentials of Immunology and Serology*. Clifton Park, NY: Delmar Cengage Learning.

Strunk, W. & White, E. (1999). *Elements of Style*, 4th ed. New York, NY: Longman.

Taber's Cyclopedic Medical Dictionary, 19th ed. (2001). Philadelphia, PA: F. A. Davis.

Tamparo, C. & Lewis, M. (2000). *Diseases of the Human Body*, 3rd ed. Philadelphia, PA: F. A. Davis.

Tamparo, C. & Lindh, W. (2008). *Therapeutic Communications for Health Professionals*, 3rd ed. Clifton Park, NY: Delmar Cengage Learning.

Tyler, L. (2002). *Tyler's Guide: The Healthcare Executive's Job Search*, 3rd ed. Chicago, IL: Health Administration Press.

U.S. Small Business Administration (1999). *ADA Guide for Small Businesses*. Washington, D.C.: U.S. Department of Justice, Civil Rights Division.

Walston-Dunham, B. (2009). *Introduction to Law*, 5th ed. Clifton Park, NY: Delmar Cengage Learning.

Weinland, J. (1957). *How to Improve Your Memory*. New York, NY: Barnes and Noble, Inc.

Werhane, P. et al. (1986). *Philosophical Issues in Human Rights*. NY: Random House.

Witt, S. (1983). *How to be Twice as Smart*. West Nyack, NY: Parker Publishing Co.

Wood & Cohen. (2000). *Payroll Records and Procedures*, 4th ed. Chicago, IL: McGraw-Hill.

IMPORTANT! READ CAREFULLY: This End User License Agreement ("Agreement") sets forth the conditions by which Cengage Learning will make electronic access to the Cengage Learning-owned licensed content and associated media, software, documentation, printed materials, and electronic documentation contained in this package and/or made available to you via this product (the "Licensed Content"), available to you (the "End User"). BY CLICKING THE "I ACCEPT" BUTTON AND/OR OPENING THIS PACKAGE, YOU ACKNOWLEDGE THAT YOU HAVE READ ALL OF THE TERMS AND CONDITIONS, AND THAT YOU AGREE TO BE BOUND BY ITS TERMS, CONDITIONS, AND ALL APPLICABLE LAWS AND REGULATIONS GOVERNING THE USE OF THE LICENSED CONTENT.

1.0 SCOPE OF LICENSE
1.1 Licensed Content. The Licensed Content may contain portions of modifiable content ("Modifiable Content") and content which may not be modified or otherwise altered by the End User ("Non-Modifiable Content"). For purposes of this Agreement, Modifiable Content and Non-Modifiable Content may be collectively referred to herein as the "Licensed Content." All Licensed Content shall be considered Non-Modifiable Content, unless such Licensed Content is presented to the End User in a modifiable format and it is clearly indicated that modification of the Licensed Content is permitted.

1.2 Subject to the End User's compliance with the terms and conditions of this Agreement, Cengage Learning hereby grants the End User, a nontransferable, nonexclusive, limited right to access and view a single copy of the Licensed Content on a single personal computer system for noncommercial, internal, personal use only. The End User shall not (i) reproduce, copy, modify (except in the case of Modifiable Content), distribute, display, transfer, sublicense, prepare derivative work(s) based on, sell, exchange, barter or transfer, rent, lease, loan, resell, or in any other manner exploit the Licensed Content; (ii) remove, obscure, or alter any notice of Cengage Learning's intellectual property rights present on or in the Licensed Content, including, but not limited to, copyright, trademark, and/or patent notices; or (iii) disassemble, decompile, translate, reverse engineer, or otherwise reduce the Licensed Content.

2.0 TERMINATION
2.1 Cengage Learning may at any time (without prejudice to its other rights or remedies) immediately terminate this Agreement and/or suspend access to some or all of the Licensed Content, in the event that the End User does not comply with any of the terms and conditions of this Agreement. In the event of such termination by Cengage Learning, the End User shall immediately return any and all copies of the Licensed Content to Cengage Learning.

3.0 PROPRIETARY RIGHTS
3.1 The End User acknowledges that Cengage Learning owns all rights, title and interest, including, but not limited to all copyright rights therein, in and to the Licensed Content, and that the End User shall not take any action inconsistent with such ownership. The Licensed Content is protected by U.S., Canadian and other applicable copyright laws and by international treaties, including the Berne Convention and the Universal Copyright Convention. Nothing contained in this Agreement shall be construed as granting the End User any ownership rights in or to the Licensed Content.

3.2 Cengage Learning reserves the right at any time to withdraw from the Licensed Content any item or part of an item for which it no longer retains the right to publish, or which it has reasonable grounds to believe infringes copyright or is defamatory, unlawful, or otherwise objectionable.

4.0 PROTECTION AND SECURITY
4.1 The End User shall use its best efforts and take all reasonable steps to safeguard its copy of the Licensed Content to ensure that no unauthorized reproduction, publication, disclosure, modification, or distribution of the Licensed Content, in whole or in part, is made. To the extent that the End User becomes aware of any such unauthorized use of the Licensed Content, the End User shall immediately notify Cengage Learning. Notification of such violations may be made by sending an e-mail to infringement@cengage.com.

5.0 MISUSE OF THE LICENSED PRODUCT
5.1 In the event that the End User uses the Licensed Content in violation of this Agreement, Cengage Learning shall have the option of electing liquidated damages, which shall include all profits generated by the End User's use of the Licensed Content plus interest computed at the maximum rate permitted by law and all legal fees and other expenses incurred by Cengage Learning in enforcing its rights, plus penalties.

6.0 FEDERAL GOVERNMENT CLIENTS
6.1 Except as expressly authorized by Cengage Learning, Federal Government clients obtain only the rights specified in this Agreement and no other rights. The Government acknowledges that (i) all software and related documentation incorporated in the Licensed Content is existing commercial computer software within the meaning of FAR 27.405(b)(2); and (2) all other data delivered in whatever form, is limited rights data within the meaning of FAR 27.401. The restrictions in this section are acceptable as consistent with the Government's need for software and other data under this Agreement.

7.0 DISCLAIMER OF WARRANTIES AND LIABILITIES
7.1 Although Cengage Learning believes the Licensed Content to be reliable, Cengage Learning does not guarantee or warrant (i) any information or materials contained in or produced by the Licensed Content, (ii) the accuracy, completeness or reliability of the Licensed Content, or (iii) that the Licensed Content is free from errors or other material defects. THE LICENSED PRODUCT IS PROVIDED "AS IS," WITHOUT ANY WARRANTY OF ANY KIND AND CENGAGE LEARNING DISCLAIMS ANY AND ALL WARRANTIES, EXPRESSED OR IMPLIED, INCLUDING, WITHOUT LIMITATION, WARRANTIES OF MERCHANTABILITY OR FITNESS FOR A PARTICULAR PURPOSE. IN NO EVENT SHALL CENGAGE LEARNING BE LIABLE FOR: INDIRECT, SPECIAL, PUNITIVE OR CONSEQUENTIAL DAMAGES INCLUDING FOR LOST PROFITS, LOST DATA, OR OTHERWISE. IN NO EVENT SHALL CENGAGE LEARNING'S AGGREGATE LIABILITY HEREUNDER, WHETHER ARISING IN CONTRACT, TORT, STRICT LIABILITY OR OTHERWISE, EXCEED THE AMOUNT OF FEES PAID BY THE END USER HEREUNDER FOR THE LICENSE OF THE LICENSED CONTENT.

8.0 GENERAL
8.1 Entire Agreement. This Agreement shall constitute the entire Agreement between the Parties and supercedes all prior Agreements and understandings oral or written relating to the subject matter hereof.

8.2 Enhancements/Modifications of Licensed Content. From time to time, and in Cengage Learning's sole discretion, Cengage Learning may advise the End User of updates, upgrades, enhancements and/or improvements to the Licensed Content, and may permit the End User to access and use, subject to the terms and conditions of this Agreement, such modifications, upon payment of prices as may be established by Cengage Learning.

8.3 No Export. The End User shall use the Licensed Content solely in the United States and shall not transfer or export, directly or indirectly, the Licensed Content outside the United States.

8.4 Severability. If any provision of this Agreement is invalid, illegal, or unenforceable under any applicable statute or rule of law, the provision shall be deemed omitted to the extent that it is invalid, illegal, or unenforceable. In such a case, the remainder of the Agreement shall be construed in a manner as to give greatest effect to the original intention of the parties hereto.

8.5 Waiver. The waiver of any right or failure of either party to exercise in any respect any right provided in this Agreement in any instance shall not be deemed to be a waiver of such right in the future or a waiver of any other right under this Agreement.

8.6 Choice of Law/Venue. This Agreement shall be interpreted, construed, and governed by and in accordance with the laws of the State of New York, applicable to contracts executed and to be wholly preformed therein, without regard to its principles governing conflicts of law. Each party agrees that any proceeding arising out of or relating to this Agreement or the breach or threatened breach of this Agreement may be commenced and prosecuted in a court in the State and County of New York. Each party consents and submits to the nonexclusive personal jurisdiction of any court in the State and County of New York in respect of any such proceeding.

8.7 Acknowledgment. By opening this package and/or by accessing the Licensed Content on this Web site, THE END USER ACKNOWLEDGES THAT IT HAS READ THIS AGREEMENT, UNDERSTANDS IT, AND AGREES TO BE BOUND BY ITS TERMS AND CONDITIONS. IF YOU DO NOT ACCEPT THESE TERMS AND CONDITIONS, YOU MUST NOT ACCESS THE LICENSED CONTENT AND RETURN THE LICENSED PRODUCT TO CENGAGE LEARNING (WITHIN 30 CALENDAR DAYS OF THE END USER'S PURCHASE) WITH PROOF OF PAYMENT ACCEPTABLE TO CENGAGE LEARNING, FOR A CREDIT OR A REFUND. Should the End User have any questions/comments regarding this Agreement, please contact Cengage Learning at Delmar.help@cengage.com.

System Requirements PC:
Windows XP/SP3, Windows Vista SP/1, SP2, or Windows 7
Hardware: CD-ROM drive, mouse
Disk Space: 256 MB RAM
20 MB free hard drive space

System Requirements Macintosh: Univeral Binary for PowerPC or Intel CPU Mac OS 10.4, 10.5, or 10.6
Hardware: CD-ROM drive, mouse
Disk Space: 256 MB RAM
20 MB free hard drive space
Note: Software will not work with Mac OS 10.3 or earlier.

Setup Instructions
PC:
1. Insert disc into CD-ROM drive. The CD installation program should start automatically. If it does not, go to step 2.
2. From My Computer, double-click the icon for the CD drive.
3. Double click the setup.exe file to start the program.

Mac
1. Insert the CD-ROM in the drive. In a moment, the Exam Practice CD icon will appear on your desktop.
2. Double click the Exam Practice CD icon to open the Finder window.
3. Double click the Install Exam Practice icon to start the installation program.
4. Click Continue to begin the installation process.
5. Read the License Agreement carefully and click Continue.
6. Click Agree to confirm that you understand the License Agreement and will agree to its terms.
7. Choose a place to install the Exam Practice program. Typically, you select your main system drive. The installer program will install the software in the Applications folder of the selected drive.
8. Click Quit to complete the installation and exit the installer program. Your software is now installed and ready to use.